The Protocol Book
for Intensive Care

The Protocol Book for Intensive Care

SIXTH EDITION

Editor
Soumitra Kumar
MD DM FCSI FACC FESC FSCAI FICC FIAE FICP
Professor and Head
Department of Cardiology
Ramakrishna Mission Seva Pratishthan
Vivekananda Institute of Medical Sciences
Kolkata, West Bengal, India

Foreword
S Padmavati

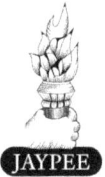

JAYPEE
JAYPEE BROTHERS MEDICAL PUBLISHERS
The Health Sciences Publisher
New Delhi | London

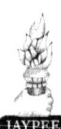

Jaypee Brothers Medical Publishers (P) Ltd

Headquarters

Jaypee Brothers Medical Publishers (P) Ltd
EMCA House, 23/23-B
Ansari Road, Daryaganj
New Delhi 110 002, India
Landline: +91-11-23272143, +91-11-23272703
+91-11-23282021, +91-11-23245672
Email: jaypee@jaypeebrothers.com

Overseas Office

JP Medical Ltd
83 Victoria Street, London
SW1H 0HW (UK)
Phone: +44 20 3170 8910
Email: info@jpmedpub.com

Corporate Office

Jaypee Brothers Medical Publishers (P) Ltd
4838/24, Ansari Road, Daryaganj
New Delhi 110 002, India
Phone: +91-11-43574357
Fax: +91-11-43574314
Email: jaypee@jaypeebrothers.com

EU GPSR Authorised Representative

Logos Europe, 9 rue Nicolas Poussin
17000, La Rochelle, France
Phone: +33 (0) 6 67 93 73 78
E-mail: Contact@logoseurope.eu

Website: www.jaypeebrothers.com
Website: www.jaypeedigital.com

© 2025, Jaypee Brothers Medical Publishers

The views and opinions expressed in this book are solely those of the original contributor(s)/author(s) and do not necessarily represent those of editor(s) or publisher of the book.

All rights reserved. No part of this publication may be reproduced, stored or transmitted in any form or by any means, electronic, mechanical, photocopying, recording or otherwise, without the prior permission in writing of the publishers.

All brand names and product names used in this book are trade names, service marks, trademarks or registered trademarks of their respective owners. The publisher is not associated with any product or vendor mentioned in this book.

Medical knowledge and practice change constantly. This book is designed to provide accurate, authoritative information about the subject matter in question. However, readers are advised to check the most current information available on procedures included and check information from the manufacturer of each product to be administered, to verify the recommended dose, formula, method and duration of administration, adverse effects and contraindications. It is the responsibility of the practitioner to take all appropriate safety precautions. Neither the publisher nor the author(s)/editor(s) assume any liability for any injury and/or damage to persons or property arising from or related to use of material in this book.

This book is sold on the understanding that the publisher is not engaged in providing professional medical services. If such advice or services are required, the services of a competent medical professional should be sought.

Every effort has been made where necessary to contact holders of copyright to obtain permission to reproduce copyright material. If any have been inadvertently overlooked, the publisher will be pleased to make the necessary arrangements at the first opportunity.

Inquiries for bulk sales may be solicited at: jaypee@jaypeebrothers.com

The Protocol Book for Intensive Care
First Edition: 2003 (by Editor)
Second Edition: 2008
Third Edition: 2010
Fourth Edition: 2014
Fifth Edition: 2018
Sixth Edition: **2025**

ISBN: 978-93-6616-503-5

Dedicated to
*My family,
friends, and
well-wishers*

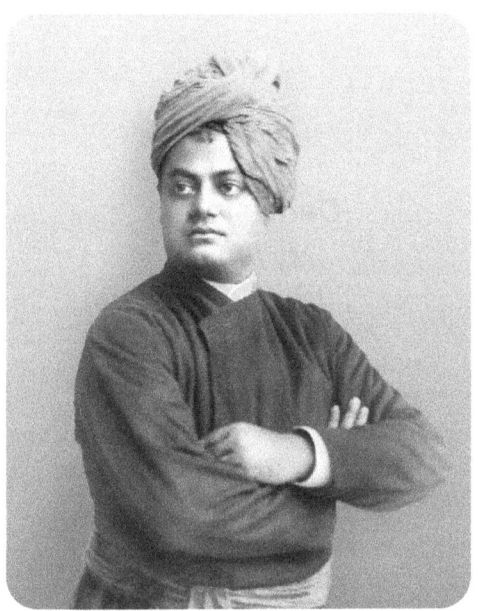

Swami Vivekananda

The secret of religion lies not in theories but in practice.
To be good and to do good—that is the whole of religion.

Contributors

Achyut Sarkar
Consultant Interventional Cardiologist
Woodland Multispecialty Hospital
Kolkata, West Bengal, India

Ajitesh Roy
Professor and Head
Department of Endocrinology
Ramakrishna Mission Seva Pratishthan
Vivekananda Institute of Medical Sciences
Kolkata, West Bengal, India

Amitava Mazumdar
Professor of Medicine
Ramakrishna Mission Seva Pratishthan
Vivekananda Institute of Medical Sciences
Kolkata, West Bengal, India

Arghya Majumder
Director and Head
Department of Nephrology
Manipal Hospitals
Kolkata, West Bengal, India

Debashis Dutta
Director
Department of Gastroenterology and Hepatology
Fortis Hospitals
Kolkata, West Bengal, India

Jayanta Roy
Director of Neurology
Manipal Hospitals
(Mukundapur Cluster)
Kolkata, West Bengal, India

Prabuddha Mukhopadhyay
Associate Professor of Medicine
Ramakrishna Mission Seva Pratishthan
Vivekananda Institute of Medical Sciences
Kolkata, West Bengal, India

Samar Ranjan Pal
Consultant
Rheumatology Unit
Ramakrishna Mission Seva Pratishthan
Vivekananda Institute of Medical Sciences
Kolkata, West Bengal, India

Contributors

Shuvanan Ray
Director
Department of Cardiology and
Cardiovascular Intervention
Fortis Hospitals
Kolkata, West Bengal, India

Soumitra Kumar
Professor and Head
Department of Cardiology
Ramakrishna Mission Seva
Pratishthan
Vivekananda Institute of Medical
Sciences
Kolkata, West Bengal, India

Sujata Majumder
Professor of Medicine
Ramakrishna Mission Seva
Pratishthan
Vivekananda Institute of Medical
Sciences
Kolkata, West Bengal, India

Sumit Sen Gupta
Consultant Pulmonologist
HP Ghosh Hospital
Kolkata, West Bengal, India

ALL INDIA HEART FOUNDATION
4874 (First Floor), Ansari Road
24, Daryaganj
New Delhi-110 002

DR. S. PADMAVATI
FRCP (Lond.) FRCPE, FACC, FAMS
PRESIDENT-All India Heart Foundation
DIRECTOR-National Heart Institute

NATIONAL HEART INSTITUTE
(WHO Collaborative Centre in Preventive Cardiology)
49, Community Centre
East of Kailash
New Delhi-110 065
E-mail : padmavat@del2.vsnl.net.in

Foreword to the First Edition

The Protocol Book represents guidelines for the diagnosis and management of common medical emergencies seen in hospitals. It covers mostly cardiac problems but also includes respiratory, gastrointestinal, renal diseases and diabetes. It has the same objectives as the American Heart Association/American College of Cardiology's *Pocket Guidelines Updates* compiled by the Special Task Forces of these organizations which are proving extremely useful for practicing physicians.

This book has been compiled by the postgraduate students of the Vivekananda Institute of Medical Sciences, Ramakrishna Mission Seva Pratishthan, Kolkata, West Bengal, India, under the guidance of senior consultants in these departments at the hospital and under the able Editorship of Dr Soumitra Kumar. The text is written in a typical 'Senior Resident' language that can be easily understood by their colleagues. The latest 'state-of-the-art' information and knowledge has been used in preparing the various sections. It is a very laudable effort on the part of the postgraduate staff.

I am sure *The Protocol Book* will prove very useful for all categories of physicians dealing with acute emergencies in hospitals.

S Padmavati
FRCP (London) FRCPE FACC FAMS
President, All India Heart Foundation
Director, National Heart Institute

Preface

The sixth edition of this treatise comes little more than 6 years after the fifth edition and its publication had to endure the challenges of the COVID period (2020-2022) when almost nothing beyond mundane items moved. While the basic structure of the book has been retained, all the chapters have been updated to incorporate as many recent developments in diagnostic and therapeutic modalities as possible. Considering the breakneck speed at which cardiology and allied specialties of medicine are progressing, there are bound to be some omissions for which the editor begs to be pardoned.

As conceived right from the first edition in 2003, the driving theme of this edition too remains "complete management" of the patient surpassing borders of individual disciplines of medicine. The intricate nature of the human body's internal milieu and working mandates a comprehensive care of the patient to ensure that he/she ultimately leaves the hospital safe and sound.

I am personally grateful to all the contributing authors of this edition for their unstinting cooperation and very warm support. I am particularly thankful to Mr B Mukherjee for his untiring support in the primary composition of the chapters. I sincerely acknowledge the sustained patronage provided by M/s Zydus Pharmaceuticals to this title since the first edition. Finally, no words are enough to express my gratitude to my family members for their passionate affection and encouragement over the last two decades.

Soumitra Kumar

Contents

1. **Acute Coronary Syndrome** 1
   Soumitra Kumar
2. **Cardiogenic Shock** 29
   Soumitra Kumar
3. **Acute Heart Failure** 50
   Soumitra Kumar
4. **Management of Chronic Heart Failure** 82
   Soumitra Kumar
5. **Syncope** 127
   Soumitra Kumar
6. **Atrial Fibrillation** 145
   Soumitra Kumar
7. **Tachycardias** 212
   Soumitra Kumar
8. **Cardiopulmonary Resuscitation** 263
   Soumitra Kumar
9. **Percutaneous Coronary Intervention in Acute Myocardial Infarction** 278
   Shuvanan Ray, Soumitra Kumar
10. **Acute Pulmonary Embolism** 304
    Soumitra Kumar
11. **Acute Cardiac Care in Pediatric Practice** 321
    Soumitra Kumar, Achyut Sarkar
12. **Hypertensive Emergencies** 336
    Soumitra Kumar
13. **Acid-base Disturbance** 353
    Sujata Majumder, Amitava Mazumdar

14. **Electrolyte Imbalance** 368
    Amitava Mazumdar, Sujata Majumder

15. **Management of Adult Severe Acute Asthma** 388
    Sumit Sen Gupta

16. **Management of Acute Exacerbation of
    Chronic Obstructive Pulmonary Disease** 405
    Sumit Sen Gupta

17. **Mechanical Ventilation** 416
    Soumitra Kumar, Sumit Sen Gupta

18. **Acute Respiratory Distress Syndrome** 447
    Sumit Sen Gupta

19. **Management of Gastrointestinal Bleeding** 462
    Debashis Dutta

20. **Stroke** 487
    Soumitra Kumar, Jayanta Roy

21. **Acute Kidney Injury** 520
    Soumitra Kumar, Arghya Majumder

22. **Endocrine Emergencies** 550
    Ajitesh Roy

23. **Rheumatological Emergencies** 582
    Samar Ranjan Pal

24. **Antimicrobial Therapy Including
    Management of Septic Shock** 597
    Prabuddha Mukhopadhyay

Index 639

CHAPTER 1

Acute Coronary Syndrome

Soumitra Kumar

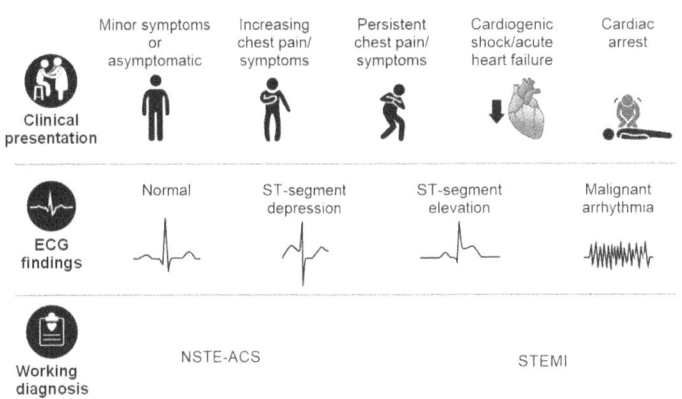

Fig. 1: The acute coronary syndrome (ACS) spectrum of ACS. (NSTE: non-ST-segment elevation; STEMI: ST-elevation myocardial infarction)

Working diagnosis	Further investigations	Final diagnosis
STEMI	hs-cTn levels	STEMI
	± Angiography	NSTEMI
NSTE-ACS	± Imaging	Unstable angina
		Non-ACS diagnosis

Fig. 2: Classification of patients presenting with suspected acute coronary Syndrome (ACS): From a working to a final diagnosis. (hs-cTn: high-sensitivity cardiac troponin; NSTE-ACS: non-ST-segment elevation acute coronary syndrome; NSTEMI: non-STEMI; STEMI: ST-elevation myocardial infarction)

Working diagnosis	STEMI	NSTE-ACS with very high-risk features	NSTE-ACS without very high-risk features
Early invasive angiography according to patient risk	Immediate angiography[a] ± PPCI or fibrinolysis if timely PPCI not feasible	Immediate[b] angiography ± PCI	Consider angiography within 24 hours for NSTE-ACS with high risk features
Further investigations	Nonimmediate angiography / Echo	Intravascular imaging / Noninvasive imaging	hs-cTn[a] levels / ECG monitoring
Further management	PCI / CABG	Long-term medical therapy	Lifestyle measures / Smoking cessation

Fig. 3: Primary percutaneous coronary intervention (PPCI) antithrombotic therapy (ATT). (hs-cTn: high-sensitivity cardiac troponin; NSTE-ACS: non-ST-segment elevation acute coronary syndrome; STEMI: ST-elevation myocardial infarction)

Notes:
[a]Results of hs-cTn measurements are not required for the initial stratification of ACS and the initial emergency management (i.e., for patients with a working diagnosis of STEMI or very high-risk NSTE-ACS) should not be delayed based on this.
[b]For patients with NSTE-ACS with very high-risk features, immediate angiography is recommended. For patients with NSTE-ACS with highrisk features, early invasive angiography (i.e., <24 hours) should be considered and inpatient invasive angiography is recommended. See Table 4 for details of recommendations.

An overview of the management and investigation of patients who present with signs and symptoms potentially consistent with acute coronary syndrome.

TIMING OF LOADING DOSE OF ORAL ANTIPLATELET THERAPY

Both aspirin andoral $P2Y_{12}$ inhibitors achieve platelet inhibition more rapidly following an oral loading dose (LD). Pretreatment refers to a strategy in which an antiplatelet drug, usually a $P2Y_{12}$ receptor inhibitor, is give before coronary angiography and, therefore, before the coronary anatomy is known. Although a potential benefit with pretreatment in the setting of acute coronary syndrome (ACS) has been hypothesized, large-scale randomized trials supporting a routine pretreatment strategy with $P2Y_{12}$ receptor

TABLE 1: ESC 2023 recommendations for clinical and diagnostic tools for patients with suspected acute coronary syndrome.

Recommendations	Class	Level
It is recommended to base the diagnosis and initial short-term risk stratification of ACS on a combination of clinical history, symptoms, vital signs, other physical findings, ECG, and hs-cTn	I	B
ECG		
Twelve-lead ECG recording and interpretation is recommended as soon as possible at the point of FMC with a target of <10 minutes	I	B
Continuous ECG monitoring and the availability of defibrillation capacity are recommended as soon as possible in all patients with suspected STEMI, in suspected ACS with other ECG changes or ongoing chest pain and once the diagnosis of MI is made	I	B
The use of additional ECG leads (V3R, V4R, and V7–V9) is recommended in cases of inferior STEMI or if total vessel occlusion is suspected and standard leads are inconclusive	I	B
An additional 12-lead ECG is recommended in cases with recurrent symptoms or diagnostics uncertainty	I	C
It is recommended to measure cardiac troponins with high sensitivity assays immediately after presentation and to obtain the results within 60 minutes of blood sampling	I	C
It is recommended to use an ESC algorithmic approach with serial hs-cTn measurements (0 h/1 h or 0 h/2 h) to rule in and rule out NSTEMI	I	B
Additional testing after 3 hours is recommended if the first two hs-cTn measurements of 0 h/1 h algorithm are inconclusive and to alternative diagnoses explaining the condition have been made	I	B
The use of established risk scores (e.g., GRACE risk score) for prognosis estimation should be considered	IIa	B
Triage for emergency reperfusion therapy: It is recommended that patients with suggested STEMI are immediately triaged for an emergency reperfusion strategy	I	A

(ACS: acute coronary syndrome; ECG: electrocardiogram; ESC: European Society of Cardiology; FMC: first medical contact; GRACE: Global Registry of Acute Coronary Events; hs-cTn: high-sensitivity cardiac troponin; NSTEMI: non-STEMI; STEMI: ST-elevation myocardial infarction)

4 Acute Coronary Syndrome

Flowchart 1: The 0 h/1 h or 0 h/2 h rule-out and rule-in algorithms during high-sensitivity cardiac troponin (hs-cTn) assays in patients presenting to the emergency department with suspected NSTEMI and without an indication for immediate invasive angiography.

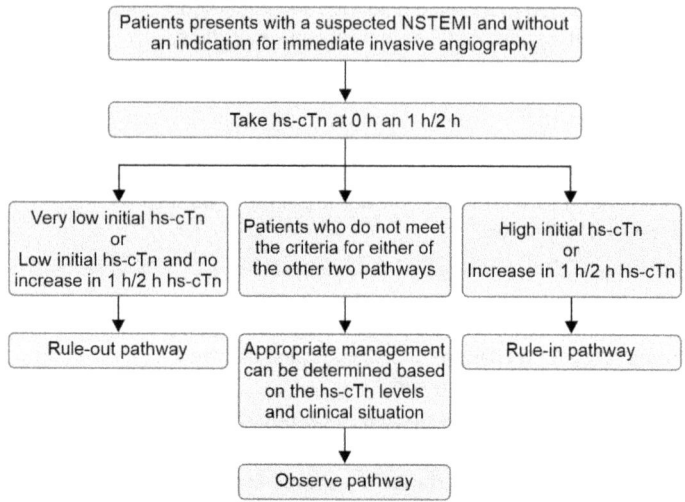

(NSTEMI: non-ST-elevation myocardial infarction)

TABLE 2: ESC 2023 Recommendations for noninvasive imaging in the initial assessment of patients with suspected acute coronary syndrome.

Recommendations	Class	Level
Emergency TTE is recommended in patients with suspected ACS presenting with cardiogenic shock or suspected mechanical complications	I	C
In patients with suspected ACS, nonelevated (or uncertain) hs-cTn levels, no ECG changes and no recurrence of pain, incorporating CCTA or a noninvasive stress imaging test as part of the initial workup should be considered	IIa	A
Emergency TTE should be considered at triage in cases of diagnostic uncertainty but this should not result in delays in transfer to the cardiac catheterization laboratory if there is suspicion of an acute coronary artery occlusion	IIa	C
Routine early CCTA in patients with suspected ACS is not recommended	III	B

(ACS: acute coronary syndrome; CCTA: computed tomography coronary angiography; ECG: electrocardiogram; ESC: European Society of Cardiology; hs-cTn: high-sensitivity cardiac troponin; TTE: transthoracic echocardiography)

TABLE 3: ESC 2023 recommendations for the initial management of patients with acute coronary syndrome.

Recommendations	Class	Level
Hypoxia: Oxygen is recommended in patients with hypoxemia (SaO$_2$ <90%)	I	C
Routine oxygen is not recommended in patients without hypoxemia (SaO$_2$ >90%)	III	A
Symptoms: Intravenous opioids should be considered to relieve pain	IIa	C
A mild tranquilizer should be considered inn very anxious patients	IIa	C
Intravenous beta-blockers: Intravenous beta-blockers (preferably metoprolol) should be considered at the time of presentation in patients undergoing PPCI with no signs of acute heart failure an SBP >120 mm Hg and no other contraindications	III	A

(ESC: European Society of Cardiology; PPCI: primary percutaneous coronary intervention; SBP: systolic blood pressure)

inhibitors are lacking. Caution in relation to pretreatment may be of particular relevance in patients at HBR [e.g., those receiving an oral anticoagulant (OAC)].

PRETREATMENT IN PATIENTS WITH SUSPECTED ST-ELEVATION MYOCARDIAL INFARCTION

The Administration of Ticagrelor in the Cath Lab or in the Ambulance for New ST-Elevation Myocardial Infarction to Open the Coronary artery (ATLANTIC) trial is the only randomized study testing the safety and efficacy of different timings of P2Y$_{12}$ receptor inhibitor anticipation in patients with a working diagnosis of ST-elevation myocardial infarction (STEMI)-undergoing PPCI. In this trial, patients were randomized to receive a ticagrelor LD either during transfer to PPCI center or immediately before angiography. The median difference between the timing of P2Y$_{12}$ receptor inhibitor loading with the two treatment strategies was 31 minutes. In this study, the pretreatment strategy failed to meet the pre-specified primary end-point of improved ST-segment elevation resolution or thrombolysis. In transient myocardial infarction (TMI) flow

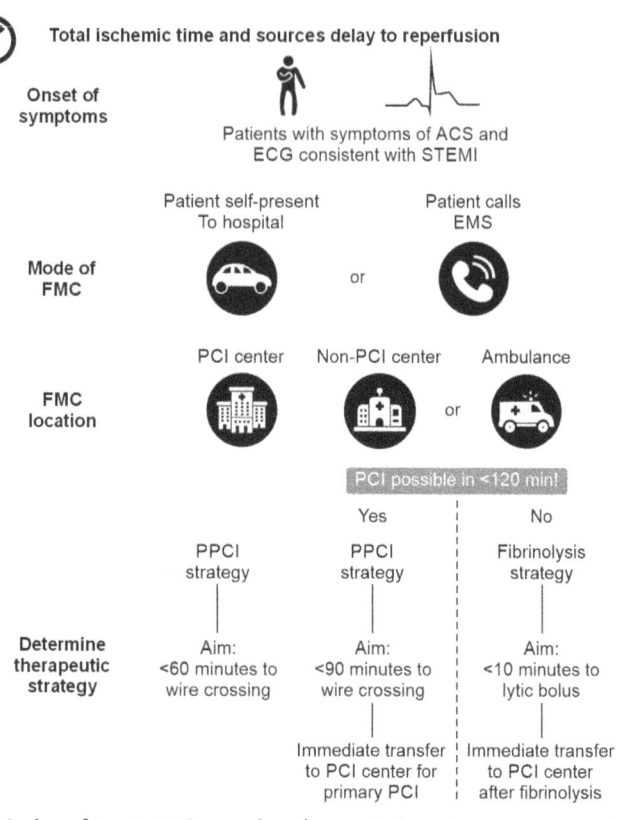

Fig. 4: Modes of presentation and pathways to invasive management and myocardial revascularization in patients presenting with STEMI. (ACS: acute coronary syndrome; ECG: electrocardiogram; EMS: emergency medical services; FMC: first medical contact; PCI: percutaneous coronary intervention; PPCI: primary percutaneous coronary interventions; STEMI: ST-segment elevation myocardial infarction)

before intervention. Rates of major and minor bleeding events were identical in both treatment arms. These results were supported by real-world data obtained from the SWEDEHEART (Swedish Web-System for Enhancement and Development of Evidence-Based Care in Heart Disease Evaluated. Accordingly to Recommended Therapies) registry in STEMI patients. Prasugrel pretreatment has not been directly investigated in patients with STEMI.

Flowchart 2: Selection of invasive strategy and reperfusion therapy in patients presenting with NSTE-ACS.

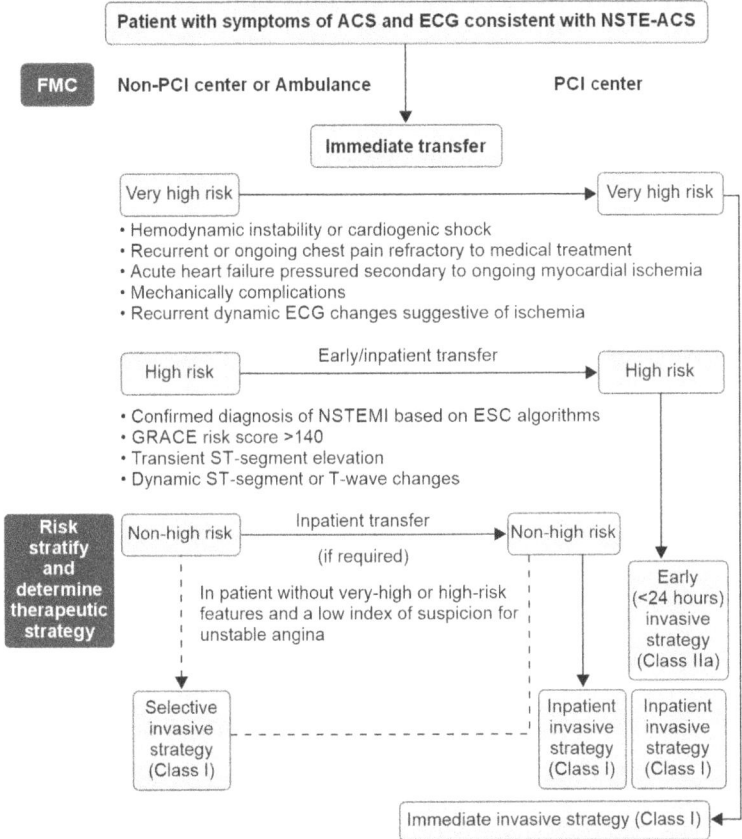

(ACS: acute coronary syndrome; ECG: electrocardiogram; ESC: European Society of Cardiology; STEMI: ST-elevation myocardial infarction; NSTEMI: non-STEMI)

PRETREATMENT IN PATIENTS WITH NON-ST ELEVATION ACUTE CORONARY SYNDROME

The randomized: A Comparison of Prasugrel at the Time of Percutaneous Coronary Intervention or as Pretreatment at the Time of Diagnosis in Patents with Non-ST Elevation Myocardial Infarction (ACCOAST) trial not only demonstrated a lack of benefit with respect to ischemic outcomes with prasugrel pre-treatment, but also

TABLE 4: ESC 2023 recommendations for reperfusion therapy and timing of invasive strategy.

Recommendations	Class	Level
Recommendations for reperfusion therapy for patients with STEMI: Reperfusion therapy is recommended in all patients with a working diagnosis of STEMI (persistent ST-segment elevation or equivalents) and symptoms of ischemia of ≤12 hours duration	I	A
A PPCI strategy is recommended over fibrinolysis of he anticipated time from diagnosis to PCI is <120 minutes	I	A
If timely PPCI (<120 minutes) cannot be performed in patients with a working diagnosis of STEMI, fibrinolytic therapy is recommended within 12 hours of symptom onset in patients without contraindications	I	A
Rescue PCI is recommended for failed fibrinolysis (i.e., ST-segment reduction <50% within 60–90 minutes of fibrinolytic administration) or in the presence of hemodynamic or electrical instability, worsening ischemia, or persistent chest pain	I	A
In patients with a working diagnosis of STEMI and a time from symptom onset >12 hours, a PPCI strategy is recommended in the presence of ongoing symptoms suggestive of ischemia, hemodynamic instability, or life-threatening arrhythmias	I	C
A routine PPCI strategy should be considered in STEMI patients presenting late (12–48 hours) after symptom onset	IIa	B
Routine PCI an occluded IA is not recommended in STEMI patients presenting >48 hours after symptom onset and without persistent symptoms	III	A

(ESC: European Society of Cardiology; PPCI: primary percutaneous coronary intervention; STEMI: ST-elevation myocardial infarction)

a substantially higher bleeding risk. In this study, the median time from first LD to the start of coronary angiography in the pretreatment group was 4.4 hours. With respect to pretreatment data for ticagrelor, the ISAR-REACT S trial showed that a ticagrelor-based strategy with routine pretreatment was inferior to a prasugrel-based strategy with a deferred LD in non-ST-segment elevation ACS (NSTE-ACS)

TABLE 5: Management of patients presenting with cardiac arrest (2025 ACC/AHA/ACEP/NAEMSP/SCAI Guidelines for management of patients with ACS).

Following achievement of return of spontaneous circulation (ROSC)

Mental Status	Awake	Comatose	Comatose	Comatose
Presence of STEMI	Yes	Yes	Yes	No
Prognostic features	–	Favorable	Unfavorable	–
Guideline recommendation	PPCI (Class I)	PPCI (Class I)	PPCI reasonable after	Immediate coronary Angiography Not Recommended (Class 3, no benefit)

(ACC: American College of Cardiology; AHA: American Heart Association; ACEP: American College of Emergency Physicians; NAEMSP: National Association of EMS Physicians; PPCI: primary percutaneous coronary intervention; SCAI: Society for Cardiovascular Angiography and Interventions; STEMI: ST-elevation myocardial infarction)

TABLE 6: ESC 2023 recommendations for transfer/interventions after fibrinolysis.

Recommendations	Class	Level
Transfer to a PCI-capable center is recommended in all patients immediately after fibrinolysis	I	A
Emergency angiography and PCI of the IRA, if indicated are recommended in patients with new-onset or persistent heart failure/shock after fibrinolysis	I	A
Angiography and PCI of the IRA if indicated are recommended between 2 and 24 hours after successful fibrinolysis	I	A

(ESC: European Society of Cardiology; IRA: infarct-related artery; PCI: percutaneous coronary intervention)

patients. The DUBIUS (Downstream Versus Upstream Strategy for the Administration of $P2Y_{12}$ Receptor Blockers) trial also attempted to address this question but was stopped early for futility as there was no difference between upstream versus down-stream oral $P1Y_{12}$ administration in patients with NSTE-ACS (both NSTEMI and UA) scheduled for coronary angiography within 72 hours of hospital admission.

TABLE 7: ESC 2023 recommendation for invasive strategy in NSTE-ACS.

Recommendations	Class	Level
An invasive strategy during hospital admission is recommended in NSTE-ACS patients with high-risk criteria or a high index of suspicion for unstable angina	I	A
A selective invasive approach is recommended in patients without very high-or high-risk NSTE-ACS criteria and with a low index of suspicion for NSTE-ACS	I	A
An immediate invasive strategy is recommended in patients with a working diagnosis of NSTE-ACS and with at least one of the following very high-risk criteria: • Hemodynamic instability or cardiogenic shock • Recurrent or refractory chest pain despite medical treatment • In-hospital life-threatening arrhythmias • Mechanical complications of MI • Acute heart failure presumed secondary to ongoing myocardial ischemia • Recurrent dynamic ST-segment or T-wave changes, particularly intermittent ST-segment elevation	I	C
An early invasive strategy within 24 hours should be considered in patients with at least one of the following high-risk criteria: • Confirmed diagnosis of NSTEMI based on current recommended ESC hs-cTn algorithms • Dynamic ST-segment or T-wave changes • Treatment ST-segment elevation • GRACE risk score >140	IIa	A

(ESC: European Society of Cardiology; GRACE: Global Registry of Acute Coronary Events; hs-cTn: high-sensitivity cardiac troponin; NSTE-ACS: non-ST-segment elevation acute coronary syndrome; NSTEMI: non-ST-elevation myocardial infarction)

SPONTANEOUS CORONARY ARTERY DISSECTION

Spontaneous coronary artery dissection (SCAD) is an infrequent cause of ACS in general but accounts for a significant proportion of ACS cases in young/middle-aged women. The pathophysiology underlying SCAD is different to that of type 1 MI and there are some differences in its management and outcomes. For these reasons, it is of paramount importance that an accurate diagnosis is established. Until evidence from ongoing prospective trials becomes available,

Acute Coronary Syndrome

TABLE 8: Dose regimen of antiplatelet and anticoagulant drugs in acute coronary syndrome patients.

I. Antiplatelets drugs

Aspirin	• LD of 150–300 mg orally or 75–250 mg IV if oral ingestion is not possible, followed by oral MD of 75–100 mg od • No specific dose adjustment in CKD patients

$P2Y_{12}$ receptor inhibitors (oral or IV)

Clopidogrel	• LD of 300–600 mg orally, followed by an MD of 75 mg od; no specific dose adjustment in CKD patients • *Fibrinolysis:* At the time of fibrinolysis an initial dose of 300 mg (75 mg for patients older than 75 years of age)
Prasugrel	LD of 60 mg orally, followed by an MD of 10 mg od. In patients with body weight <60 kg, an MD of 5 mg od is recommended. In patients aged ≥75 years, prasugrel should be used with caution, but a MD of 5 mg od should be used if treatment is deemed necessary. No specific dose adjustment in CKD patients. Prior stroke is a contraindication for prasugrel
Ticagrelor	LD of 180 mg orally, followed by an MD of 90 mg bid.; no specific dose adjustment in CKD patients
Cangrelor	• Bolus of 30 mg/kg IV followed by 4 µg/kg/min infusion for at least 2 hours or the duration of the procedure (whichever is longer). In the transition from cangrelor to a thienopyridine, the thienopyridine should be administered immediately after discontinuation of cangrelor with an LD (clopidogrel 600 mg or prasugrel 60 mg); to avoid a potential DDI, prasugrel may also be administered 30 minutes before the cangrelor infusion is stopped • Ticagrelor (LD 180 mg) should be administered at the time of PCI to minimize the potential gap in platelet inhibition during the transition phase

GP IIb/IIIa receptor inhibitors (IV)

Eptifibatide	• Double bolus of 180 µg/kg IV (given at a 10-minute interval) by an infusion of 2.0 µg/kg/min for up to 18 hours • For CrCl 30–50 mL/min; first LD, 180 µg/kg IV bolus (max 22.6 mg); maintenance of infusion 1 µg/kg/min (max 7.5 mg/h). Second LD (if PCI), 180 µg/kg IV bolus (max 22.6 mg) should be administered 10 minutes after the

Contd...

Contd...

	first bolus. Contraindicated in patients with end-stage renal disease and with prior ICH, ischemic stroke within 30 days, fibrinolysis, or platelet count <100,000/mm^3
Tirofiban	• Bolus of 25 µg/kg IV over 3 minutes, followed by an infusion of 0.15 µg/kg/min continued for up to 18 hours • Contraindicated in patients with prior ICH, ischemic stroke within 30 days, fibrinolysis, or platelet count <100,000/min^3
II. Anticoagulant drugs	
UFH	• *Initial treatment:* IV bolus 70–100 U/kg followed by IV infusion titrated to achieve an aPTT of 60–80s • *During PCI:* 70–100 U/kg IV bolus or according to ACT in case of UFH pretreatment
Enoxaparin	• *Initial treatment:* For treatment of ACS 1 mg/kg bid subcutaneously for a minimum of 2 days and continued until clinical stabilization. In patients whose CrCl is below 30 mL/min (by Cockcroft—Gault equation), the enoxaparin dosage should be reduced to 1 mg per kg od • *During PCI:* For patients managed with PCI, if the last dose of enoxaparin was given <8 hours before balloon inflation, no additional dosing is needed. If the last SC administration was given more than 8 hours before balloon inflation, an IV bolus of 0.3 mg/kg enoxaparin sodium should be administered
Bivalirudin	• *During PPCI:* 0.75 mg/kg IV bolus followed by IV infusion of 1.75 mg/kg/h for 4 hours after the procedure • In patients whose CrCl is below 30 mL/min (by Cockcroft–Gault equation), maintenance infusion should be reduced to 1 mg/kg/h
Fondaparinux	• *Initial treatment:* 2.5 mg/d subcutaneously • *During PCI:* A single bolus of UFH is recommended • Avoid if CrCl <20 mL/min

(ACS: acute coronary syndrome; ACT: activated clotting time; aPPT: activated partial thromboplastin time; bid: bis in die (twice a day); CKD: chronic kidney disease; CrCl: creatinine clearance; DDI: drug-drug interactions; ICH: intracranial hemorrhage; IV: intravenous; LD: loading dose; MD: maintenance dose; od: once a day; PPCI: primary percutaneous coronary intervention; SC: subcutaneous; UFH: unfractionated heparin)

TABLE 9: Recommended default antithrombotic therapy regimens in acute coronary syndrome patients without an indication for oral anticoagulation.

STEMI

Anticoagulation	PPCI UFH (Class I)	PPCI Enoxaparin (Class IIa)	PPCI Bivalirudin (Class IIa)	PPCI Fondaparinux (Class III)
Routine antiplatelet pretreatment		ACS (Aspirin) (Class I)	PPCI P2Y$_{12}$ inhibitor (Class IIa)	

Invasive coronary angiography

Choice of P2Y$_{12}$ inhibitor	ACS Prasugrel Ticagrelor If prasugrel and ticagrelor are unavailable, contraindicated, or cannot be tolerated Clopidogrel (Class I)	Proceeding to PCI Prasugrel >Ticagrelor (Class IIa)

NSTE-ACS

Anticoagulation	Angiography <24 hours	Angiography <24 hours	Angiography >24 hours
Routine antiplatelet pretreatment	UFH (Class I)	Enoxaparin (Class IIa)	Fondaparinux (Class I)

NSTE-ACS P2Y$_{12}$ inhibitor (Class III)

Choice of P2Y$_{12}$ inhibitor	Proceeding to PCI Prasugrel >Ticagrelor (Class IIa)

Default DAPT beyond the first 12 months after ACS	Time (months)	1 2 6 9 12 ↓	Aspirin

Contd...

14 Acute Coronary Syndrome

Contd...

(ACS: acute coronary syndrome; DAPT: dual antiplatelet therapy; NSTE-ACS: non-ST-segment elevation acute coronary syndrome; NSTEMI: non-ST-elevation myocardial infarction; PCI: percutaneous coronary intervention; PPCI: primary percutaneous coronary intervention; UFH: unfractionated heparin)

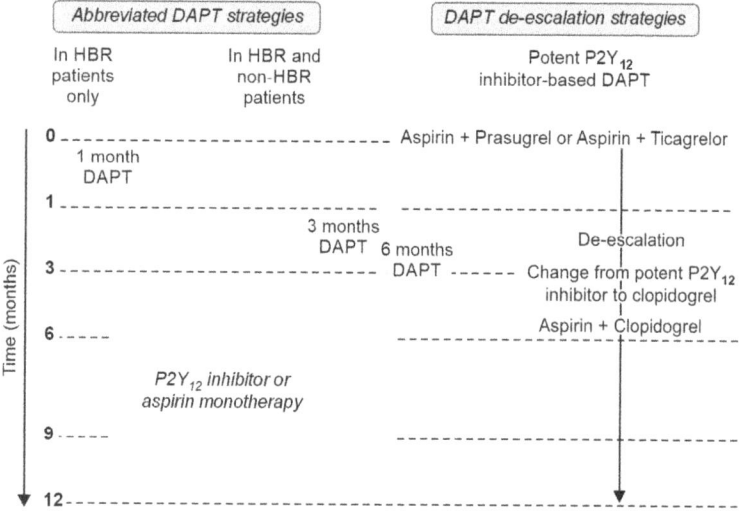

Flowchart 3: Antiplatelet strategies to reduce bleeding risk in the first 12 months after ACS.

(ACS: acute coronary syndrome; DAPT: dual antiplatelet therapy)

patients with SCAD should receive the same pharmacological therapy as other ACS.

▪ INTRAVASCULAR IMAGING IN SCAD

There are no RCTs to guide management strategies in patients with SCAD. The use of intravascular imaging is based on observations reported from clinical cohort studies and expert opinion. In cases of diagnostic uncertainty after angiography, the use of intracoronary imaging with OCT or IVUS has to be carefully considered.

TABLE 10: ESC 2023 recommendations for antiplatelet and anticoagulant therapy in acute coronary syndrome.

Recommendations	Class	Level
Antiplatelet therapy:		
Aspirin is recommended for all patients without contraindications at an initial oral LD of 150–300 mg (or 75–250 mg IV) and an MD of 75–100 mg od for long-term treatment	I	A
In all ACS patients, a $P2Y_{12}$ receptor inhibitor is recommended in addition to aspirin given as an initial oral LD followed by an MD for 12 months unless there is HBR	I	A
A proton pump inhibitor in combination with DAPT is recommended in patients at high risk of gastrointestinal in patients at high risk of gastrointestinal bleeding	I	A
Prasugrel is recommended in $P2Y_{12}$ receptor inhibitor-native patients proceeding to PCI (60 mg LD, 10 mg od MD, and 5 mg od MD for patients aged ≥75 years or with a body weight <60 kg)	I	B
Ticagrelor is recommended irrespective of the treatment strategy (invasive or conservative) (10 mg LD, 90 mg bid. MD)	I	B
Clopidogrel (300–600 mg LD, 75 mg od MD) is recommended when prasugrel or ticagrelor are not available, cannot be tolerated or are contraindicated	I	C
It patient presenting with ACS stop DAPT to undergo CABG, it is recommended they resume APT after surgery for at least 12 months	I	C
Prasugrel should be considered in preference to ticagrelor for ACS patients who proceed to PCI	IIa	B
GP IIb/IIIa receptor antagonists should be considered if there is evidence of no-reflow or a thrombotic complication during PCI	IIa	C
In $P2Y_{12}$ receptor inhibitor-naive patients undergoing PCI cangrelor may be considered	IIb	A
In older ACS patients, especially if HBR clopidogrel as the $P2Y_{12}$ receptor inhibitor may be considered	IIb	B
Pretreatment with a $P2Y_{12}$ receptor inhibitor may be considered in patients undergoing a primary PCI strategy	IIb	B

Contd...

Contd...

Recommendations	Class	Level
Pretreatment with a $P2Y_1$ receptor inhibitor may be considered in NSTE-ACS patients who are not expected to undergo an early invasive strategy (<24 hours) and do not have HBR	IIb	C
Pretreatment with a GP IIb/IIIa receptor antagonist is not recommended	III	A
Routine pretreatment with a $P2Y_{12}$ receptor inhibitor in NSTE-ACS patients in whom coronary anatomy is not known and early invasive management (<24 hours) is planned is not recommended	III	A

(ACS: acute coronary syndrome; APT: antiplatelet therapy; CABG: coronary artery bypass graft; DAPT: dual antiplatelet therapy; ESC: European Society of Cardiology; HBR: high bleeding risk; LD: loading dose; MD: maintenance dose; NSTE: non-ST-segment elevation; PCI: percutaneous coronary intervention)

TABLE 11: ESC 2023 recommendations for anticoagulation therapy.

Recommendations	Class	Level
Anticoagulation therapy:		
Parenteral anticoagulation is recommended for all patients with ACS at the time of diagnosis	I	A
Routine use of a UFH bolus (weight-adjusted IV bolus during PCI of 70–100 IU/kg) is recommended in patients undergoing	I	C
Intravenous enoxaparin at the time of PCI should be considered in patients pre-treated with subcutaneous enoxaparin	IIa	B
Discontinuation of parenteral anticoagulation should be considered immediately after an invasive procedure	IIa	C
Patients with STEMI:		
Enoxaparin should be considered an alternative to UFH patients with STEMI undergoing PPCI	IIa	A
Bivalirudin with a full-dose pos PCI infusion should be considered as an alternative to UFH in patients with STEMI undergoing PPCI	IIa	A
Fondaparinux is not recommended in patients with STEMI undergoing PPCI	III	B

Contd...

Acute Coronary Syndrome

Contd...

Recommendations	Class	Level
Patients with NSTE-ACS:		
For patients with NSTE-ACS in whom early invasive angiography (i.e., within 24 hours) is not anticipated, fondaparinux is recommended	I	B
For patients with NSTE-ACS in whom early invasive angiography (i.e., within 24 hours) is anticipated enoxaparin should be considered as an alternative to UFH	IIa	B
Combining antiplatelets and OAC:		
As the default strategy for patients with atrial fibrillation and CHA2-DS-VASc score ≥1 in men and ≥2 in women, after up to 1 week of triple antithrombotic therapy following the ACS event, dual anti thrombotic therapy using a NOAC at the recommended done for stroke prevention and a single oral antiplatelet agent (preferably clopidogrel) for up to 12 months is recommended	I	A
During PCI, a UFH bolus is recommended in any of the following circumstances: • If the patient is on a NOAC • If the INR is <2.5 in VKA-related patients	I	C
In patients with an indication for OAC with VKA in combination with aspirin and/or clopidogrel, careful regulation of the dose intensity of VKA with a target INR of 2.0–2.5 and a time in the therapeutic range >70% should be considered	IIa	II
When rivaroxaban is used and concerns about HBR prevail over ischemic stroke, rivaroxaban 15 mg od should be considered in preference to rivaroxaban 20 mg od for the duration of concomitant SAPT or DAPT	IIa	B
In patients at HBR, dabigatran 110 mg bid should be considered in preference to dabigatran 150 mg bid for the duration of concomitant SAPT or DAPT, to mitigate bleeding risk	IIa	B
• In patients requiring anticoagulation and treated medically, a single antiplatelet agent in addition to an OAC should be considered for up to 1 year • In patients treated with an OAC aspirin plus clopidogrel for longer than 1 week and up to 1 month should be	IIa	B

Contd...

Contd...

Recommendations	Class	Level
considered in those with high ischemic risk or with other anatomical/procedural characteristics that are judged to outweigh the bleeding risk		
In patients requiring OAC withdrawing antiplatelet therapy at 6 months while continuing OAC may be considered	IIb	B
The use of ticagrelor or prasugrel as part of triple antithrombotic therapy is not recommended	III	C

(DAPT: dual antiplatelet therapy; ESC: European Society of Cardiology; HBR: high bleeding risk; NOAC: nonvitamin K antagonist oral anticoagulant; NSTE-ACS: non-ST-segment elevation acute coronary syndrome; PCI: percutaneous coronary intervention; PPCI: primary percutaneous coronary intervention; SAPT: single antiplatelet therapy; STEMI: ST-elevation myocardial infarction; OAC: oral anticoagulant; UFH: unfractionated heparin; VKA: vitamin K antagonist)

BOX 1: Suspected strategies to reduce bleeding risk related to percutaneous coronary intervention.

- Anticoagulant doses adjusted to body weight and renal function, especially in women and older patients
- Radial artery approach as default vascular access
- Proton pump inhibitors in patients on dual antiplatelet therapy at higher-than-average risk of gastrointestinal bleeds (i.e., history of gastrointestinal ulcer/hemorrhage, anticoagulant therapy chronic nonsteroidal anti-inflammatory drug/corticosteroid use), or two or more of:
    – Age ≥65 years
    – Dyspepsia
    – Gastroesophageal reflux disease
    – Helicobacter pylori infection
    – Chronic alcohol use
- In patients on OAC:
    – PCI performed without interruption of VKAs or NOACs
    – In patients on VKAs, do not administer UFH if INR >25
    – In patients on NOACs, regardless of the timing of the last administration of NOACs, add-low-dose parenteral anticoagulation (e.g., enoxaparin 0.5 g/kg (IV or UFH 60 IU/kg)
- Aspirin is indicated but avoid pre-treatment with $P2Y_{12}$ receptor inhibitors
- GP IIb/IIIa receptor inhibitors only for bailout or periprocedural complications

(NOAC: nonvitamin K antagonist oral anticoagulant; OAC: oral anticoagulant; PCI: percutaneous coronary intervention; UFH: unfractionated heparin; VKA: vitamin K antagonist)

Acute Coronary Syndrome

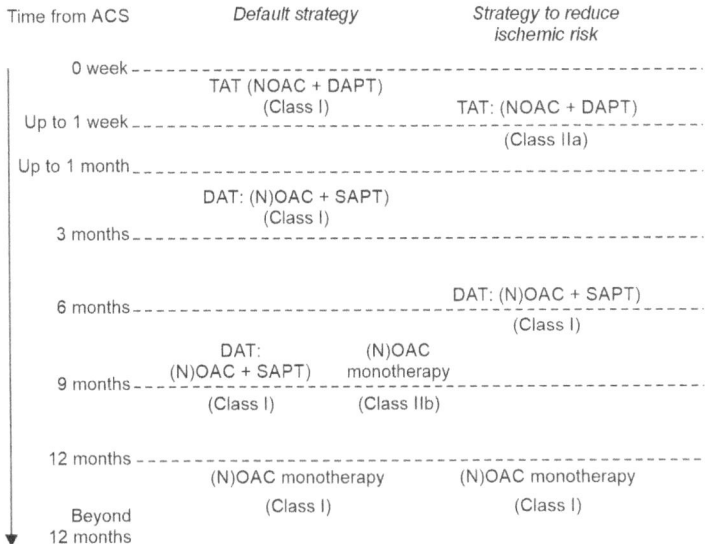

Fig. 5: Patients with ACS and an indication for OAC. (DAPT: dual antiplatelet therapy; NOAC: nonvitamin K antagonist oral anticoagulant; SAPT: single antiplatelet therapy; OAC: oral anticoagulant)

TABLE 12: ESC 2023 recommendations for fibrinolytic therapy.

Recommendations	Class	Level
Fibrinolytic therapy:		
When fibrinolysis is the reperfusion strategy, it is recommended to initiate this treatment as soon as possible after diagnosis in the prehospital setting (aim for target of <10 minutes to lytic bolus)	I	A
A fibrin-specific agent (i.e., tenecteplase, alteplase, or reteplase) is recommended	I	B
A half-dose of tenecteplase should be considered in patients >75 years of age	IIa	B
Antiplatelet co-therapy with fibrinolysis:		
Aspirin and clopidogrel are recommended	I	A
Anticoagulation co-therapy with fibrinolysis:		
Anticoagulation is recommended in patients treated with fibrinolysis until revascularization (if performed) or for the duration of hospital stay (up to 8 days)	I	A

Contd...

Contd...

Recommendations	Class	Level
Enoxaparin IV followed by SC is recommended as the preferred anticoagulant	I	A
When enoxaparin is not available, UFH is recommended as a weight-adjusted IV bolus, followed by infusion	I	B
Patients treated with streptokinase, an IV bolus of fondaparinux followed by an SC dose 24 hours later should be considered	IIa	B
(ESC: European Society of Cardiology; UFH: unfractionated heparin)		

TABLE 13: Doses of fibrinolytic agents and antithrombotic co-therapies (2017 ESC Guidelines for STEMI).

Doses of fibrinolytic therapy

Streptokinase	1.5 million units over 30–60 minutes IV
Alteplase (tPA)	15 mg IV bolus 0.75 mg/kg over 30 min (up to 50 mg) then 0.5/kg IV over 60 minutes (up to 35 mg)
Reteplase (rPA)	10 units + 10 units IV bolus given 30 minutes apart
Tenecteplase (TNK tpA)	Single IV bolus
	30 mg if <60 kg
	35 mg if 60-<70 kg
	40 mg if 80 to <90 kg
	50 mg if >90 kg

It is recommended to reduce to half dose in patients >75 years of age

Doses of antiplatelet co-therapies:

Aspirin	Starting dose of 150–300 mg orally (or 75–150 mg IV if oral ingestion is not possible) followed by a maintenance dose of 75–100 mg/day
Clopidogrel	Loading dose of 300 mg orally followed by maintenance dose of 75 mg/day

In patients >75 years of age, loading dose of 75 mg followed by a maintenance dose of 75 mg/day

Contd...

Acute Coronary Syndrome

Contd...

Doses of anticoagulant co-therapies	
Enoxaparin	In patients, <75 years of age 30 mg IV bolus followed 15 minutes later by 1 mg/kg SC every 12 hours until revascularization or hospital discharge for a maximum of 8 days. The first two SC doses should not exceed 100 mg per injection

- In patients >75 years of age no IV bolus; start with first SC dose of 0.75 mg/kg with a maximum of 75 mg per injection for the first two SC doses
In patients with eGFR <30 mL/min/1.73 m² regardless of age the SC doses are given once every 24 hours
- UFH 60 IU/kg/bolus with a maximum of 4,000 IU followed by an IV infusion of 12 IU/kg with a maximum of 1,000 IU/h for 24–48 hours. Target APTT 50–70s or 1.5–2.0 times that of control to be monitored at 3,6,12 and 24 hours
- Fondaparinux: 2.5 mg IV bolus followed by a SC dose of 2.5 mg once daily up to 8 days or till hospital (only for streptokinase) discharge

(ESC: European Society of Cardiology; STEMI: ST-elevation myocardial infarction; UFH: unfractionated heparin)

Flowchart 4: Coronary Angiography and PCI after Fibrinolytic therapy.

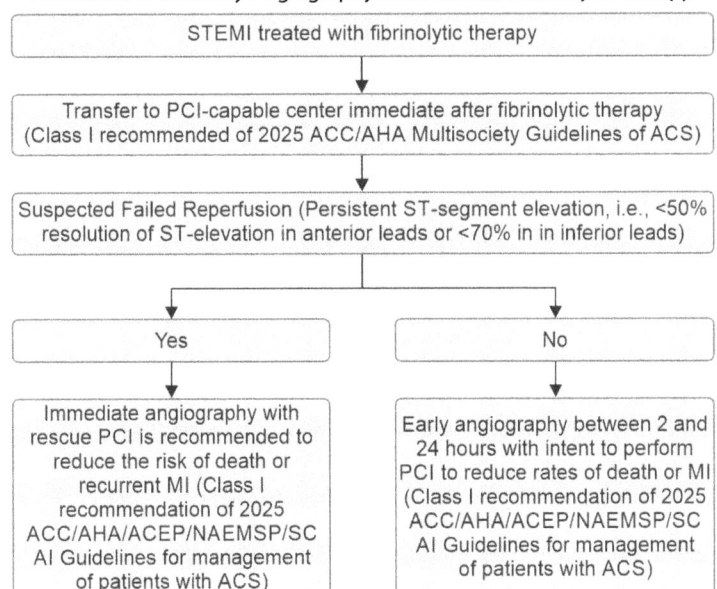

(ACC: American College of Cardiology; AHA: American Heart Association; ACEP: American College of Emergency Physicians; NAEMSP: National Association of EMS Physicians; PCI: percutaneous coronary intervention; SCAI: Society for Cardiovascular Angiography and Interventions; STEMI: ST-elevation myocardial infarction)

Flowchart 5: Patient with ACS undergoing PCI of IRA with an angiographically significant stenosis in ≥1 non-IRA.

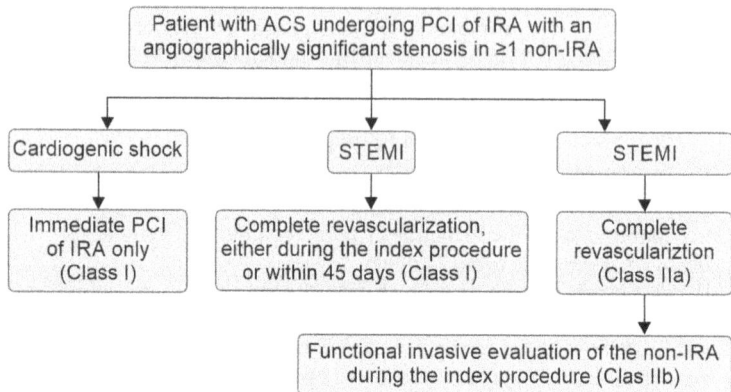

(ACS: acute coronary syndrome; IRA: infarct-related artery; NSTE: non-ST-segment elevation; PCI: percutaneous coronary intervention)

TABLE 14: ESC 2023 recommendations for technical aspects of invasive strategies.

Recommendations	Class	Level
• Radial access is recommended as the standard approach, unless there are over-riding procedural considerations	I	A
• Percutaneous coronary intervention (PCI) with stent deployment in the IRA during the index procedure is recommended in patients		
Undergoing primary PCI (PPCI)	I	A
Drug-eluting stents are recommended in preference to bare metal stents in all cases	I	A
In patients with spontaneous coronary artery dissection, PCI is recommended only for patients with symptoms and signs of ongoing myocardial ischemia, a large area of myocardium in jeopardy, and reduced antegrade flow	I	C
Intravascular imaging should be considered to guide PCI	IIa	A
Coronary artery bypass grafting should be considered in patients with an occluded IRA when PPCI is not feasible/unsuccessful and there is a large area of myocardium in jeopardy	IIa	C
Intravascular imaging (preferably optical coherence tomography) may be considered in patients with ambiguous culprit lesions	IIb	C
The routine use of thrombus aspiration is not recommended	III	A

TABLE 15: Adjunctive pharmacological management after ACS.

(a) Nitroglycerine SL	• 0.4 µg sublingual every 5 minutes for up to three doses • IV start at 10 µg/min and titrate to pain relief and hemodynamic tolerability • Avoid if suspected RV infarction or SBP <90 mm Hg
(b) Morphine	2–4 mg IV. May repeat if needed every 5–15 minutes up to 10 mg total dose
(c) Fentanyl	25–50 µg; may repeat if needed up to 100 µg total dose (Both morphine and fentanyl may delay effects of oral $P2Y_{12}$ therapy)
(d) Beta-blocker	In all patients without contraindication, early (<24 hours) initiation of oral beta-blocker therapy to reduce the risk of reinfarction and ventricular arrhythmia (Class I recommendation of 2025 ACC/AHA/Multisociety ACS Guidelines)
(e) ACEi or ARB	• In high-risk patients with ACS (LVEF ≤40%, hypertension, diabetes mellitus, or STEMI with anterior location) an oral ACEi or an ARB is indicated to reduce all-cause mortality and MACE (Class I recommendation of 2025 ACC/AHA/Multisociety ACS Guidelines) • In ACS patients who are not considered high-risk, an oral ACEi or an ARB is reasonable to reduce MACE (Class 2a recommendation of 2025 ACC/AHA/Multisociety ACS Guidelines)
(f) MRA	In patients with ACS and LVEF ≤40% and with HF symptoms and/or diabetes mellitus, a MRA is indicated to reduce all-cause mortality and MACE (Class I recommendation of 2025 ACC/AHA/Multisociety ACS Guidelines)
(g) Lipid lowering treatment	• In patients with ACS, high-intensity statin therapy is recommended to reduce the risk of MACE (Class I recommendation of 2025 ACC/AHA/multisociety ACS Guidelines) • In patients with ACS, the concurrent initiation of ezetimibe in combination with maximally tolerated statin may be considered to reduce the risk of MACE (Class 2b recommendation of 2025 ACS/AHA/ACS Multisociety Guidelines)

Contd...

Contd...

- In patients with ACS who are statin intolerant, nonstatin lipid lowering therapy is recommended to lower LDL and reduce the risk of MACE (Class I recommendation of 2025 ACC/AHA/Multisociety ACS Guidelines)
- In patients with ACS who are already on maximally tolerated statin therapy with LDL ≥70 mg/dL, nonstatin lipid lowering therapy like ezetimibe, evolocumab, alirocumab, inclisiran, or bempedoic acid should be added to further reduce the risk of MACE (Class I recommendation of 2025 ACC/AHA/Multisociety Guidelines)
- It is reasonable to add a nonstatin therapy if the LDL-cholesterol level is 55–69 mg/dL (Class 2a recommendation of 2025 ACC/AHA/Multisociety Guidelines)

(ACC: American College of Cardiology; ACEi: angiotensin-converting enzyme inhibitor; ACS: acute coronary syndrome; ARB: angiotensin receptor blocker; AHA: American Heart Association; LDL: low-density lipoprotein; LVEF: left ventricular ejection fraction; MACE: major adverse cardiovascular event; MRA: mineralocorticoid receptor antagonist; STEMI: ST-elevation myocardial infarction)

REVASCULARIZATION IN SCAD

Conservative medical management, as opposed to PCI, is generally recommended for patients with SCAD. In an international case series, coronary complications following PCI occurred in >30% of patients. In a pooled analysis of three SCAD-PCI cohorts including 215 patients (94% female) drawn from Dutch, Spanish, and UK registries, and a matched cohort of conservatively managed SCAD patients ($n = 221$). PCI was associated with complications in ≈40% of cases (in during 13% with serious complications). PCI is recommended only for SCAD with associated symptoms and signs of ongoing myocardial ischemia, a large area of myocardium in jeopardy, and reduced antegrade low. Useful strategies for these patients may include minimal plain balloon angioplasty to restore flow, followed by a conservative strategy, targeted stenting to heal the proximal and distal ends of the dissection, and/or extended stent lengths to prevent propagation of the hematoma. In patients with

SCAD, CABG is recommended when dissection affects the left main or two proximal vessels, if PCI is not feasible or unsuccessful, and if there are symptoms and signs of ongoing myocardial ischemia.

MYOCARDIAL INFARCTION WITH NONOBSTRUCTIVE CORONARY ARTERIES

Myocardial infarction with nonobstructive coronary arteries (MINOCA) refers to the clinical situation when a patient presents with symptoms suggestive of ACS, demonstrates troponin elevation, and has nonobstructive coronary arteries at the time of coronary

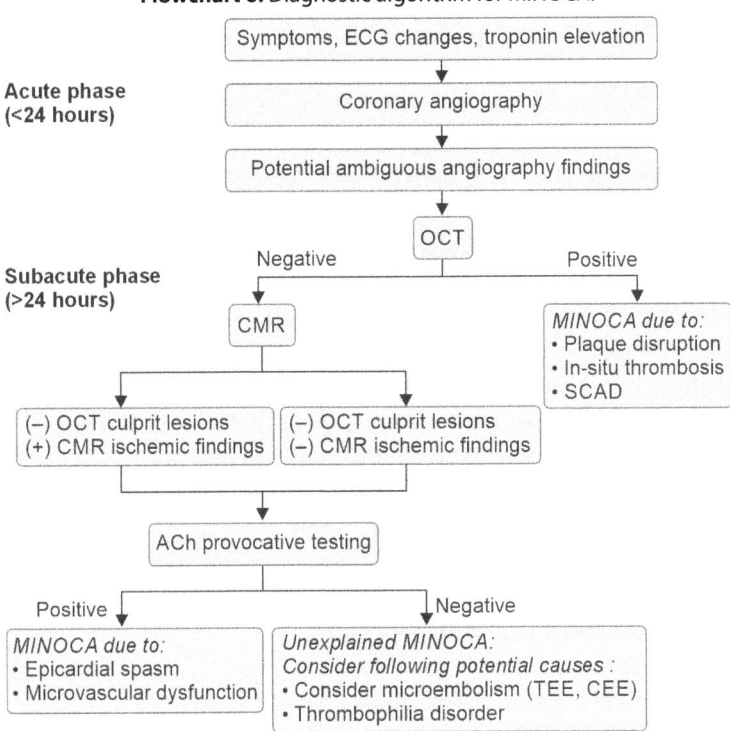

Flowchart 6: Diagnostic algorithm for MINOCA.

(Ach: acetylcholine; CMR: cardiac magnetic resonance; ECG: electrocardiogram; LV: left ventricular; MI-CAD: myocardial infarction with obstructive coronary artery disease; MINOCA: myocardial infarction with nonobstructive coronary arteries; OCT: optical coherence tomography; SCAD: spontaneous coronary artery dissection)

angiography (defined as coronary artery stenosis <50% in any major epicardial vessel). The reported prevalence of NONOCA varies widely across studies (from around 1 to 14% of patients with ACS undergoing angiography). MINOCA can be considered as an umbrella term that encompasses a heterogeneous group of underlying causes. This includes both coronary and noncoronary pathologies, with the latter including both cardiac and extracardiac disorders.

MANAGEMENT OF MINOCA PATIENTS

As previously addressed, the term MINOCA should constitute a "working diagnosis", aimed at identifying underlying causes to optimize treatments and promote prevention of further infarction events. We have also discussed the fundamental role of cardiac magnetic resonance (CMR) in allowing us to arrive at a definitive diagnosis in about 90% of cases. However, only 44% of MINOCA patients present with an ischemic pattern on CMR, even when plaque destruction has already been documented on OCT.

In three observational studies, it has been shown that treatment with Angiotensin-converting enzyme (ACE) inhibitors and angiotensin receptor blockers (ARBs) has beneficial effect on the outcome of these patients. The SWEDEHEART study, mentioned in the previous section, showed a 23% reduction in major adverse cardiovascular event (MACE) in patients treated with statins, an 18% reduction in patients treated with ACE inhibitors and ARBs, and a 14% reduction in patients treated with metoprolol (a beta-blocker). No significant reduction in MACE has been demonstrated with dual antiplatelet therapy (DAPT).

According to a recent statement from the AHA (American Heart Association), the optimal strategy for correct management of patients with MINOCA should include:
- Supportive care in emergencies
- A working diagnosis approach for patient evaluation
- Cardioprotective therapy regardless of the underlying cause of MINOCA
- Targeted therapies

The AHA guidelines primarily focus on evidence of targeted therapies for the cause in the overall treatment of MINOCA, particularly for MINOCA with ischemic presentation. Any patient with atherosclerosis, modifiable risk factors for CAD (such as smoking, hypertension, diabetes mellitus, and hyperlipidemia), should be aggressively treated through aspirin intake as a treatment for the prevention of atherosclerotic plaque erosion, given the similar pathogenetic mechanism to that of AMI-CAD. Recent studies conducted on patients with AMI have also highlighted an increased benefit from the intake of $P2Y_{12}$ receptor inhibitors concurrently with aspirin.

For MINOCA patients with vasospastic angina, calcium channel blockers and nitrates are used as first-line treatment. In case of refractory forms of vasospastic angina, a combination therapy of dihydropyridine and nondihydropyridine calcium channel blockers or the addition of nicorandil (a potassium channel activator) can be considered. In the group of patients with MINOCA due to microcirculatory dysfunction, dipyridamole and ranolazine are indicated, promoting vasodilation. Potential benefits can also be obtained from drugs such as imipramine and aminophylline. Physical exercise for cardiac rehabilitation plays a very important role in the management of cardiovascular diseases, as it reduces both mortality and possible adverse cardiovascular events. He et al. have demonstrated that engaging in physical activity three times a week, for about 20–30 minutes, improves the survival and health of MINOCA patients; therefore, it becomes essential to empower the patient about the benefits of consistent physical exercise.

Currently, there are no studies on the treatment of SCAD, however, an observational study recommends the use of beta-blockers. The use of DAPT in patients with SCAD is still controversial as it carries an increased risk of bleeding. However, a study has suggested the possibility of administering clopidogrel to SCAD patients if the intimal lesion is in a prothrombotic stage. From a study conducted on 72 patients with Takotsubo syndrome, it emerged that these patients benefit from a combination therapy of antithrombotic and heart failure therapy for the first 2 months after the acute event. According to the Inter Tak group, if coronary atherosclerosis is also present, aspirin and statins should be added.

COMPLICATIONS
Heart Failure

Acute heart failure (HF) may occur as a complication of ACS, Acute HF as a result of ACS significantly increases the risk of other in-hospital complications, including worsening of renal function, respiratory failure, pneumonia, and death. De novo acute HF complicating ACS should be distinguished from preexisting HF exacerbated by ACS. This can be challenging and the presence of acute HF may impede the straightforward diagnosis of ACS. Patients with ACS and acute HF are more likely to present with resting dyspnea and clinical signs/symptoms of fluid over-load. In some clinical scenarios, increased troponin levels in patients with acute HF may reflect myocardial injury due to HF rather than myocardial necrosis due to ischemia.

Patients with ACS complicated by acute HF require urgent and coordinated management of both conditions. The management of acute HF should follows current recommendations included in the ESC Guidelines on HF and ancillary documents. The use of diuretics, vasodilators, inotropic, agents, and vasopressors should be considered according to the established algorithms. Mechanical circulatory support may also be considered in selected cases. Invasive respiratory support and/or renal replacement therapy may be required in some circumstances vide chapters on cardiogenic shock and acute heart failure.

SUGGESTED READING

1. Bergmark BA Mathenge N, Merlini PA, Lawrence-Wright MB, Giugliano RP. Acute Coronary Syndrome. Lancet. 2022;399(10332):1347-58.
2. Byrne RA, Rossello X, Coughlan JJ, Barbato E, Berry C, Chieffo A, et al. 2023 ESC Guidelines for management of acute coronary syndrome. Eur Heart J. 2023;44(38):3720-826.
3. Kumbhani DJ, Cibotti-Sun M, Moore MM. The 2025 ACC/AHA/ACEP/NAEMSP/SCAI Guideline for the Management of Patients with Acute Coronary Syndrome (ACC/AHA/Multisociety ACS Guideline). JACC. 2025.
4. Vranckx P, Valgimigli M, Aleksie M. shaping the future of acute coronary syndrome management: A look back at 2024. Eur Heart J Acute Cardiovasc Care. 2025;14(1):40-3.

CHAPTER 2

Cardiogenic Shock

Soumitra Kumar

DEFINITION

Cardiogenic shock (CS) is generally defined as a state of critical end-organ hypoperfusion and hypoxia due to primary cardiac disorders. Diagnosis of CS is made on the basis of clinical criteria of end-organ hypoperfusion such as cold extremities, oliguria, or altered mental status and in addition, biochemical manifestations of inadequate tissue perfusion, such as increased arterial lactate, and increased creatinine are taken into account.

Definitions applied in the European Society of Cardiology (ESC) guidelines and selected major randomized trials are enumerated further **(Boxes 1 to 3)**.

> **BOX 1:** Clinical parameters.
>
> *SHOCK trial:* SBP <90 mm Hg for ≥30 minutes spontaneous or maintained >90 mm Hg with vasopressor support
>
> *TRIUMPH trial:* Refractory PCI or demonstration of infarct-related artery (IRA) spontaneous patency with SBP <100 mm Hg despite vasopressors (dopamine ≥7 μg/kg/min or norepinephrine or epinephrine ≥0.15 μg/kg/min)
>
> *IABP-SHOCK II:*
> - SBP <90 mm Hg for ≥30 minutes or catecholamines to maintain SBP >90 mm Hg
> - Clinical pulmonary congestion
>
> *CULPRIT SHOCK:*
> - SBP <90 mm Hg for >30 minutes spontaneous or >90 mm Hg with support by catecholamines
> - Clinical signs of pulmonary congestion
> - Signs of impaired organ perfusion (as detailed below)
>
> *ESC heart failure guidelines:* SBP <90 mm Hg with adequate volume
>
> (ESC: European Society of Cardiology; PCI: percutaneous coronary intervention; SBP: systolic blood pressure; TRIUMPH: treating resistant hypertension using lifestyle modification to promote health)

BOX 2: Markers of impaired end-organ perfusion.

- *SHOCK trial:*
  - Clinical criteria
    - Cool extremities
    - Heart rate >60 beats/min
  - Hemodynamic criteria
    - Urine output <30 mL/h
    - Cardiac index ≤2.2 L/min/m^2
    - PCWP ≥15 mm Hg
- *TRIUMPH trial:*
  - Clinical or hemodynamic criteria for elevated LV filling pressure LVEF <40%
- *IAEF-SHOCK II trial:*
  - Clinical criteria
    - Altered mental status
    - Cold/clammy skin and extremities
  - Hemodynamic criteria
    - Urine output <30 mL/h
    - Lactate >2 mmol/L
- *CULPRIT-SHOCK trial:*
  - Clinical criteria
    - Altered mental status
    - Cold/clammy skin and extremities
  - Hemodynamic criteria
    - Urine output <30 mL/h
    - Lactate >2.0 mmol/L
- *ESC HF guidelines:*
  - Clinical criteria
    - Cold extremities
    - Oliguria
    - Mental confusion/dizziness
    - Narrow pulse pressure
  - Laboratory criteria
    - Metabolic acidosis
    - Elevated lactate
    - Elevated creatinine

(ESC: European Society of Cardiology; HF: heart failure; PCWP: pulmonary capillary wedge pressure; LV: left ventricular; LVEF: left ventricular ejection fraction)

Identifying the preshock state is vitally important since it may reduce mortality by preventing progression to CS. The best validated score to predict development of CS is ORBI (Observatoire Regional Breton sur l'Infarctus/du myocarde) **(Tables 1 and 2)**.

> **BOX 3:** SCAI clinical expert consensus statement on classification of cardiogenic shock.
>
> *Stage A:* Currently no signs/symptoms of CS but being "At risk" for its development
> *Stage B:*
> - Preshock:
>   – Clinical evidence of relative hypotension or tachycardia without hypoperfusion being at "Beginning" of CS
>
> *Stage C:*
> - Classic CS:
>   – Manifest CS with hypoperfusion requiring intervention (inotropes, vasopressors, or MCS excluding ECMO) beyond volume resuscitation to restore perfusion
>
> *Stage D:* CS signals deteriorating to "Doom". Similar to stage C but getting worse and failing to respond to initial interventions
>
> *Stage E:* Patients in "Extremis" such as those experiencing cardiac arrest with ongoing cardiopulmonary resuscitation and/or ECMO cardiopulmonary resuscitation
>
> (CS: cardiogenic shock; ECMO: extracorporeal membrane oxygenation; MCS: mechanical circulatory support; SCAI: Society for Cardiovascular Angiography and Interventions)

TABLE 1: ORBI score.

Variable	Points
Age >70 years	2
Previous stroke/TIA	2
Presentation as cardiac arrest	3
Anterior myocardial infarction	1
First medical contact to PPCI delay >90 minutes	2
Killip class II on admission	2
Killip class III on admission	6
Heart rate >90 beats/min on admission	3
SBP <125 mm Hg and PP <45 mm Hg on admission	4
Glycemia >10 mmol/l on admission	3
Culprit lesion of left main	5
Post PPCI TIMI flow <3	5

(ORBI: Observatoire Regional Breton sur l'Infarctus/du myocarde; PPCI: primary percutaneous coronary intervention; PP: pulse pressure; SBP: systolic blood pressure; TIA: transient ischemic attack; TIMI: thrombolysis in myocardial infarction)

TABLE 2: Risk categories.

Category	Score	Observed incidence of CS
Low	0–7	1.3
Low to intermediate	8–10	6.6
Intermediate to high	11–12	11.7
High	≥13	31.8

(CS: cardiogenic shock)

TABLE 3: IABP–SHOCK II risk score.

Variable	Points
Age 73 years	1
History of stroke	2
Glucose >19/mg/dL	1
Creatinine >1.5 mg/dL	1
Lactate <5 mmol/L	2
TIMI for <3 after PCI	2

(IABP: intra-aortic balloon pump; PCI: percutaneous coronary intervention; TIMI: thrombolysis in myocardial infarction)

TABLE 4: IABP–SHOCK II risk score categories.

Category	Points	Short-term mortality in cardiogenic shock trial population
Low	0–2	28%
Intermediate	3–4	42.9%
High	5–9	77.3%

(IABP: intra-aortic balloon pump)

Currently, there is only one CS score in the setting of classical CS derived from IABP—SHOCK II trial with both internal and external validation **(Tables 3 and 4)**.

Broadly speaking, CS has two etiological groups:
1. Acute myocardial infarction (AMI) leading to CS (50–60%)
2. Advanced heart failure leading to CS (20–30%)

Accordingly, the "Shock-Team" should be orchestrated as mentioned in **Table 6**.

TABLE 5: Potential hemodynamic presentations of CS.

		Volume status	
		Wet	**Dry**
Circulation Peripheral	Cold	Classic cardiogenic shock (↓CI; ↑SVRI; ↑PCWP)	Euvolemic cardiogenic shock (↓CI; ↑SVRI; ↔PCWP)
	Warm	Vasodilatory cardiogenic shock or Mixed shock (↓CI; ↓/↔SVRI; ↑PCWP)	Vasodilatory shock (Not cardiogenic shock) (↑CI; ↓SVRI; ↓PCWP)

(CI: cardiac index; CS: cardiogenic shock; PCWP: pulmonary capillary wedge pressure; SVRI: systemic vascular resistance index)

TABLE 6: Arrangement of Shock-Team.

Acute MI CS team	Advanced HF CS team
1. Interventional cardiologist	1. Advanced HF specialist
2. Cardiac surgeon	2. Interventional cardiologist
3. Critical care intensivist	3. Cardiac surgeon
4. Advanced HF specialist	4. Critical care intensivist
5. Critical care nursing team	5. Critical care nursing team
6. Perfusion team	6. Palliative care
7. Respiratory specialists	7. Perfusion team
8. Physical and occupational therapists	8. Respiratory specialists
9. Palliative care	9. Physical and occupational therapist

(HF CS: heart failure cardiogenic shock; MI CS: myocardial infarction cardiogenic shock)

CARDIOGENIC SHOCK SPECIFIC PREPAREDNESS PLAN

- Parallel palliative care and curative care interventions—tailored to patient's values and preferences
- Multiple intravenous drug infusion facility
- Hemodynamic monitoring
- Artificial nutrition
- Mechanical ventilation
- Hemodialysis

> **BOX 4:** Etiologies of cardiogenic shock.
>
> *Myocardial:*
> - *Acute myocardial infarction:*
>   - >40% loss of left ventricular mass
>   - <40% loss of left ventricular mass with arrhythmia or vasodilation
>   - Right ventricular infarction
>   - *Mechanical complication:*
>   - Papillary muscle rupture
>   - Ventricular septal rupture
>   - Free wall rupture
> - *Acute decompensated heart failure:*
>   - Chronic heart failure (established etiology) with decompensation
>   - *Acute heart failure first presentation:*
>   - Chronic ischemia
>   - Dilated cardiomyopathy
>   - Myocarditis
>   - Stress induced cardiomyopathy (Takotsubo)
>   - *Pregnancy associated heart disease:*
>   - Peripartum cardiomyopathy
>   - Coronary artery dissection
>   - Endocrine disorders (hypo-/hyperthyroidism and pheochromocytoma)
> - Postcardiotomy shock:
>   - Prolonged cardiopulmonary bypass
>   - Insufficient cardioprotection
> - Dynamic outflow tract obstruction
> - Post cardiac arrest stunning
> - Myocardial depression in setting of septic shock or SIRS
> - Myocardial contusion
>
> (SIRS: systemic inflammatory response syndrome)

- Mechanical circulatory support device application
- Family support and counseling

American College of Cardiology/American Heart Association (ACS/AHA) indicates for pulmonary artery catheterization in acute myocardial infarction (AMI) are as follows:

Class I:
- Severe or progressive congestive heart failure (CHF) or pulmonary edema
- CS or progressive hypotension
- Suspected mechanical complications of acute infarction

TABLE 7: Considerations for initial critical care monitoring in patients with CS.

Monitoring parameters	Frequency	Comment/Rationale
Noninvasive monitoring		
Telemetry, pulse oximetry, respiratory rate	Continuous	High incidence of arrhythmias, ventricular failure, and pulmonary edema
Critical care unit monitoring	1:1 nurse-to-patient ratio	High incidence of hemodynamic deterioration and multisystem organ failure
Invasive monitoring		
Arterial BP monitoring	Continuous	Consider continuing until vasoactive medications have been discontinued for 12–24 h
CVP	Continuous	• A central line is required for delivery of vasoactive medications, single-point-in-time • CVP measurements may be unreliable measures of fluid status, but longitudinal • CVP trends may provide information on trends in fluid status
Central venous saturation	Every 4 h	Trends in central venous oxygen saturation in patients with a central line can be used to help monitor trends in cardiac output
Urine output	Every hour	Urine output and serum creatinine monitoring are markers of renal perfusion and acute kidney injury
PAC or noninvasive cardiac	Selected use	Consider using early in the treatment course in patients not responsive to initial therapy or in cases of diagnostic or therapeutic uncertainty
Laboratory investigations		
Complete blood counts	Every 12–24 h	Consider more frequently in patients with CS with, or at high risk for bleeding

Contd...

Contd...

Monitoring parameters	Frequency	Comment/Rationale
Serum electrolyte	Every 6–12 h	Frequency should be tailored to risks or presence of renal failure and electrolyte dyscrasias
Serum creatinine	Every 12–24 h	Urine output and serum creatinine monitoring are the markers of renal perfusion and acute kidney injury
Liver function tests	Daily	Monitoring for congestive hepatopathy and hypoperfusion
Lactate	Every 1–4 h	Lactate clearance is a marker of resolving end-organ hypoperfusion, and lack of clearance is associated with a higher risk of mortality
Coagulation laboratories	Every 4–6 hours for those on anticoagulants until therapeutically stable, every 2–hours if patient is not on anticoagulants	Altered drug elimination and frequent Use of mechanical support devices often necessitate antithrombotic monitoring

(BP: blood pressure; CS: cardiogenic shock; CVP: central venous pressure; PAC: pulmonary artery catheter)

TABLE 8: Critical care complication prevention bundles in patients with CS.

Bundle	Target	Components
ABCDE bundle	Delirium, weakness, and Trials Ventilation liberation	• Daily awakening and spontaneous breathing trials • Assessment and management of delirium • Early and progressive mobility
Ventilator bundle	Ventilator-associated pneumonia	• Head of bed elevation • Sedation protocols targeting light sedation with RAAS or SAS scores • Daily sedation vacation if light sedation contraindicated

Contd...

Contd...

Bundle	Target	Components
		• Chlorhexidine oral rinse
		• Endotracheal tube with subglottic secretion drainage
Central line bundle	Central line-associated bloodstream infection	• Hand hygiene • Maximal barrier precautions • Chlorhexidine skin antisepsis • Optimal catheter site selection (avoidance of femoral approach) • Ultrasound-guided central line placement • Daily review of line necessity
Stress ulcer prophylaxis	Stress ulcer	• Proton pump inhibitor or H_2 blocker in patients without enteral nutrition • In enterally fed patients, the risk of prophylaxis should be balanced with risk of ventilator-associated pneumonia
Deep vein	Venous thromboembolism	Routine venous thromboembolism prophylaxis in thrombosis patients not on anticoagulants prophylaxis

(ABCDE: awakening and breathing coordination; delirium monitoring/management, and early exercise mobility; CS: cardiogenic shock; RAAS: Richmond Agitation-Sedation Scale; SAS: Sedation-Agitation Scale)

Class II:
Hypotension which does not respond promptly to fluid administration in a patient without pulmonary congestion.

ANTIPLATELET THERAPY IN CARDIOGENIC SHOCK

Cardiogenic shock is a potent predictor of stent thrombosis. Hence, means to enhance potency, consistency and rapidity of antiplatelet therapy in AMI with CS (AMICS) may justify preferential use of third generation oral P2Y12 inhibitors instead of clopidogrel, i.e., ticagrelor or prasugrel, administration of crushed ticagrelor via

TABLE 9: Utility of echocardiogram in cardiogenic shock.

Clinical question	Information
Ventricular function	Predominantly left, right, or biventricular involvement
Etiology of shock	*Acute myocardial infarction:* • Extent of infarction/myocardium in jeopardy • Status of the nonculprit infarct zone • Presence of mechanical complications *Acute valvular insufficiency/obstruction (native/prosthetic):* • Etiology: Endocarditis; degenerative valve disease • Location and hemodynamic consequences *Dynamic left ventricular tract obstruction takotsubo cardiomyopathy cardiac tamponade:* • Circumferential versus localized effusion • Route of pericardiocentesis if indicated *Acute pulmonary embolism:* • Right ventricular function • Presence of clot in transition/patent foramen ovale *Acute aortic syndrome:* • Nature and extent of dissection • Degree of aortic insufficiency • Presence of pericardial effusion
Hemodynamics	• Volume assessment as gauged by inferior vena cava • Estimated pulmonary artery systolic pressure • Estimated left atrial pressure
Therapeutic guidance	• Guide vasoactive support • Monitor response to therapy • Mechanical circulatory support decisions: Single or biventricular support • Catheter position and guidance
Hemodynamic formulas to assess RV function		
Cardiac filling pressure	RA/PCWP	>0.63 (RVF after LVAD) >0.88 (RVF in acute MI)
PA pulsatility index	(PASP-PADP)/RA	<1.85 (RVF after LVAD) <1.0 (RVF in Acute MI)
Pulmonary vascular resistance	MPA-PCWP/CO	>3.6 (RVF after LVAD)

Contd...

Contd...

Transpulmonary gradient	MPA-PCWP	Undetermined
Diastolic pulmonary gradient	PAD-PCWP	Undetermined
RV stroke work	(mPAP-RA) × SV × 0.0136	<15 (RVF after LVAD) <10 (RVF after acute MI)
RV stroke work index	(mPAP-RAV/SV index)	<0.3–0.6 (FVF after LVAD)
Pulmonary artery compliance	SV (PASP-PADP)	<2.5 (RVF in chronic heart failure)
Pulmonary artery	PASP/SV	Undetermined

(LVAD: left ventricular assist device; MI: myocardial infarction; mPAP: mean PA pressure; PA: pulmonary artery; PASP: pulmonary artery systolic pressure; PADP: pulmonary artery diastolic pressure; PCWP: pulmonary capillary wedge pressure; RA: right atrial; RVF: right ventricular failure; SV: stroke volume)

TABLE 10: Potential cardiogenic shock care pathway.

Step 1	*Resuscitation and medical therapy:* • Inotropes/vasopressors • Mechanical ventilation/ultrafiltration • Etiology-specific medical therapy
Step 2	*Revascularization (in acute coronary syndrome only):* • PCI • CABG • Fibrinolysis
Step 3	*Temporary mechanical circulatory support (MCS):* • IABP • Peripheral VAD • ECMO • Implantable VAD
Step 4	Durable VAD
Step 5	Transplant Destination VAD

(CABG: coronary artery bypass grafting; ECMO: extracorporeal membrane oxygenation; IABP: intra-aortic balloon pump; PCI: percutaneous coronary intervention; VAD: ventricular assist device)

TABLE 11: Hemodynamic effects of common vasoactive medications in CS.

Medication	Usual infusion dose	Receptor binding				Hemodynamic effects
		α_1	β_1	β_2	Dopamine	
Vasopressors/inotropes						
Dopamine	0.5–2 µg/kg/min	–	+	–	+++	↑CO
	5–10 µg/kg/min	+	+++	+	++	↑CO, ↑SVR
	10–20 µg/kg/min	+++	++	–	++	↑SVR, ↑CO
Norepinephrine	0.05–0.4 µg/kg/min	++++	++	+	–	↑SVR, ↑CO
Epinephrine	0.01–0.5 µg/kg/min	++++	++++	+++	–	↑CO, ↑↑SVR
Phenylephrine	0.1–10 µg/kg/min	++++	–	–	–	↑↑SVR
Vasopressin	0.02–0.04 U/min	Stimulates V_1 receptors in vascular smooth muscle				↑↑SVR, ↔PVR
Inodilators						
Dobutamine	2.5–20 µg/kg/min	–	++++	++	–	↑↑CO, ↓SVR, ↓PVR
Isoproterenol	2.0–20 µg/min	–	++++	++++	–	↑↑CO, ↓SVR, ↓PVR
Milrinone	0.125–0.75 µg/kg/min	–	–	–	PDE-3 inhibitor	↑CO, ↓SVR, ↓PVR
Enoximone	2–10 µg/kg/min	–	–	–	PDE-3 inhibitor	↑CO, ↓SVR, ↓PVR
Levosimendan	0.05–0.2 µg/kg/min	Myofilament Ca^{2+} sensitizer, PDE-3 inhibitor				↑CO, ↓SVR, ↓PVR

(CO: cardiac output; CS: cardiogenic shock; PDE-3: phosphodiesterase-3; PVR: pulmonary vascular resistance; SVR: systemic vascular resistance)

Cardiogenic Shock

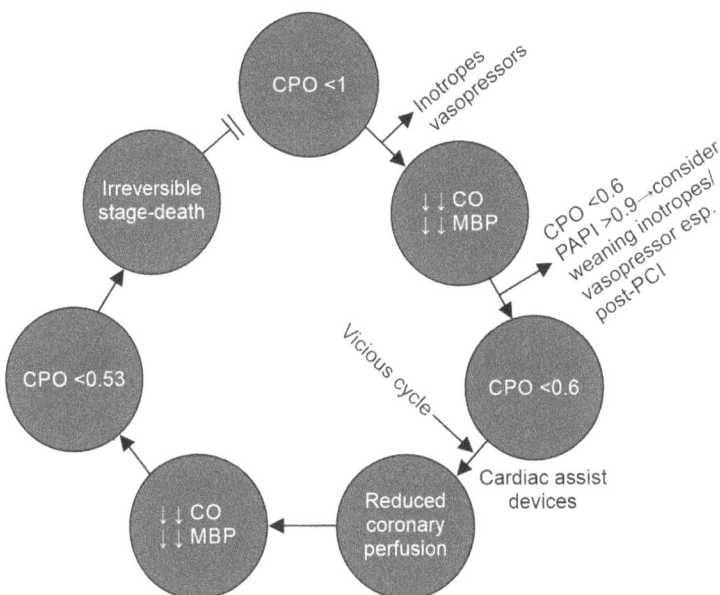

Fig. 1: The course of hemodynamic compromise. (CO: cardia output; CPO: cardiac power output = $\frac{MAP \times CO}{451}$; dPAP: diastolic pulmonary artery pressure; PAPI: pulmonary artery pulsatility index = $\frac{sPAP - dPAP}{RA}$; MAP: mean arterial pressure; MBP: mean blood pressure; PCI: percutaneous coronary intervention; sPAP: systolic pulmonary artery pressure)

TABLE 12: Initial Vasoactive Management in types of CS.

Cause of presentation of CS	Hemodynamic setting	Vasoactive management consideration
Classic wet and cold	Low CI and high SVR ↑LVEDP arrhythmias	• *Norepinephrine:* If ↑HR or arrhythmias • *Dopamine:* If ↓HR—higher risk of arrhythmias • Consider after revascularization (MI only)
Euvolemic cold and dry	Low LVEDP, low CI, high SVR	• *Norepinephrine:* If ↑HR or arrhythmias • *Dopamine:* If ↓HR—higher risk of arrhythmias • Fluid boluses if low LVEDP • Consider after revascularization (MI only)

Contd...

Contd...

Cause of presentation of CS	Hemodynamic setting	Vasoactive management consideration
Vasodilatory warm and wet or mixed (cardiogenic and vaso-dilatory)	Low SVR	Norepinephrine—consider hemodynamics guided Rx
RV shock	RV systolic dysfunction AV dissociation	• Fluid boluses • Maintain RV preload, ↓RV afterload (PVR) • Pacer to maintain • AV synchrony or correct bradycardia • Norepinephrine, dopamine or vasopressin • Inodilators (dobutamine) • Inhaled pulmonary vasodilatory
Normointensive shock	SBP >90 mm Hg Relatively high SVR	Inodilator (dobutamine)
Aortic stenosis	• Low CI in an afterload-dependent state • Preserved LVEF or reduced	• Inotropes if LVEF is ↓(phenylephrine or vasopressin) • Echocardiography or PAC-guided dobutamine titration • SAVR/TAVR/BAV
Aortic regurgitation	• ↑LVEDP • High heart rate	• Maintain elevated HR • →↓DFT and ↓LVEDP • SAVR
Mitral stenosis	Low CI, low preload high rate/HF	• Slowing heart rate and maintaining AV synchrony (Esmolol/Amiodarone) • Improve preload • BMV/SMVR
Mitral regurgitation	Low forward CI ↑LVEDP	• Norepinephrine or dopamine • →inotrope once BP↑ • Reduce afterload • IABP/temporary MCS • SMVR/repair or mitral clip procedure

Contd...

Cardiogenic Shock

Contd...

Cause of presentation of CS	Hemodynamic setting	Vasoactive management consideration
Post-MI VSR (wet and cold shock)	Low CI and high SVR ↑LVEDP	• IABP/temporary MCS • Norepinephrine, dopamine as for wet and cold shock • Surgery/Percutaneous device closure
Dynamic LVOT obstruction	↑Contractility ↓CI	• Fluid boluses (↑preload) • ↑Afterload (phenylephrine or vasopressin) • ↓Contractility (Esmolol) • Maintain AV synchrony (amiodarone) • Induce ventricular dyssynchrony (RV pacing) • Avoid inotropes (dobutamine and dopamine)
Bradycardia (atropine/ isoproterenol/ dopamine)	Low HR	• Chronotropic agents • Temporary pacing
Pericardial tamponade	↓Preload ↓CI	• Fluid bolus • Pericardiocentesis

(AV: atrioventricular; BAV: bicuspid aortic valve; CS: cardiogenic shock; CI: cardiac index; DFT: diastolic filling time; HR: heart rate; IABP: intra-aortic balloon pump; LVEDP: left ventricular end-diastolic pressure; LVEF: left ventricular ejection fraction; LVOT: left ventricular outflow tract; MCS: mechanical circulatory support; MI: myocardial infarction; PAC: pulmonary artery catheter; PVR: pulmonary vascular resistance; RV: right ventricular; SAVR: surgical aortic valve replacement; SMVR: surgical mitral valve repair; SVR: systemic vascular resistance; TAVR: transcatheter aortic valve replacement)

gastric tube, and parenteral use of cangrelor alone or in combination with ticagrelor. Adjunctive use of glycoprotein IIb/IIIa inhibitors may also further reduce platelet reactivity. However, in patients in whom large caliber access is created for MCS devices, this may have bleeding issues. Rapid reversibility of cangrelor despite bowel, liver, and kidney dysfunction is a point in favor of safety.

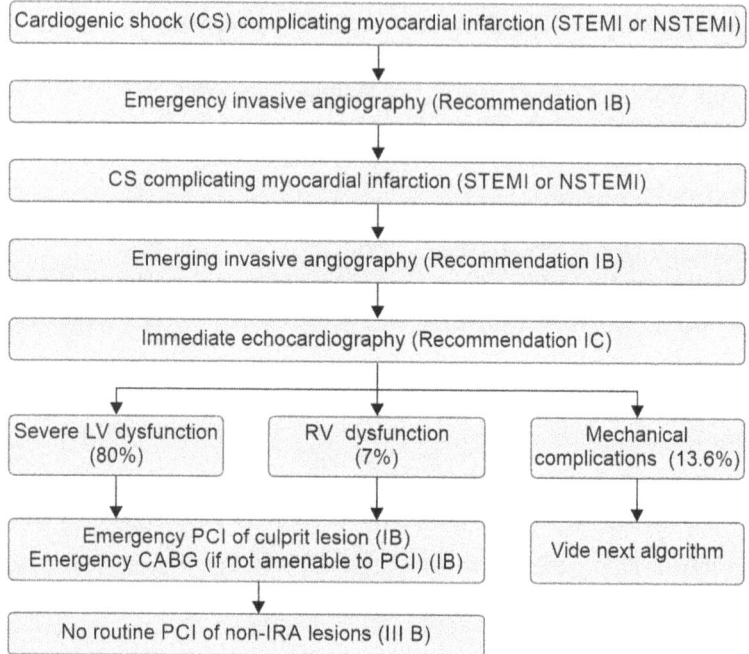

Flowchart 1: Treatment algorithm for patients with CS complicating myocardial infarction.

(CABG: coronary artery bypass grafting; IRA: infarct-related artery; LV: left ventricular; NSTEMI: non-ST-elevation myocardial infarction; PCI: percutaneous coronary intervention; RV: right ventricular; STEMI: ST-elevation myocardial infarction)

MANAGEMENT OF MULTIVESSEL DISEASE IN CARDIOGENIC SHOCK

The CULPRIT-SHOCK trial showed a significant reduction in 30-day mortality or reveal replacement therapy (primary end point) with a strategy of culprit lesion-only PCI (with an option for staged revascularization of additional lesions) compared with multivessel PCI [45% vs. 55.4%; relative risk 0.83 (95% confidence interval 0.71–0.96) driven basically by an absolute 8.21% reduction in mortality].

In vast majority of patients with AMICS, PCI should be limited to the culprit lesion with scope of staged revascularization of other lesions. However, it should be noted that few patients in the CULPRIT-SHOCK trial received MCS.

Contd...

Cause of presentation of CS	Hemodynamic setting	Vasoactive management consideration
Post-MI VSR (wet and cold shock)	Low CI and high SVR ↑LVEDP	• IABP/temporary MCS • Norepinephrine, dopamine as for wet and cold shock • Surgery/Percutaneous device closure
Dynamic LVOT obstruction	↑Contractility ↓CI	• Fluid boluses (↑preload) • ↑Afterload (phenylephrine or vasopressin) • ↓Contractility (Esmolol) • Maintain AV synchrony (amiodarone) • Induce ventricular dyssynchrony (RV pacing • Avoid inotropes (dobutamine and dopamine)
Bradycardia (atropine/ isoproterenol/ dopamine)	Low HR	• Chronotropic agents • Temporary pacing
Pericardial tamponade	↓Preload ↓CI	• Fluid bolus • Pericardiocentesis

(AV: atrioventricular; BAV: bicuspid aortic valve; CS: cardiogenic shock; CI: cardiac index; DFT: diastolic filling time; HR: heart rate; IABP: intra-aortic balloon pump; LVEDP: left ventricular end-diastolic pressure; LVEF: left ventricular ejection fraction; LVOT: left ventricular outflow tract; MCS: mechanical circulatory support; MI: myocardial infarction; PAC: pulmonary artery catheter; PVR: pulmonary vascular resistance; RV: right ventricular; SAVR: surgical aortic valve replacement; SMVR: surgical mitral valve repair; SVR: systemic vascular resistance; TAVR: transcatheter aortic valve replacement)

gastric tube, and parenteral use of cangrelor alone or in combination with ticagrelor. Adjunctive use of glycoprotein IIb/IIIa inhibitors may also further reduce platelet reactivity. However, in patients in whom large caliber access is created for MCS devices, this may have bleeding issues. Rapid reversibility of cangrelor despite bowel, liver, and kidney dysfunction is a point in favor of safety.

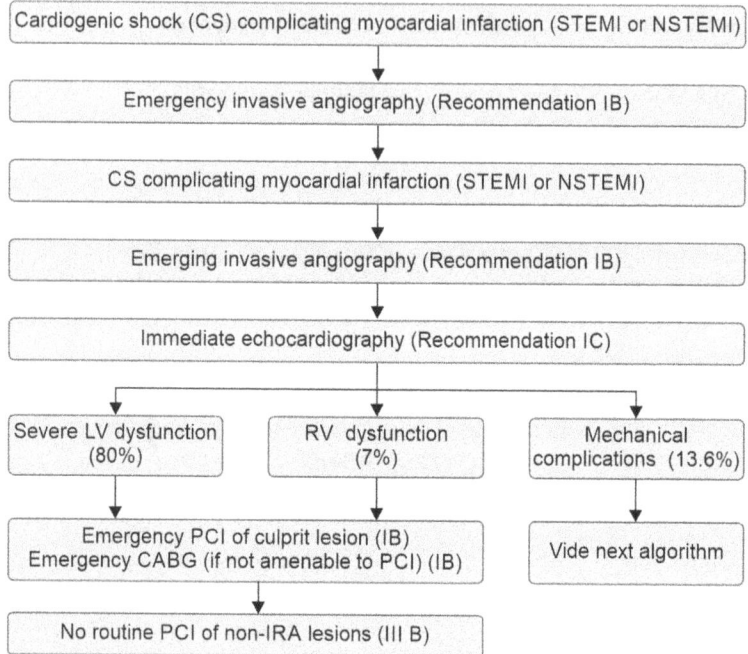

Flowchart 1: Treatment algorithm for patients with CS complicating myocardial infarction.

(CABG: coronary artery bypass grafting; IRA: infarct-related artery; LV: left ventricular; NSTEMI: non-ST-elevation myocardial infarction; PCI: percutaneous coronary intervention; RV: right ventricular; STEMI: ST-elevation myocardial infarction)

MANAGEMENT OF MULTIVESSEL DISEASE IN CARDIOGENIC SHOCK

The CULPRIT-SHOCK trial showed a significant reduction in 30-day mortality or reveal replacement therapy (primary end point) with a strategy of culprit lesion-only PCI (with an option for staged revascularization of additional lesions) compared with multivessel PCI [45% vs. 55.4%; relative risk 0.83 (95% confidence interval 0.71–0.96) driven basically by an absolute 8.21% reduction in mortality].

In vast majority of patients with AMICS, PCI should be limited to the culprit lesion with scope of staged revascularization of other lesions. However, it should be noted that few patients in the CULPRIT-SHOCK trial received MCS.

Flowchart 2: Mechanical complications following myocardial infarction.

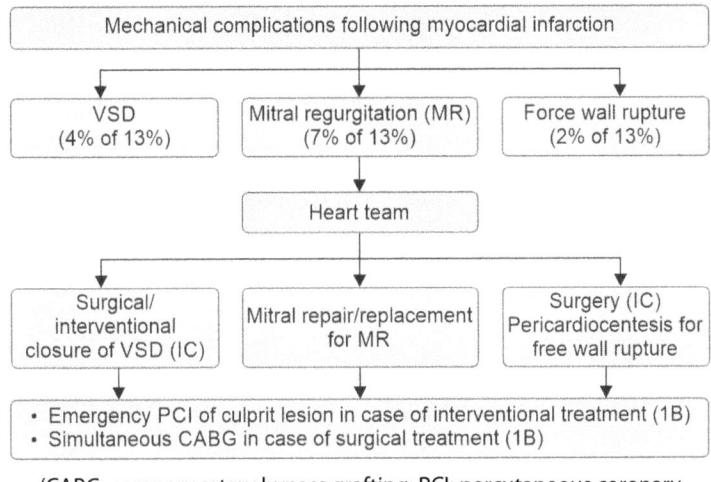

(CABG: coronary artery bypass grafting; PCI: percutaneous coronary intervention; VSD: ventricular septal defect)

As the recent Korea Acute Myocardial Infarction National Health Registry data has suggested that multivessel PCI in CSI was associated with a lower risk of all-cause death culprit-artery only PCI at 3 years. Hence, the role of multivessel PCI in AMI CS continues to be debated.

A meta-analysis by Bertaina et al. which included 11 observational studies and one randomized controlled trial (RCT) (the CULPRIT-SHOCK trial) showed that multivessel PCI was not associated with increased mortality compared to culprit-only PCI but did produce higher rates of acute kidney injury (AKI). A study by Lemor et al. demonstrated that in patients with multivessel coronary artery disease (CAD) presented with AMICS treated with early MCS, revascularization of nonculprit lesions was associated with similar hospital survival and AKI when compared with culprit-only PCI. They concluded that selective nonculprit PCI can be safely performed in AMICS in patients supported with mechanical circulatory support.

While deciding on intervention culprit vessels, operators should bear in mind a multitude of factors such as TIMI flow grade, presence of a chronic total occlusion (CTO), size and distribution of the vessel in question, underlying hemodynamics, availability of suitable MCS, and skilled manpower.

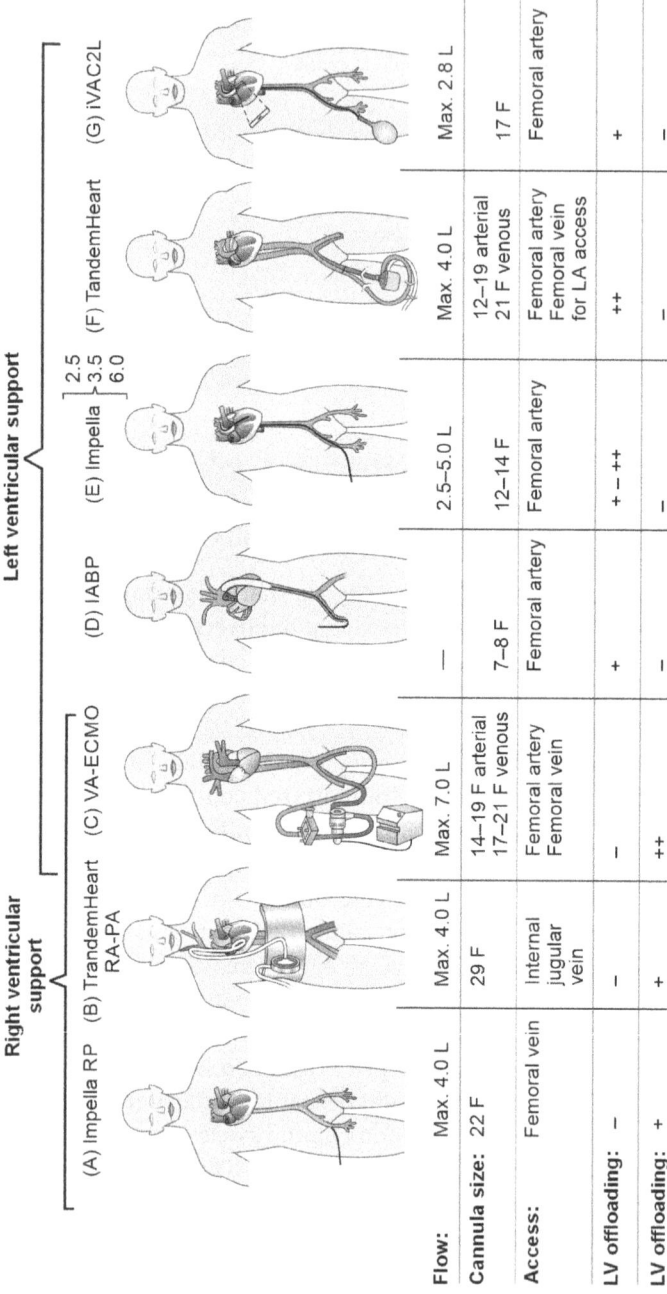

Fig. 2: Routine scheme of use of percutaneous mechanical support devices for cardiogenic shock.
(IABP: intra-aortic balloon pump; LA: left atrium; LV: left ventricular)

CARDIAC INTENSIVE CARE IN CARDIOGENIC SHOCK

The role of cardiac intensive care cannot be overstated in CS and management. This includes relentless monitoring of vital parameters and titration of therapies based on evolving data, anticipation, and management of complications, collaboration, and shared decision making by a multidisciplinary shock team, including escalation or de-escalation of MCS. A study of Jin NA, et al. showed that presence of a dedicated cardiac intensivist reduce cardiac intensive care unit (CICU) mortality rates in critical cardiac patients acquiring cardiac ICU treatment.

CARDIAC ARREST IN CARDIOGENIC SHOCK

Cardiac arrest is common among patients with AMICS and confers an increased risk of mortality that in independent of shock stage. Outcomes are exponentially influenced by a variable extent of hypoxic-ischemic encephalopathy. Those patients with AMICS suffering cardiac arrest, whose spontaneous circulation fails to result, have the highest risk of multiorgan failure and mortality. SHOCK-COOL trial, a trial of mild hypothermia in AMICS, was a negative trial.

However, AMCS should not be used indiscriminately. A collaborative meta-analysis by Thiele et al. compared Tandem Heart or Impella MCS vs. Control (IABP) in terms of 30-day mortality and device-related complications, e.g., bleeding and leg ischemia. No significant difference was observed in terms of 30-day mortality and leg ischemia. However, rate of bleeding was significant increased with MCS compared to IABP. Acute MCS significantly increased mean arterial pressure and decreased arterial lactate and PCWP. Hence, this collaborative meta-analysis does not support the unselected use of active MCS in patients with CS complicating AMI. However, greater benefit may be expected in setting other than in AMI (e.g., patients with shock complicating end-stage heart failure if cardiac transplantation may be an option).

Cardiogenic Shock

Flowchart 3: Approach to cardiogenic shock in the era of acute mechanical circulatory support (AMCS).

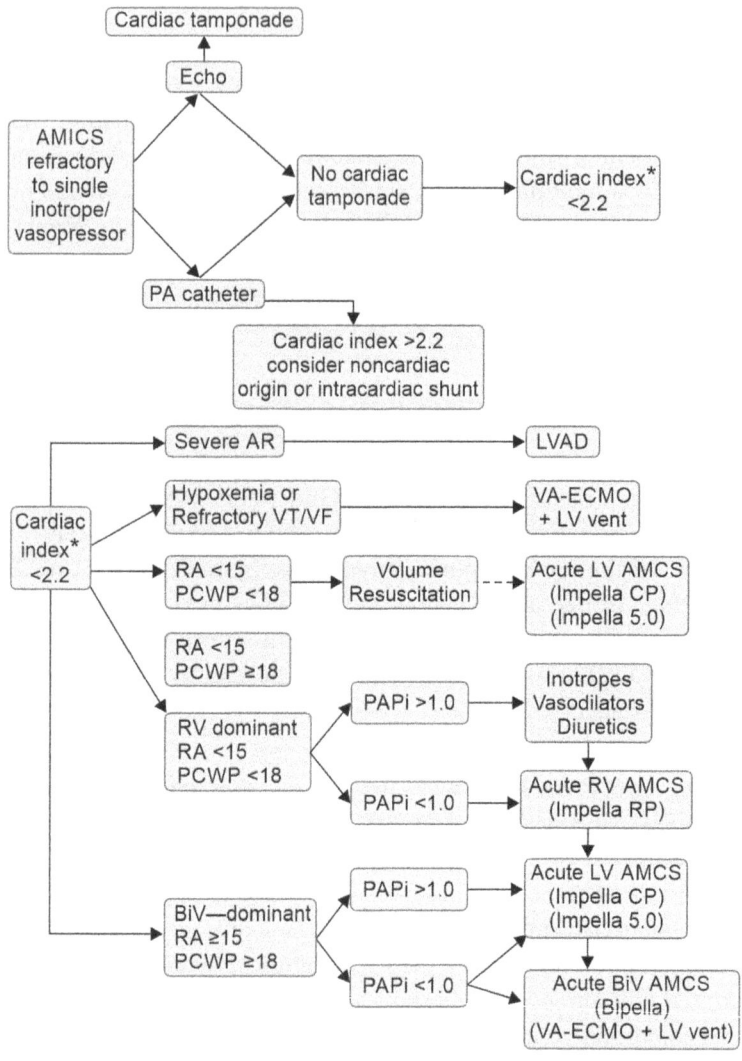

(AR: aortic regurgitation; AMICS: acute myocardial infarction cardiogenic shock; BiV: biventricular; LV: left ventricular; LVAD: left ventricular assist device; PA: pulmonary artery; PAPi: pulmonary artery pulsatility index; PCWP: pulmonary capillary wedge pressure; RA: right atrium; RV: right ventricular; VA-ECMO: venoarterial extracorporeal membrane oxygenation; VF: ventricular fibrillation; VT: ventricular tachycardia)

SUGGESTED READING

1. Henry TD, Pina IL, Kapur NK, Dangas GA on behalf of American Heart Association. Invasive management of acute myocardial infarction complicated by cardiogenic shock: a scientific statement from the American Heart Association. Circulation. 2021;143(15):e815-e829.
2. Lemor A, Basir MB, Patel K, Kolski B, Kaki A, Kapur NK, et al. Multivessel versus Culprit-vessel Percutaneous Coronary Intervention in Cardiogenic Shock. J Am Coll Cardiol Intv. 2020;13:1171-8.
3. Thile H, Jobs A, Ouwencel DM, Henriques JPS, Seyfarth M, Desch S, et al. Percutaneous short-term active mechanical support devices in cardiogenic shock: a systematic renin, and collaborative meta-analysis of randomized trials. Eur Heart J. 2017;38(47):3523-31.
4. Thiele H, Ohman EM, Waha-Thiele de, Zeymer U, Desch S. Management of cardiogenic shock complicating myocardial infarction: an update 2019. Eur Heart J. 2019;40(32):2671-83.

CHAPTER 3

Acute Heart Failure

Soumitra Kumar

Acute heart failure (AHF) is defined as a new onset or recurrence of heart failure (HF) symptoms and signs requiring emergency therapeutic interventions. It may occur as the first manifestation of HF, or more frequently as an acute decompensation of chronic HF.

Different AHF classification criteria have been proposed, mainly reflecting the clinical heterogeneity of the syndrome {e.g., hemodynamic status [wet/dry-warm/cold] or according to clinical scenario [decompensated heart failure, acute right heart failure, acute pulmonary edema, cardiogenic shock (CS)]} **(Table 1)**.

■ DIAGNOSTIC WORKUP OF ACUTE HEART FAILURE

Rapid Clinical Assessment

The most common symptoms (reflecting pulmonary and/or systemic congestion) include dypnea during exercise or at rest, orthopnea, fatigue, and reduced exercise tolerance. Clinical signs usually include peripheral edema, jugular vein distension, the presence of a third heart sound, and pulmonary rales.

Symptoms and signs such as cold and clammy skin, altered mental status, and oliguria indicate peripheral hypoperfusion—impending CS.

Search for Reversible Causes

Management starts with the search for specific causes of AHF. These include acute coronary syndrome (ACS), hypertensive emergency, rapid arrhythmias or severe bradycardia/conduction disturbances, acute mechanical causes (i.e., acute valve regurgitation), acute pulmonary embolism (PE), infections, and tamponade. Dietary and fluid restriction and medication noncompliance should also be ascertained at this time.

TABLE 1: Different AHF classification.

	Acutely decompensated heart failure	Acute pulmonary edema	Isolated right ventricular failure	Cardiogenic shock
Description	Progressive fluid retention in patients with history of HF	Lung congestion and acute respiratory failure	RV dysfunction and/or precapillary pulmonary hypertension	Severe cardiac dysfunction with marked hypotension (SBP <90 mm Hg) despite adequate LV filling pressure
Onset	Gradual (days)	Rapid (hours)	Gradual/rapid	Gradual/rapid
Main clinical presentation	Wet and warm (rarely wet and cold)	Wet and warm (rarely wet and cold)	Wet and cold	Wet and dry
Heart rate	↑	↑	Usually ↓	↑
SBP	Variable	Variable	→	→
Cardiac index	Variable	Variable	→	→
Hypoperfusion	+/−	+/−	+	+
PCWP	↑↑	↑↑	→	↑↑
Main treatment	• Diuretics • Inotropic agents/vasopressors (If peripheral hypoperfusion/hypotension) • Short-term MCS or RRT if needed	• O₂ (CPAP/NIV) Diuretics • Vasodilators • Inotropic agents/vasopressors (If peripheral hypoperfusion/hypotension) • Short-term MCS or RRT if needed	• Diuretics for congestion • Inotropic agents/vasopressors (If peripheral hypoperfusion/hypotension) • Short-term MCS or RRT if needed	• Inotropic agents/vasopressors • Short-term MCS or RRT if needed

(CPAP: continuous positive airway pressure; HF: heart failure; LV: left ventricle; MCS: mechanical circulatory support; NIV: non-invasive ventilation; PCWP: pulmonary capillary wedge pressure; RRT: renal replacement therapy; RV: right ventricle; SBP: systolic blood pressure; ↑: increase; ↓: decrease)

TABLE 2: Data from AHF registries.

Registry	ESC-HF pilot'	EHFS II	EAHFE	ESC-EORP-HFA HF-LT	ALARM-HF	REPORT-HF
Region	Europe	Europe	Spain	Europe	International	International
Number of patients	1,892 (AHF)	3,580	13,971	7,865 (AHF)	4,953	18,102
Time period	2004–2005	2004–2005	Different time points (2007/2009/2014/2016)	2011-ongoing	2006–2007	2014–2017
Demographics						
Age, years	69 (±13)	69.9 (±12)	80 (±10)	69 ±12.9	66–70 (median) 38%	67 (57–77)
Female	37.4%	39%	55.5%	37.1%		39%
Previous HF diagnosis	N/A	62.9%	60.4%	70.3%	63.8%	57%
Medical history						
CAD	50.7%	53.6%	29.4%	53.4% previous MI, 20.3% PCI, 10% CABG	N/A	48%
Hypertension	61.8%	62.5%	83.5%	N/A		64%
AF	43.7%	38.7%	48.9%	N/A		31%

Contd...

Contd...

Registry	ESC-HF pilot'	EHFS II	EAHFE	ESC-EORP-HFA HF-LT	ALARM-HF	REPORT-HF
DM	35.1%	32.8%	42.2%	39%		37%
CKD	26%	16.8%	26.2%	26.3%		20%
LVEF	64.5% (<45%) 35.5% (≥45%)	29.9% (<30%) 35.8% (30–44%) 34.3% (≥45%)	21.6% (reduced) 14.3% (mid-range) 56.1% (preserved)	51.1% (reduced) 25.1% (mid-range) 23.8% (preserved)	74% (<45%) 26% (≥45%)	50% (<40%) 17% (40–49%) 31% (≥50%) 9% missing
Length of stay, days	N/A	9 (6–14)	9.3 (±8.6)	10.7 (±25.4)	6 (4–10)	8 (5–12)
In-hospital mortality	3.8%	6.7%	7.8%	5.3%	12%	N/A
Postdischarge mortality	17.2% (1 year)	N/A	10.2% (30 days) 30.3% (1 year)	22.2% (1 year)	N/A	20% (1 year)
Postdischarge readmissions	31.9% (1 year, all-cause) 24.8% (1 year, HF)	N/A	16.9% (30-day readmissions)	43.6% (1 year, all-cause) 25.6% (1 year, HF)	N/A	38% (all-cause) 22% (HF hospitalization) 39% (death or HF hospitalization)

Flowchart 1: Flow of management of acute heart failure patients.

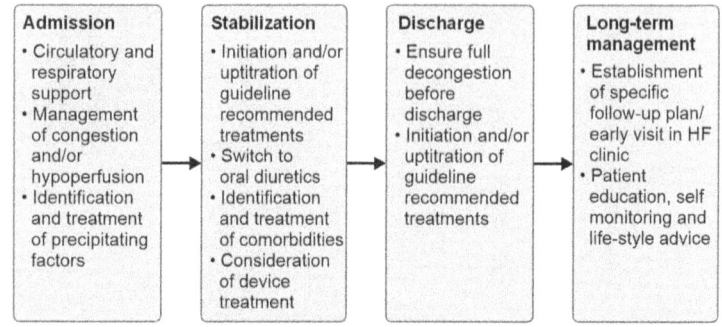

Flowchart 2: Triaging of AHF.

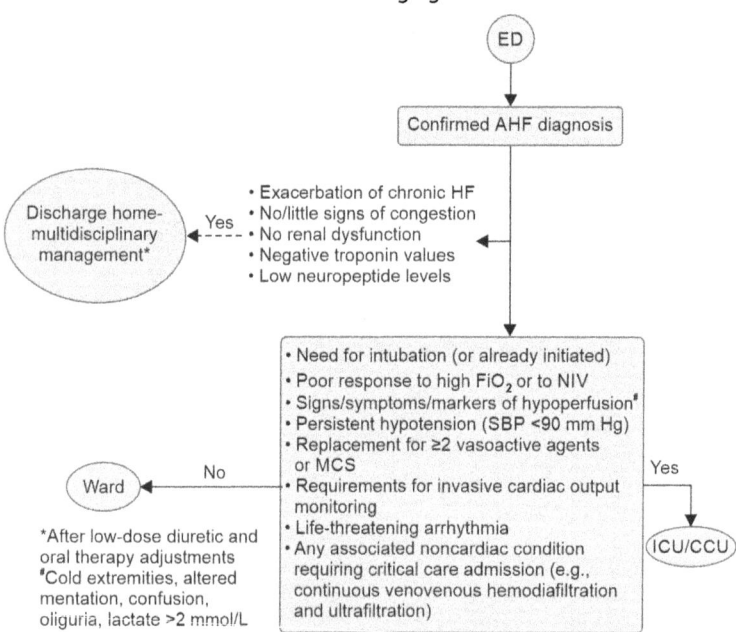

(AHF: acute heart failure; ED: emergency department; ICU/CCU: intensive cardiology unit/critical care unit; MCS: mechanical circulatory support; NIV: noninvasive ventilation; SBP: systolic blood pressure)

After exclusion of these conditions, which need to be treated/corrected urgently, management of AHF should be tailored according to clinical presentation.

Acute Heart Failure

Flowchart 3: Diagnostic workup of AHF.

Emergency department

Check for SARS-CoV-2: Clinical and lab markers, rapid antigen testing/polymerase chain reaction, vaccination status

Patient history, signs and symptoms suspected of AHF

Key Lab tests
NT-proBNP ≥300 pg/mL or BNP ≥100 pg/mL
Troponin I or T: Myocardial ischaemia, myocardial infarction
D-dimer: Aortic dissection, pulmonary embolism, Thrombosis

Additional diagnostic tests
Coronary angiography: ACS
Chest CT: pneumonia, pneumothorax
Angio CT: acute aortic syndromes, pulmonary embolism, artery disease
TOE: atrial fibrillation (pre cardioversion), endocarditis, acute aortic syndromes.
Abdominal ultrasound: ascites + other pathological findings

Key diagnostic tests
ECG: ACS, arrhythmias
Focus Cardiac Ultrasound (FoCUS): HFrEF (≤40%), HFmrEF (41–49%), HFPEF (≥50%) + other abnormalities
Lung ultrasound: B-lines, pleural effusion
Chest X-ray: pneumonia, pulmonary edema, pneumothorax, widened medistinum

Additional Labs
Red blood cell count: Blood loss, bleeding, anemia
White blood cell count: Infection, inflammation (SIRS)
C-reactive protein: Inflammatory response
Procalcitonin: Differential diagnosis between SIRS and sepsis
Creatine kinase: Reperfusion injury, rhabdomyolysis
AST/ALT: Liver disease, liver ischemia
Creatinine, BUN: Renal failure
TSH: Tyroid disfunction
Lactate: Bowel ischemia, metabolic disorder
Glucose: Diabetes mellitus
Arterial blood gases: Respiratory insufficiency

Acute heart failure confirmed

(ACS: acute coronary syndrome; ALT: alanine aminotransferase; AST: aspartate aminotransferase; BUN: blood urea nitrogen; BNP: brain natriuretic peptide; CT: computed tomography; ECG: electrocardiogram; TOE: transesophageal echocardiogram; TSH: thyroid-stimulating hormone)

TABLE 3: Triggers of AHF and summary of appropriate management.

Triggers	Laboratory workup	Invasive/Noninvasive workup	Management approach
ACS	hs-cTn (I or T)	• ECG • TTE • Coronary angiography	• Immediate primary PCI (or CABG in selected cases) is recommended • Centers without 24/7 PCI availability must transfer the patient immediately
Arrhythmias	Electrolytes, TFTs	• ECG • TTE • Interrogation of ICD (in selected patients)	• Electrical cardioversions recommended in patients hemodynamically compromised by AF/SMVT and in whom urgent restoration of sinus rhythm is required to improve the patient's clinical condition rapidly • ALS/defibrillation in VF/VT without pulse • Pacing is recommended in patients hemodynamically compromised by severe bradycardia or heart block to improve the patient's clinical condition
Acute myocarditis	hs-cTn (I or T), PCR, ESR, WBC count	ECG + TTE CCT/coronary angiography endomyocardial biopsy in patients presenting with severe heart failure on cardiogenic shock	• Patients presenting with severe heart failure or cardiogenic shock should immediately be referred to hub centers • CMRI should be performed within 2/3 weeks from the onset of symptoms when the patient is hemodynamically stable

Contd...

Acute Heart Failure

Flowchart 3: Diagnostic workup of AHF.

Emergency department

Check for SARS-CoV-2: Clinical and lab markers, rapid antigen testing/polymerase chain reaction, vaccination status

---

Patient history, signs and symptoms suspected of AHF

Key Lab tests	Additional diagnostic tests
NT-proBNP ≥300 pg/mL or BNP ≥100 pg/mL *Troponin I or T:* Myocardial ischaemia, myocardial infarction *D-dimer:* Aortic dissection, pulmonary embolism, Thrombosis	*Coronary angiography:* ACS *Chest CT:* pneumonia, pneumothorax *Angio CT:* acute aortic syndromes, pulmonary embolism, artery disease *TOE:* atrial fibrillation (pre cardioversion), endocarditis, acute aortic syndromes. *Abdominal ultrasound:* ascites + other pathological findings
Key diagnostic tests *ECG:* ACS, arrhythmias *Focus Cardiac Ultrasound (FoCUS):* HFrEF (≤40%), HFmrEF (41–49%), HFPEF (≥50%) + other abnormalities *Lung ultrasound:* B-lines, pleural effusion *Chest X-ray:* pneumonia, pulmonary edema, pneumothorax, widened medistinum	**Additional Labs** *Red blood cell count:* Blood loss, bleeding, anemia *White blood cell count:* Infection, inflammation (SIRS) *C-reactive protein:* Inflammatory response *Procalcitonin:* Differential diagnosis between SIRS and sepsis *Creatine kinase:* Reperfusion injury, rhabdomyolysis *AST/ALT:* Liver disease, liver ischemia *Creatinine, BUN:* Renal failure *TSH:* Tyroid disfunction *Lactate:* Bowel ischemia, metabolic disorder *Glucose:* Diabetes mellitus *Arterial blood gases:* Respiratory insufficiency

---

Acute heart failure confirmed

(ACS: acute coronary syndrome; ALT: alanine aminotransferase; AST: aspartate aminotransferase; BUN: blood urea nitrogen; BNP: brain natriuretic peptide; CT: computed tomography; ECG: electrocardiogram; TOE: transesophageal echocardiogram; TSH: thyroid-stimulating hormone)

TABLE 3: Triggers of AHF and summary of appropriate management.

Triggers	Laboratory workup	Invasive/Noninvasive workup	Management approach
ACS	hs-cTn (I or T)	• ECG • TTE • Coronary angiography	• Immediate primary PCI (or CABG in selected cases) is recommended • Centers without 24/7 PCI availability must transfer the patient immediately
Arrhythmias	Electrolytes, TFTs	• ECG • TTE • Interrogation of ICD (in selected patients)	• Electrical cardioversions recommended in patients hemodynamically compromised by AF/SMVT and in whom urgent restoration of sinus rhythm is required to improve the patient's clinical condition rapidly • ALS/defibrillation in VF/VT without pulse • Pacing is recommended in patients hemodynamically compromised by severe bradycardia or heart block to improve the patient's clinical condition
Acute myocarditis	hs-cTn (I or T), PCR, ESR, WBC count	ECG + TTE CCT/coronary angiography endomyocardial biopsy in patients presenting with severe heart failure on cardiogenic shock	• Patients presenting with severe heart failure or cardiogenic shock should immediately be referred to hub centers • CMRI should be performed within 2/3 weeks from the onset of symptoms when the patient is hemodynamically stable

Contd...

Contd...

Triggers	Laboratory workup	Invasive/Noninvasive workup	Management approach
Endocarditis	ESR, CRP, blood culture, auto-immunity testing in selected cases	• TTE + TOE • CCT/total-body CT scan	Patients presenting with severe heart failure or cardiogenic shock should be referred early and managed in a reference center with immediate surgical facilities
Acute aortic syndromes	D-dimer	• TTE + CTA (1st choice) • TTE + TOE (2nd choice)	D-dimer is highly sensitive to rule out classical AAD within the first 6 hours of symptom onset in low-moderate-risk patients
Mechanical cause (free wall rupture ventricular septal defect, acute mitral regurgitation, cardiac tamponade)	hs-cTn (I or T) D-dimer	TTE	Prompt intervention/surgery is needed; transfer to Hub center
Pulmonary embolism	D-dimer, hs-cTn, ABG	• ECG + TTE • CTPA • Compression ultrasonography	If hemodynamically unstable, transfer to ICU

Contd...

Contd...

Triggers	Laboratory workup	Invasive/Noninvasive workup	Management approach
Hypertension emergency	FBC, creatinine, electrolytes, LDH, hepatoglobin, hs-cTn, pregnancy test in women of child-bearing age	• Chest X-ray • TTE • CT or MRI brain in suspected nervous system involvement • CTA in suspected acute aortic disease	Patients with severe hypertension associated with AHF require an urgent reduction of BP with IV drug administration
Pneumonia	FBC, ESR, CRP, PCT	• Chest X-ray • Chest CT	Admission to an ICU for patients with hypotension requiring vasopressors or respiratory failure requiring mechanical ventilation
COPD exacerbation or asthma	ABG, PCR, PCT	• Chest X-ray • Chest CT	Admission to an ICU for patients with hypotension requiring vasopressors or respiratory failure requiring mechanical ventilation
Thyroid dysfunction	TFTs	• ECG • TTE	Management of myxedema coma and thyroid storm requires both medical and supportive therapies and should be treated in an ICU setting

(ABG: arterial blood gases; ALS: advanced life support; CABG: coronary artery bypass graft surgery; CCT: cardiac computer tomography; CRP: C-reactive protein; CT: computer tomography; CTA: computed tomography angiography; CTPA: CT pulmonary angiogram; ECG: electrocardiogram; ESR: erythrocyte sedimentation rate; FBC: full blood count; hs-Tn: high-sensitive troponins; ICD: implantable cardioverter defibrillator; ICU: intensive care unit; MRI: magnetic resonance imaging; PCI: percutaneous coronary intervention; PCT: procalcitonin; RBC: red blood cells; TFTs: thyroid function tests; TOE: transesophageal echocardiogram; TTE: transthoracic echocardiogram; SMVT: sustained monomorphic ventricular tachycardia)

Check for SARS-CoV-2 Infection

At the time of hospital admission, it is advisable to search for clinical and laboratory clues, suggesting COVID-19 infection; perform SARS-CoV2 rapid antigen testing/polymerase chain reaction, and check for COVID-19 vaccination status.

Laboratory Workup

Neuropeptides

Cardiovascular biomarkers play a crucial role in the diagnostic-prognostic process of AHF. Upon presentation to the ED, plasma neuropeptide (NP) levels (BNP, NT-proBNP, or MR-proANP) should be measured (point-of-case assay) in all patients with acute dyspnea. Due to the strong link with hemodynamic intracardiac stress, they may help to differentiate between cardiac and noncardiac causes of acute dyspnea.

Cut-offs for AHF are BNP <100 pg/mL, NT-proBNP <300 pg/mL, and MR-proANP <120 pg/mL, with normal NP concentrations, making the diagnosis of AHF extremely unlikely.

However, there are many causes of elevated NP-levels both cardiovascular (CV) and non-CV that might reduce their diagnostic accuracy. These causes include AF, increase age, and acute or chronic kidney disease. Conversely, NP concentrations may be disproportionately low in obese patients, in patients with preleft ventricle causes of HF (i.e., mitral stenosis and acute mitral regurgitation), or pericardial diseases.

As a note, NT-proBNP instead of BNP should be tested in patients taking sacubitril-valsartan. It should also be highlighted that NP levels are strong predictors of readmissions and death.

Troponin

In addition to ACS, elevated high-sensitivity troponin I/T (hsTnI/T) levels may be observed in most non-ACS AHF patients and an associated with worse in-hospital and postdischarge outcomes.

Others

Further laboratory tests [i.e., BUN (or urea), creatinine, electrolytes, glucose, complete blood count, procalcitonin, PCR, and D-dimer] may be useful to detect and/or to confirm clinically suspected comorbidities and/or end-organ damage.

Peripheral Oxygen Saturation/Arterial Blood Gas

Peripheral oxygen saturation (SpO2) should be measured routinely at the time of AHF patient presentation and continuous monitoring may be needed in the first hours or days.

Routine arterial blood gas (ABG) is not needed. Specific indications for ABG are: Respiratory distress [defined as acute increase in the work of breathing or significant tachypnea (RR >25 breaths/min)], documented hypoxemia (SpO_2 <90%) not responsive to supplemented oxygen, and evidence of acidosis or elevated lactate levels. In the case of respiratory failure, ABG may show PaO_2 <60 mmHg, $PaCO_2$ >45 mmHg, or PaO_2/FiO_2 <300 mm Hg. Of note, venous sample might acceptably indicate pH and CO^2.

Electrocardiogram

Routine admission electrocardiogram (ECG) is recommended since it can exclude ACS and arrhythmias. In this regard, careful attention should be paid to ECG changes suggestive of myocardial ischemia. Tachyarrhythmias [i.e., AF (present in 20–30% patients), ventricular tachycardia], or bradyarrhythmias (i.e., advanced atrioventricular blocks) are also a common trigger for AHF.

Chest X-ray

Chest X-ray may reveal lung congestion and/or pleural effusion. Furthermore, it may identify noncardiac-disease causes of the patient's symptoms (i.e., pneumonia, pneumothorax, and widened mediastinum).

Lung Ultrasound

Lung ultrasound (LUS) has emerged as a valuable modality to detect and monitor pulmonary congestion in patients with AHF in a low-cost, portable, real-time, and radiation-free manner.

It outperforms the diagnostic accuracy of the chest radiograph in the detection of pleural water (pleural effusion) and lung water (pulmonary congestion as multiple B-lines).

B-lines are well-defined (laser-like), hyperechoic, vertical comet-tail artifacts that arise strictly from the pleural line, move in sync with lung sliding and spread to the edge of the screen without fading and erasing A lines. The number of lines is proportional to the severity of congestion and identifies the cardiogenic origin of dyspnea with 85% sensitivity and 92% specificity.

The B profile is useful to track dynamic changes in pulmonary congestion in responses to treatment, and its persistence at predischarge or in clinically stable outpatients with HF is predictive of HF hospitalization or death.

The amount of pleural effusion can be scored as trivial (<2 mm), small (2 to 15 mm), moderate (15–25 mm), or large (>25 mm). Furthermore, LUS represents a guide to thoracentesis in patients with AHF and at least moderate pleural effusion.

As a note, the evaluation of "lung sliding" (a horizontal, to-and-fro movement, beginning at the pleural line and synchronous with respiration) is helpful in the differential diagnosis of several parenchymal lung diseases that are present as comorbidities in HF or as causes of dyspnea suspected to be cardiac in origin. For instance, "lung sliding" disappears in pneumothorax and it is reduced or abolished in the case of pneumonia, acute respiratory distress syndrome (ARDS), or pleural adhesions.

Chest Computed Tomography Angiography

Computed tomography angiography (CTA) can be used as a one-step imaging modality (dual rule-out strategy) to exclude PE or AAS. It can be performed with most CT equipment. Furthermore, with state-of-the-art CT equipment, synchronizing image acquisition with the cardiac cycle, it is possible to perform the so-called Triple Rule-Out strategy (TRO). This protocol allows the heart and the coronary arteries to be imaged, allowing the exclusion of ACS in a clinical context where this diagnosis might not be straightforward. The main drawbacks of CTA are the administration of iodinated contrast agent, which may cause acute kidney injury or allergic reactions, even though the amount of contrast material currently required to perform the scan is quite low compared to the past (i.e., using state-of-the-art CT technology, 50 mL). Furthermore, the use of ionizing radiation should be avoided in younger patients, especially women.

Transesophageal Echocardiogram

Transesophageal echocardiogram (TEE) may be performed in suspected endocarditis and acute aortic syndrome (AAS). Furthermore, it may be useful to better define heart valve abnormalities and to detect intracardiac shunt and thrombi. Absolute contraindications include: Unrepaired tracheoesophageal fistula, esophageal obstruction/stricture, perforated hollow viscus, active gastric/esophageal bleeding, poor airway control, severe respiratory depression, and uncooperative, unsedated patient.

High-resolution Chest Computed Tomography

High-resolution chest computed tomography (chest HR-CT) should be considered when pulmonary parenchymal component is suspected among patients presenting with AHF.

Computed tomography can also identify signs of pulmonary edema, such as interlobular septal thickening, fissural thickening, peribronchovascular thickening, perihilar or bat-wing appearance of edema, increased artery-to-bronchus ratio, pleural effusion, and cardiac enlargement in more advanced HF.

Furthermore, high-resolution CT provides an effective modality to evaluate patients with suspected COVID-19.

Coronary Angiography

In AHF patients with a clinical picture related to ACS, an immediate coronary angiography, along with revascularization (if needed), should be performed.

IN-HOSPITAL THERAPEUTIC INTERVENTIONS

The main goals of treatment in AHF consist of alleviating symptoms, improving congestion and organ perfusion, restoring oxygenation, and preventing thromboembolism.

Pharmacologic

Diuretics

The cornerstone of AHF treatment is represented by diuretics with intravenous (IV) loop diuretics (e.g., furosemide, bumetanide, or

TABLE 4: Diuretics.

Drug	Mechanism of action	Dose	Adverse reaction	Notes
Diuretics				
Used in hypervolemia to relief symptoms of congestion				
Loop diuretics				
• Frusemide • Torsemide • Bumetanide	Sulfonamide loop diuretics. Inhibit contransport system (Na$^+$/K$^+$/2Cl$^-$) of thick ascending limb of loop of Henle. Abolish hypertoxicity of medulla, preventing concentration of urine. Associated with increased PGE (vasodilatory effect on afferent arteriole). Increase Ca^{2+} excretion	Initial dose, diuretic-naïve • Furosemide; 20–40 mg IV • Torsemide; 10–20 mg IV • Bumetanide; 0.5–1 mg IV Initial dose, for those on chronic diuretics: 1–2 times the daily oral chronic dose as intermitten IV boluses or continuous IV infusion adjust dose to relieve symptoms, reduce volume excess, and avoid hypotension	Ototoxicity Hypokalemia, hypomagnesemia, dehydration, allergy, metabolic alkalosis, nephritis, gout	Monitor symptoms, urine output, and renal function, regularly during therapy. Consider continuous infusion in diuretic-resistant patients. A satisfactory diuretic response can be defined as a urine sodium content >50–70 mEq/L/h and/ or by a urine output >100–150 mL/h during the first 6 hours
Thiazide diuretics				
Hydrochlorothiazide	Inhibit NaC1 reabsorption in early	• Hydrochlorothiazide: Start with 25 mg PO	Hyperkalemic metabolic alkalosis,	Use with caution in patients with

Contd...

Contd...

Drug	Mechanism of action	Dose	Adverse reaction	Notes
chlorthalidone, metolazone	distal convolute tubule. Decrease Ca^{2+} excretion	once or twice daily (dose range: 12.5–200 mg/day) • *Chlorthalidone:* Start with 24 mg PO once daily (dose range: 12.5–200 mg/day) • *Metolazone:* Start with 1.25–5 mg PO 1–7 times/week (dose range: 1.25–20 mg/day)	hyponatremia, hyperglycemia, hyperlipidemia, hyperuricemia, hypercalcemia, and sulfa allergy	severe renal disease, hepatic impairment, or progressive liver disease |//

Potassium-sparing diuretics

| Spironolactone, Eplerenone, Amiloride, Triamterene | • Spironolactone and eplerenone are competitive aldosterone receptor antagonists in cortical collecting tubule
• Amiloride blocks Na^+ channels at the same part of the tubule | • *Spironolactone:* Start with 12.5–25 mg PO daily (target dose: 25–50 mg PO daily)
• *Eplerenone:* Start with 25 mg PO once daily (target dose: 50 mg PO once daily)
• *Amiloride:* Start with 5 mg PO once daily (dose range: 1.25–20mg/daily) | Hyperkalemia (can lead to arrhythmias), endocrine effects with spironolactone (e.g., gynecomastia and antiandrogen effects) | Monitor serum potassium |

torasemide) used as first-line therapy in patients with AHF and congestion.

The use of an IV dose of diuretics at least equal to the preexisting oral dose is recommended in those already receiving oral diuretics, and 20–40 mg IV furosemide (or equivalent) in those who are not on regular oral diuretics.

Furosemide can be given as 2–3 daily boluses or as a continuous infusion. Daily single bolus administrations are discouraged for the possibility of post-dosing sodium retention.

The diuretic response is evaluated by measuring the urinary volume output and/or spot urinary sodium content, with a satisfactory diuretic response defined as a urine sodium content >50–70 mEq/L at 2 hours and/or by a urine output >100–150 mL/h during the first 6 hours.

If there is an insufficient diuretic response, the loop diuretic IV dose can be doubled. Transition to oral treatment should be started when the patient's clinical condition is stable.

In patients with resistant edema, dual treatment with a loop diuretic and an oral thiazide-like diuretic (e.g., metolazone) may be considered to achieve adequate diuresis (so-called "sequential nephron blockade").

Which loop diuretic to use?
Furosemide is the most commonly used loop diuretic in both in- and out-patients. However, there are important and possibly, clinically significant differences in the pharmacokinetics of oral furosemide, bumetanide, and torsemide.

There have been a few head-to-head comparisons of loop diuretics in patients with HF.

The TRANSFORM (Effect of Torsemide vs. Furosemide After Discharge on All-Cause Mortality in Patients Hospitalized With Heart Failure) trial randomized 2,859 patients to either oral furosemide or torsemide at the point of discharge following admission with HF, the dose of which was determined by the treating clinician.

There was no benefit of one treatment over the other in subgroup analysis.

Regardless, given the high event rate and neutral findings, it is probable that the type of loop diuretic used is not important.

What dose to use?
The Diuretic Optimization Strategies Evaluation (DOSE) trial attempted to clarify the optimal diuretic dosing strategy for patients admitted to hospital with HF and the best mode of administration (bolus vs. continuous infusion). Patients were randomized to either low dose (usual dose of oral loop diuretic) versus high dose (2.5× usual dose of oral loop diuretic) and to either continuous infusion or twice daily bolus administration of loop diuretic.

The trial was neutral in that neither dosing nor administration strategy was superior in respect to the primary endpoints, but there were a number of interesting, clinically relevant findings.

The results suggest that high-dose treatment (2.5× the oral dose on admission) induces a greater diuresis than does low-dose treatment, without a greater risk of adverse effects and that continuous infusion may cause similar diuresis to bolus dosing but without the need for treatment intensification. Due to the short half-life of IV loop diuretics, bolus dosing may allow for a period between doses during which renal sodium resorption may increase (and diuresis decrease). Other studies have found a greater diuresis and greater improvements in clinical congestion with continuous infusions over bolus dosing.

Poor "natriuretic response" (low urine sodium concentration after administration of IV loop diuretic) is associated with a greater risk of worsening renal function, inadequate treatment of congestion, loop diuretic resistance, and poor prognosis in patients treated with IV loop diuretic. Natriuretic-guided dosing of loop diuretics—increasing dose of loop diuretic to achieve a given urine sodium concentration—has featured in ESC HF recommendations since 2019, but the efficacy of natriuresis-guided diuretic treatment was not assessed in a randomized controlled trial (RCT) until 2023.

In the PUSH-AHF trial, 310 patients admitted to the hospital with HF were randomized to either natriuresis-guided therapy or standard care.

Unsurprisingly, titrating loop diuretic dose based on urine sodium concentration was associated with greater natriuresis compared to standard therapy. Urine output at 24 and 48 hours was also greater in the natriuresis-guided arm.

Natriuresis-guided treatment was stopped after 24 hours, and, perhaps as a result, the differences in natriuresis and urine output were lost after 72 hours of treatment. There was no difference in the adverse event rate, length of hospitalization, readmission with HF, or mortality between the two groups.

It is unlikely that natriuresis-guided treatment will become the standard care for most HF specialists in busy healthcare systems.

Angiotensin-converting enzyme inhibitors (ACEis), sacubitril valsartan, mineralocorticoid receptor antagonists (MRAs), and sodium-glucose cotransporter 2 inhibitors, all have either a mild diuretic effect or reduce the need for loop diuretic treatment.

Diuretic withdrawal in patients with no or minimal congestion who are receiving optimal disease-modifying therapy is associated with improvements in renal function and reduction in plasma renin concentration without worsening symptoms or an increased risk of hospitalization during short-term follow-up. However, diuretic withdrawal will not be suitable for all euvolemic patients.

One small study of medication withdrawal (including diuretics) in stable out-patients with HF with reduced ejection fraction (HFREF) found worsening symptoms and doubling of serum natriuretic peptide concentration after 48 hours. In the only RCT of diuretic withdrawal in stable out-patients with HFREF, all of whom had New York Heart Association (NYHA) class I symptoms and were receiving less than 80 mg of furosemide equivalents per day, one in four needed to restart loop diuretic during 90-day follow-up. For those without congestion, the optimal dose may be that which prevents the recurrence of congestion, which will vary between patients and may change over time.

Vasodilators

Intravenous vasodilators may be considered to relieve AHF symptoms when SBP is >110 mm Hg.

They may be started at low doses and uptitrated to achieve clinical improvement and BP control. Nitrates are generally administered with an initial bolus followed by continuous infusion. However, these agents should be avoided in patients with concurrent obstructive valvular disease (i.e., severe aortic stenosis) or restrictive physiology (i.e., hypertrophic cardiomyopathy).

TABLE 5: Vasodilators.

Drug	Mechanism of action	Dose	Adverse reactions	Notes
Vasodilators				
Used for relief of dyspnea in patients without hypotension (SBP >110 mm Hg), potentially useful in severely congested patients with hypertension or severe mitral valve regurgitation complicating LV dysfunction				
Nitroglycerine Isosorbide dinitrate	Vasodilate by increasing NO in vascular smooth muscle that leads to increase of cGMP and smooth muscle relaxation (veins > arteries)	• *Nitroglycerine*: Start with 10–20 μg/min, increase up to 200 μg/min IV • *Isosorbide dinitrate*: Start with 1 mg/h, increase up to 10 mg/h IV	• Hypotension, reflex tachycardia, headache • Tolerance in continuous use	Contraindicated in right ventricular infarction, hypertrophic cardiomyopathy, severe aortic stenosis and with concurrent PDE-5 inhibitor use
Nitroprusside	• Short-acting vasodilator (arteries = veins) • Increases cGMP via direct release of NO	Start with 0.3 μg/kg/min and increase up to 5 μg/kg/min IV	Hypotension, isocyanate toxicity, and light sensitivity	Contraindicated in right ventricular infarction, hypertrophic cardiomyopathy, severe aortic stenosis, and with concurrent PDE-5 inhibitor use

(cGMP: cyclic guanosine monophosphate; IV: intravenous; NO: nitric oxide; PDE: phosphodiesterase; SBP: systolic blood pressure)

Acute Heart Failure

Opiates

Although the routine use of opiates (i.e., morphine) in AHF is not recommended, they may be considered in selected patients, particularly in case of severe pain, anxiety, or in the setting of palliation.

Digoxin

Digoxin is mostly indicated (boluses of 0.25-0.5 mg IV if not used previously, followed by an oral or IV dose of 0.25 mg at least 12 hours after the initial dose) in patients with AF and rapid ventricular rate (>110 beat/min) despite β-blockers.

Caution should be taken in the elderly or in patients with factors affecting digoxin metabolism (i.e., renal failure and drug interaction).

Furthermore, unless the risk of toxicity outweighs the benefit, discontinuation of digoxin is generally discouraged. In this regard, an association between withdrawal of therapy and worsening HF has been well documented.

Anticoagulants

Acute heart failure patients are at high risk of deep venous thrombosis (DVT) and PE as a direct consequence of higher venous pressures and lower cardiac output. In this regard, current guidelines support the use of thromboprophylaxis [e.g., low-molecular-weight heparin (LMWH) given at 4,000-5,000 units daily, or 2,500-3,000 units twice daily subcutaneously] in all appropriate hospitalized AHF patients, unless contraindicated.

In addition, oral anticoagulation [preferring new oral anticoagulants (NOACs) to vitamin K antagonists (VKAs), except in patients with mechanical heart valves or moderate-severe mitral stenosis] is recommended in AHF patients with paroxysmal, persistent, or permanent AF with a CHA2DS2-VASc score 2 in men and 3 in women. The HAS-BLED score should be considered to identify patients at high risk of bleeding [HAS-BLED (Hypertension, Abnormal renal and liver function, Stroke, Bleeding, Labile INR, Elderly, Drugs or alcohol) score ≥3] for early and more frequent clinical assessments and follow-up.

TABLE 6: Inotropes/vasopressors.

Drug	Mechanism of action	Dose	Adverse reactions	Notes
Inotropes/Vasopressors				
Used for maintenance of systemic perfusion and preservation of end organ function in patients with severe systolic dysfunction presenting with hypotension (<90 mm Hg) or low cardiac output in the presence of congestion and organ hypoperfusion				
Dobutamine	Agonist of both beta-1 and beta-2 adrenergic receptors with variable effects on the alpha receptors	Continuous IV infusion rate of 2–20 µg/kg/min	Hypotension, increased myocardial oxygen demand, and phlebitis	Continuously monitor ECG and blood pressure. Dobutamine is preferred over milrinone in patients who are acutely unstable or hypotensive, or those with renal insufficiency
Dopamine	Agonist of both, adrenergic and dopaminergic receptors	Infusion rate of 3–5 µg/kg/min; inotropic (beta+); >5 µg/kg/min: (beta+), vasopressor (alpha+)	Arrhythmias, tachycardia	Continuously monitor ECG and blood pressure. Clinical effects are dose-related; low doses increase renal blood flow/urine output, intermediate doses also increase cardiac contractility and chronotropy, and high doses result in vasoconstriction
Milrinone	PDE inhibitor (increases cAMP)	*Bolus:* 25–75 µg/kg over 10–20 minutes then infusion rate of 0.375–0.75 µg/kg/min continuous IV infusion	Tachycardia, ventricular arrhythmias, and hypotension	Continuously monitor ECG and blood pressure. Not recommended in acutely worsened ischemic heart failure

Contd...

Contd...

Drug	Mechanism of action	Dose	Adverse reactions	Notes
Levosimendan	Cardiac Ca^{2+} channels sensitizer. Activator of K^+ channels of vascular smooth muscle cells	Optional bolus: 2 µg/kg over 10 minutes; infusion rate of 0.1 µg/kg/min, which can be decreased to 0.05 or increased to 0.2 µg/kg/min	Tachycardia, ventricular arrhythmias, and hypotension	Continuously monitor ECG and blood pressure. Bolus not recommended in hypotensive patients
Norepinephrine	Potent agonist of the beta-1 and the alpha-1 receptors	Infusion rate of 0.2–1.0 µg/kg/min	End-organ hypoperfusion and tissue necrosis, arrhythmias	Continuously monitor ECG and blood pressure
Epinephrine	Full beta receptor agonist	Infusion rate of 0.05–0.5 µg/kg/min. A bolus of 1 mg can be given IV during resuscitation, repeated every 3–5 minutes	End-organ hypoperfusion and tissue necrosis, arrhythmias	Continuously monitor ECG and blood pressure. Use should be restricted to patients with persistent hypotension despite adequate cardiac filling pressures and the use of other vasoactive agents, as well as for resuscitation protocols

(cAMP: cyclic adenosine monophosphate; ECG: electrocardiogram; IV: intravenous; PDE: phosphodiesterase)

Inotropes/Vasopressors

Inotropes [including sympathomimetics/synthetic catecholamines (e.g., dobutamine and adrenaline), phosphodiesterase inhibitors (e.g., milrinone and enoximone), and, more recently, Ca^{2+} sensitizers (e.g., levosimendan)] should be reserved for patients with LV systolic dysfunction, low cardiac output, and low SBP (e.g., <90 mm Hg), resulting in poor vital organ perfusion.

Inotropes improve myocardial contractility, but, especially in the case of the sympathomimetics, also increase myocardial O_2 consumption. As a direct consequence they may trigger supraventricular and ventricular tachyarrhythmias. In this regard, it should be underlined that all patients under inotrope treatment require close monitoring of cardiac rhythm and hemodynamic parameters.

Of note, while inotropes have been shown to improve symptoms and signs of congestion, these agents have failed to reveal any improvement in mortality in patients with AHF.

FUTURE DIRECTIONS

In the EMPULSE trial, early initiation of sodium-glucose cotransporter-2 (SGLT-2) inhibitor, empagliflozin, in patients hospitalized for AHF led to a statistically significant clinical benefit at 90 days with fewer deaths, improvement in quality of life, lower NT-pro BNP levels, and weight loss. The ADVOR trial has reported that, when used in combination with loop diuretic, acetazolamide (a carbonic anhydrase inhibitor) can lead to a greater incidence of successful decongestion.

Istaroxime, a novel compound with inotropic and lusitropic positive properties and a dual mechanism of action (activation of the sarcoplasmic reticulum Ca^{2+}/ATPase 2a (SERCA2a) and inhibition of the Na^+/K^+-ATPase) has been shown to increase SBP without activating the adrenergic system, and to improve pulmonary capillary wedge pressure and diastolic cardiac function.

Furthermore, in AHF patients, early administration (within 16 hours) of serelaxin, a peptide involved in cardiovascular adaptations during pregnancy, has been shown to be associated with a reduction in 5-day worsening HF and markers of renal dysfunction.

TABLE 7: Summary of studies on sacubitril/valsartan in AHF.

Study design	No. of patients	Key findings
Exploratory analysis of PIONEER-HF assessing the clinical composite end point of HF hospitalization or CV death	881	Patients on sacubitril/valsartan had significantly lower risk for CV death or HF rehospitalization (HR 0.58; 95% CI: 0.39–0.87; $p = 0.007$, 8 weeks later
Secondary analysis of the open-label extension of PIONEER-HF		From week 8 to 12 patients who switched from enalapril to sacubitril/valsartan had a greater decline to NT-proBNP (−37.4%; 95% CI: −28.1–45.6; $p < 0.001$; comparing changes in two group)
Secondary analysis of the PIONEER-HF		Black patients admitted for AHF had a similar improvement to while patients in NT-proBNP levels
Open-label randomized controlled trial		Proportion of patients achieving target dose at 10 weeks was 45.4% in the predischarge group and 50.7% in the postdischarge group. Early litimation of sacubitril/valsartan was safe and Well tolerated. Patients were more likely to achieve target dose if they were <65 years old, had SBP >120 mm Hg at baseline, de-novo HF and an estimated glomerular filtration rate >60 mL/min/1.73 m^2)
Subgroups analysis of the TRANSITION study		Achievement of target doses was higher in patients withed novo HF compared to prior HFrEF patients De novo patients had greater decrease in NT-proBNP levels at week 10
Post-hoc analysis of the TRANSITION study		In-hospital initiation of sacubitril/valsartan led to a significantly greater reduction of NT-proBNP at discharge compared to patients who initiated postdischarge (28% vs. 4%, $p < 0.001$)

TABLE 8: Selection of studies of novel medical therapies for acute decompensated heart failure.

	First author	Key findings
β-blockers	Gattis et al.	A 60-day postdischarge, 91.2% of patients randomized to predischarge carvedilol were on β-blocker compared in 73.4% randomized in postdischarge initiation ($p < 0.0001$). Serious adverse events did not differ between the two groups
	Fonarrow et al.	At 60–90 day postdischarge, continuation of β-blocker was associated with lower risk for mortality or readmission (OR: 0.69; 95% CI: 0.52–0.92, $p = 0.012$) compared with no β-blocker
SGLT2-inhibitors	Damman et al.	In patients with AHF, initiation of empagliflozin no significant difference in dyspnea, diuretic response, change in natriuretic peptides, and length of stay was noted
		Reduced combined endpoint of in-hospital worsening HF, rehospitalization for HF and death at 60 days was observed compared to placebo [4 (10%) vs. 13 (33%); $p = 0.014$]
		Empagliflozin increased urine output until day 4 of hospitalization [difference 3,449 (95% CI: 578–6,321) mL; $p < 0.01$]
	Cox et al.	Patients with T2DM hospitalized for AHF who continued empagliflozin as part of their in-hospital antihyperglycemic regimen had better glycemic control with less hypoglycemic episodes, increased urine output, and lower NT-proBNP levels
		Adverse events, length of stay, and in-hospital mortality did not differ between the two groups

Contd...

Contd...

	First author	Key findings
	NCT04363697	Patients who continued SGLT-2 inhibitors during hospitalization had fewer rehospitalization compared to the discontinued group (24% vs. 39%, $p = 0.008$) with a hazard ratio of 0.29 (95% CI: 0.10–0.85)
	ClinicalTrials.gov	In very old patients with T2DM hospitalized with AHF, continuing empagliflozin reduced NT-proBNP (1699 ± 522 vs. 2303 ± 598 pg/mL, $p = 0.021$) and increased urine output
	Ferreira et al.	Canagliflozin initiation before discharge in T2DM patients with AHF reduced NT-proBNP and readmission rated for HF (22.2% vs. 37.3%; HR: 0.45; 95% CI: 0.21–0.96; $p < 0.039$)
MRAs	Test et al.	High-dose spironolactone in patients with AHF did not significantly reduce NT-proBNP compared to usual care. No significant difference on 3-day all-cause mortality or HF hospitalization was observed
	Jankowska et al.	Percentage of HF readmissions was significantly lower in the MRA group than in the no MRA group (18.7% vs. 24.8%; HR: 0.70; 95% CI: 0.60–0.86; $p < .001$)
		No significant difference in mortality was found between the two groups (15.6% vs. 15.8%; HR: 0.98; 95% CI: 0.821.18; $p = 0.85$)
Ferric carboxymaltose	MacMurray and Packer	Treatment with ferric carboxymaltose in patients with iron deficiency stabilized after an episode of AHF reduced the risk for HF hospitalizations (RR 0.8, 95% CI: 0.64–1, 0 = 0.05)

Transition to Oral Treatments and Predischarge Management

Once hemodynamic stabilization during AHF hospitalization is achieved, HFrEF medications should be initiated/uptitrated. Switching from intravenous to oral diuretics is often challenging. Right heart catheterization provides the most robust information concerning volume status; however, it is invasive and its use is not as broad as the use of noninvasive clinical and laboratory parameters such as symptoms, weight, and daily urine output. Intensive diuretic treatment often results in hypovolemia, which poses additional barriers in optimizing guideline-directed medical therapy (GDMT). Novel data for initiation of HFrEF treatments before discharge are presented below and most important studies in the field are summarized further.

Based on existing evidence, in-hospital initiation of sacubitril/valsartan appears to be safe and is well-tolerated by most patients. Hospitalization for AHF is a window of opportunity for switching from ACEis to sacubitril/valsartan as this strategy improves overall patient adherence and eventually short- and long- term prognosis.

Recently, the EMPA-RESPONSE-AHF study, a randomized, double-blind, placebo controlled, multicenter pilot study investigated the safety and efficacy of empagliflozin inpatients with AHF. According to their findings, while there was not a significant difference in the primary endpoint (change in dyspnea, diuretic response, change in natriuretic peptides, and length of stay), initiation of empagliflozin was safe, in terms of renal function and systolic blood pressure and led to a reduction of in-hospital worsening, death and hospital readmission within 60 days. A few recent real-world prospective studies support that continuation of SGLT2 inhibitors in diabetic patients admitted for AHF comprises a safe strategy, even in very old patients, results in greater NT-proBNP reduction and leads to fewer adverse events although larger randomized controlled studies are warranted to verify this hypothesis..

Several larger RCTs evaluating safety and efficacy of SGLT2 inhibitors in AHF are currently on going: DICTATE-AHF, DAPA ACT HF-TIMI 68, Dapagliflozin Heart Failure Readmissions, and EMPULSE.

Acute Heart Failure

The efficacy and safety of early initiation of eplerenone in patients with AHF were evaluated by a multicenter, double-blind RCT, the EARLIER trial. The study demonstrated that early eplerenone initiation was safe; however, no difference in the incidence of cardiovascular death or first readmission for HF was observed. Finally, a subanalysis of the EAHFE study evaluating outcomes of patients with HFpEF discharged on neurohormonal antagonists after an acute decompensated heart failure (ADHF) hospitalization showed that MRAs alone or in combination with other antineurohormonal drugs did not result in reduction of 1-year all-cause mortality or all-cause death and HF readmissions at 90-day postdischarge. In conclusion, based on existing evidence, there is no clear advantage other than a guideline-directed therapy is initiated, and this likely improves adherence to treatment.

Intravenous Iron Supplementation

The AFFIRM-HF trial, a large, randomized, double-blind RCT, demonstrated that in patients with ejection fraction (EF) <50% and iron deficiency stabilized after an episode of AHF, ferric carboxymaltose was safe and effective and reduced the risk of HF readmissions; however, it did not affect the risk of cardiovascular death. A recent substudy of AFFIRM-HF additionally demonstrated improvement in quality of life lasting up to 24-month postadministration. Based on these findings, ferric carboxymaltose received a IIa recommendation for predischarge administration by the 2021 ESC guidelines on HF. Recently, a retrospective study evaluated intravenous sodium ferric gluconate complex administration in patients with ADHF, including patients with HFpEF. The study did not show a benefit in readmission rates compared to patients who did not receive iron supplementation. Three more clinical trials, HEART-FID (NCT03037931), FAIR-HF2 (NCT03036462), and IRON-MAN (NCT02642562), are expected to shed light on the role of ferric carboxymaltose in heart failure.

Beta-blockers

A randomized clinical trial, IMPACT-HF, showed that predischarge initiation of carvedilol led to a significantly higher percentage of treatment attainment at 60-day postrandomization and data from the large observational OPTIMIZE-HF registry showed a 31% lower risk for mortality and rehospitalization at 60–90 days for patients who maintained β-blockers during hospitalization. Based on existing evidence, β-blockers should not be routinely withdrawn in case of AHF admission, and attempts to initiate and/or uptitrate β-blocker treatment should be made once patient is hemodynamically stable.

Strategies of Initiation of Guideline-directed Medical Therapy

In the setting of AHF, for example, initial interruption of ACEi may be required upon admission while, generally, β-blockers should be maintained throughout the hospital stay. Once hemodynamic stabilization has occurred, angiotensin receptor-neprilysin inhibitor (ARNI) and SGLT2 inhibitors should be promptly initiated followed by MRAs before discharge, ensuring that all patients without contraindications will leave hospital with all four lifesaving treatments.

Nonpharmacologic

Mechanical Ventilation

Noninvasive consists of applying positive intrathoracic pressure (PIP) to conscious patients through different interfaces, and can be either continuous positive airway pressure (CPAP) or bilevel positive airway pressure (BIPAP).

It should be highlighted that NIV has to be started as soon as possible in patients with respiratory distress [respiratory rate (RR) >25 breaths/min, SpO_2 <90%] to improve gas exchange and reduce the rate of endotracheal intubation.

Absolute contraindications to NIV include:
- Cardiac or respiratory arrest
- Anatomical abnormality (unable to fit the interface)
- Inability to keep patent airway (uncontrolled agitation, coma, or obtunded mental status)
- Refractory hypotension

If there is only hypoxemia, CPAP is the treatment of choice. In cases of hypoxemia and hypercapnia, BiPAP is preferred. CPAP is generally started at a pressure of 5 cmH$_2$O, which is increased in a stepwise manner up to 10 cmH$_2$O. In BiPAP, it is reasonable to start with an expiratory positive airway pressure (EPAP) of 5 cmH$_2$O and an inspiratory positive airway pressure (IPAP) of 10-14 cmH$_2$O. EPAP and IPAP can be adjusted further according to the effect on oxygenation and ventilation, respectively.

The response to NIV should be assessed after 60 minutes, and thereafter on a continuous basis. Signs of NIV failure are patient fatigue, progressive worsening of level of consciousness, hemodynamic instability, persistent tachypnea (>35 breaths/min), and progressive worsening of respiratory failure with acidosis, hypoxemia, or hypercapnia. Endotracheal intubation and mechanical ventilation are only required in a minority of AHF patients, as most of them will respond to NIV.

Criteria for endotracheal intubation are the following:
- Cardiac or respiratory arrest
- Progressive worsening of altered mental status
- Progressive worsening of pH, PaCO$_2$ or PaO$_2$ despite NIV
- Progressive signs of fatigue during NIV
- Need to protect the airway
- Persistent hemodynamic instability
- Agitation or intolerance to NIV with progressive respiratory failure

Electric Cardioversion

Atrial fibrillation (AF) patients presenting with a rapid ventricular rate and acute hemodynamic instability (i.e., acute pulmonary edema, ongoing myocardial ischemia, symptomatic hypotension, or CS) require prompt intervention, and emergency electrical cardioversion should be attempted without delay. In this setting, amiodarone may also be considered in order to control heart rate (HR) response.

Mechanical Circulatory Support

Short-term mechanical circulatory support (MCS) (which increases cardiac output and supports end organ damage) may be implemented as a bridge to recovery (BTR), bridge to decision (BTD), or bridge to transplant (BTT). Intra-aortic balloon pump (IABP) is not routinely recommended (vide chapter on Cardiogenic Shock for more details).

Renal Replacement Therapy

Ultrafiltration (i.e., hemodialysis) may be indicated in case of refractory congestion nonresponsive to diuretics. It may be considered if the following criteria are met:
- Oliguria unresponsive to fluid resuscitation measures
- Severe hyperkalemia (K^+ >6.5 mmol/L)
- Severe academia (pH <7.2)
- Serum urea level >25 mmol/L (>150 mg/dL)
- Serum creatinine >300 mmol/L (>3.4 mg/dL) that is worsening

Daily Patient Monitoring

Daily patient monitoring includes:
- Weight check along with completion of an accurate fluid balance chart
- Standard noninvasive monitoring of HR, RR, blood pressure (BP)
- Renal function and electrolyte measurement

Invasive monitoring with pulmonary artery catheter failed to show any positive influence on in-patient or follow-up outcomes of patients admitted with AHF, and should be carefully used for selected patients.

Predischarge

Once hemodynamic stabilization is achieved with IV therapy, treatment should be optimized before discharge according to current HF guidelines in order to (1) relieve congestion, (2) treat comorbidities, (3) initiate or restart oral optical medical treatment (OMT).

Indicators of good response to initial therapy that might be considered in discharge include:
- Patient reported subjective improvement
- Resting HR <100 beats/min
- Lack of orthostatic changes in BP

- Adequate urine output
- SpO$_2$ >95 in room air
- Decreased body weight

SUGGESTED READING

1. Arrigo M, Jessup M, Mullens W, Reza N, Shah AM, Sliwa K, et al. Acute heart failure. Nat Rev Dis Primer. 2020;6:16.
2. Bozkurt B, Coats AJS, Tsutsui H, Abdelhamid CM, Adamopoulos S, Albert N, et al. Universal definition and classification of heart failure: A report of the Heart Failure Society of America, Heart Failure Association of the European Society of Cardiology, Japanese Heart Failure Society and Writing Committee of the Universal Definition of Heart Failure: Endorsed by the Canadian Heart Failure Society, Heart Failure Association of India, Cardiac Society of Australia and New Zealand, and Chinese Heart Failure Association. Eur J Heart Fail. 2021;23:352-80.
3. Chioncel O, Mebazaa A, Harjola VP, Coats AJ, Piepoli MF, Crespo-Leiro MG, et al. Clinical phenotypes and outcome of patients hospitalized for acute heart failure: the ESC Heart Failure Long-Term Registry. Eur J Heart Fail. 2017;19(10):1242-54.
4. Felker GM, Teerlink JR. Diagnosis and management of acute heart failure. In: Zipes DP, Libby P, Bonow R, Mann LD, Tomaselli GF (Eds). Braunwald's Heart Disease a Textbook of Cardiovascular Medicine, 11th edition. Elsevier: Philadelphia, PA, USA; 2019. pp. 462-89.
5. McDonagh A, Metra M, Adamo M, Gardner RS, Baumbach A, Böhm M, et al. 2021 ESC Guidelines for the diagnosis and treatment of acute and chronic heart failure. Eur Heart J. 2021;42:3599-726.

CHAPTER 4

Management of Chronic Heart Failure

Soumitra Kumar

DEFINITION OF HEART FAILURE

Heart failure (HF) is not a single pathological diagnosis, but a clinical syndrome consisting of cardinal symptoms (e.g., breathlessness, ankle swelling, and fatigue) that may be accompanied by signs (e.g., elevated jugular venous pressure, pulmonary crackles, and peripheral edema). It is due to a structural and/or functional abnormality of the heart that results in elevated intracardiac pressures and/or inadequate cardiac output at rest and/or during exercise. Identification of the etiology of the underlying cardiac dysfunction is mandatory in the diagnosis of HF as the specific pathology can determine subsequent treatment. Most commonly, HF is due to myocardial dysfunction, either systolic, diastolic, or both. However, pathology of the valves, pericardium, and endocardium, and abnormalities of heart rhythm and conduction can also cause or contribute to HF.

TERMINOLOGY

Heart Failure with Preserved, Mildly Reduced, and Reduced Ejection Fraction

Traditionally, HF has been divided into distinct phenotypes based on the measurement of left ventricular ejection fraction (LVEF). The rationale behind this relates to the original treatment trials in HF that demonstrated substantially improved outcomes in patients with LVEF <40%. However, HF spans the entire range of LVEF (a normally distributed variable), and measurement by echocardiography is subject to substantial variability.

Patients with noncardiovascular (CV) disease, e.g., anemia, pulmonary, renal, thyroid, or hepatic disease may have symptoms and signs very similar to those of HF, but in the absence of cardiac

TABLE 1: Definition of heart failure with reduced ejection fraction, mildly reduced ejection fraction, and preserved ejection fraction.

Type of HF		HFrEF	HFmrEF	HFpEF
Criteria	1	Symptoms ± Signs[a]	Symptoms ± Signs[a]	Symptoms ± Signs[a]
	2	LVEF ≤40%	LVEF 41–49%[b]	LVEF ≥50%
	3	–	–	Objective evidence of cardiac structural and/or functional abnormalities consistent with the presence of LV diastolic dysfunction/raised LV filling pressures, inducing raised natriuretic peptides[c]

[a]Signs may not be present in the early stages of HF (especially in HFpEF) and in optimally treated patients.
[b]For the diagnosis of HFmrEF, the presence of other evidence of structural heart disease (e.g., increased left atrial size, LV hypertrophy or echocardiographic measures of impaired LV filling) makes the diagnosis more likely.
[c]For the diagnosis of HFpEF, the greater the number of abnormalities present, the higher the likelihood of HFpEF.
(HF: heart failure; HFmrEF: heart failure with mildly reduced ejection fraction; HFpEF: heart failure with preserved ejection fraction; HFrEF: heart failure with reduced ejection fraction; LV: left ventricle; LVEF: left ventricular ejection fraction)

dysfunction, they do not fulfill the criteria for HF. However, these pathologies can coexist with HF and exacerbate the HF syndrome.

Right Ventricular Dysfunction

Heart failure can also be a result of right ventricular (RV) dysfunction. RV mechanics and function are altered in the setting of either pressure or volume overload. Although the main etiology of chronic RV failure is LV dysfunction-induced pulmonary hypertension, there are a number of other causes of RV dysfunction [e.g. MI, arrhythmogenic right ventricular cardiomyopathy (ARVC), or valve disease]. The diagnosis is determined by a quantitative assessment of global RV function, most commonly by echocardiography, using at least one of the following measurements: Fractional area change (FAC); tricuspid annular plane systolic excursion (TAPSE), and Doppler tissue imaging-derived systolic S′ velocity of the tricuspid annulus.

HISTORY

- Dyspnea, orthopnea, and paroxysmal nocturnal dyspnea (PND)
- Fatigue and weakness
- Abdominal symptoms, e.g., anorexia, nausea, pain, and fullness of abdomen
- Cerebral symptoms, e.g., (in severe HF) headache, insomnia, anxiety, confusion, and impairment of memory

CLINICAL EXAMINATION

Look for:
- Cyanosis, icterus, malar flush, cachexia, edema, coldness of extremities, raised JVP, tachycardia, and pulsus alternans
- Hypotension
- Bilateral pulmonary rales
- Wheeze
- Pleural effusion
- Hepatomegaly, ascites
- Cardiomegaly, gallop sound
- S_3, S_4

OUTLINE OF TREATMENT OF CHRONIC HEART FAILURE

Stage A:
- Life-style modification:
  - Regular exercise Smoking Cessation
  - Discourage alcohol intake and illicit drug use
- Treat hypertension, lipid disorders, and metabolic syndrome
- Angiotensin-converting enzyme inhibitor (ACEI) or angiotensin receptor blocker (ARB) in appropriate patients, e.g., for vascular disease or diabetes

Stage B:
- All measures under stage A
- ACEI or ARB in appropriate patients

Management of Chronic Heart Failure

TABLE 2: Recommended diagnostic tests in all patients with suspected chronic heart failure (ESC Guidelines 2021).

Recommendations	Class[a]	Level[b]
BNP/NT-proBNP	I	B
12-lead ECG	I	C
Transthoracic echocardiography	I	C
Chest radiography (X-ray)	I	C
Routine blood tests for comorbidities, including full blood count, urea and electrolytes, thyroid function, fasting glucose and HbA1c, lipids, iron status (TSAT and ferritin)	I	C

aClass of recommendation.
bLevel of evidence.
(BNP: B-type natriuretic peptide; ECG: electrocardiogram; HbA1c: glycated hemoglobin; NT-proBNP: N-terminal pro-B-type natriuretic peptide; TSAT: transferrin saturation.)

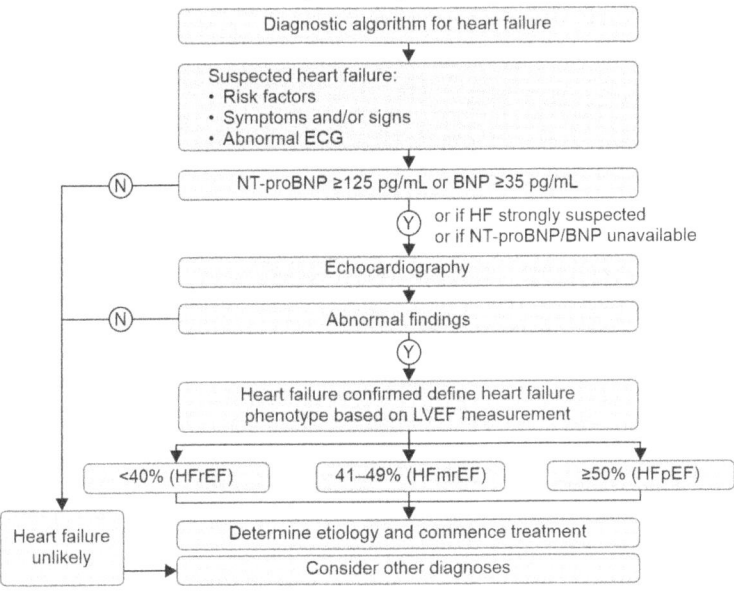

Flowchart 1: The diagnostic algorithm for heart failure.

(BNP: B-type natriuretic peptide; ECG: electrocardiogram; HFmrEF: heart failure with mildly reduced ejection fraction; HFpEF: heart failure with preserved ejection fraction; HFrEF: heart failure with reduced ejection fraction; LVEF: left ventricular ejection fraction; NT-proBNP: N-terminal pro-B type natriuretic peptide)

TABLE 3: Causes of elevated concentrations of natriuretic peptides.

Cardiac	Noncardiac
• Heart failure • ACS • Pulmonary embolism • Myocarditis • Left ventricular hypertrophy • Hypertrophic or restrictive cardiomyopathy • Valvular heart disease • Congenital heart disease • Atrial and ventricular tachyarrhythmias • Heart contusion • Cardioversion, ICD shock • Surgical procedures involving the heart • Pulmonary hypertension	• Advanced age • Ischemic stroke • Subarachnoid hemorrhage • Renal dysfunction • Liver dysfunction (mainly liver cirrhosis with ascites) • Paraneoplastic syndrome • COPD • Severe infections (including pneumonia and sepsis) • Severe burns • Anemia • Severe metabolic and hormone abnormalities (e.g., thyrotoxicosis, diabetic ketosis)

(ACS: acute coronary syndrome; COPD: chronic obstructive pulmonary disease; ICD: implantable cardioverter-defibrillator)

TABLE 4: Recommendations for specialized diagnostic tests for selected patients with chronic heart failure to detect reversible/treatable causes of heart failure (ESC Guidelines 2021).

Recommendations	Class	Level
CMR		
CMR is recommended for the assessment of myocardial structure and function those with poor echocardiogram acoustic windows	I	C
CMR is recommended for the characterization of myocardial tissue in suspected infiltrative disease, Fabry disease, inflammatory disease (myocarditis), LV noncompaction, amyloid sarcoidosis, iron overload/hemochromatosis	I	C
CMR with LGE should be considered in DCM to distinguish between ischemic and nonischemic myocardial damage	IIa	C
Invasive coronary angiography (in those who are considered eligible for potential coronary revascularization)		
Invasive coronary angiography is recommended in patients with angina despite pharmacological therapy or symptomatic ventricular arrhythmias	I	C
Invasive coronary angiography may be considered in patients with HFrEF with an intermediate to high pretest probability of CAD and the presence of ischemia in noninvasive stress tests	IIb	B

Contd...

Management of Chronic Heart Failure

Contd...

Recommendations	Class	Level
Noninvasive testing		
CTCA should be considered in patients with a low to intermediate pretest probability of CAD or those with equivocal noninvasive stress tests in order to rule out coronary artery stenosis	IIa	C
Noninvasive stress imaging (CMR, stress echocardiography, SPECT, PET) may be considered for the assessment of myocardial ischemia and viability in patients with CAD who are considered suitable for coronary revascularization	IIb	B
Exercise testing may be considered to detect reversible myocardial ischemia and investigate the cause of dyspnea	IIb	C
Cardiopulmonary exercise testing		
Cardiopulmonary exercise testing is recommended as a part of the evaluation for heart transplantation and/or MCS	I	C
Cardiopulmonary exercise testing should be considered to optimize prescription of exercise training	IIa	C
Cardiopulmonary exercise testing should be considered to identify the cause of unexplained dyspnea and/or exercise intolerance	IIa	C
Right heart catheterization		
Right heart catheterization is recommended in patients with severe HF being evaluated for heart transplantation or MCS	I	C
Right heart catheterization should be considered in patients where HF is thought to be due to constrictive pericarditis, restrictive cardiomyopathy, congenital heart disease, and high output states	IIa	C
Right heart catheterization should be considered in patients with probable pulmonary hypertension, assessed by echo in order to confirm the diagnosis and assess its reversibility before the correction of valve/structural heart disease	IIa	C
Right heart catheterization may be considered in selected patients with HFpEF to confirm the diagnosis	IIb	C
EMB		
EMB should be considered in patients with rapidly progressive HF despite standard therapy when there is a probability of a specific diagnosis, which can be confirmed only in myocardial samples	IIa	C

(CAD: coronary artery disease; CMR: cardiac magnetic resonance; CTCA: computed tomography coronary angiography; DCM: dilated cardiomyopathy; EMB: endomyocardial biopsy; HF: heart failure; HFpEF: heart failure with preserved ejection fraction; HFrEF: heart failure with reduced ejection fraction; LGE: late gadolinium enhancement; LV : left ventricular; MCS: mechanical circulatory support; PET: positron emission tomography; SPECT: single-photon emission computed tomography)

TABLE 5: Stages of heart failure (ACC/AHA Guidelines 2022).

Stages	Definition and criteria
Stage A: At Risk for HF	At risk for HF but without symptoms, structural heart disease, or cardiac biomarkers of stretch or injury (e.g., patients with hypertension, atherosclerotic CVD, diabetes, metabolic syndrome and obesity, exposure to cardiotonic agents, genetic variant for cardiomyopathy, or positive family history of cardiomyopathy)
Stage B: Pre-HF	No symptoms or signs of HF and evidence of one of the following: *Structural heart disease* • Reduced left or right ventricular systemic function • Reduced ejection fraction, reduced strain • Ventricular hypertrophy • Chamber enlargement • Wall motion abnormalities • Valvular heart disease *Evidence for increased filling pressures* • By invasive hemodynamic measurements • By noninvasive imaging suggesting elevated filling pressures (e.g., Doppler echocardiography) *Patients with risk factors and* • Increased levels of BNPs or • Persistently elevated cardiac troponin in the absence of competing diagnoses resulting in such biomarker elevations such as acute coronary syndrome, CKD, pulmonary embolus, or myopericarditis
Stage C: Symptomatic HF	Structural heart disease with current or previous symptoms of HF
Stage D: Advanced HF	Marked HF symptoms that interfere with daily life and with recurrent hospitalizations despite attempts to optimize GDMT

(BNP: B-type natriuretic peptide; CKD: chronic kidney disease; CVD: cardiovascular disease; GDMT: guideline-directed medical therapy; HF: heart failure)

Management of Chronic Heart Failure

Flowchart 2: Diagnostic algorithm for heart failure.

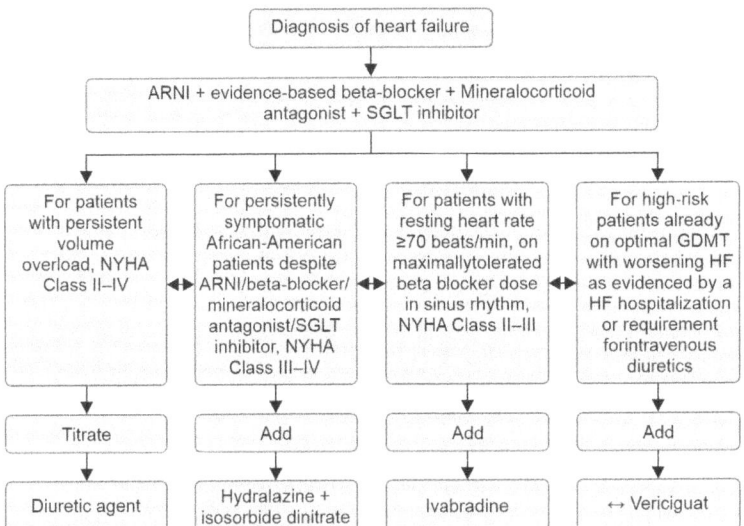

TABLE 6: Recommendations for renin–angiotensin–system inhibition with ACEI or ARB or ARNi.

COR	LOE	Recommendations
1	A	1. In patients with HFrEF and NYHA class II to III symptoms, the use of ARNi is recommended to reduce morbidity and mortality
1	A	2. In patients with previous or current symptoms of chronic HFrEF, the use of ACEI is beneficial to reduce morbidity and mortality when the use of ARNI is not feasible
1	A	3. In patients with previous or current symptoms of chronic HFrEF who are intolerant to ACEI because of cough or angioedema and when the use of ARNI is not feasible, the use of ARB is recommended to reduce morbidity and mortality
Value statement: High value (A)		4. In patients with previous or current symptoms of chronic HFrEF, in whom ARNI is not feasible, treatment with an ACEI or ARB provides high economic value
1	B-R	5. In patients with chronic symptomatic HFrEF NYHA class II or III who tolerate an ACEI or ARB, replacement by an ARNi is recommended to further reduce morbidity and mortality

TABLE 7: Recommendation for beta-blockers.

COR	LOE	Recommendations
1	A	1. In patients with HFrEF, with current or previous symptoms, use of 1 of the 3 beta-blockers proven to reduce mortality (e.g., bisoprolol, carvedilol, and sustained-release metoprolol succinate) is recommended to reduce mortality and hospitalizations
Value statement: High value (A)		2. In patients with HFrEF, with current or previous symptoms, beta-blocker therapy provides high economic value

TABLE 8: Recommendation for mineralocorticoid receptor antagonists (MRAs).

COR	LOE	Recommendations
1	A	1. In patients with HFrEF and NYHA class II to IV symptoms, an MRA (spironolactone or eplerenone) is recommended to reduce morbidity and mortality, if eGFR is >30 mL/min/1.73 m^2 and potassium is <5.0 mEq/L. Careful monitoring of potassium, renal function, and diuretic closing should be performed at initiation and closely monitored thereafter to minimize risk of hyperkalemia and renal insufficiency
Value statement: High value (A)		2. In patients with HFrEF and NYHA class II to IV symptoms, MRA therapy provides high economic values
3: Harm	B-NR	3. In patients taking MRA whose serum potassium cannot be maintained at <5.5 mEq/L, MRA should be discontinued to avoid life-threatening hyperkalemia

TABLE 9: Recommendation for SGLT2i.

COR	LOE	Recommendations
1	A	1. In patients with symptomatic chronic HFrEF, SGLT2i are recommended to reduce hospitalization for HF and cardiovascular mortality, irrespective of the presence of type 2 diabetes
Value statement: intermediate value (A)		2. In patients with symptomatic chronic HFrEF, SGLT2i therapy provides intermediate economic value

Management of Chronic Heart Failure

TABLE 10: Recommendation for other drug treatment.

COR	LOE	Recommendation
2	B-R	1. In patients with HF Class II–IV symptoms, omega-3 polyunsaturated fatty acid (PUFA) supplementation may be reasonable to use as adjunctive therapy to reduce mortality and cardiovascular hospitalizations
2B	B-R	2. In patients with HF who experience hyperkalemia (serum potassium level ≥5.5 mEq/L) while taking a renin–angiotensin–aldosterone system inhibitor (RAAS), the effectiveness of potassium binders (patiromer, sodium zirconium cyclosilicate) to improve outcomes by facilitating continuation of RAASi therapy is uncertain
3: No Benefit	B-R	3. In patients with chronic HFrEF without a specific indication [e.g., venous thromboembolism (VTE), AF, a previous thromboembolic event, or a cardioembolic source), anticoagulation is not recommended

- Beta-blockers in appropriate patients
- Implantable defibrillators in selected patient

Heart Failure with Mildly Reduced Ejection Fraction

Diagnosis

The diagnosis of heart failure with mildly reduced ejection fraction (HFmrEF) requires the presence of symptoms and/or signs of HF, and a mildly reduced EF (41–49%). The presence of elevated natriuretic peptides (NPs) [B-type natriuretic peptide (BNP) >35 pg/mL or NT-proBNP >125 pg/mL] and other evidence of structural heart disease [e.g. increased left atrial (LA) size, left ventricular hypertrophy (LVH) or echocardiographic measures of LV filling] make the diagnosis more likely but are not mandatory for diagnosis if there is certainty regarding the measurement of LVEF.

There is a substantial overlap of clinical characteristics, risk factors, patterns of cardiac remodeling, and outcomes among the LVEF categories in HF. Patients with HFmrEF have on average, features that are more similar to heart failure with reduced ejection fraction (HFrEF) than heart failure with preserved ejection fraction (HFpEF), in thay they are more commonly men, younger, and are more likely to have coronary artery disease (CAD) (50–60%), and less

TABLE 11: Evidence-based doses of disease-modifying drugs in key randomized trials in patients with heart failure with reduced ejection fraction.

	Starting dose	Target dose
ACEI:		
Captopril	6.25 mg bid	50 mg tid
Enalapril	2.5 mg bid	10–20 mg bid
Lisinopril	2.5–5 mg od	20–35 mg od
Ramipril	2.5 mg bid	5 mg bid
Trandolapril	0.5 mg od	4 mg od
ARNI:		
Sacubitril/valsartan	49/51 mg bid	97/103 mg bid
Beta-blockers:		
Bisoprolol	1.25 mg od	10 mg od
Carvedilol	3.125 mg bid	25 mg bid
Metoprolol (CR/XL)	12.5–25 mg od	200 mg od
Nebivolol	1.25 mg od	10 mg od
MRA:		
Eplerenone	25 mg od	50 mg od
Spironolactone	25 mg od	50 mg od
SGLT2i:		
Dapagliflozin	10 mg od	50 mg od
Empagliflozin	25 mg od	50 mg od
Other agents:		
Candesartan	4 mg od	32 mg od
Losartan	50 mg od	150 mg od
Valsartan	40 mg bid	160 mg bid
Ivabradine	5 mg bid	75 mg bid
Vericiguat	2.5 mg od	10 g od
Digoxin	62.5 µg od	250 µg od
Hydralazine/Isosorbide dinitrate	37.5 mg tid/20 mg tid	75 mg tid/40 mg tid

TABLE 12: Contraindications and cautions for sacubitril/valsartan for specific patient populations.

Contraindications	Cautions
A. Sacubitril/Valsartan	

• Within 36 hours of ACE inhibitor use
• Any history of angioedema
• Pregnancy
• Lactation (no data)
• Severe hepatic impairment (Child-Pugh class C)
• Concomitant aliskiren use in patients with diabetes
• Known hypersensitivity to either ARBs or ARNIs
	• *Kidney impairment:*
	  – Mild-to-moderate (eGFR 30–59 mL/min/1.73 m^2): No starting dose adjustment required
	  – Severe (eGFR <30 mL/min/1.73 m^2): Reduce starting dose to 24 mg/26 mg twice daily; double the dose every 2–4 weeks to target maintenance dose of 97 mg/103 mg twice daily, as tolerated
	• *Hepatic impairment:*
	  – Mild (Child-Pugh class A): No starting dose adjustment required
	  – Moderate (Child-Pugh class B): Reduce starting dose to 24/26 mg twice daily; double the dose every 2–4 weeks to target maintenance dose of 97/103 mg twice daily, as tolerated
	• Renal artery stenosis
	• Systolic blood pressure <100 mm Hg
	• Volume depletion

B. SGLT inhibitors	

• Not approved for use in patients with type 1 diabetes due to increased risk of diabetic ketoacidosis
• Known hypersensitivity to drug
	• For HF care, dapagliflozin or sotagliflozin, eGFR <25 mL/min/1.73 m^2
	• Pregnancy
	• Increased risk of mycotic genital infections
	• May contribute to volume depletion. Consider altering diuretic agent dose if applicable
	• Ketoacidosis in patients with diabetes:
	  – Temporary discontinuation for at least 3 days before scheduled surgery is recommended to avoid potential risk for ketoacidosis
	  – Assess patients who present with signs and symptoms of metabolic acidosis for ketoacidosis, regardless of blood glucose level
	• *Acute kidney injury and impairment in kidney function:* Consider temporarily discontinuing in settings of reduced oral intake or fluid losses
	• *Urosepsis and pyelonephritis:* Evaluate patients for signs and symptoms of urinary tract infections and treat promptly, if indicated

Contd...

Contd...

Contraindications	Cautions
	• *Necrotizing fasciitis of the perineum (Fournier gangrene):* Rare, serious, life-threatening cases have occurred in both female and male patients; assess patients presenting with pain or tenderness, erythema, or swelling in the genital or perineal area, along with fever or malaise
C. Ivabradine	
• HFpEF • Presence of angina with normal EF • Hypersensitivity • Severe hepatic impairment (Child-Pugh class C) • Acute decompensated HF • Blood pressure <90/50 mm Hg • Sick sinus syndrome without a pacemaker • Sinoatrial node block • Second- or third-degree block without a pacemaker • Persistent AF or flutter • Atrial pacemaker dependence	• Sinus node disease • Cardiac conduction defects • Prolonged QT interval • Resting heart rate <60 beats/min
D. Vericiguat	
• Patients with concomitant use of other soluble guanylate cyclase stimulators • Pregnancy	• Patients with anemia • Patients with symptomatic hypotension • Concomitant use with PDE-5 inhibitors is not recommended due to the potential for hypotension

Management of Chronic Heart Failure

Flowchart 3: Comprehensive management of HFrEF.

To reduce mortality-for all patients			
ACE-I/ARNI	BB	MRA	SGLT2i

To reduce HF hospitalization/mortality-for selected patients	
Volume overload	
Diuretics	
SR with LBBB ≥150 ms	SR with LBBB 130–149 ms or non LBBB ≥150 ms
CRT-P/D	CRT-P/D
Ischaemic aetiology	Non-ischaemic aetiology
ICD	ICD

Atrial fibrillation	Atrial fibrillation		Coronary artery disease	Iron deficiency
Anticoagulation	Digoxin	PVI	CABG	Ferric carboxymaltose
Aortic stenosis	Mitral regurgitation	Heart rate SR >70 bpm	Black Race	ACE-WARNI intolerance
SAVR/TAVI	TEE MV repair	Ivabradine	Hydralazine/ISDN	ARB

For selected advanced HF patients		
Heart transplantation	MCS as BTT/BTC	Long-term MCS as DT

To reduce HF hospitalization and improve QOL - for all patients
Exercise rehabilitation
Multi-professional disease management

likely to have atrial fibrillation (AF) and noncardiac comorbidities. However, ambulatory patients with HFmrEF have a lower mortality than those with HFrEF more akin to those with HFpEF.

Patients with HFmrEF may include patients whose LVEF has improved from <40% or declined from ≥50%.

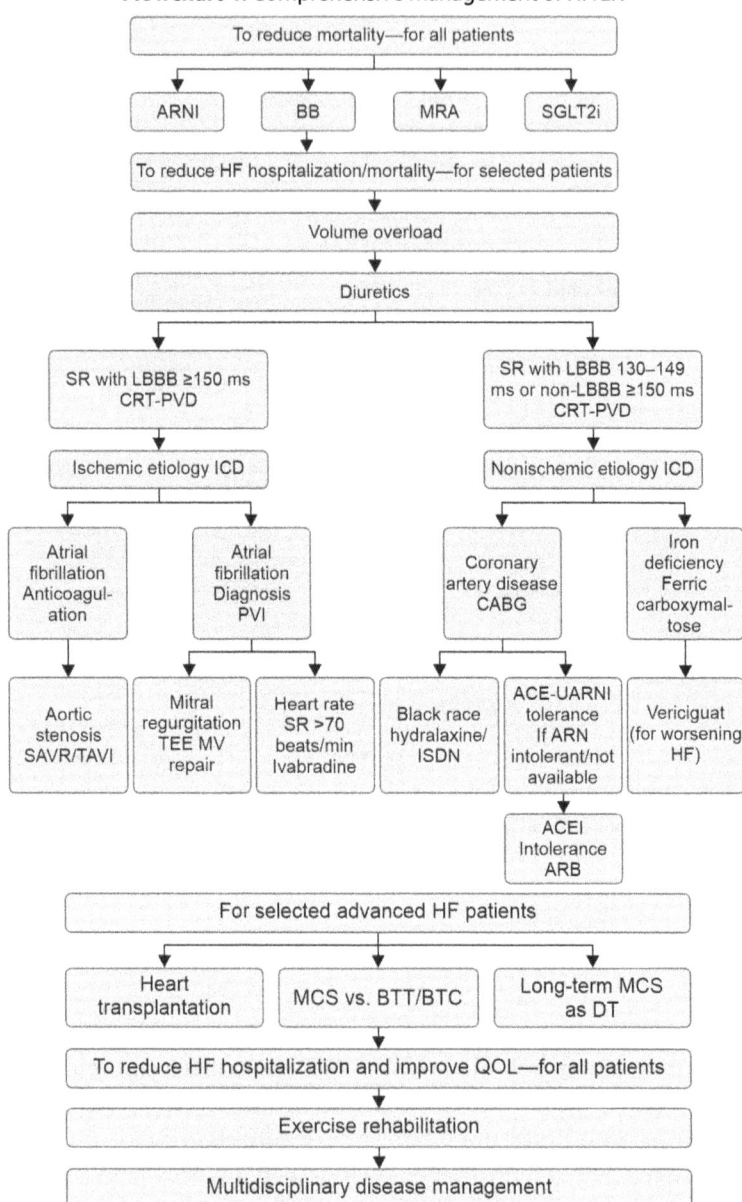

Flowchart 4: Comprehensive management of HFrEF.

TABLE 13: ICDs and CRTs (2022 AHA/ACC/HFSA Heart Failure Guideline).

Recommendations for ICDs and CRTs
Referenced studies that support the recommendations are summarized in the Online Data Supplements
Recommendations for renin–angiotensin–system inhibition with ACEI or ARB or ARNI
Referenced studies that support the recommendations are summarized in the Online Data Supplements

COR	LOE	Recommendations
1	A	1. In patients with nonischemic DCM or ischemic heart disease at least 40 days post-MI with LVEF ≤35% and NYHA class II or III symptoms on chronic GDMT, who have reasonable expectation of meaningful survival for >1 year, ICD therapy is recommended for primary prevention of SCD to reduce total mortality
Value statement: High value (A)		2. A transvenous ICD provides high economic value in the primary prevention of SCD particularly when the patient's risk of death caused by ventricular arrhythmia is deemed high and the risk of nonarrhythmic death (either cardiac or noncardiac) is deemed low based on the patient's burden of comorbidities and functional status
1	B-R	3. In patients at least 40 days post-MI with LVEF ≤30% and NYHA class I symptoms while receiving GDMT, who have reasonable expectation of meaningful survival for >1 year, ICD therapy is recommended for primary prevention of SCD to reduce total mortality
1	B-R	4. For patients who have LVEF ≤35%, sinus rhythm, left bundle branch block (LBBB) with a QRS duration ≥150 ms, and NYHA class II, III, or ambulatory IV symptoms on GDMT, CRT is indicated to reduced total mortality, reduce hospitalizations, and improve symptoms and QOL
Value statement: High value (B-NR)		5. For patients who have LVEF ≤35%, sinus rhythm, a non-LBBB pattern with a QRS duration ≥150 ms, and NYHA class II, III, or ambulatory class IV symptoms on GDMT, CRT can be useful to reduce total mortality, reduce hospitalizations, and improve symptoms and QOL

Contd...

Contd...

COR	LOE	Recommendations
2a	B-R	6. For patients who have LVEF ≤35%, sinus rhythm, a non-LBBB patients with a QRS duration ≥150 ms, and NYHA class II, III, or ambulatory class IV symptoms on GDMT, CRT can be useful to reduce total mortality, reduce hospitalizations, and improve symptoms and QOL
2a	B-R	7. In patients with high-degree or complete heart block and LVEF of 36–50%, CRT is reasonable to reduce total mortality, reduce hospitalization, and improve symptoms and QOL
2a	B-NR	8. For patients who have LVEF ≤35%, sinus rhythm, LBBB with a QRS duration of 120–149 ms and NYHA class II, III, or ambulatory IV symptoms on GDMT, CRT can be useful to reduce total mortality, reduce hospitalizations, and improve symptoms and QOL
2a	B-NR	9. In patients with AF and LVEF ≤35% on GDMT, CRT can be useful to reduce total mortality, improve symptoms and QOL, and increase LVEF, if (a) the patient require ventricular pacing or otherwise meets CRT criteria and (b) atrioventricular nodal ablation or pharmacological rate control will allow near 100% ventricular pacing with CRT
2a	B-NR	10. For patients of GDMT who have LVEF ≤35% and are undergoing placement of new or replacement device implantation with anticipated requirement for significant (>40%) ventricular pacing, CRT can be useful to reduce total mortality, reduce hospitalizations, and improve symptoms and QOL
2a	B-NR	11. In patients with genetic antithrombogenic cardiomyopathy with high-risk features of sudden death, with EF ≤45%, implantation of ICD is reasonable to decrease sudden death
2b	B-NR	12. For patients who have LVEF ≤35%, sinus rhythm, a non-LBBB pattern with QRS duration of 120–149 ms, and NYHA class III or ambulatory class IV on GDMT, CRT may be considered to reduce total mortality, reduce hospitalizations, and improve symptoms and QOL

Contd...

Management of Chronic Heart Failure

Contd...

COR	LOE	Recommendations
2b	B-NR	13. For patients who have LVEF ≤30%, ischemic cause of HF, sinus rhythm, LBBB with a QRS duration ≥150 ms, and NYHA class I symptoms on GDMT, CRT may be considered to reduce hospitalizations and improve symptoms and QOL
3: No Benefit	B-NR	14. In patients with QRS duration <120 ms, CRT is not recommended
3: No Benefit	B-NR	15. For patients with NYHA class I or II symptoms and non-LBBB pattern with QRS duration <150 ms, CRT is not recommended
3: No Benefit	C-LD	16. For patients whose comorbidities or frailty limit survival with good functional capacity to <1 year, ICD and cardiac resynchronization therapy with defibrillation are not indicated

Heart Failure with Mildly Reduced Ejection Fraction is not All Alike

This study confirms that among HF patients with mildly reduced EF, different phenotypes with differing disease trajectories coexist. It also suggests that clinical prognosis (and, probably, the risk of EF deterioration) of patients diagnosed with HFmrEF is worse, compared with those who improve from reduced EF to mildly reduced EF. Further research with larger groups is required to identify predictors of EF deterioration and assess the potential role of intensification of neurohormonal modulation in preventing it **(Flowchart 7)**.

Recommendation	Class	Level
An SGLT2i (dapagliflozin or empagliflozin) is recommended in patients with HFmrEF to reduce the risk of HF hospitalization or CV death	I	A

Other Drugs

In the DIG trial, for those with HFmrEF in SR, there was a trend fewer hospitalizations for HF in those assigned to digoxin, but no reduction

Flowchart 5: Algorithm for CRT indications in patients with cardiomyopathy or HFrEF.

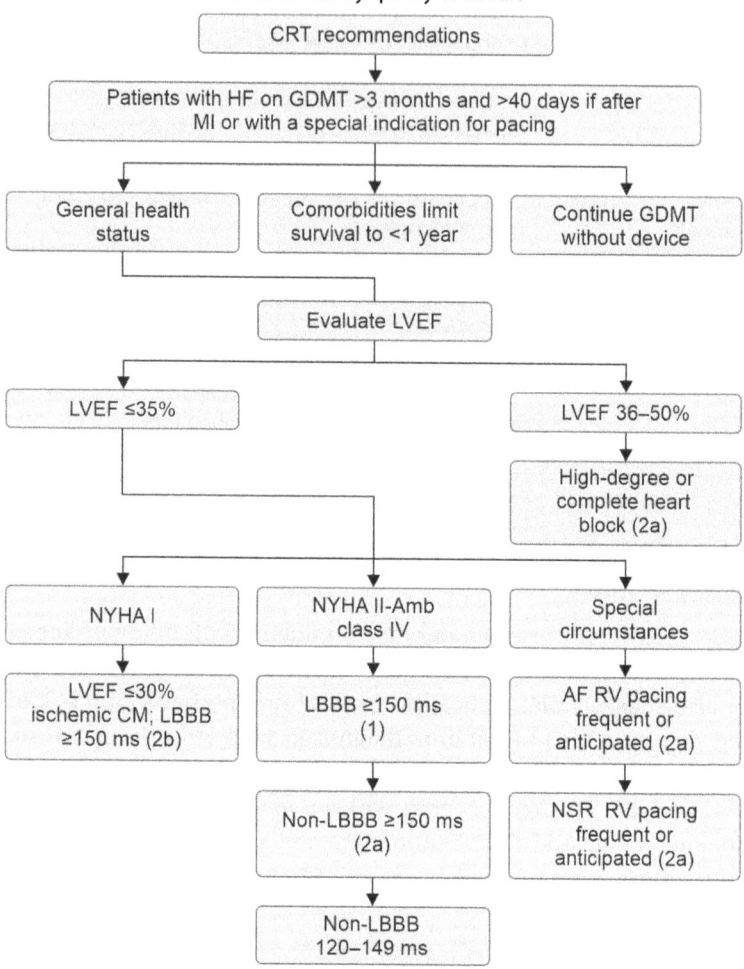

(AF: atrial fibrillation; Amb: ambulatory; CM: cardiomyopathy; GDMT: guideline-directed medical therapy; HB: heart block; HF: heart failure; HFrEF: heart failure with reduced ejection fraction; LBBB: left bundle branch block; LV: left ventricular; LVEF: left ventricular ejection fraction; NSR: normal sinus rhythm; NYHA: New York Heart Association; RV: right ventricular)

in mortality and a trend to an excess of CV deaths. Therefore, there are insufficient data to recommend its use.

There are also insufficient data on ivabradine in HFmrEF to draw any conclusions.

Management of Chronic Heart Failure

TABLE 14: Recommendations for revascularization for CAD.

COR	LOE	Recommendations
1	B-R	1. In selected patients with HF, reduced EF (EF ≤35%), and suitable coronary anatomy, surgical revascularization plus GDMT is beneficial to improve symptoms, cardiovascular hospitalizations, and long-term all-cause mortality

TABLE 15: Recommendations for valvular heart disease.

COR	LOE	Recommendations
1	B-R	1. In patients with HF, VH should be managed in a multidisciplinary manner in accordance with clinical practice guidelines for VHD to prevent worsening of HF and adverse clinical outcomes
1	C-LD	2. In patients with chronic severe secondary MR and HFrEF, optimization of GDMT is recommended before any intervention for secondary MR related to LV dysfunction

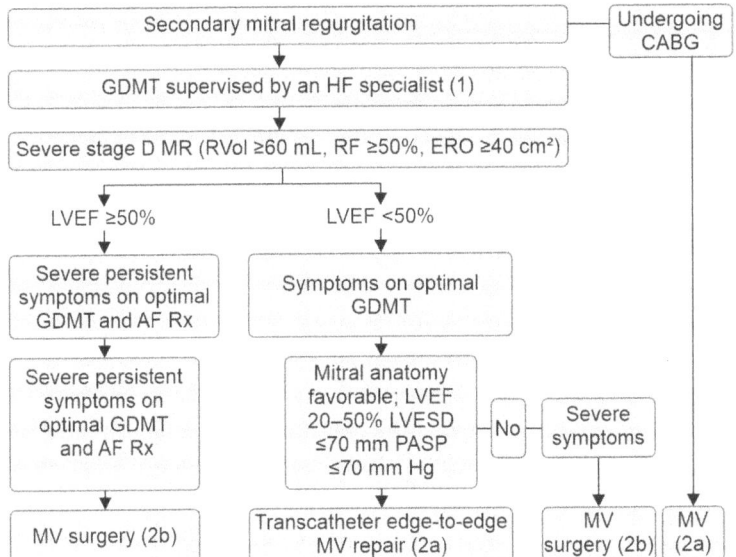

Flowchart 6: Treatment approach in secondary mitral regurgitation.

(AF: atrial fibrillation; CABG: coronary artery bypass graft; ERO: effective regurgitant orifice; GDMT: guideline-directed medical therapy; HF: heart failure; LVEF: left ventricular ejection fraction; LVESD: left ventricular end-systolic diameter; MR: mitral regurgitation; MV: mitral valve; PASP: pulmonary artery systolic pressure; RF: regurgitant fraction; RVol: regurgitant volume; Rx: medication)

Flowchart 7: Diagnostic and treatment algorithm of cardiac amyloidosis.

```
History, ECG, echocardiogram, cardiac MRI suggestive of
cardiac amyloidosis (see text)
        ↓
Check for monoclonal light chains
        ↓
Presence of a monoclonal light chain?
   ↓ Yes          ↓ No
```

- Yes branch: Hematology-oncology consultation and consider heart or other biopsy → Amyloid on heart biopsy?
  - No evidence of amyloid → Cardiac amyloidosis unlikely
  - Evidence of amyloid → AL-CM / ATTR-CM
    - AL-CM → Treatment by hematologist oncologist
    - ATTR-CM → Perform TTR gene sequencing (0)

- No branch: Check Tc-99m-PYP scan (1)
  - Yes → Perform TTR gene sequencing (0)
  - No → Tc-99m-PYP amyloidosis-unlikely → No → Cardiac amyloidosis

TTR gene sequencing results: ATTRv-CM / ATTRwt-CM

ATTRv-CM:
- Referral to genetic counselor
- Potential screening of family members
- TTR silencer therapy if neuropathy

Treatment:
- HFrEF → Individualize therapy (see text)
- NYHA I–III symptoms → Tafamidis (0)
- Atrial fibrillation → Anticoagulation regardless of CHA$_2$DS$_2$-VASc score (2)

(AL-CM: amyloid cardiomyopathy; ATTR-CM: transthyretin amyloid cardiomyopathy; ATTRv: variant transthyretin amyloidosis; ATTRwt: wild-type transthyretin amyloidosis; CHA$_2$DS$_2$-VASc: congestive heart failure, hypertension, age ≥75 years, diabetes mellitus, stroke or transient ischemic attack (TIA), vascular disease, age 65 to 74 years, sex category; ECG: electrocardiogram; H/CL: heart to contralateral chest; HFrEF: heart failure with reduced ejection fraction; IFE: immunofixation electrophoresis; MRI: magnetic resonance imaging; NYHA: New York Heart Association; PYP: pyrophosphate; Tc: technetium; TTR: transthyretin)

TABLE 16: ESC 2021 Heart Failure Guidelines (2022 AHA/ACC/HFSA Heart Failure Guideline).

Recommendations	Class	Level
Intravenous iron supplementation is recommended in symptomatic patients with HFrEF and HFmrEF, and iron deficiency, to alleviate HF symptoms and improve quality of life	I	A
Intravenous iron supplementation with ferric carboxymaltose or ferric derisomaltose should be considered in symptomatic patients with HFrEF and HFmrEF, and iron deficiency, to reduce the risk of HF hospitalization	IIa	A

BOX 1: ESC definition of advanced heart failure.

All these criteria must be present despite optimal guideline-directed treatment:
1. Severe and persistent symptoms of HF [NYHA class III (advanced) or IV]
2. Severe cardiac dysfunction defined by ≥1 of these:
   - LVEF ≤30%
   - Isolated RV failure
   - Nonoperable severe valve abnormalities
   - Nonoperable severe congenital heart disease
   - EF ≥40%, elevated natriuretic peptide levels and evidence of significant diastolic dysfunction
3. Hospitalizations or unplanned visits in the past 12 months for episodes of:
   - Congestion requiring high-dose intravenous diuretics or diuretic combinations
   - Low output requiring inotropes or vasoactive medications
   - Malignant arrhythmias
4. Severe impairment of exercise capacity with inability to exercise or low 6-minute walk test distance (<300 meter) or peak
   - VO_2 (<12–14 mL/kg/min) estimated to be of cardiac origin
   - Criteria 1 and 4 can be met in patients with cardiac dysfunction (as described in criterion 2) but also have substantial limitations as a result of other conditions (e.g., severe pulmonary disease, noncardiac cirrhosis, and renal disease). The therapeutic options for these patients may be more limited

(EF: ejection fraction; ESC: European Society of Cardiology; HF: heart failure; LVEF: left ventricular ejection fraction; NYHA: New York Heart Association; RV: right ventricular; VO_2, oxygen consumption/oxygen uptake)
Source: Adapted with permission from Crespo-Leiro et al.

Flowchart 8: Management of patients with HFmrEF.

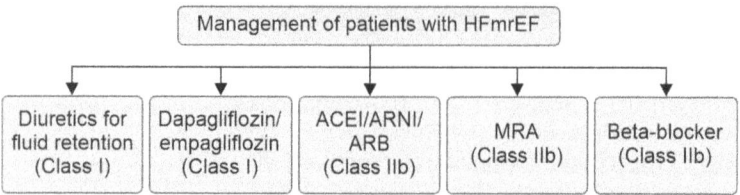

(ACEI: angiotensin-converting enzyme inhibitor; ARB: angiotensin receptor blocker; ARNI: angiotensin receptor-neprilysin inhibitor; HFmrEF: heart failure with mildly reduced ejection fraction; MRA: mineralocorticoid receptor antagonist)

BOX 2: Clinical indicators of advanced heart failure.

- Repeated hospitalizations or emergency department visits for HF in the past 12 months
- Need for intravenous inotropic therapy
- Persistent NYHA functional class III–IV symptoms despite therapy
- Severely reduced exercise capacity (peak VO_2, <14 mL/kg/min or <50% predicted, 6-minute walk test distance <300 meter, or inability to walk 1 block on level ground because of dyspnea or fatigue)
- Intolerance to RAASi because of hypotension or worsening renal function
- Intolerance to beta blockers as a result of worsening HF or hypotension
- Recent need to escalate diuretics to maintain volume status, often reaching daily furosemide equivalent dose >160 mg/day or use of supplemental metolazone therapy
- Refractory clinical congestion
- Progressive deterioration in renal or hepatic function
- Worsening right HF or secondary pulmonary hypertension
- Frequent SBP ≤90 mm Hg
- Cardiac cachexia
- Persistent hyponatremia (serum sodium, <134 mEq/L)
- Refractory or recurrent ventricular arrhythmias, frequent ICD shocks
- Increased predicted 1-year mortality (e.g., >20%) according to HF survival models (e.g., MAGGIC, SHFM)

(HF: heart failure; ICD: implantable cardioverter-defibrillator; MAGGIC: Meta-analysis Global Group in Chronic Heart Failure; NYHA: New York Heart Association; RAAS: renin-angiotensin aldosterone system inhibitors; SBP: systolic blood pressure; SHFM: Seattle Heart Failure Model; VO_2: oxygen consumption/oxygen uptake)

Management of Chronic Heart Failure

TABLE 17: INTERMEDICS profile.

Profile description	Features
1. Critical cardiogenic shock	Life-threatening hypotension and rapidly escalating inotropic/pressor support, with critical organ hypoperfusion often confirmed by worsening acidosis and lactate levels
2. Progressive decline	"Dependent" on inotropic support but nonetheless shows signs of continuing deterioration in nutrition, renal function, fluid retention, or other major status indicator. Can also apply to a patient with refractory volume overload, perhaps with evidence of impaired perfusion, in whom inotropic infusions cannot be maintained because of tachyarrhythmias, clinical ischemia, or other intolerance
3. Stable but inotrope dependent	Clinically stable on mild–moderate doses of intravenous inotropes (or has a temporary circulatory support device) after repeated documentation of failure to wean without symptomatic hypotension, worsening symptoms, or progressive organ dysfunction (usually renal)
4. Resting symptoms on oral therapy at home	Patient who is at home on oral therapy but frequently has symptoms of congestion at rest or with activities of daily living (dressing or bathing). He or she may have orthopnea, shortness of breath during dressing or bathing, gastrointestinal symptoms (abdominal discomfort, nausea, and poor appetite), disabling ascites, or severe lower extremity edema
5. Exertion intolerant	Patient who is comfortable at rest but unable to engage in any activity, living predominantly within the house or housebound
6. Exertion limited	Patient who is comfortable at rest without evidence of fluid overload but who is able to do some mild activity. Activities of daily living are comfortable, and minor activities outside the home such as visiting friends or going to a restaurant can be performed, but fatigue results within a few minutes or with any meaningful physical exertion
7. Advanced NYHA class III	Patient who is clinically stable with a reasonable level of comfortable activity, despite a history of previous decompensation that is not recent. This patient is usually able to walk more than a block. Any decompensation requiring intravenous diuretics or hospitalization within the previous month should make this person a Patient Profile 6 or lower

(ICD: implantable cardioverter-defibrillator; INTERMACS: Interagency Registry for Mechanically Assisted Circulatory Support; NYHA: New York Heart Association)

TABLE 18: Recommendation for specialty referral for advanced HF (2022 AHA/ACC).

COR	LOE	Recommendation
1	C-LD	1. In patients with advanced HF, when consistent with the patient's goals of care, timely referral for HF specialty care is recommended to review HF management and assess suitability for advanced HF therapies (e.g., LVAD, cardiac transplantation, palliative care, and palliative inotropical)

TABLE 19: Nonpharmacological management: Advanced HF (2022 AHA/ACC/HFSA Heart Failure Guideline).

Recommendation for nonpharmacological management: Advanced HF

COR	LOE	Recommendation
2b	C-LD	1. For patients with advanced HF and hyponatremia, the benefit of fluid restoration to reduce congestive symptoms is uncertain

TABLE 20: Ionotropic support (2022 AHA/ACC/HFSA Heart Failure Guideline).

Recommendations for inotropic support
Referenced studies that support the recommendations are summarized in the Online Data Supplements

COR	LOE	Recommendations
2a	B-NR	1. In patients with advanced (stage D) HF refractory to GDMT and device therapy who are eligible for and awaiting MCS or cardiac transplantation, continuous intravenous inotropic support is reasonable as "bridge therapy"
2b	B-NR	2. In select patients with stage D HF, despite optimal GDMT and device therapy who are ineligible for either MCS or cardiac transplantation, continuous intravenous inotropic support may be considered as palliative therapy for symptom content and improvement in functional status
3: Harm	B-R	3. In patients with HF, long-term use of either continuous or intermittent intravenous inotropic agents, for reasons other than palliative care or as a bridge to advanced therapies, is potentially harmful

TABLE 21: Intravenous inotropic agents used in the management of HF.

Inotropic agent	Bolus	Dose (µg/kg) Infusion (/min)	CO	HR	SVR	Effects PVR	Adverse effects
Adrenergic agonists							
Dopamine	NA	8–10	↑	↑	↑↑	↑↑	T, HA, N, tissue necrosis
		10–15	↑	↑	↑		
Dobutamine	NA	2.5–20	↑	↑	↑↑	↑↑	↑/↓BP, HA, T, N, F hypersensitivity
PDE3 inhibitor							
Milrinone	NR	0.125–0.75	↑	↑	↓	↓	T, ↓BP
Vasopressors							
Epinephrine	NR	5–15 µg/mm	↑	↑	↑(↓)	↑↑	HA, T
		15–20 µg/min	↑	↑↑	↑↑	↑↑	HA, T
Norepinephrine	NR	0.5–30 µg/min	↑↑	↑	↑↑	↑↑	↓HR, tissue necrosis

TABLE 22: Indications and contraindications to mechanical support.

Indications (combination of these)	Contraindications
• Frequent hospitalizations for HF • NYHA class IIIb to IV functional limitations despite maximal therapy • Intolerance of neurohormonal antagonists • Increasing diuretic requirement • Symptomatic despite CRT • Inotropic dependence • Low peak VO_2 (<14–16) • End-organ dysfunction attributable to low cardiac output	• Absolute • Irreversible hepatic disease • Irreversible renal disease • Irreversible neurological disease • Medical nonadherence • Severe psychosocial limitations • Relative • Age >80 years for destination therapy • Obesity or malnutrition • Musculoskeletal disease that impairs rehabilitation • Active systemic infection or prolonged intubation • Untreated malignancy • Severe PVD • Active substance abuse • Impaired cognitive function • Unmanaged psychiatric disorder • Lack of social support

(CRT: cardiac resynchronization therapy; HF: heart failure; NYHA: New York Heart Association; VO_2: oxygen consumption; PVD: peripheral vascular disease)

Devices

While post hoc analyses of landmark cardiac resynchronization therapy (CRT) trials suggest that CRT may benefit patients with LVEF >35%, trials of CRT for HFmrEF were abandoned due to poor recruitment. There are no substantial trial of implantable cardioverter-defibrillator (ICDs) for primary prevention of ventricular arrhythmias for HFmrEF; trials conducted more than 20 years ago suggested no benefit from ICD implantation for secondary prevention of ventricular arrhythmias for HFmrEF. Therefore, there is insufficient evidence to advise CRT or ICD therapy in patients with HFmrEF. In HF patients with an LVEF ≥40%, the implantation of an interatrial shunt device was found to be safe, and this device is subject to investigation in a larger study before any recommendation on their use in HFpEF or HFmrEF can be given.

TABLE 23: Recommendations for mechanical circulatory support (2022 AHA/ACC/HFSA Heart Failure Guideline).

Referenced studies that support the recommendations are summarized in the Online Data Supplements

COR	LOE	Recommendations
1	A	1. In selected patients with advanced HFrEF with NYHA class IV symptoms who are deemed to be dependent on continuous intravenous inotropes or temporary MCS, durable LVAD implantation is effective to improve functional status QOL, and survival
2a	B-R	2. In select patients with advanced HFrEF who have NYHA class IV symptoms despite GDMT, durable MCS can be beneficial to improve symptoms, improve functional class, and reduce mortality
Value statement: Uncertain value (B-NR)		3. In patients with advanced HFrEF who have NYHA class IV symptoms despite GDMT, durable MCS devices provide low to intermediate economic value based on current costs and outcomes
2a	B-NR	4. In patients with advanced HFrEF and hemodynamic compromise and shock, temporary MCS, including percutaneous and extracorporeal ventricular assist devices, is reasonable as a "bridge to recovery" or "bridge to decision"

Heart Failure with Preserved Ejection Fraction

Clinical Characteristics of Patients with Heart Failure with Preserved Ejection Fraction

Heart failure with preserved ejection fraction differs from HFrEF and HFmrEF in that HFpEF patients are older and more often female. AF, chronic kidney disease (CKD), and non-CV comorbidities are more common in patients with HFpEF than in those with HFrEF.

There are numerous potential causes of HFpEF. The pathophysiology of various HFpEF syndromes differs, and thus they require distinct therapies. Red flags for the potential presence of CA include low normal BP in patients with a history of hypertension, intolerance to beta-blockers or ACEI, history of bilateral carpal

TABLE 24: Objective evidence of cardiac structural, functional, and serological abnormalities consistent with the presence of left ventricular diastolic dysfunction/raised left ventricular filling pressure.

Parameter	Threshold	Comments
• LV mass index • Relative wall thickness	≥95 g/m² (Female), ≥115 g/m² (Male)	Although the presence of concentric LV remodeling or hypertrophy is supportive, the absence of LV hypertrophy does not exclude the diagnosis of HFpEF
LA volume index	>34 mL/m² (SR)	In the absence of AF or valve disease, LA enlargement reflects chronically elevated LV filling pressure (in the presence of AF, the threshold is >40 mL/m²)
E/e' ratio at rest	>9	Sensitivity 78%, specificity 59% for the presence of HFpEF by invasive exercise testing, although reported accuracy has varied. A higher cut-off of 13 had lower sensitivity (46%) but higher specificity (86%)
NT-proBNP BNP	>125 (SR) or >365 (AF) pg/mL >35 (SR) or >105 (AF) pg/mL	Up to 20% of patients with invasively proven HFpEF have NPs below diagnostic thresholds, particularly in the presence of obesity
PA systolic pressure TR velocity at rest	>35 mm Hg >2.8 m/s	Sensitivity 54%, specificity 85% for the presence of HFpEF by invasive exercise testing

(AF: atrial fibrillation; BNP: B-type natriuretic peptide; E/e' ratio: early filling velocity on transmitral Doppler/early relaxation velocity on tissue Doppler; HFpEF: heart failure with preserved ejection fraction; LA: left atrial; LV: left ventricular; NP: natriuretic peptide; NT-proBNP: N-terminal pro-B-type natriuretic peptide; PA: pulmonary artery; SR: sinus rhythm; TR: tricuspid regurgitation)

tunnel syndrome, low voltage on ECG and echocardiographic features such as thickening of the septum, posterior wall, or RV wall, enlarged atria, a small pericardial effusion, or valve thickening. Furthermore, it is important to exclude other conditions that might mimic the HFpEF syndrome (e.g., lung disease, anemia, obesity, and deconditioning).

Diagnosis of Heart Failure with Preserved Ejection Fraction

This simplified diagnostic approach starts with assessment of pretest probability (see clinical characteristics above). The diagnosis should include the following:
- Symptoms and signs of HF
- An LVEF ≥50%.

Objective evidence of cardiac structural and/or functional abnormalities consistent with the presence of LV diastolic dysfunction/raised LV filling pressures, including raised natriuretic peptides (NPs).

In the presence of AF, the threshold for LA volume index is >40 mL/m2. Exercise stress thresholds include E/e' ratio at peak stress ≥15 or tricuspid regurgitation (TR) velocity at peak stress >3.4 m/s. LV global longitudinal strain <16% has a sensitivity of 62% and a specificity of 56% for the diagnosis of HFpEF by invasive testing.

If resting echocardiographic and laboratory markers are equivocal, a diastolic stress test is recommended. The confirmatory test for the diagnosis of HFpEF is invasive hemodynamic exercise testing.

An invasively measured pulmonary capillary wedge pressure (PCWP) of ≥15 mm Hg (at rest) or ≥25 mm Hg (with exercise) or LV end-diastolic pressure ≥16 mm Hg (at rest) is generally considered diagnostic. However, instead of an exercise PCWP cut-off, some have used an index of PCWP to cardiac output for the invasive diagnosis of HFpEF. Recognizing that invasive hemodynamic exercise testing is not available in many centers worldwide, and is associated with risks, its main use is limited to the research setting. In the absence of any disease-modifying treatments, the current guidelines do not mandate gold standard testing in every patient to make the diagnosis, but emphasize that the greater the number of objective noninvasive markers of raised LV filling pressures, the higher the probability of a diagnosis of HFpEF.

The diagnosis of HFpEF remains challenging. Several diagnosis criteria have been proposed by societies and in clinical trials. These criteria vary widely in their sensitivities and specificities for diagnosing HFpEF. More recently, two score-based algorithms (H2FPEF and HFA-PEFF) have been proposed to aid the

TABLE 25: Diagnostic scores for heart failure with preserved ejection fraction.

			Biomarker	
	Functional	**Morphological**	**Sinus rhythm**	**Atrial fibrillation**
Major criteria (2 points)	• Septal e' <7 cm/s • Lateral e' <10 cm/s • Average E/e' ≥15 • TR velocity >2.8 m/s	• LAVI >34 mL/m² • LVMi ≥149/122 g/m² • RWT > 0.42	• NT-proBNP >220 pg/mL • BNP >80 pg/mL	• NT-proBNP >660 pg/mL • BNP >240 pg/mL
Minor criteria (1 point)	• Average E/e' 9–14 • GLS <16	• LAVI 29–34 mL/m² • LVMi >115/95 g/m² • RWT >0.42 • LV wall thickness ≥12 mm	• NT-proBNP 125–220 pg/mL • BNP 35–80 pg/mL	• NT-proBNP 365–660 pg/mL • BNP 105–240 pg/mL

≥5 points: HFpEF

2–4 points: Echo stress test or Invasive hemodynamic measurement

Stress echo → Invasive hemodinamic measurements

- Average E/e' 215: 2 points
- Average E/e' 215 and TR velocity >2.8 m/s: 3 points
- No criteria fulfilled

At Rest: LVEDP ≥16 mm Hg; PCPW ≥15 mm Hg
During exercise: PCPW ≥25 mm Hg

→ HFpEF

HFA-PEFF SCORE

	Variable	**Values (points)**
H₂	Heavy Hypertensive	BMI > 30 kg/m² (2) Two or more antihypertensive medicines (1)
F	Atrial fibrillation	Paroxysmal or persistent (3)
P	Pulmonary hypertension	PAPs >35 mm Hg (1)
E	Elder	Age >60 years (1)
F	Filling pressure	Doppler echocardiographic E/e' >9 (1)

Total points: 0 1 2 3 4 5 6 7 8 9
Probability of HFpEF: 0.2 0.3 0.4 0.5 0.6 0.7 0.8 0.9 0.95

H₂FPEF SCORE

diagnosis. While the generalizability of the scores has been tested in various trial and observational cohorts, their diagnostic performance has varied.

Both scores assign a substantial proportion of suspected HFpEF patients in intermediate likelihood, wherein additional diagnostics are proposed. Thus, depending on which score is used, different patients will be referred for additional testing or allocated as having HFpEF. Furthermore, physicians may not have been access to all the specialized tests recommended by the specific diagnostic algorithms. This limits the broad clinical applicability of the scores and demonstrates the ongoing diagnostic uncertainty in HFpEF.

Treatment of Heart Failure with Preserved Ejection Fraction

- *Goals of therapy:* For patients with HFpEF, the goals of treatment are to reduce HF severity and increase functional status. There is no clear evidence that pharmacologic therapy, diet, or other therapies reduce the risk of mortality in patients with HFpEF.
- *Exercise, diet, weight loss, and cardiac rehabilitation:* In patients with HFpEF, participation in structured exercise programs, cardiac rehabilitation, and dietary interventions is safe and can lead to small improvements in exercise tolerance.

MANAGEMENT AND ASSOCIATED CONDITIONS

Atrial fibrillation: Patients with HFpEF and AF are managed according to clinical practice guidelines that apply to all patients with HF.

There are no prospective trials of revascularization in patients with HFpEF. In a single-center study of patients with HFpEF, revascularization was associated with higher survival and a lower rate of progression to HFrEF.

Myocardial ischemia: Coronary artery disease is common among patients with HFpEF.

MANAGEMENT OF VOLUME OVERLOAD

Patients with HFpEF and volume overload require diuretic therapy. The usual approach to therapy is the treatment with a loop diuretic. In patients with mild volume overload who are likely to benefit from sodium-glucose co-transporter 2 (SGLT2) inhibitor therapy, the diuretic effect of an SGLT2 inhibitor agent may adequately treat volume overload.

In patients resistant to diuresis, the approach to diuretic use typically involves higher doses, changing agents, or use of multiple agents.

PHARMACOTHERAPY

Initial therapy (SGLT2 inhibitor): In patients with HFpEF (LVEF ≥50%) who have New York Heart Association (NYHA) class II to III symptoms, treatment with an SGLT2 or suggested inhibitor (algorithm 1) can be initiated. In patients who cannot take an SGLT2 inhibitor (e.g., cost and risk of infection), it is reasonable to initiate therapy with a mineralocorticoid receptor antagonist (MRA). SGLT2 inhibitor therapy reduces the risk of HF hospitalization by a small amount and is one of few therapies with a beneficial effect in patients with HFpEF. Start an SGLT2 inhibitor before adding other therapies.

Dosing: We prefer to use empagliflozin 10 mg daily or dapagliflozin 10 mg daily.

In a meta-analysis that included two trials (DELIVER and EMPEROR-PRESERVED), composed of patients with either HFpEF or HFmrEF, treatment with an SGLT2 inhibitor reduced the rate of HF hospitalization [8.6 vs. 11.8%; hazard ratio (HR): 0.74, 95% confidence interval (CI): 0.67-0.83] but not the rate of all-cause death (14.1 vs. 14.3%; HR: 0.97, 95% CI: 0.88-1.06) compared with placebo. Treatment with an SGLT2 inhibitor was associated with a nonsignificant reduction in CV death (6.2 vs. 7.1%; HR: 0.88, 95% CI: 0.77-1.00). More patients treated with an SGLT2 inhibitor had either an improvement in or a lower rate of deterioration of quality of life. The rates of serious adverse events were similar between groups.

Additional therapy for patients with obesity (GLP-1 agonist): In patients with HFpEF and obesity [body mass index (BMI) ≥30 kg/m^2], therapy with a glucagon-like peptide (GLP-1) receptor agonist and lifestyle interventions alone is suggested. The dose is semaglutide .4 mg subcutaneously weekly. Therapy with a GLP-1 receptor agonist typically continues indefinitely. Semaglutide can be used in combination with an SGLT2 inhibitor.

Trials (STEP-HFpEF and STEP-HFpEF DM) suggest that therapy with a GLP-1 receptor agonist decreases the risk of hospitalization and improves quality of life when compared with placebo in both diabetic and nondiabetic patients with HFpEF and obesity.

Secondary therapies: Patients optimally treated with an SGLT2 inhibitor with or without a GLP-1 receptor agonist and who have ongoing HF symptoms may be treated with an MRA. In similar patients who cannot take an MRA, sacubitril-valsartan is another option for therapy and may be more effective in subgroups of patients with factors such as lower LVEF and recent hospitalization for HF. Since the efficacy of these agents is uncertain, we avoid use of both agents in patients with risk factors for hyperkalemia and avoid sacubitril-valsartan in patients at risk for hypotension. The dosing and evidence for these therapies include.

- *Mineralocorticoid receptor antagonists:* To initiate an MRA, the patient's serum potassium should be ≤4.7 mEq/L and eGFR must be ≥30 mL/min/1.73 m^2. To increase the MRA dose, the patient's serum potassium should be ≤4.7 mEq/L.

    For spironolactone tablets, the initial dose is 12.5 mg once daily, which is titrated as tolerated every 2 weeks to the maximum tolerated dose. The goal dose is 25–50 mg, provided there is no dose-limiting hyperkalemia, worsening kidney function, or hypotension.

    For eplerenone, the initial dose is 25 mg once daily, which is titrated in 4 weeks to 50 mg, as tolerated.

- The evidence on the efficacy of MRAs is limited to one trial that showed a small effect on reducing HF hospitalizations and no clear effect on mortality. In a trial (TOPCAT) that included 3,445 patients with symptomatic HF, an LVEF ≥45% (median 56%), who were randomly assigned to either spironolactone or placebo, hospitalization for HF was less frequent in the spironolactone group compared with the placebo group (12.0% vs. 14.2%; HR: 0.83, 95% CI: 0.69-0.99). The rates of all-cause death and all-cause hospitalizations were similar on the spironolactone and placebo groups. Compared with the control group, the spironolactone group had a higher rate of hyperkalemia (19 vs. 9%) and a higher rate of increased creatinine levels (10% vs. 7%).

In subgroup analyses focused on regional effects, the efficacy of spironolactone was greater in the Americas (primary outcome 27% vs. 32% with placebo) compared with Russia and Georgia (9% vs. 8% with placebo). In addition, compliance was higher in the Americas compared with Russia and Georgia (canrenone levels 30% vs. 3%, respectively). These differences suggest poorer adherence to the trial procedures outside of the Americas and raise questions about the veracity of the HFpEF diagnosis in this cohort as well.

Finerenone

Treatment of Heart Failure with Preserved Ejection Fraction

Recent FINEARTS-HF trial tested the nonsteroidal MRAs, namely Finerenone, in patients with heart failure and mildly reduced or preserved ejection fraction (LVEF ≥40%). Patients were randomly assigned I a 1:1 ratio to receive Finerenone (at a maximum dose of 20 or 40 mg once daily) or matching placebo, in addition to usual therapy. Over a medium follow-up of 32 months, 1,083 primary outcome events (composite of total worsening HF events and death from CV causes) occurred in 3,003 patients in finerenone group and 1,283 events in 2,998 patients in the placebo group (HR: 0.84%; 95% CI: 0.74–0.95; p = 0.007). Total number of worsening HF events was 842 in the finerenone group and 1,024 in placebo group (HR: 0.82; p = 0.006) and CV mortality was 8.1% and 8.7%, respectively (HR: 0.93). Finerenone was associated with an increased risk of hyperkalemia and a reduced risk of hypokalemia.

Thus, in patients with HFmrEF and HFpEF, finerenone resulted in a significantly lower rate of a composite of total worsening HF events and death from CV causes.

Sacubitril Valsartan

Dosing: The starting dose of sacubitril-valsartan is 24/26 mg twice daily. The dose can be increased to a maximum of 97/103 mg (twice daily, as tolerated).

The PARAGON-HF trial compared clinical outcomes with sacubitril-valsartan versus valsartan in 4,796 patients with NYHA class II–IV HF, LVEF ≥45% (median 57%), and elevated NP levels.

At a median follow-up of 35 months, there was a nonsignificant reduction in HF hospitalizations in the sacubitril-valsartan group (10 vs. 12 events per 100 patient years; rate ratio 0.85, 95% CI: 0.72–1.00), and the rate of all-cause mortality was similar between groups (14% and 15%). Patients in the sacubitril-valsartan group had a higher incidence of hypotension and angioedema and a lower incidence of hyperkalemia and adverse kidney outcomes (death from kidney failure, end-stage kidney disease, or a decrease in eGFR of ≥50% from baseline). The mean systolic blood pressure at 8 months was 4.5 mm Hg lower (95% CI: 3.6–5.4) in the sacubitril-valsartan group.

One limitation of the trial was the inclusion of patients with an LVEF <50% (25% of the sample), who do not meet the definition of HFpEF.

Other Therapies

- *ACE inhibitors:* ACE inhibitors are not used as a primary treatment for HFpEF, though many patients with HFpEF may have an indication for treatment with an ACE inhibitor (e.g., diabetes and acute myocardial infarction).
- *Angiotensin II receptor blockers (ARBs):* ARB monotherapy is not used as a primary treatment for HFpEF; sacubitril-valsartan is likely more effective than ARB monotherapy based on the results of the PARAGON-HF trial, as described above. However, ARB monotherapy is a first-line therapy for the treatment of hypertension in many patients with diabetes or CKD.
- *Beta blockers:* These are not used as a primary treatment for HFpEF, but beta-blockers may be used to treat chronic coronary syndromes to control heart rate in AF, or to treat hypertension.
- *Calcium channel blockers:* In patients with HFpEF, calcium channel blockers are generally used as a third- or fourth-line therapy for hypertension.

Device-Based Therapies

- *Implantable hemodynamic monitoring:* For highly selected patients with HFpEF, who have refractory NYHA class II–III HF symptoms and multiple hospitalizations despite traditional chronic disease management, a remote, wireless, PA pressure monitoring device is an option. The use of this device is highly individualized based on the patient's comorbidities and disease severity, as well as their values and preferences.

Trials that tested the efficacy of PA pressure monitoring show that hemodynamic monitoring may reduce HF admissions. However, these studies were not limited to patients with HFpEF and had methodologic issues.

- *Interatrial shunt device:* In patients with HFpEF, placement of an interatrial shunt device can reduce LA pressure at rest and during exercise. However, we do not routinely perform this procedure in patients with HFpEF; a trial that studied the long-term effects of this procedure did not show a benefit and suggested possible harm.

  In a trial that included 626 patients with an LVEF ≥40% and a PCWP ≥25 mm Hg during exercise, patients were randomly assigned to placement of an interatrial shunt device or to a sham procedure. After 24 months of observation, the rates of death (1% in both groups), stroke (1 vs. 0 events in the sham procedure group), worsening HF (0.28 vs. 0.25 events per patient year), and change in quality-of-life scores (KCCQ at 12 months 10 vs. 9 points) were similar between the two groups. While the risk of safety events was nonsignificantly higher in the shunt device group (38 vs. 31%), the risk of serious events (i.e., cardiac death, myocardial infarction, cardiac tamponade, or cardiac surgery) was higher in the shunt device group (4 vs. 1%).

- *Pacing:* In patients with HFpEF, trials of pacing interventions were either not effective or had positive effects and small sample size. Thus, patients with HFpEF should only undergo pacemaker implantation or pacemaker programing appropriate for any existing rhythm abnormality.

Prognosis of Heart Failure with Preserved Ejection Fraction

Morbidity: Morbidity outcomes in HFrEF and HFpEF are similar. These include the rate and frequency of hospitalization for HF, symptomatic status as measured by abnormalities in myocardial oxygen consumption, 6-minute walk distance, Minnesota Living with Heart Failure questionnaire scores, and other quality-of-life indicators. Therefore, patients with HFpEF have a morbidity burden equivalent to that in patients with HFrEF.

TABLE 26: Comparison of the advantages and disadvantages of different diagnostic tools in HFpEF.

	Pros	Cons
Natriuretic peptides (BNP, NT-proBNP)	• Very high negative predictive value • Time efficient	• Not widely available • Expansive
Invasive diagnostic tools (right heart catheterization)	• Gold standard • Useful for addressing presence of pulmonary hypertension	• Invasive • Time consuming • Expensive • Not widely available
Cardiopulmonary exercise test	• Useful for addressing different causes of dyspnea • Not invasive	• Not widely available • Hard to interpret
Echocardiography	• Widely available • Useful in phenotyping • Time efficient (ejection fraction)	• Not useful for more precise diagnostic purpose • Limited correlation with prognosis • Time consuming (GLS, 3D echo)
Lung ultrasound	• Useful for defining the congestion status and guide therapy • Time efficient	• Limited data available • Hard to interpret

Mortality: The prognosis of patients with HFpEF (i.e., symptomatic HF) is less well defined than that of patients with HFrEF. Population-based data from hospitalized patients have shown similar mortality rates in patients with HFpEF and HFrEF.

Dosing: The starting dose of sacubitril-valsartan is 24/26 mg twice daily. The dose can be increased to a maximum of 97/103 mg twice daily, as tolerated.

Lung Ultrasound

Lung ultrasound (LUS) is a straightforward and expeditious technique for evaluating pulmonary congestion among patients diagnosed with HF. It is widely accessible, particularly within acute care environments. However, in outpatient primary care settings,

> **BOX 3:** Current approaches to worsening heart failure.
> *Worsening HF:*
> - *Conceptual definition:* Severe and dynamic condition, characterized by significant clinical and hemodynamic deterioration; it is a transversal, novel, and multimodal concept, regardless of LVEF, HF etiology, and clinical presentation
> - *Clinical definition:* HF symptoms and signs exacerbation, hospitalizations, and emergency department entries due to HF, urgent outpatient visits and the need of diuretic administration and/or increase in dose, despite OMT
> - *Subclinical worsening:* Increase of myocardial stress markers (i.e., NT-proBNP and cardiac troponins), worsening of imaging, CIEDs and invasive device parameters, in absence of detectable HF symptoms and signs worsening
> - *Perspectives:* Need of more accurate WHF predictors able to better stratify patients; standardization of WHF definition (i.e., prognostic models and risk scores); improvement of management strategies to prevent worsening episodes, achieving a personalized approach

its feasibility is limited due to the constrained proficiency of general practitioners and the uneven dissemination of ultrasound equipment. LUS involves the measurement of vertical hyperechoic reverberation artifacts originating from the pleural line, extending uninterrupted to the screen's base, and exhibiting synchronous motion with lung sliding. These phenomena are categorized as "B-lines"; they are identified through scanning along the intercostal spaces, preferably utilizing a curvilinear transducer. Different epidemiological studies have demonstrated its diagnostic utility in assessing extravascular lung congestion and correctly identifying patients with HF. B-lines and pleural effusion are the diagnostic hallmarks of increased extravascular lung congestion. Compared to chest X-rays, lung ultrasound demonstrated higher sensitivity, specificity, and accuracy for identifying lung congestion in HF regardless.

Advances in Remote Monitoring Technologies for Heart Failure Management Insights from CardioMEMS and Other Emerging Devices

CardioMEMS is an innovative and safe technology that consists of an implantable device placed in the pulmonary artery of the

TABLE 27: Summary of drugs studied in WHF with trials and their main findings.

Drug	Trials and main findings
Levosimendan	• *LevoRep trial:* Intermittent levosimendan infusion did not significantly improve patients' functional capacity and quality of life • *LION-HEART trial:* Intermittent levosimendan administration was effective in decreasing the serum concentration of NT-proBNP and was associated with improvement in clinical symptoms • *LAICA study:* Repetitive levosimendan infusion is effective in reducing the HF hospitalization rate and HF worsening in patients with advanced HF • *LeoDOR trial:* Repetitive levosimendan administration in patients with a recent HF hospitalization did not result in posthospitalization clinical stability
Vericiguat	*VICTORIA trial:* The primary composite of death from cardiovascular causes or first hospitalization for HF was lower in those who received Vericiguat
Omecamtiv mecarbil	• *GALACTIC-HF trial:* The primary composite endpoint of hospitalization or urgent visit for HF and death from cardiovascular causes is reduced in patients treated with OM • *METEORIC-HF trial:* OM did not increase exercise capacity after 20 weeks of treatment • *COSMIC-HF trial:* Guiding the administration of OM through drug pharmacokinetic is associated with reduction in ventricular diameter and cardiac function improvement
Sotagliflozin	• *SOLOIST-WHF trial:* The primary endpoint, a combination of total number of cardiovascular deaths, hospitalizations, and urgent visits for HF, resulted lower, and the benefits of an early initiation of sotagliflozin, before or immediately after hospital discharge, was highlighted • *SCORED trial:* Sotagliflozin reduced the composite endpoint of HF hospitalization, urgent ambulatory visit, and cardiovascular death, along with major incidence of adverse events

TABLE 28: Summary of drugs with diuretic properties studied in WHF with trials and their main findings.

Drug	Trials and main findings
SGLT2i	• *EMPAG-HF:* In patients with acute decompensated HF, the early initiation of empagliflozin on top of standard diuretic improves urinary output • *EMPA-RESPONSE-AHF:* In acute HF patients, the use of empagliflozin is associated with reduction in WHF, death and rehospitalization, and increased urinary output • *EMPULSE trial:* Starting empagliflozin in patients admitted for AHF is associated with early and effective decongestion • *DAPA-RESPONSE-AHF:* In patients with acute HF, dapagliflozin is associated with diuresis and symptoms improvement
Acetazolamide	*ADVOR trial:* In patients with acute decompensated HF, the addition of acetazolamide on top of furosemide is associated with increased rate of decongestion
HCTZ	*CLOROTIC trial:* Patients treated with HCTZ on top of intravenous furosemide show significant weight loss and better 24-hour urinary output, but no difference in terms of dyspnea
Finerenone	• *FIDELIO-DKD:* Finerenone reduces the risk of kidney disease progression and cardiovascular events, including HF hospitalization, in patients with diabetes mellitus and chronic kidney disease • *FIGARO-DKD:* Finerenone reduces the incidence of new HF and improved HF outcomes in patients with diabetes mellitus and chronic kidney disease, regardless of HF presence • *ARTS-HF:* Finerenone determines a significant reduction in NT proBNP levels in patients with WHF and diabetes mellitus and/or chronic kidney disease

left lower lobe. It measures pulmonary artery pressure (PAP) and wirelessly transmits these data to a healthcare provider. This real-time monitoring allows prompt adjustments in medication and treatment plans, mostly concerning changes in diuretic dose, in order to prevent HF exacerbations and hospitalizations; its role in HF management was stated in the latest HF guidelines with a class IIb, level B recommendation. Patients with high PAP are more susceptible to decompensation, and different studies have explored the role of home telemonitoring (HTM) in this scenario.

When Pharmacological Therapy is not Enough: Cardiac Contractility Modulation and Baroreceptor Activation Therapy

In recent years, a new implantable device has shown promising effects in the HF setting. Cardiac contractility modulation (CCM) represents a device-based therapy suitable for a wide range of HF patients that do not meet the criteria for CRT. This device is reserved for those with LVEF between 25% and 45% who remain symptomatic (NYHA II-IV) despite optimal medical therapy (OMT) and who do

TABLE 29: Summary of invasive monitoring systems and device therapy used in WHF: for these systems, the main trials and their main findings are described.

Device	Trials and main findings
CardioMEMS	• *CHAMPION trial:* Significant reduction in HF hospital admissions in patients with daily PAP monitoring through CardioMEMS was observed • *MONITOR-HF trial:* CardioMEMS improves the QoL of HF patients with a significant increase in KCCQ-12 score • *EMBRACE-HF trial:* A prompt reduction in PAP in patients treated with empagliflozin and monitored with CardioMEMS was observed
V-LAP	*VECTOR-HF study:* A significant correlation was found between the mean LA pressure and mean PCWP
CCM	*FIX-HF-4 study and FIX-HF-5:* CCM is safe and effective in improving exercise tolerance and QoL, while reducing HF hospitalizations
BAT	*BeAT-HF study and HOPE4HF study:* BAT therapy significantly improves QoL, exercise capacity, and reduced NT-proBNP levels

(BAT: baroreflex activation therapy; CCM: cardiac contractility modulation; HF: heart failure; LA: left atrial; KCCQ-12: Kansas City cardiomyopathy questionnaire; NT-proBNP: N-terminal pro B-type natriuretic peptide; PAP: pulmonary artery pressure; PCWP: pulmonary capillary wedge pressure; QoL: quality of life)

Flowchart 9: Potential upcoming pharmacological approaches for chronic heart failure: New drugs and cardiovascular targets.

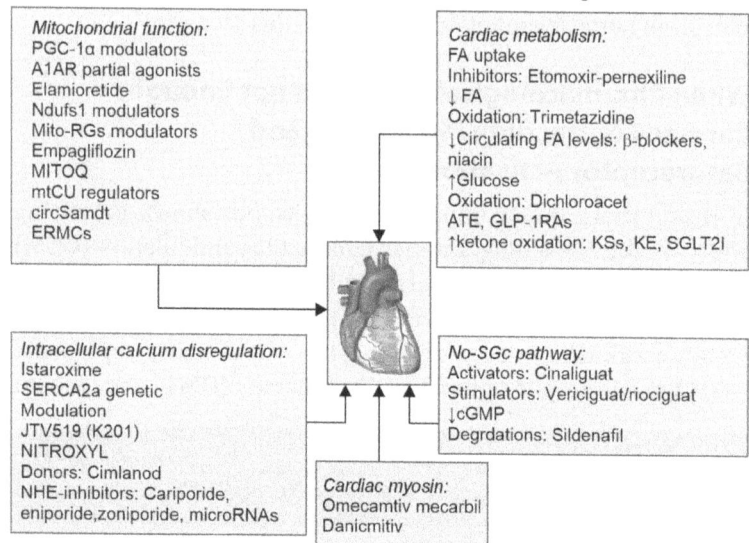

(FA: fatty acid; SGc: soluble guanylate cyclase; SGLT2i: sodium-glucose cotransporter 2 inhibitor; NHE-1: Na H$^+$ exchanger; PGC-1α: peroxisome proliferator-activated receptor γ coactivator 1α; Ndufs1 NADH: ubiquinone oxidoreductase core subunit S1; mtCU: Ca^{2+} uniporter; SERCA2: sarcoplasmic–endoplasmic reticulum Ca^{2+} ATPase 2; mPTP: mitochondrial permeability transition pore; A1AR: adenosine A1 receptor; MitoQ: mitoquinone)

not have a left bundle branch block (LBBB) morphology. The CCM device physically resembles a pacemaker, as it is constituted by a generator and two leads; the generator, containing the battery and electronic circuits, similar to any other cardiac implantable electronic device (CIED) generator, can be positioned in the left or right pectoral region, in a pocket located under the skin. Two ventricular active fixation leads complete the CCM structure: During the implantation procedure, these two leads are inserted through the subclavian vein and must be screwed into the RV septum. However, the CCM function differs from pacemakers as it generates an electrical signal specifically and exclusively during the absolute refractory period of the myocardium for 5–7 hours a day. It does not capture the myocardium in order to obtain heart contractions, because impulses are delivered during the nonexcitatory period, but acts at the intracellular level. Chronic HFrEF induces a phenotypic transition in cardiomyocytes toward a fetal pattern, with a subsequent enhanced expression of BNP and reduced levels of protein kinase A (PKA). Low levels of PKA determine low phosphorylation of phospholamban with inhibition of sarco-/endoplasmic reticulum Ca^{2+}ATPase (SERCA2a) channels. Chronic HF is also characterized by low synthesis of SERCA2A and ryanodine receptor 2 channels (RYR2). The common final effect is the reduced availability of intracellular Ca^{2+} with a resulting reduction in myocardial contractility.

Cardiac contractility modulation manages to enhance Ca^{2+} handling through the upregulation of RYR2 and SERCA2a, restoring the function of the Na^+/Ca^{2+} exchanger and normalizing the levels of phospholamban phosphorylation. These different actions enhance cellular Ca^{2+} availability and improve myocardial contractility without increasing myocardial oxygen consumption, but they do not directly influence the LVEF. Instead of pacemakers, CCM can be compared to levosimendan for its effect on the enhancement of myofilament calcium sensitivity.

Baroreflex activation therapy (BAT) consists of a device implanted to electrically stimulate the baroreceptors responsible for autonomic nervous system modulation. The device typically includes a lead or electrode that is placed near the baroreceptor region and connected to a pulse generator, which is implanted under the skin. The pulse generator delivers controlled electrical impulses to the baroreceptor area, mimicking the signals that the body's natural baroreflex would produce. The electrical stimulation of the baroreceptors leads to various physiological effects, including a reduction in sympathetic nervous system activity (which tends to increase heart rate and blood pressure) and an increase in parasympathetic activity (which tends to decrease heart rate and promote relaxation). As a result, blood pressure is lowered, and the overall CV system experiences a more balanced regulation. The Barostim Neo device has shown promising results in safely improving clinical symptoms and NYHA functional class in patients with worsening HF. The BeAT-HF study and the HOPE4HF study, for instance, have revealed that BAT therapy significantly improved QoL and exercise capacity, and reduced NT-proBNP levels.

SUGGESTED READING

1. Heindenreich PA, Bozkurt B, Aguilar D, Allen LA, Byun JJ, Colvin MM, et al. 2022 AHA/ACC/HFSA Guideline for the Management of Heart Failure: A Report of the American College of Cardiology/American Heart Association Joint Committee on Clinical Practice Guidelines. Circulation. 2022;145(18):18;e895-e1032.
2. Maddox TM, Januzzi JL, Allen LA, Breathett K, Brouse S, Butler J, et al. 2024 ACC Expert Consensus Decision Pathway for Treatment of Heart Failure with Reduced Ejection Fraction: A Report of the American College of Cardiology Solution Set Oversight Committee. J Am Coll Cardiol. 2024;83(15):1444-88.
3. McDonagh TA, Metre M, Adamo M, Gardner RS, Baumbach A, Böhm M, et al. 2021 ESC Guidelines for the diagnosis and treatment of acute and chronic heart failure: Developed by the Task Force for the diagnosis and treatment of acute and chronic heart failure of the European Society of Cardiology (ESC). With the special contribution of the Heart Failure Association (HFA) of the ESC. Eur Heart J. 2022;24(1):4-131.
4. McDonagh TA, Metra M, Adamo M, Gardner RS, Baumbach A, Böhm M, et al. 2023 Focused Update of the 2021 ESC Guidelines for the diagnosis and treatment of acute and chronic heart failure: Developed by the task force for the diagnosis and treatment of acute and chronic heart failure of the European Society of Cardiology (ESC). With the special contribution of the Heart Failure Association (HFA) of the ESC. Eur Heart J. 2024;26(1):5-17.
5. Sapna F, Raveena F, Chandio M, Bai K, Sayyar M, Varrassi G, et al. Advancements in Heart Failure Management: A Comprehensive Narrative Review of Emerging Therapies. Cureus. 2023;15(10):e46486.

5 CHAPTER

Syncope

Soumitra Kumar

DEFINITION

Syncope is one of the causes of transient loss of consciousness (TLOC). TLOC is defined as a state of real or apparent loss of consciousness (LOC) with loss of awareness, characterized by amnesia for the period of unconsciousness, abnormal motor control, loss of responsiveness, and a short duration.

Syncope is defined as TLOC due to cerebral hypoperfusion, characterized by a rapid onset, short duration, and spontaneous complete recovery.

INCIDENCE

Incidence is between 4 and 37% of general population, accounting for 3% of emergency department visits and 1% of hospital admissions.

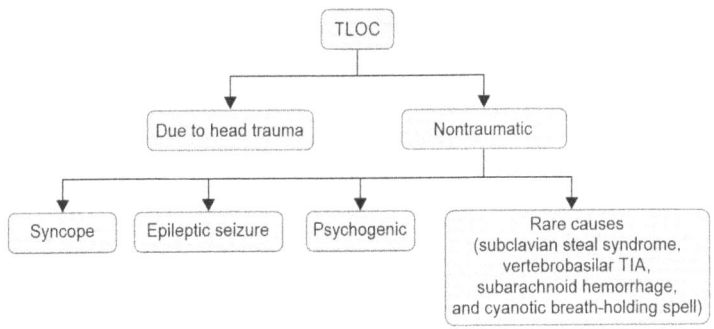

Flowchart 1: Classification of transient loss of consciousness (TLOC).

(TIA: transient ischemic attack)

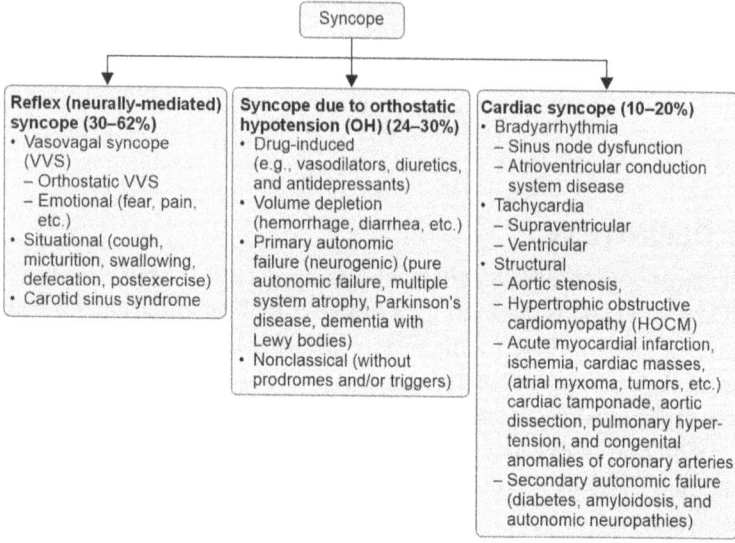

Flowchart 2: Classification of syncope.

HISTORY TAKING

Meticulous history taking concerning present and previous attacks, as well as eye-witness accounts, in person or through a telephone interview is the first and most important step in establishing syncope as a cause of TLOC and also differentiating from epileptic seizure.

ELECTROCARDIOGRAM

Beyond careful history taking and physical examination, which should include supine and standing blood pressure (BP) measurements, an electrocardiogram ECG should be the starting point of the diagnostic evaluation of TLOC. Diagnostic clues on electrocardiogram are enlisted in **Table 1**.

TABLE 1: Diagnostic clues on electrocardiogram.

Parameter	Indications
• Short PR interval – Delta wave (WPW syndrome)	Supraventricular tachycardia/AF
• Bundle branch block – Prolonged PR interval block	Advanced AV block or complete AV

Contd...

Contd...

Parameter	Indications

• Sinus bradycardia
  – Sinus pause
  – Brady–tachy syndrome
	Ventricular tachycardia

• Intraventricular conduction delay
  – Myocardial infarction/ischemia
  – LV or RV enlargement
  – Complex VPCs
  – Long QTc
  – TU abnormality
	Ventricular fibrillation

• RBBB + ST elevation in V1/V2 (Brugada syndrome)	Ventricular fibrillation
• T-wave inversion in V1-V3 sharp wide deflection (epsilon wave) following S in V1 (arrhythmogenic RV dysplasia)	Ventricular tachycardia (LBBB with left axis deviation)
• T-wave alternans	Ventricular fibrillation

(AF: atrial fibrillation; AV: atrioventricular; LV: left ventricle; LBBB: left bundle branch block; RV: right ventricle; RBBB: right bundle branch block; VPC: ventricular premature complexes; WPW: Wolf–Parkinson–White syndrome)

BOX 1: Important historical facts for syncope.

Prior to the episode:
- *Activity:* During or after exercise, during or after standing up; while in supine position; during or immediately after micturition/defecation, coughing, or swallowing
- *Prodromal signs:* Dizziness, pallor, diaphoresis, blurred vision, warmth, and light-headedness
- *Circumstances:* Prolonged standing, warm or crowded environment, postprandial, experiencing fear or pain, neck movements, instrumentation

At onset of the episode:
- *Associated symptoms:* Palpitations; chest pain; radiating pain to arms, jaw or back; ripping/tearing back pain; abdominal pain; dyspnea; pleuritic chest pain; sudden headache neck pain; paralysis; melena, diarrhea; fever; and weakness
- *Timing of symptoms:* Prolonged sudden

Contd...

Contd...

- *Witness information:*
  - *Fall/injury:* Mechanism of falling (sudden, stumping, or keeling over), losing consciousness first, and head trauma
  - *Duration of loss of consciousness:* Seconds or minutes
  - *Movements:* No movement, jerking, or tonic/clonic movements, and duration of movements
  - *Associated symptoms:* Skin color (pallor, cyanosis, and flushing) and breathing pattern (snoring)

After the episode:
- *Mental status:* Confusion and length of recovery time
- *Associated symptoms*
  - Palpitations, chest pain; radiating pain to arms, jaw, or back; ripping/tearing back pain; abdominal pain; dyspnea; pleuritic chest pain; sudden headache; and paralyses and melena
  - Diarrhea, fever, weakness, incontinence of urine or feces, and tongue bite
  - Diaphoresis, nausea, vomiting, fatigue, muscle aches, and injury

Past medical history:
- *Family history:* Sudden death, fainting, and congenital heart disease
- *Cardiovascular history:* Structural heart disease, coronary artery disease/myocardial infarction, and dysrhythmias
- *Neurological history:* Parkinsonism epilepsy
- *Metabolic disorders:* Diabetes
- *Medications (including drugs of abuse):* Prescribed, over-the-counter, and recreational
- *Previous events:* Previous syncope, associated symptoms, and diagnosis

TABLE 2: Differentiation between syncope and epileptic seizures.

Clinical features	Syncope	Epileptic seizure
Identification of trigger	Very frequent	Rare
Nature of trigger	Variable between pain, standing, emotions for vasovagal syncope or situational triggers, e.g., cough, micturition, etc.	Best known trigger is flashing light; others are rare and variable
Prodromes	• Presyncope • Light-headedness • Palpitation	Epileptic auras include déjà vu, epigastric sensation or unpleasant smell

Contd...

Contd...

Clinical features	Syncope	Epileptic seizure
Nature of myoclonus	<10, asynchronous, asymmetrical, and of irregular amplitude	20–100 synchronous, symmetrical, and hemilateral
	Starts after onset of LOC	Onset most coincides with LOC
		Long-lasting automatisms such as lip smoking or chewing
Tongue bite	Rare, tip of tongue	Side of tongue (bilateral)
Duration of unconsciousness	10–30 seconds	May be several minutes
Confusional state post-attack	No understanding of situation for <10 seconds mostly, full alertness and awareness later. Children may fall asleep after a syncope	Memory deficit, i.e., repeated questions without imprinting for many minutes. Postictal fatigue and sleep is very common
Incontinence	Not uncommon	Common

(LOC: loss of consciousness)

SYNCOPE IN THE ATHLETIC PATIENTS

Syncope in an athletic patient is a common symptom but should always raise the possibility of cardiac pathology. Although most cases of syncope in athletic patients are reflex syncope and considered benign, neurally-mediated syncope, if occurs when an athlete is in a physically dangerous circumstance (such as driving, motorsports, and road cycling), may still be life-threatening.

Syncope during exertion is often caused by underlying heart disease [such as hypertrophic cardiomyopathy (HCM), right ventricular outflow tract tachycardia, ion channel defects, arrhythmogenic right ventricular cardiomyopathy, coronary anomalies, etc.] and may be a harbinger of sudden cardiac death.

Syncope in an athlete requires a thorough evaluation including a detailed and focused history and physical examination with the addition of case-dependent diagnostic tests. Ultimately, the purpose of this evaluation is to distinguish between life-threatening and non-life-threatening causes of syncope.

TABLE 3: Risk stratification of syncope.

Parameter	High-risk	Low-risk
Clinical history	New onset of chest discomfort, breathlessness, abdominal pain, or headache	Associated with prodrome typical of reflex syncope (e.g., light-headedness feeling of warmth, sweating, nausea, vomiting, etc.)
	Syncope during exertion or when supine	After sudden unpleasant sensory signal or in crowded, hot place
	Sudden onset palpitation immediately followed by syncope	During meal or postprandial
	High risk (only if associated with structural heart disease or ECG)	Triggered by cough, defecation or abnormal micturition
	No warning symptoms or short (<10 seconds) prodrome	With head rotation or pressure on carotid sinus
	Family history of SCD at young age	Standing from supine/sitting position
	Syncope in the sitting position	
Past history Features	Severe structural or coronary artery disease (heart failure, low LVEF or previous myocardial infarction)	Long history (years) of recurrent syncope
		Absence of structural heart disease
Physical examination	• Unexplained systolic BP on presentation <90 mm Hg • Suggestion of gastrointestinal bleeding • Persistent low heart rate <40 beats/min in awake state • Nonspecified systolic murmur	Normal examination

Contd...

Contd...

Parameter	High-risk	Low-risk
ECG	• ECG changes suggestive of acute ischemia • Advanced AV block (Mobitz type II AV block or third-degree AV block) • Slow AF (<40 bpm) • Persistent sinus bradycardia (<40 bpm) or SA block or sinus pauses >3 seconds in awake state and in absence of physical training • Bundle branch block, intraventricular conduction disturbance, pathological Q-waves, LV hypertrophy • Sustained or nonsustained VT • Type 1 Brugada pattern • QTc >460 ms in repeated 12-lead	Normal ECG • High risk only if history is consistent with arrhythmic syncope • Mobitz type 1 AV block • First degree AV block with markedly prolonged PR-interval • Asymptomatic mild sinus bradycardia (40–50 bpm) • Paroxysmal SVT or AF • Pre-excited QRS complex • Atypical Brugada pattern • Short QTc interval (≤340 ms) • Negative T-waves in right precordial leads epsilon-waves suggestive of ARVC

(AF: atrial fibrillation; AV: atrioventricular; ARVC: arrhythmogenic right ventricular cardiomyopathy; BP: blood pressure; ECG: electrocardiogram; LV: left ventricle; LVEF: left ventricular ejection fraction; SA: sinoatrial; SCD: sudden cardiac death; SVT: supraventricular tachycardia; VT: ventricular tachycardia)

Flowchart 3: Course of action in emergency department (ED) following risk-stratification of syncope.

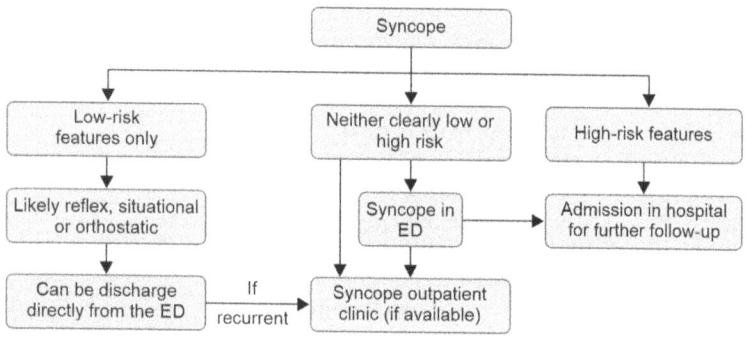

DIAGNOSTIC TESTS

Active Standing

- Intermittent determination by sphygmomanometer of BP and heart rate (HR) while supine and during active standing for 3 minutes at initial syncope evaluation (Recommendation: IC)
- Continuous beat-to-beat BP and HR measurement may be preferred when short-lived BP variations are suspected, such as initial orthostatic hypotension (OH) (Recommendation: IIb).

Diagnostic Criteria

- Syncope due to OH is confirmed when there is a fall in systolic BP from baseline value ≥20 mm Hg or diastolic BP ≥10 mm Hg or a decrease in systolic BP <90 mm Hg that reproduces spontaneous symptoms and OH is considered likely when with same BP findings, symptoms (from history) are wholly or partially consistent with OH.
- Postural orthostatic tachycardia syndrome (POTS) should be considered likely when there is an orthostatic HR increase (>30 bpm or >120 bpm within 10 minutes of active standing) in the absence of OH that reproduces spontaneous symptoms.

Basic Autonomic Function Tests

- *Valsalva maneuver* should be considered for the assessment of autonomic function in patients with suspected neurogenic OH

(Recommendation: IIaB). Absence of a BP overshoot and an absence of an HR increase during Valsalva is pathognomonic for neurogenic OH. Degree of hypotension and/or lack of compensation during forced expiration usually correlates with degree of autonomic dysfunction (primary or secondary). In contrast, a pronounced BP fall beyond that is normally expected during forced expiration with preserved chronotropic response and is suggestive of suspected situational syncope.

- **Deep breathing tests** should be considered for assessment of autonomic function in patients with suspected neurogenic OH (Recommendation: IIaB). HR variability during deep breathing (or expiratory/inspiratory index) ≥15 bpm is normal in healthy individuals aged >50 years. Blunted or absent variation is indicative of parasympathetic dysfunction.
- *Ambulatory blood pressure monitoring (ABPM)* is recommended in suspected autonomic failure to detect nocturnal hypertension (Recommendation: IB) and degree of OH and supine hypertension in daily life (Recommendation: IIaC).

Flowchart 4: Approach to a patient with suspected autonomic failure.

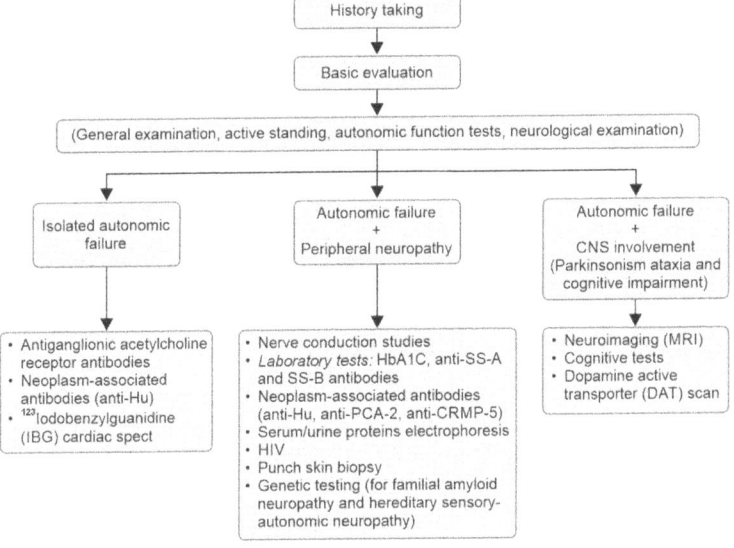

(CNS: central nervous system; HIV: human immunodeficiency virus; HbA1C: glycated hemoglobin; MRI: magnetic resonance imaging)

Carotid Sinus Massage

Carotid sinus massage (CSM) is indicated in patients >40 years of age with syncope of unknown origin compatible with a reflex syncope (Recommendation: IB).

Diagnostic Criteria

Carotid sinus syndrome (CSS) is confirmed if there is a ventricular pause lasting >3 seconds and/or a fall in systolic BP of >50 mm Hg with reproduction of spontaneous symptoms and if patients have clinical features compatible with a reflex mechanism of syncope. Main complications of CSM are transient ischemic attacks (TIAs) or strokes (0.24%). Response to CSM can be cardioinhibitor (ventricular pause ≥3.0 seconds), vasodepressive [Fall in systolic blood pressure (SBP) ≥50 mm Hg], or mixed.

Tilt Testing

Tilt testing is useful for reproduction of delayed OH or POTS, which could not be detected by active standing because of its delayed onset. Tilt testing may be helpful in separating syncope from psychogenic pseudosyncope (PPS).

Tilt-table Test

Tilt-table test is a valuable diagnostic test in the evaluation of cause of syncope with positive response suggesting susceptibility to neurally-mediated syncope.

TABLE 4: Summary of Newcastle protocols for head-up tilt-table testing.

Tilt-test description	Method
Passive drug-free tilt	40 minutes at 70°
Isoproterenol (µg) tilt	5 minutes tilt, 5 minutes supine; 6 minutes 1 µg/min supine; 5 minutes 1 µg/min at 70° infusion; discontinued, supine; 2 minutes, 5 minutes 3 µg/min Supine; 5 minutes 3 µg/min at 70°
GTN tilt	2 metered doses sublingual GTN spray supine 5 minutes then 20 minutes at 70°
(GTN: glyceryl trinitrate)	

Syncope

Patients should remain supine for 20 minutes before testing. Isoprotereno and glyceryl trinitrate (GTN) tilts should follow nondiagnostic passive drug-free tilt where history is suggestive of vasovagal syncope. Tilt should be terminated if symptom reproduction with concomitant hypotension/bradycardia or adverse event develops.

- Indications:
  - If a neurocardiogenic cause is suspected
  - Recurrent syncope with cause being not found in patients of any age group
  - Treating other potential causes is ineffective.
- Response to TTT in different situations:
  - Neurocardiogenic: Sudden hypotension with/without bradycardia
  - Dysautonomic: Gradual parallel decline in systolic and diastolic blood pressure
  - Psychogenic: No change in HR, BP, EEG, and transcranial blood flow
  - POTS: An excessive HR response to maintain a low normal

Electrocardiographic Monitoring

The ECG monitoring is indicated only when there is a high pretest probability of detecting an arrhythmia based on clues seen as a resting 12-lead ECG. Various modalities of ECG monitoring are:

- Immediate in-hospital monitoring (in bed or telemetry) is indicated in high-risk patients (Recommendation: IC).
- Holter monitoring should be considered in patients suffering from frequent syncope or presyncope (≥1 episode per week).
- External loop recorders should be considered early after the index event, in patients who have ≤4 weeks of interval between events (Recommendation: IIaB).
- Remote (at home) telemetry has been developed recently. External implantable device systems have been developed that provide continuous ECG recording or 24-hour loop memory with real-time wireless transmission to a service center. This modality is said to increase diagnostic yield.

- Implantable loop recorders (ILRs) are indicated early in patients with recurrent syncope of undetermined origin, even in absence of high-risk criteria (Recommendations: IA).

  Implantable loop recorders are also indicated in patients with high-risk criteria after comprehensive evaluation fails to identify a specific cause of syncope (Recommendation: IA).

  Implantable loop recorders should be considered with suspected or certain reflex syncope but with frequent or severe syncopal episodes (Recommendation: IIaB).

Echocardiography

Echocardiography is indicated both for diagnosis and risk stratification in patients with suspected structural heart disease (Recommendation: IB).

Exercise echocardiography (2D and Doppler) is indicated in standing, sitting, or semisupine position to detect provocable left ventricular outflow tract (LVOT) obstruction in patients with HCM, history of syncope, and resting or provoked peak instantaneous LVOT gradient <50 mm Hg (Recommendation: IB).

Exercise Testing

Exercise testing is indicated in patients who have experienced syncope during or shortly after exertion (Recommendation: IC). Advanced atrioventricular (AV)-block or ventricular tachyarrhythmia (VT) immediately after exercise may establish the cause.

Coronary Angiography

Same indications should be followed as in patients without syncope since angiography alone is not diagnostic of the cause of syncope.

Electrophysiologic Study

- Electrophysiologic study (EPS) is indicated with syncope and previous myocardial infarction or other scar-related conditions. EPS is indicated when syncope remains unexplained after noninvasive evaluation (Recommendation: IB). Induction of sustained monomorphic VT is diagnostic (Recommendation: IB).

- EPS is indicated in syncope and bifascicular bundle branch block (BBB) when syncope remains unexplained after noninvasive evaluation (Recommendation: IIaB). In this situation, there is a presence of either a baseline H-V interval of ≥70 ms or induction of second or third-degree His-Purkinje block during incremental atrial pacing or with pharmacological stress (ajmaline, procainamide, or disopyramide) (Recommendation: IB).
- EPS may be considered in patients with syncope and asymptomatic sinus bradycardia in selected instances when noninvasive tests (e.g., ECG monitoring) fail to show a definite correlation between syncope and bradycardia (Recommendation: IIbB). Prognostic value of a prolonged sinus node recovery time (SNRT) is not well-specified. An abnormal response is defined as ≥1.6 or 2 seconds for SNRT or ≥525 ms for corrected SNRT.

Adenosine Triphosphate Test

Low predictive value of the test does not support its routine use in patients for cardiac pacing but rather its positivity suggests that it can be used to confirm suspicion of asystolic syncope by means of prolonged ECG monitoring.

TREATMENT OF SYNCOPE

Three general principles should be considered:
1. Bradycardia is a frequent mechanism of syncope. Cardiac pacing is the most powerful therapy for bradycardia but its utility is less if hypotension is a concomitant problem.
2. Management of patients at high risk of sudden cardiac death (SCD) requires careful assessment of the individual patient's risk.
3. Syncopal recurrences often reduce spontaneously after medical assessment even if specific therapy has not been instituted. The reason for this decrease is not known. In general, syncope recurs in <50% of patients within 1–2 years.

Treatment of syncope due to tachyarrhythmias:
- Catheter ablation is indicated in patients with syncope due to supraventricular tachycardia (SVT) or ventricular tachycardia (VT) in order to prevent syncope recurrence (Recommendation: IB).

Flowchart 5: Practical decision pathway for reflex syncope.

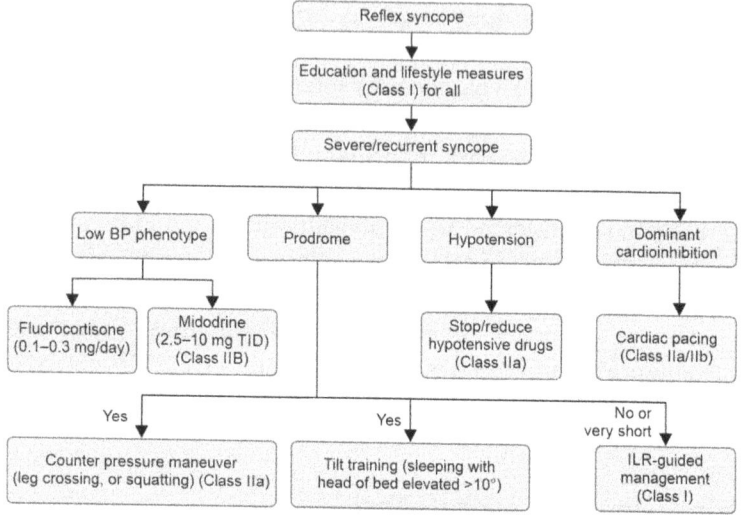

(BP: blood pressure; ILR: implantable loop recorder)

Flowchart 6: Decision pathway for pacing in reflex syncope.

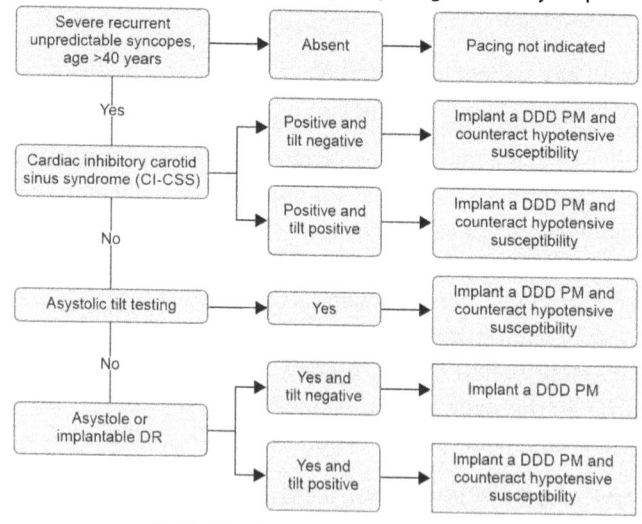

(DDD-PM: dual chamber pacemaker)

Flowchart 7: Syncope due to orthostatic hypotension.

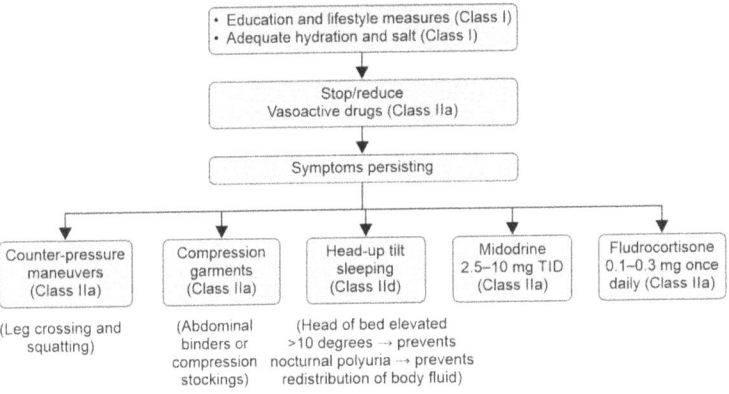

Flowchart 8: Approach to syncope due to intrinsic cardiac sinus node dysfunction (SND) or atrioventricular (AV) block.

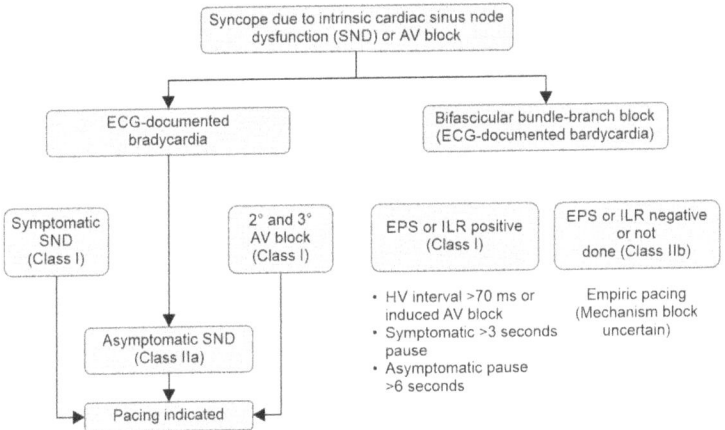

(ECG: electrocardiography; EPS: electrophysiologic study; ILR: implantable loop recorder)

- An implantable cardioverter defibrillator (ICD) is indicated in patients with syncope due to VT and an ejection fraction ≤35% (Recommendation: IA).
- An ICD is indicated in patients with syncope and previous myocardial infarction who have VT induced during EPS (Recommendation: IC)

Flowchart 9: Approach to a patient with sinus node dysfunction.

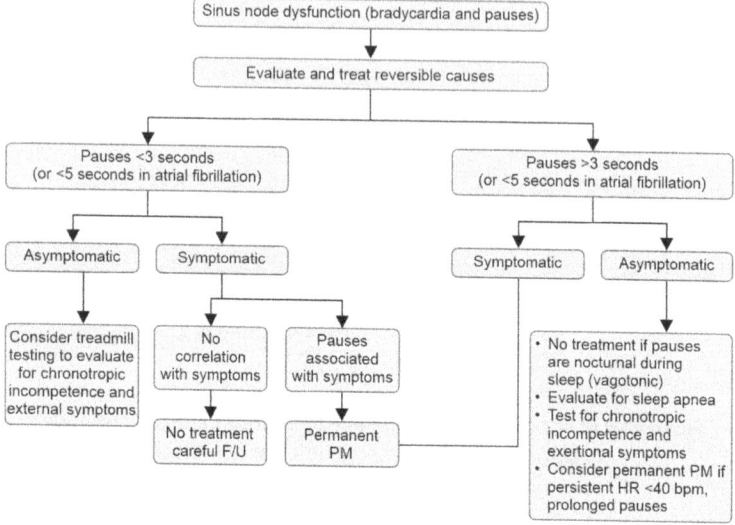

(HR: heart rate; PM: pacemaker)

Flowchart 10: Approach to a patient with 2:1 atrioventricular (AV) block.

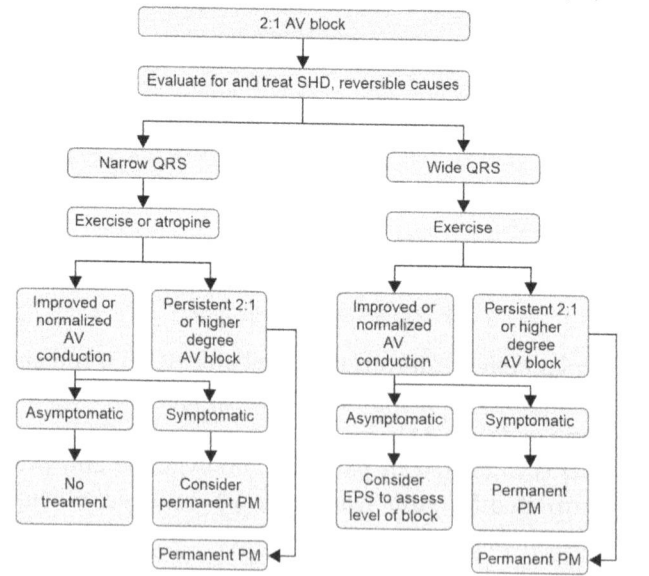

(EPS: electrophysiology study; PM: pacemaker; SHD: structural heart disease)

Syncope

Flowchart 11: Approach to bifascicular bundle branch block and unexplained syncope.

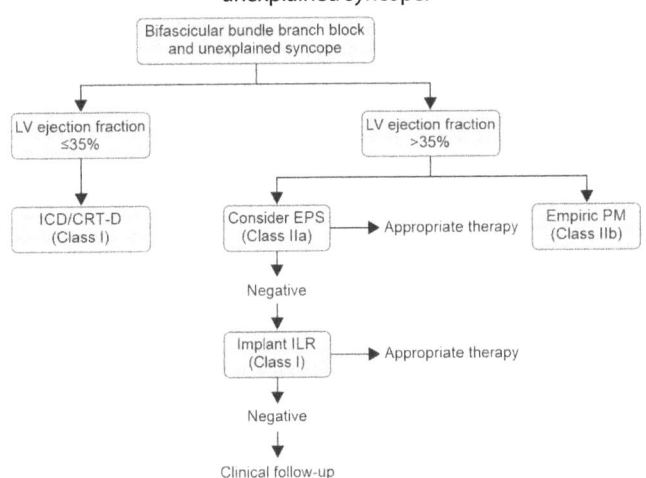

(LV: left ventricle; CRT-D: cardiac resynchronization therapy with a defibrillator; EPS: electrophysiology study; ICD: implantable cardioverter defibrillator; ILR: implantable loop recorder)

Flowchart 12: Approach to cardiac tachyarrhythmia syncope.

(ICD: implantable cardioverter defibrillator; SVT: supraventricular tachycardia; VT: ventricular tachycardia)

- An ICD should be considered in patients with an ejection fraction >35% with recurrent syncope due to VT when catheter ablation and pharmacologic therapy have failed or could not be performed (Recommendation: IIaC).
- Antiarrhythmic drug therapy, including rate-control drugs, should be considered in patients with syncope due to SVT or VT (Recommendation: IIaC).

Treatment of unexplained syncope in patients at high risk of sudden cardiac death:
- ICD therapy is recommended to reduce SCD in patients with symptomatic heart failure (NYHA Class II–III) and left ventricular ejection fraction (LVEF) ≤35% after ≥3 months of optimal medical therapy, who are expected to survive ≥1 year with good functional status (Recommendation: IA).
- In patients with hypertrophic cardiomyopathy and unexplained syncope, ICD implantation is recommended if decisions are made according to European Society of Cardiology (ESC) Risk-SCD score (Recommendation: IB).
- ICD implantation may be considered in patients with arrhythmogenic right ventricular cardiomyopathy (ARVC) and a history of unexplained syncope (Recommendation: IIb,c).
- ICD implantation in addition to beta-blockers should be considered in long QT syndrome patients who experience unexplained syncope while receiving an adequate dose of beta-blockers (Recommendation: IIaB).
- ICD implantation should be considered in patients with a spontaneous diagnostic Brugada type-1 ECG pattern and a history of unexplained syncope (Recommendation: IIaC).

SUGGESTED READING

1. Benditt DG, Can I. Initial evaluation of "syncope and collapse" the need for a risk stratification consensus. J Am Coll Cardiol. 2010;55(8):722-4.
2. Brignole M, Moya A, de Lange PJ, Deharo JC, Elliott PM, Fanciulli A, et al. ESC Scientific Document Group. 2018 ESC guidelines for the diagnosis and management of syncope. Eur Heart J. 2018;39(21):1883-948.
3. Marrison VK, Fletcher A, Parry SW. The older patients with syncope: practicalities and controversies. Int J Cardiol. 2012;155(1):9-13.
4. Patel PR, Quinn JV. Syncope: a review of emergency department management and disposition. Clin Exp Emerg Med. 2015;2(2):67-74.
5. Priori SS, Biomström-Lundgvist C, Mazzanti A, Blom N, Borggrefe M, Camm J, et al.; ESC Scientific Document Group. 2015 ESC Guidelines for the management of patients with ventricular arrhythmias and prevention of sudden cardiac death: The Task Force for the Management of Patients with Ventricular Arrhythmias and the Prevention of Sudden Cardiac Death of the European Society of Cardiology (ESC). Endorsed by Association for European Paediatric and Congenital Cardiology (AEPC). Eur Heart J. 2015;36(41):2793-867.

6
CHAPTER

Atrial Fibrillation

Soumitra Kumar

Atrial fibrillation (AF) is the most common clinically significant cardiac arrhythmia affecting 1–2% of the general population increasing with age.

DEFINITION

Atrial fibrillation is defined as cardiac arrhythmia with the following characteristics:
- Irregular R-R interval
- No distinct P wave
- Atrial cycle length (if visible) is variable and <200 ms (>300 bpm)

TABLE 1: Definitions.

Term	Definition
Atrial fibrillation (AF)	It is a supraventricular tachyarrhythmia with uncoordinated atrial activation and ineffective atrial contraction. *Electrocardiographic characteristics include:* (1) irregular R-R intervals (when atrioventricular conduction is present, (2) absence of distinct P waves, and (3) irregular atrial activity also known as fibrillatory waves. AF can be documented by, for example, 12-lead ECG, rhythm strips, wearables, and intracardiac electrocardiac electrograms, but will always require visual confirmation that the diagnosis is accurate
Clinical AF	With the increasing availability of wearable devices and other continuous monitoring technologies, the distinction between clinical and subclinical AF has become increasingly blurred, thus the writing committee felt the term clinical AF has become less useful. Yet the term was kept because most of the evidence from randomized trials that have led to guideline recommendations for the treatment of AF is referred to as "Clinical AF". These trials required electrocardiographic documentation of the arrhythmia for inclusion and most patients presented for clinical evaluation and/or therapy of the arrhythmia

Contd...

Contd...

Term	Definition
Subclinical AF	Subclinical AF refers to this arrhythmia identified in individuals who do not have symptoms attributable to AF and in whom there are no previous ECGs documenting AF
	This includes AF identified by implanted devices (pacemakers, defibrillators, or implantable loop recorders) or wearable monitors
Atrial high-rate episodes	These are defined as atrial events exceeding the programmed defection rate that is set by the device.
	These are recorded by implanted devices but require visual inspection to confirm AF and exclude other atrial arrhythmias, artifacts, or oversensing
AF burden	AF burden encompasses both frequency and duration and refers to the amount of AF that an individual has. AF burden has been defined differently across studies. For the purpose of the guideline, AF burden will be defined as the durations of an episode or as a percentage of AF burden during the monitoring period depending on how it was defined in the individual studies.
First detected AF	The first documentation of AF, regardless of previous symptoms AF
Paroxysmal AF	AF that is intermittent and terminates within ≤7 days of onset.
Persistent AF	AF that is continuous and sustains for >7 days and requires intervention. Of note, patients with persistent AF who, with therapy, become paroxysmal should still be defined as persistent as this reflects their original pattern and is more useful to predict outcomes and define substrate
Long-standing persistent AF	AF that is continuous for >12 months in duration
Permanent AF	A term that is used when the patient and clinician make a joint decision to stop further attempts to restore and/or maintain sinus rhythm. Acceptance of AF represents a therapeutic decision and does not represent an inherent pathophysiological attribute of AF

Contd...

Contd...

Term	Definition
No longer used	
Chronic AF	This historical term has had variable definitions and should be abandoned. It has been replaced by the "persistent", "long-standing persistent", and "permanent" terminology
Valvular and nonvalvular AF	The distinction between "valvular: and "nonvalvular AF" remains a matter of debate. Their definitions may be confusing. Recent trials comparing vitamin K antagonists with nonvitamin K antagonist oral anticoagulants in AF were performed among patients with so-called "nonvalvular" AF. These trials have all allowed native valvular heart disease other than mitral stenosis (mostly moderate and severe) and prosthetic heart valves to be included. We should no longer consider the classification of AF as "valvular" or "nonvalvular" for the purpose of defining the etiology of AF since the term was specific to eligibility of stroke risks reduction therapies. Valvular and nonvalvular terminology should be abandoned
Lone AF	This term has been used in the past to identify AF in younger patients without structural heart disease who are at a lower risk for thromboembolism. This term does not enhance patient care, is not currently used, and should be abandoned

Among nonanticoagulated patients, stroke risk was lower with paroxysmal than nonparoxysmal AF, and a greater total AF burden (but not the longest AF episode) was independently associated with higher thromboembolic event rates. Clinical AF burden may influence the response to rhythm control therapy. The presence of >6 hours of AF per week (especially when progressing to >24 hours weekly) was associated with increased mortality, especially in women.

Systems used for AF screening:
- Patient (or medical professional) initiated oscillometric blood pressure cuff
- Pulse palpitation auscultation

- Patient (or medical professional) initiated intermittent electrocardiogram (ECG) rhythm strip using smartphone or dedicated connectable device
- Semicontinuous photoplethysmogram on a smartwatch or wearable
- Patient initiated photoplethysmogram on smartphone
- Intermittent smartwatch ECG initiated by semicontinuous photoplethysmogram with prompt notification of irregular rhythm or symptoms
- Wearable belts for continuous recordings
- Stroke with hospital telemetry monitoring
- Long-term Holter
- 1–2-week continuous ECG patches
- Implantable cardiac monitors

ATRIAL FIBRILLATION SCREENING

Risks:
- Abnormal results may cause anxiety.
- ECG misinterpretation results may lead to over-diagnosis and overtreatment.
- ECG may detect other abnormalities (true or false positive) that may lead to invasive tests and treatment that have the potential for serious harm (e.g., angiography/revascularization with bleeding, contrast-induced nephropathy, and allergic reactions to the contrast)

Benefits:
- Prevention of:
  - Stroke/SE using OAC patients at risk
  - Subsequent onset of symptoms
- *Prevention/reversal of:*
  - Electrical/mechanical atrial remodeling
  - AF-related hemodynamic derangements
  - Atrial and ventricular tachycardia-induced cardiomyopathy
- *Prevention/reduction of:*
  - *AF-related mortality:* hospitalization, mortality

TABLE 2: EHRA symptom scale of AF.

Score	Symptoms	Description
1	None	AF does not cause any symptoms
2a	Mild	Normal daily activity not affected by symptoms related to AF
2b	Moderate	Normal daily activity not affected by symptoms to AF, but patient troubled by symptoms
3	Severe	Normal daily activity affected by symptoms related to AF
4	Disabling	Normal daily activity discontinued

(AF: atrial fibrillation; EHRA: European Heart Rhythm Association)

- *Reduction of:*
  - The outcomes associated with conditions/diseases associated with AF that are discovered and treated as a consequence of the examinations prompted by AF detection

Imaging in Atrial Fibrillation

Noninvasive multimodality imaging can provide all needed information.

In selected patients, transesophageal echocardiography (TOE) can be used to evaluate valvular heart disease (VHD) or left atrial appendage (LAA) thrombus; CT coronary angiography can be performed for assessment of CAD; CT/MRI of the brain can be performed when stroke is suspected. Specific predictors of stroke have been suggested such as LA dilation, spontaneous LA contrast, reduced LA strain, LAA thrombus, low peak LAA velocity (<20 cm/s), and LAA nonchicken wing configuration (on CT).

Anatomical imaging provides the LA size, shape, and fibrosis. Most accurate assessment of LA dilation is obtained by CMR or CT. For routine assessment, two-dimensional (2D) or (preferably) three-dimensional (3D) transthoracic echocardiography is used. The 3D echocardiographic normal volume values are 15–42 mL/m^2 for men and 15–39 mL/m^2 for women. Assessment of LA fibrosis with LGE-CMR has been described but only rarely applied in clinical practice. Functional imaging includes TDI and strain. TDI measures the velocities of the myocardium in diastole and systole, whereas LA strain reflects active LA contraction. The PA-TDI interval reflects the atrial electromechanical delay [total LA conduction time, the time interval between the P-wave on the ECG, and the A' (atrial peak velocity) on TDI] and reflects LA strain. LA wall infiltration by epicardial fat is a potential early marker of inflammation and can be detected with CT or cardiac MRI. Before AF ablation, the pulmonary vein anatomy can be visualized with CT or CMR.

INITIAL ACUTE CARE OF ATRIAL FIBRILLATION AND ATRIAL FLUTTER

Initial acute care of AF and atrial flutter (AFL) depends on hemodynamic stability.

Unstable AF/AFL:
- Begin resuscitation and consider other conditions contributing to instability (ID).
- If instability is due to AF/AFL, immediate direct current cardioversion (DCCV) is recommended (IB).

Stable AF/AFL:
- *For ED patients:* Screen for early cardioversion in the emergency department (IIA)
- Special management considerations for patients with comorbid cardiac disease, including heart failure with reduced ejection fraction (HFrEF), are discussed later in the chapter.
- Prescribe medications to control heart rate (HR), as summarized later in the chapter.
- If the patient's HR or symptoms are not controlled with rate control medications, consider a rhythm control strategy (IB)
  - In some cases, if a rhythm control strategy is appropriate/desired, EP consultation may be helpful
  - DCCV may be required, as discussed later in the chapter.
- Consider anticoagulation based on CHA_2DS_2-VASc score, as shown in details in following sections. Discharge planning and follow-up should be last step.

TABLE 3: Three validated risk models for stroke.

Risk factor	CHA$_2$DS$_2$-VASc	ATRIA	GARFIELD
Age ≥85 years		6	0.98
Age ≥75 years	2	5	0.59
Age 65–74 years	1	3	0.20
Female sex	1	1	
Hypertension	1	1	0.16
Renal disease		1	0.35
Diabetes	1	1	0.21
Current smoking			0.48
Congestive heart failure	1	1	0.23
Previous stroke or TIA	2	2–8*	0.80
Vascular disease	1		0.20
Dementia			0.51
Previous bleeding			0.30
Proteinuria		1	
Low-risk score	0	0–5	0–0.89
Intermediate-risk score	1	6	0.90–1.59
High-risk score	≥2	7–15	≥1.60
C-index (11)	0.63	0.66	—
C-index (13)	0.67	—	0.71

*8 points if age <65 years, 4 points if age 65–74 years, 2 points if age 75–84 years, and 3 points if ≥85 years.

ATRIA indicates anticoagulation and risk factors in atrial fibrillation; anemia, renal disease, elderly (age ≥75 years) any previous bleeding, hypertension; CHA$_2$DS$_2$-VASc, indicates congestive heart failure, hypertension, age ≥75 years (doubled), diabetes mellitus, prior stroke or transient ischemic attack or thromboembolism (doubled), vascular disease, age 65 to 74 years, sex category; GARFIELD-AF: Global Anticoagulant Registry in the Field-Atrial Fibrillation; and TIA: transient ischemic attack.

TABLE 4: Some best-known published clinical scores with potential advantages.

Year of publication, source name	Source components	Potential advantages
2001 CHADS$_2$	CHF, hypertension, age (≥65 years is 1 point, ≥75 years is 2 points), diabetes, stroke/TIA (2 points)	CHADS$_2$ was superior to existing risk classification schemes *AFI scheme:* C-statistic, 0.68 (0.65–0.71) *SPAF-III scheme:* C-statistic, 0.74 (0.71–0 76) *CHADS$_2$ score:* C-statistic, 0.82 (0.80–084)
2010 CHA$_2$DS$_2$-VASc$_2$	CHF. hypertension, age ≥75 years, diabetes, stroke or TIA, vascular disease, age 65-74 y, female sex	Most commonly used and studied, superior to CHADS$_2$ score. C-statistic, 0.606 (0.513–0.699) for CHA$_2$DS$_2$-VASc score vs. 0.561 (0.450–0.672) for CHADS$_2$ score Improved compared with original CHADS$_2$ score
2013 ATRIA	Age (65–74 years is 3 points, 75–84 years is 5 points, ≥85 years is 6 points), hypertension, diabetes, CHF, proteinuria, GFR <45 mL/min/1.73 m^2, sex	Includes more age categories, renal function, and proteinuria More patients were classified as low or high risk but not as well tested in general
2017 GARFIELD- AF	Web-based, uses routinely collected clinical data, and includes a total of 16 questions	Web-based tool for predicting stroke and mortality includes the effect of the different anticoagulants, bleeding risk, and mortality to facilitate shared decision-making on the potential benefits/risks of anticoagulation

Contd...

Atrial Fibrillation

Contd...

Year of publication, source name	Source components	Potential advantages
2016 MCHA$_2$DS$_2$-VASc	Expanded lower threshold for age to 50 years (1 point for age 50–74 years)	Validated in Asian cohort. Can further identify Asian AF patients who may derive benefits from stroke prevention. In 1 study, MCHA$_2$DS$_2$-VASc was superior to CHA$_2$DS$_2$-VASc; C-statistics = 0.708 (0.703–0.712) vs. 0.689 (0.684–0.694)

Notes:
- ATRIA indicates Anticoagulation and Risk Factors in Atrial Fibrillation: anemia, renal disease, elderly (age ≥75 y), any previous bleeding, hypertension; CHADS$_2$, congestive heart failure, hypertension, age >75 y, diabetes, stroke/transient ischemia attack/thromboembolism,
- CHA$_2$DS$_2$-VASc indicates congestive heart failure, hypertension, age ≥75 y (doubled), diabetes mellitus, prior stroke or transient ischemic attack or thromboembolism (doubled), vascular disease, age 65–74 y, sex category; CHF, congestive heart failure
- GARFIELD-AF indicates Global Anticoagulant Registry in the Field-Atrial Fibrillation

(GFR: glomerular filtration rate; SPAF: stroke prevention atrial fibrillation; TIA: transient ischemic attack)

Additional risk factors that increase risk of stroke not included in CHA$_2$DS$_2$-VASc:

- Higher AF burden/long duration
- Persistent/permanent AF versus paroxysmal
- Obesity [body mass index (BMI) ≥30 kg/m^2]
- Hypertrophic cardiomyopathy (HCM)
- Poorly controlled hypertension
- Estimated glomerular filtration rate (eGFR) (<45 mL/h)
- Proteinuria (>150 mg/24 h or equivalent)
- Enlarged left atrium (LA) volume (≥73 mL) or diameter (≥4.7 cm)

Atrial Flutter (AFL) and Macroreentrant AT: They occur in many of the same situations as AF. Typical AFL, also known as "cavortricuspid isthmus (CTI)-dependent AFL," involves a macroreentrant circuit around the tricuspid annulus traversing the CTI on the right side of the heart. This is the arrhythmia associated with the classic ECG finding of sawtooth flutter waves in the inferior leads when the circuit goes in the counterclockwise direction. The same circuit in the clockwise direction is called "reverse typical AFL". If the flutter involves a different circuit than tricuspid valve/isthmus, then it is called "atypical" AFL, which is also known as "noncavotricuspid isthmus-dependent macroreentrant atrial flutter was previously

TABLE 5: Clinical risk factors in the HAS-BLED score.

	Risk factors and definitions	Points awarded
H	Uncontrolled hypertension SBP > 160 mm Hg	1
A	Abnormal renal and/or hepatic function Dialysis, transplant, serum creatinine >200 μmol/L, cirrhosis, bilirubin > 2 × upper limit of normal, AST/ALT/ALP >3 × upper limit of normal	1 point for each
S	Stroke Previous ischemic or hemorrhagic[a] stroke	1
B	Bleeding history or predisposition Previous major hemorrhage or anemia or severe thrombocytopenia	1
L	Labile INR[b] TTR < 60% in patient receiving VKA	1
E	Elderly Aged > 65 years or extreme frailty	1
D	Drugs or excessive alcohol drinking Concomitant use of antiplatelet or NSAID and/or excessive[c] alcohol per week	1 point for each
	Maximum score	

[a]Hemorrhagic stroke would also score 1 point under the "B" criterion.
[b]Only relevant if patient is receiving a VKA.
[c]Alcohol excess or abuse refers to a high intake (e.g., >14 units per week), where the clinician assesses there would be an impact on health or bleeding risk.
(ALP: alkaline phosphatase; ALT: alanine aminotransferase; AST: aspartate aminotransferase; INR: international normalized ratio; NSAID: nonsteroidal anti-inflammatory drug; SBP: systolic blood pressure; TTR: time in therapeutic range; VKA: vitamin K antagonist)

classified as either type I or type II. That terminology is no longer used.

Direct Oral Anticoagulants Laboratory Monitoring

- *Hb/Hematocrit:* HAS-BLED ≥ 3—every 3 months
  HAS-BLED 0-2—every <3 months

Flowchart 1: Approach to patient with atrial fibrillation eligible for oral anticoagulation.

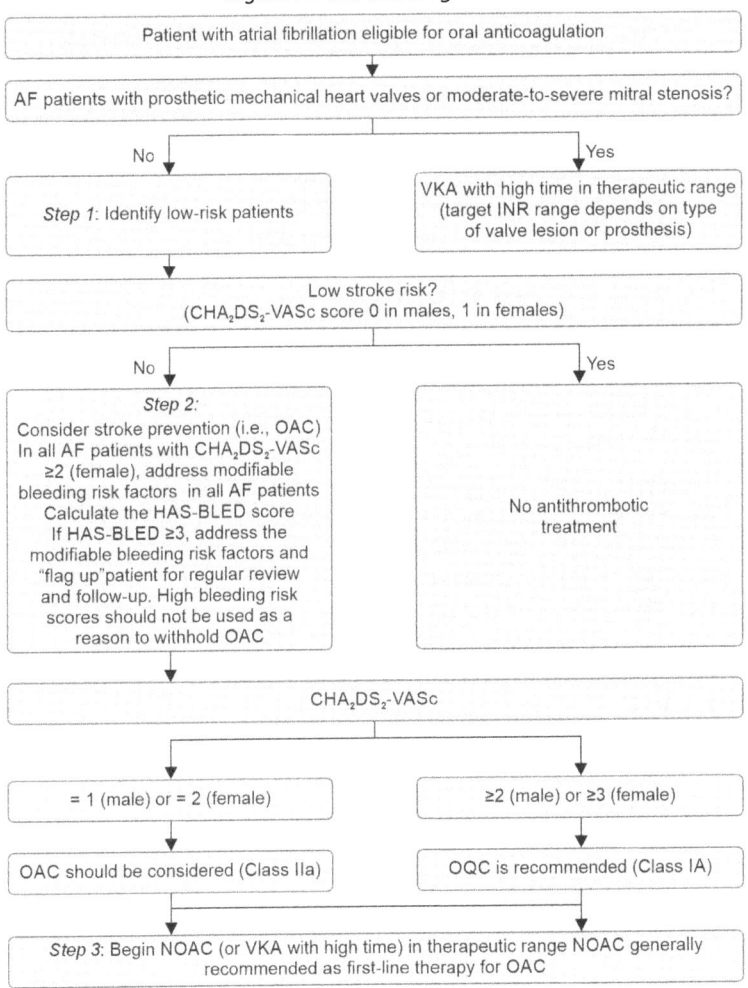

- *Renal function:* Creatinine clearance (CrCl) >60 mL/min, every 6 months
  CrCl 30-60 mL/min, every 3 months
  CrCl <30 mL/min, every 1-2 months
- *Liver function test:* *No liver disease:* Every 12 months, mild decrease (Child-Pugh A), Every 6 months, moderate liver disease (Every 3 months), Severe liver disease (Child-Pugh C), every 1-2 months

TABLE 6: 2023 ACC/AHA/ACCP/HRS guidelines.

Guidelines	Strength of recommendation
• For a formal risk-score-based assessment of bleeding risk, the HAS-BLED score should be considered to help address modifiable bleeding risk factors and to identify patients at high risk of bleeding (HAS-BLED score ≥3) for early and more frequent clinical review and follow-up	IIA
• Stroke and bleeding risk reassessment at periodic intervals is recommended to inform treatment decisions (e.g., initiation of OAC in patients no longer at low risk of stroke) and address potentially modifiable bleeding risk factors	I
• In patients with AF initially at low risk of stroke, first reassessment of stroke risk should be made at 4–6 months after the index evaluation	IIa
• If a VKA is used, a target INR of 2.0–3.0 is recommended with individual TTR ≥70%	I
• In patients on VKAs with low time in INR therapeutic range (e.g., TTR < 70%), recommended options are:	
– Switching to a NOAC but ensuring good adherence and persistence with therapy or	I
– Efforts to improve TTR (e.g., education/counseling and more frequent INR checks)	IIa
• Antiplatelet therapy alone (monotherapy or aspirin in combination with clopidogrel) is not recommended for stroke prevention in AF	III

Contd...

Atrial Fibrillation

Contd...

Guidelines	Strength of recommendation
• Estimated bleeding risk, in the absence contra-indications to OAC, should not in itself guide treatment decisions to use OAC for stroke prevention	III
• Clinical pattern of AF (i.e., first detected, paroxysmal, persistent, long-standing persistent, permanent) should not condition the indication to thromboprophylaxis	III
Recommendations for occlusion or exclusion of the LAA	
• LAA occlusion may be considered for stroke prevention in patients with AF and contraindications for long-term anticoagulant treatment (e.g., intracranial bleeding without a reversible cause)	
• Surgical occlusion or exclusion of the LAA may be considered for stroke prevention in patients with AF undergoing cardiac surgery	

ANTICOAGULATION SUMMARY

(Note: Paroxysmal AF/AFL is associated with increased risk for cardioembolic stroke, similar to persistent and permanent AF/FL)

- Patients who may be candidates for DCCV during this admission should be treated with immediate anticoagulation. Patients who will not be treated with DCCV during this admission usually do not require immediate anticoagulation, although it should be started before discharge. Patients with AF should be anticoagulated, according to their CHA_2DS_2-VASc score.
- Most patients treated with cardioversion should receive post-DCCV anticoagulation for at least 4 weeks (patients who are cardioverted within 48 hours of the onset of AF/FL and who have a CHA_2DS_2-VASc score of 0 in men or 1 in women may not require post-DCCV anticoagulation, especially if bleeding risk is elevated).
- DOAC's are the preferred agents unless the patient has moderate or severe mitral stenosis, a mechanical heart valve, or inadequate

Flowchart 2: Acute management of unstable atrial fibrillation and atrial flutter (AF/AFL).

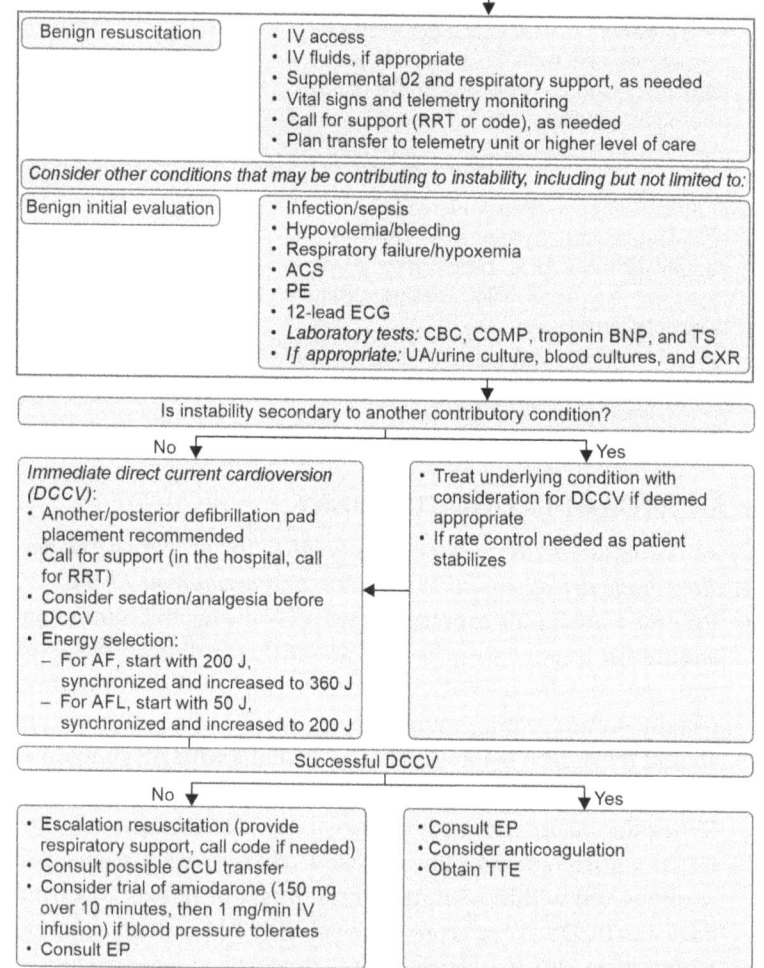

(ACS: acute coronary syndrome; BNP: brain natriuretic peptide; CBC: complete blood count; CCU: cardiac care unit; COMP: comprehensive metabolic panel; CXR: chest X-ray; ECG: electrocardiogram; EP: electrophysiology; HR: heart rate; IV: intravenous; J: Joules; PE: pulmonary embolism; RRT: rapid response team; SBP: systolic blood pressure; TSH: thyroid stimulating hormone; UA: urinalysis)

TABLE 7: OACs pharmacokinetics characteristics and dosing.

Class	VKA	Direct Thrombin Inhibitor	Factor Xa Inhibitor		
Metabolism	S-isomer: CYP2C9 R-isomer: CYP1A2, CYP2C19, and CYP3A4	Minimal	CYP3A4/5	CYP3A4	Minimal CYP3A4
P-glycoprotein substrate	No	Yes	Yes	Yes	Yes
Excretion	0% renal; very little warfarin excreted unchanged in urine	80% renal	66% renal and 28% feces	27% renal, 73% biliary and intestinal	50% renal, 50% liver and biliary/intestinal
Half-life	20–60 h	12–17 h	5–9 h	12 h	10–14 h
Renal dosing adjustment based on actual body weight	N/A	CrCl >30 mL/min: 150 mg twice daily; CrCl 15–30 mL/min: 75 mg twice daily	CrCl >50 mL/min: 20 mg daily with the biggest meal; CrCl 15–50 mL/min: 15 mg daily with the biggest meal	If any 2 of the following: age ≥80 y, body weight ≤60 kg, SCr ≥1.5 mg/dL: 2.5 mg twice daily; else 5 mg twice daily	CrCl >50–≤95 mL/min: 60 mg once daily; CrCl 15–50 mL/min: 30 mg once daily
Appropriate use based on liver function (Child-Pugh score)† Child-Pugh A (mild)	Not mentioned in the labeling	No dose adjustment needed	No dose adjustment needed	No dose adjustment needed	No dose adjustment needed
Child-Pugh B (moderate)		Use with caution	Avoid use	Use with caution	Use with caution
Child-Pugh C (severe)		Avoid use	Avoid use	Avoid use	Avoid use

renal function. In these cases, a warfarin-based regimen is usually preferred.
- When prescribing anticoagulants, always consider the patient's bleeding risk.
- If the patient has a contraindication to anticoagulation or opts out of this therapy, this should be documented in detail in the medical record.
- Obtain neurology consult prior to initiation of anticoagulation for patients with recent ischemic stroke within the prior 2 weeks.
- When starting an anticoagulation drug, consider discontinuing antiplatelet medications if they are prescribed for primary prophylaxis or secondary prophylaxis of stable disease (e.g., no ACS or stent placement within the last year).

RATE CONTROL SUMMARY

- Note that negative inotropes (beta-blockers and calcium channel blockers) are contraindicated in patients with decompensated HFrEF with hypoperfusion, and beta-blockers should be dosed properly (start low and titrate slowly) in patients with compensated HFrEF.
- Goal is for HR <110 bpm at rest and adequate symptom control.
- Use oral agents, preferentially, and titrate them often (e.g., every 6 hours) to goal. Oral metoprolol or bisoprolol is the drug of choice in most patients (unless there is a contraindication). Oral diltiazem is an alternative.
- If more rapid rate control is desired, use noncontinuous (bolus) IV therapy with metoprolol or diltiazem. Continuous IV therapy should not be frequently required.

TABLE 8: Silent AF and Stroke of Undetermined Cause (2023 ACC/AHA/ACC/HRS Guidelines)

Strength of recommendation	Recommendations
2a	In patients with stroke or TIA of undetermined cause, initial cardiac monitoring and, if needed, extended monitoring with an implantable loop recorder are reasonable to improve detection of AF

TABLE 9: Oral anticoagulation for device-detected atrial high-rate episodes among patients without a previous diagnosis of AF (2023 ACC/AHA/ACC/HRS Guidelines).

Strength of recommendation	Recommendations
2a	For patients with a device-detected atrial high-rate episode (AHRE) lasting ≥24 hours and with a HA_2DS_2-VASc score ≥2 or equivalent stroke risk, it is reasonable to initiate oral anticoagulation with a SDM framework, that considers episode duration and individual patient risk
2b	For patients with a device-detected AHRE lasting between 5 minutes and 24 hours and with a CHA_2DS_2-VASc score ≥3 or equivalent stroke risk, it may be reasonable to initiate anticoagulation within a SDM framework that considers episode duration and individual patient risk
3: No benefit	Patients with a device-detected AHRE lasting <5 minutes and without another indication for oral anticoagulation should not receive oral anticoagulation

- Patients admitted on a continuous drip for rate control should be converted to an oral agent as soon as possible.
- If HR is difficult to control with one agent, change to (or add) another. In some cases, second-line rate control medications may be necessary. If heart rate and/or symptoms remain difficult to control after 48 hours, consider a rhythm-control strategy.

SPECIAL SITUATIONS

For patients on DOAC with creatinine clearance lower than the values in **Table 18**, few clinical data exist. Consider holding for an additional 1–3 days, especially for high bleeding risk procedures.

The number of days is the number of full days before the day of surgery in which the patient does not take any dose of anticoagulant. The drug is also not taken on the day of surgery. For example, in the case of holding a twice-daily drug for 1 day, if the drug is taken at 8 PM, and surgery is at 8 AM, at the time of surgery, it will be 36 hours since the last dose was taken.

TABLE 10: Consideration of oral anticoagulation for device-detected atrial high-rate episodes (AHREs) according to patient stroke risk by CHA2DS2-VASc score and episode duration.

	Low risk HA$_2$DS$_2$-VASc = 0 (men)	Intermediate risk CHA$_2$DS$_2$-VASc = 1 (men)	High risk CHA$_2$DS$_2$-VASc = ≥2 (men)
Short, rare AHREs	(A)	"Innocent bystander"	Observe for high AHRE burden or AF development
AHRE = 6 min 5.5 hours	Observe for AF development		ARTESIA and NOAH will provide some evidence. A study-level meta-analysis of NOAH AFNETs and ATRESIA trials provides high-quality consistent evidence that oral coagulation with edoxaban or apixaban reduces the risk of stroke with device-related AF and increases risk of major bleeding.
AHRE >5.5 hours	Periodic assessment patient risk • Other OAC indication? • Changes in CHADS-VASC over time?	(B)	
AHRE >24 hours	• Changes in CHADS-VASC over time?	?	Anticoagulation indicated if true. AF document by ECG or if certainty of AF is high
AHRE >24 hours HF	• Consider data from commander • Compass to refine patient risk?		(C)

Increasing patient risk →

A = Low risk or with short and infrequent AHREs, which does not require anticoagulation

B = Intermediate risk and AHREs lasting >6 minutes to 24 hours are an uncertain population pertaining to anticoagulation requirement

C = Patients with high-risk with longer AHRE/CAF episodes are reasonable candidates for anticoagulation

(AF: atrial fibrillation; AHRE; atrial high-rate episode; ARTESiA: Apixaban for the Reduction of Thrombo-Embolism in Patients With Device-Detected Subclinical Atrial Fibrillation trial; COMMANDER HF: A Study to Assess the Effectiveness and Safety of Rivaroxaban in Reducing the Risk of Death, Myocardial Infarction, or Stroke in Participants With Heart Failure and Coronary Artery Disease Following an Episode of Decompensated Heart Failure; COMPASS: Cardiovascular Outcomes for People Using Anticoagulation Strategies; ECG: electrocardiogram; NOAH-AFNET: non-vitamin K antagonist Oral anticoagulants in patients with Atrial High rate episodes trial; OAC: oral anticoagulation; SCAF: subclinical atrial fibrillation. Female sex is treated as a modifier in the computation of the CHA$_2$DS$_2$-VASc score)

Atrial Fibrillation

TABLE 11: Situations in which long-term anticoagulation is contraindicated and situations when it remains reasonable.

Long-term anticoagulation contraindicated	Long-term anticoagulation is still reasonable
• Severe bleeding due to a nonreversible cause • involving the gastrointestinal, pulmonary, or genitourinary systems • Spontaneous intracranial/intraspinal bleeding due to a nonreversible cause • Serious bleeding related to recurrent falls when cause of falls is not treatable	• Bleeding involving the gastrointestinal, pulmonary, or genitourinary systems that is treatable • Bleeding related to isolated trauma • Bleeding related to procedural complications

TABLE 12: Percutaneous approaches to occlude the LA AF (2023 ACC/AHA/ACC/HRS guidelines).

COR	LOE	Recommendations
2a	B-NR	In patients with AF, a moderate-to-high risk of stroke (CHA$_2$DS$_2$VASc score ≥2) and a contraindication to long-term oral anticoagulation due to a non-reversible cause such as percutaneous LAAO (pLAAO) is reasonable
2b	B-R	In patients with AF and a moderate-to-high risk of stroke and a high risk of major bleeding on oral anticoagulation pLAAO may be a reasonable alternative to oral anticoagulation based on patient preference, with careful consideration of procedural risk and with the understanding that the evidence for oral anticoagulation is more extensive

TABLE 13: Cardiac surgery—LAA exclusion/excision (2023 ACC/AHA/ACC/ARS guidelines).

Strength of recommendation	Recommendations
1	In patients with AF undergoing cardiac surgery with a CHA$_2$DS$_2$-VASc score ≥2 or equivalent stroke risk, surgical LAA exclusion, in addition to continued anticoagulation, is indicated to reduce the risk of stroke and systemic embolism

Contd...

Contd...

Strength of recommendation	Recommendations
1	In patients with AF undergoing cardiac surgery and LAA exclusion, a surgical technique resulting in absence of flow across the suture line and a stump of <1 cm as determined by intraoperative transesophageal echocardiography should be used
2b	In patients with AF undergoing cardiac surgery with CHA_2DS_2-VASc score ≥2 or equivalent stroke risk, the benefit of surgical LAA exclusion in the absence of continued anticoagulation to reduce the risk of stroke and systemic embolism is uncertain

TABLE 14: Active bleeding on anticoagulant therapy and reversal drugs (2023 ACC/AHA/ACC/HRS guidelines).

Strength of recommendation	Recommendations
1	In patients with AF receiving dabigatran who develop life-threatening bleeding, treatment with idaucizumab is recommended to rapidly reverse dabigatran's anticoagulation effect
2a	In patients with AF screening dabigatran who develop life-threatening bleeding, treatment with activated prothrombin complex concentrate (PCC) is reasonable to reverse dabigatran's anticoagulation effect if idarucirumab is unavailable
	In patients with AF receiving factor Xa inhibitors who develop life-threatening bleeding, treatment with either andexanet alfa (apixaban or rivaroxaban, edoxaban) or 4-factor prothrombin complex concentrate is recommended to rapidly reverse factor Xa inhibitor's anticoagulation effect
1	In patients with AF receiving warfarin who develop life-threatening bleeding, treatment with 4-factor prothrombin complex concentrate is recommended to rapidly reverse factor Xa inhibitor's anticoagulation effect
	In patients with AF who develop major gastrointestinal bleeding, resumption of oral anticoagulation therapy may be reasonable after correction of reversible causes of bleeding and reassessment of its long-term benefits and risks with a multidisciplinary SXM

TABLE 15: Recommendations for active bleeding on anticoagulant therapy and reversal drugs.

Strength of recommendation	Recommendations
1	In patients with AF receiving dabigatran who develop life-threatening bleeding, treatment with idarucizumab is recommended to rapidly reverse dabigatran's anticoagulation effect
	In patients with AF receiving dabigatran who develop life-threatening bleeding, treatment with activated prothrombin complex concentrate (PCC) is reasonable to reverse dabigatran's anticoagulation effects if idarucizumab is unavailable
	In patients with AF receiving factor Xa inhibitors who develop life-threatening bleeding, treatment with either andexanet alfa apixaban or rivaroxaban, endoxaban or 4-factor prothrombin complex concentrate is recommended to rapidly reverse factor Xa inhibitor's anticoagulation effect
2a	In patients with AF receiving warfarin who develop life-threatening bleeding, treatment with 4-factor prothrombin complex concentrate (if available) in addition to intravenous vitamin K is recommended to rapidly achieve INR correction over fresh frozen plasma and intravenous vitamin K treatment
1	In patients with AF who develop major gastrointestinal bleeding resumption of oral anticoagulation therapy may be reasonable after correction of reversible causes of bleeding and reassessment of its long-term benefits and risks with a multidisciplinary team approach during SXM with patients

- Historical data have reported that in patients with mitral stenosis and AF, stroke risk was nearly 18-fold higher than in an age-, sex-, and hypertension-matched population without AF. More recently, stroke or systemic embolism rates ranged between 0.4 and 4 per 100 patient-years among anticoagulated patients and were highest in those with previous embolism. Warfarin

TABLE 16: Reversal agents for oral anticoagulants.

	Idarucizumab	Andexanet alfa	4-Factor PCC	Activated PCC
Class	Humanized monoclonal antibody fragment binding to dabigatran and neutralizing anticoagulation effects	A recombinant modified human factor Xa protein binding and sequestering the factor Xa inhibitors	• PCC: Coagulation factors II, VII, IX, and X • Anticoagulation proteins C and S	Nonactivated factors II, IX, and X and activated VII
Approved indications	Reversal of dabigatran effects for emergency surgery/urgent procedures, life-threatening or uncontrolled bleeding	Reversal of apixaban or rivaroxaban For life-threatening or uncontrolled bleeding	The urgent reversal for acute major bleeding or need for an urgent surgery/invasive procedure in patients receiving VKAs	Control and prevention of bleeding episodes, preoperative management, prophylaxis to prevent or reduce bleeding frequency in patients with hemophilia A and B
Off-label indications	N/A	Edoxaban-associated life-threatening bleeding	Reversal of factor Xa inhibitors in patients requiring urgent procedure or with life-threatening bleeding	Dabigatran-associated life-threatening bleeding

Contd...

	Idarucizumab	Andexanet alfa	4-Factor PCC	Activated PCC
Dosing	5 g (2 separate vials of 2.5 g/vial) intravenous infusion over 5 minutes. Additional 5 g may be given if reappearance of bleeding with elevated coagulation parameters has been observed or patients require second emergency surgery/procedure and elevated coagulation parameters	• Low-dose regimen: 400-mg bolus at a target rate of 30 mg/min followed by 4 mg/min for up to 120 min • High-dose regimen: 800-mg bolus at a target rate of 30 mg/min followed by 8 mg/min for up to 120 minutes The recommended dosing is based on apixaban or rivaroxaban dose, and time since the patient's last dose of apixaban or rivaroxaban	• Warfarin reversal based on pretreatment INR (units of factor IX): – INR 2–<4: 25 units/kg (up to 2,500 units) – INR 4–6: 35 units/kg (up to 3,500 units) – INR >6: 50 units/kg (up to 5,000 units) • Oral factor Xa inhibitors: 2,000 units once or 25–50 units/kg	Dabigatran-associated life-threatening bleeding: 50 units/kg once
Onset of action	Within 5 minutes	Within 2 minutes	Within 10 minutes	Within 30 minutes
Duration of action	12–24 hours	2 hours	8 hours	12 hours
Monitoring	Coagulation parameters (aPTT, diluted thrombin time, or ecarin clotting time) between 12 and 24 hours to assess redistribution of dabigatran from peripheral to plasma	Current commercial anti-Xa activity assays are unsuitable for measuring factor Xa activities after andexanet alfa use	Warfarin reversal: Repeat INR within 30 minutes after the administration	N/A

Contd...

	Idarucizumab	Andexanet alfa	4-Factor PCC	Activated PCC
Additional information	Risk of serious reactions (hypoglycemia, hypophosphatemia, metabolic acidosis, increase in uric acid, acute liver failure) in patients with hereditary fructose intolerance (due to sorbitol excipient 4 g in each 5 g of idarucizumab). No procoagulant effect based on endogenous thrombin potential	No FDA indication for other factor Xa inhibitors other than apixaban or rivaroxaban. Andexanet alfa may interfere with the anticoagulation effect of heparin *US black box warning:* Serious and life-threatening adverse events (arterial and venous thromboembolism, myocardial infarction, ischemic stroke, cardiac arrest, and sudden deaths)	• May not be indicated for patients with thromboembolic events in the previous 3 months It includes heparin • Administer intravenous vitamin K 10 mg over 10–20 min in addition to 4-factor PCC	• It does not include heparin coagulation parameters, does not correlate with the drug's efficacy • Not effective to reverse factor Xa inhibitors

(aPTT: activated partial thromboplastin time; FDA: US Food and Drug Administration; PCC: prothrombin complex concentrate; VKA: vitamin K antagonists)

TABLE 17: Management of patients with AF and intracerebral hemorrhage (ICH) [2023 ACC/AHA/ACC/HRS Guidelines].

Strength of recommendation	Recommendations
2a	In patients with AF and conditions associated with very high risk of thrombotic events (>5%/year), such as rheumatic heart disease or a mechanical heart valve, early (1–2 weeks) resuscitation of anticoagulation after ICH is reasonable to reduce the risk of thromboembolic events
2b	In patients with AF and ICH, delayed (4–8 weeks) resumption of anticoagulation may be considered to balance the risks of thromboembolic and hemorrhagic complications after careful risk–benefit assessment
2b	In patients with AF and conditions associated with high risk of recurrent ICH (e.g., cerebral amyloid angiopathy) anticoagulation-sparing strategies (e.g., LAAO) may be considered to reduce the risk of recurrent hemorrhage)

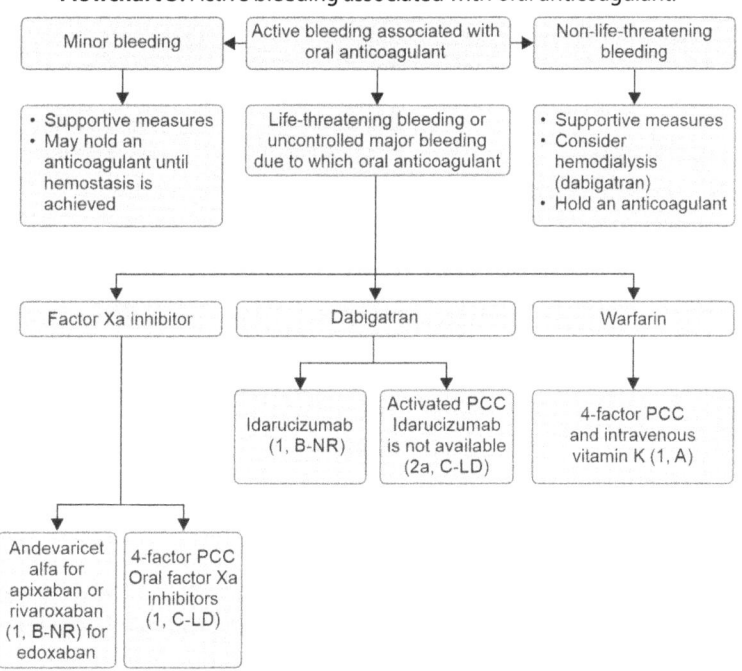

Flowchart 3: Active bleeding associated with oral anticoagulant.

TABLE 18: Risk factors for thromboembolic complications and recurrent ICH.

Factors associated with high risk of thromboembolism	Factors associated with high risk of recurrent ICH
Mechanical heart valve	Suspected cerebral amyloid angiography
Rheumatic valve disease	Lobar intraparenchymal hemorrhage
Previous history of stroke/thromboembolism	Older age
Hypercoagulable state (e.g., active malignancy,	>10 cerebral micro-bleeds on MRI genetic thrombophilia)
High CHA_2DS_2-VASc score (>5)	• Disseminated cortical superficial siderosis on MRI • Poorly controlled hypotension • Previous history of spontaneous ICH • Genetic/acquired coagulopathy • Untreated symptomatic vascular malformation or aneurysm

TABLE 19: Timing of discontinuation of OACs in patients with AF scheduled to undergo an invasive procedure or surgery in whom anticoagulation is to be interrupted.

Anticoagulated	Low bleeding risk procedure	High bleeding risk procedure
Apixaban (CrCl >25 mL/min)	1 day	2 days
Dabigatran (CrCl >50 mL/min)	1 day	2 days
Dabigatran (CrCl 30–50 mL/min)	2 days	4 days
Edoxaban (CrCl >15 mL/min)	1 day	2 days
Rivaroxaban (CrCl >30 mL/min)	1 day	2 days
Warfarin	5 days for a target INR <1.5; 2–3 days for a target INR <2	5 days

(AF: atrial fibrillation; CrCl: creatinine clearance; DOAC: direct oral anticoagulation; INR: international normalized ratio; OAC: oral anticoagulant)

is generally prescribed, but it has been questioned whether a DOAC may be an alternative. A retrospective cohort study from Korea examined 2,230 individuals with mitral stenosis and AF

Flowchart 4: Management of periprocedural anticoagulation in patients with AF.

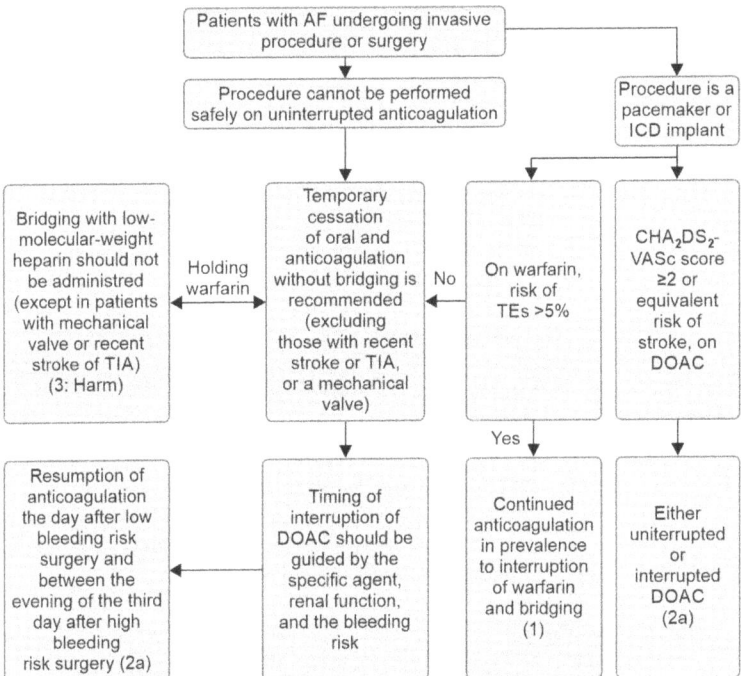

(DOAC: direct oral anticoagulant; ICD: implantable cardioverter-defibrillator; TE: thromboembolism; TIA: transient ischemic attack)

TABLE 20: Recommendations for AF complicating ACS or percutaneous coronary intervention (PCI) (2023 ACC/AHA/ACC/HRS guidelines).

Strength of recommendation	Recommendations
1	In patients with AF and an increased risk for stroke who undergo PCI, DOACs are preferred over VKAs in combination with APT to reduce the risk of clinically relevant bleeding
1	In most patients with AF who take oral anticoagulation and undergo PCI, early discontinuation of aspirin (1–4 weeks) and continuation of dual antithrombotic therapy with OAC and a P2Y12 inhibitor is referred over triple therapy (OAC P2Y12 inhibitor, and aspirin) to reduce the risk of clinically relevant bleeding

TABLE 21: Recommendation for chronic coronary disease (CCD) and AF (2023 ACC/AHA/ACC/HRS guidelines).

Strength of recommendation	Recommendations
1	In patients with AF and CCD (beyond 1 year after revascularization or CAD not requiring coronary revascularization) without history of stent thrombosis, oral anticoagulation monotherapy is recommended over the combination therapy of OAC and single APT (aspirin or P2Y12 inhibitor) to decrease the risk of major bleeding)

TABLE 22: Recommendation for peripheral artery disease (PAD) and AF (2023 ACC/AHA/ACC/HRS guidelines).

Strength of recommendation	Recommendations
2a	In patients with AF and concomitant stable PAD, monotherapy oral anticoagulation is reasonable over dual therapy (anticoagulation plus aspirin or P2Y12 inhibitors) to reduce the risk of bleeding

TABLE 23: Chronic kidney disease (CKD)/kidney failure and AF (2023 ACC/AHA/ACC/HRS guidelines).

Strength of recommendation	Recommendations
1	For patients with AF at elevated risk for stroke and CKD stage 3, treatment with warfarin or, preferably, evidence-based doses of direct thrombin or factor Xa inhibitors is recommended to reduce the risk of stroke
2a	For patients with AF at elevated risk for stroke and CKD stage 4, treatment with warfarin or labeled doses of DOACs is reasonable to reduce the risk of stroke
2b	For patients with AF at elevated risk for stroke and who have end-stage CKD (CrCl <15 mL/min) or are on dialysis, it might be reasonable to prescribe warfarin (INR 2.0–3.0) or an evidence-based dose of apixaban for oral anticoagulation to reduce the risk of stroke

TABLE 24: Recommended doses of currently approved DOACs according to renal function.

DOAC	CrCl (mL/min)			
	>95	51–95	31–50	15–30	<15 or on dialysis
Apixaban	5 or 2.5 mg twice daily*	5 or 2.5 mg twice daily*	5 or 2.5 mg twice daily*	5 or 2.5 mg twice daily*	5 or 2.5 mg twice daily*
Dabigatran	150 mg twice daily	150 mg twice daily	150 mg twice daily	75 mg twice daily	Contraindicated
Edoxaban	Contraindicated	60 mg once daily	30 mg once daily	30 mg once daily	Contraindicated
Rivaroxaban	20 mg once daily	20 mg once daily	15 mg once daily	15 mg once daily	15 mg once daily[†]

Note that other, nonrenal considerations such as drug interactions may also apply. The gray area indicates doses not studied in the pivotal clinical trials of these agents.

*If at least 2 of the following are present: Serum creatinine ≥1.5 mg/dL, age ≥80 years, or body weight ≤60 kg, the recommended dose is 2.5 mg twice daily. The ARISTOTLE trial excluded patients with either a creatinine of >2.5 mg/dL or a calculated CrCl <25 mL/min.

[†]Rivaroxaban is not recommended for other indications in patients with a CrCl <15 mL/min, but such a recommendation is not made for the AF indication. However, pharmacokinetic data are limited.

(AF: atrial fibrillation; ARISTOTLE: apixaban for reduction in stroke and other thromboembolic events in atrial fibrillation; CrCl: creatinine clearance; DOAC: direct oral anticoagulant) who were prescribed either warfarin or a DOAC, using propensity matching on 10 clinical variables. Thromboembolic events in the DOAC group were 2.22% per year compared with 4.19% per year in the warfarin group (HR, 0.28; 95% CI, 0.18–0.45). However, in the INVICTUS (the investigation of rheumatic AF treatment using VKAs, rivaroxaban or aspirin studies) RCT, patients with AF, rheumatic heart disease, and mitral stenosis had a mean survival time to a primary outcome event of stroke, systemic embolism, MI, or death from vascular or unknown cause of 1,675 days if treated with a VKA compared with 1,599 days if treated with rivaroxaban [difference, −76 days (95% CI, −121 to −31; $p <0.001$)].

- Although patients with moderate-to-severe mitral stenosis or mechanical valve were excluded from DOAC trials, other forms of VHD were allowed, such as aortic stenosis or mitral regurgitation. Bioprosthetic valves and valve repair were allowed in the edoxaban (ENGAGE AF) and apixaban (ARISTOTLE) trials, and valve repair in the rivaroxaban (ROCKET AF) trial. A systematic review of patients with VHD (other than moderate-to-severe mitral stenosis or mechanical valve) concluded that DOACs were safe. A meta-analysis confirmed that DOACs decreased the risk of stroke/systemic embolism compared with warfarin in patients with (HR, 0.70; 95% CI, 0.58–0.86) and without VHD (HR, 0.84; 95% CI, 0.75–0.95). However, for patients with mechanical heart valves, the RE-ALIGN (Randomized, Phase II Study to Evaluate

TABLE 25: AF in VHD (2023 ACC/AHA/ACC/HRS guidelines).

Strength of recommendation	Recommendations
1	In patients with rheumatic mitral stenosis or mitral stenosis of moderate or greater severity and history of AF, long-term anticoagulation with warfarin is recommended over DOACs, independent of the CHA_2DS_2-VASc score to prevent cardiovascular events, including stroke or death
1	In patients with AF and valve disease other than moderate-to-greater mitral stenosis or a mechanical heart valve, DOACs are recommended over VKAs

the Safety and Pharmacokinetics of Oral Dabigatran Etexilate in Patients After Heart Valve Replacement) trial was started but was halted during phase II after enrolling subjects due to increased thromboembolism and bleeding in the dabigatran arm. PROACT Xa (A Trial to Determine if Participants with an On-X.

Aortic Valve can be maintained safely on Apixaban) was also terminated early due to higher thromboembolic events with apixaban in patients who were >3 months after mechanical On-X aortic valves.

- In patients who have not responded to an antiarrhythmic drug due to a high burden of recurrent AF or adverse effects from the medication, RCTs have consistently demonstrated lower risk of

Flowchart 5: Anticoagulation for typical (CTI-dependent) AFL (2023 ACC/AHA/ACC/HRS guidelines).

```
                        Typical
                    (CTI-dependent)
                         AFL
       ┌─────────────────┼─────────────────┐
       ▼                 ▼                 ▼
  Rate control      Unsuccessful      Successful
  or rhythm         typical AFL       typical AFL
  control with      ablation          ablation
  antiarrhythmic    (without plans
  therapy           for re-do
                    ablation)
       ▼                 │                 │
  Anticoagulation   ┌────┴────┐      ┌─────┴─────┐
  according to      Known prior     No known
  same risk         history of AF   prior history
  profile                           of AF
  as AF (1)              ▼          ┌──┴──┐
                    Anticoagulation High-risk  Low-risk
                    according to   thromboem- thromboem-
                    same risk profile bolic profile bolic profile
                    as AF (1)           │              │
                                   Consider       Monitor off
                                   anticoagulation anticoagula-
                                   if high-risk   tion (clinical
                                   features for   follow-up
                                   development    and
                                   of AF (2b)     arrhythmia
                                                  monitoring)
                                                  (1)
```

recurrent symptomatic AF after ablation when compared to using another antiarrhythmic medication. As an example, in STOP-AF, patients who had failed ≥1 antiarrhythmic drug (approximately 70% and 30% for 1 or 2 failed drugs, respectively) were randomized to either another antiarrhythmic drug or catheter ablation. At 1 year follow-up, catheter ablation was associated with a treatment success rate of 70% compared with 7% in the drug arm. Similarly, in the ThermoCool (NaviStar ThermoCool

TABLE 26: Rate control (2023 ACC/AHA/ACC/HRS guidelines). Broad considerations for rate control.

Strength of recommendation	Recommendations
1	In patients with AF with rapid ventricular response who are hemodynamically stable, beta-blockers or nondihydropyridine calcium channel blockers (verapamil and diltiazem; provided that EF >40%) are recommended for acute rate control
2a	In patients with AF with rapid ventricular response in whom beta-blockers and nondihydropyridine calcium channel blockers are ineffective or contraindicated, digoxin can be considered for acute rate control, either alone or in combination with the aforementioned agents
2a	In patients with AF with rapid ventricular response, the addition of intravenous magnesium to standard rate-control measures is reasonable to achieve and maintain rate control
2b	In patients with AF with rapid ventricular response who are critically ill and/or in decompensated HF in whom beta-blockers and nondihydropyridine calcium channel blockers are ineffective or contraindicated, intravenous amiodarone may be considered for acute rate control
3: Harm	In patients with AF with rapid ventricular response and known moderate or severe LV systolic dysfunction with or without decompensated HF, intravenous nondihydropyridine calcium channel blockers should not be administered

TABLE 27: Consider the risk of cardioversion and stroke when using amiodarone as a rate-control agent. Rate control (2023 ACC/AHA/ACC/HRS Guidelines). Broad considerations for rate control.

Strength of recommendations	Recommendations
1	In patients with AF, SDM, where the patient is recommended to discuss rhythm-versus rate-control strategies (taking into consideration clinical presentation, comorbidity burden, medication profile, and patient preferences), discuss therapeutic options for assessing long-term benefits
2a	In patients with AF without HF who are candidates for select rate-control strategies, heart rate target should be guided by underlying patient symptoms, in general aiming at a resting heart rate of <100–110 bpm

TABLE 28: Pharmacological agents for rate control in patients with AF.

	Intravenous administration	Oral maintenance dose	Special note
Beta-blockers			
Metoprolol tartrate	2.5-5 mg bolus over 2 min; up to 3 doses	25–200 mg, twice daily	
Metoprolol succinate	N/A	50–400 mg daily or twice daily in divided doses	
Atenolol	N/A	25–100 mg daily	Renally eliminated
Bisoprolol	N/A	2.5–10 mg daily	
Carvedilol	N/A	3.125–25 mg twice	
Daily Esmolol	500 μg/kg bolus over 1 min, then 50–300 μg/kg/min	N/A	
Nadolol	N/A	10–240 mg daily	
Propranolol times	1 mg over 1 min; repeat as needed every 2 min; up to doses	10–40 mg, 3–4 daily	

Contd...

Contd...

	Intravenous administration	Oral maintenance dose	Special note
Nondihydropyridine calcium channel blockers			
Diltiazem	0.25 mg/kg (actual body weight) IV over 2 min. May repeat 0.35 mg/kg continuous infusion	120–300 mg daily (ER)	Avoid in HFrEF
Diltiazem	0.25 mg/kg (actual body weight) IV over 2 min May repeat 0.35 mg/kg continuous infusion	120–300 mg daily (ER)	Avoid in HFrEF
Verapamil	5–10 mg over ≥2 min (may repeat twice); then 5 mg/h continuous infusion (max 20 mg/h)	180–480 mg daily (ER)	Avoid in HFrEF
Digitalis glycoside			
Digoxin	0.25–0.5 mg over several min; repeat doses of 0.25 mg every 6 hours (maximum 1.5 mg/24 h)	0.0625–0.25 mg daily	Renally eliminated increased mortality at plasma concentrations exceeding 1.2 mg/mL
Other			
Amiodarone	150–300 mg IV over 1 h, then 10–50 mg/h over 24 hours	100–200 mg daily (generally IV form used for rate control)	Loading dose 6–10 g administered over 2–4 weeks; can combine IV and oral dosing to complete

(AF: atrial fibrillation; ER: extended release; HFrEF: heart failure with reduced ejection fraction; IV: intravenous; N/A: not applicable)

catheter for the radiofrequency ablation of symptomatic paroxysmal atrial fibrillation) trial, patients with paroxysmal AF who had failed antiarrhythmic medication were randomized to catheter ablation or another antiarrhythmic drug. After 9 months,

TABLE 29: Long-term rate control (2023 ACC/AHA/ACC/HRS guidelines).

Strength of recommendation	Recommendations
1	In patients with AF, beta-blockers or nondihydropyridine calcium channel blockers (diltiazem and verapamil) are recommended for long-term rate control with the choice of agent according to underlying substrate and comorbid conditions
2a	For patients with AF in whom measuring serum digoxin levels is indicated, it is reasonable to target levels <1.2 ng/mL
2a	In patients with AF and HF symptoms, digoxin is reasonable for long-term rate control in combination with other rate-controlling agents, or as monotherapy, if other agents are not preferred, not tolerated or contraindicated
3: Harm	In patients with AF and LVEF <40%, nonhydropyridine calcium channel-blocking drugs should not be administered given their potential to exacerbate HF
3: Harm	In patients with permanent AF who have risk factors for cardiovascular events, dronedarone should not be used for long-term rate control

Flowchart 6: Acute rate control in AF with rapid ventricular rate (RVR) (2023 ACC/AHA/ACC/HRS guidelines).

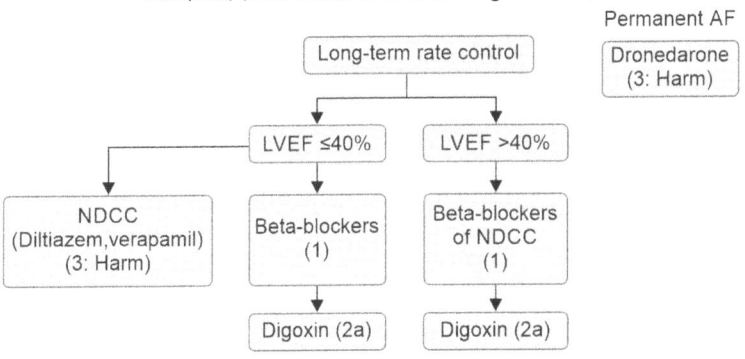

(AF: atrial fibrillation; LVEF: left ventricular ejection fraction; NDCC: nondihydropyridine calcium channel blocker)

TABLE 30: Atrioventricular nodal ablation (AVNA) (2023 ACC/AHA/ACC/HRS guidelines).

Strength of recommendation	Recommendations
1	In patients with AF and a persistently rapid ventricular response who undergo AVNA, initial pacemaker lower rate programming should be 80–90 bpm to reduce sudden death
2a	In patients with AF and uncontrolled rapid ventricular response refractory to rate-control medications (who are not candidates for or in whom rhythm control has been unsuccessful), AVNA can be useful to improve symptoms and QOL
1	In patients with AF who are planning to undergo AVNA, implantation of a pacemaker before the ablation (i.e., before or same day of ablation) is recommended to ensure adequacy of the pacing leads before performing ablation
2b	In patients with AF with normal EF undergoing AVNA, conduction system pacing of the His bundle or left bundle area may be reasonable

TABLE 31: Rhythm control (2023 ACC/AHA/ACC/HRS Guidelines). Goal of therapy with rhythm control.

Strength of recommendation	Recommendations
1	In patients with reduced LV function and persistent high burden AF, a trial of rhythm control should be recommended to evaluate whether AF is contributing to the reduced LV function
2a	In patients with symptomatic AF, rhythm control can be useful to improve symptoms
2a	In patients with a recent diagnosis of AF (<1 year), rhythm control can be useful to reduce hospitalizations, stroke, and mortality
2a	In patients with AF and HF, rhythm control can be useful for improving symptoms and improving outcomes, such as mortality and hospitalizations for HF and ischemia

Contd...

Atrial Fibrillation

Contd...

Strength of recommendation	Recommendations
2a	In patients with AF, rhythm-control strategies can be useful to reduce the likelihood of AF progression
2a	In patients with AF where symptoms associated with AF are uncertain, a trial of rhythm control (e.g., cardioversion or pharmacological therapy) may be useful to determine if any symptoms are attributable to AF
2b	In patients with AF, rhythm-control strategies may be useful to reduce the likelihood of development of dementia or worsening cardiac structural abnormalities

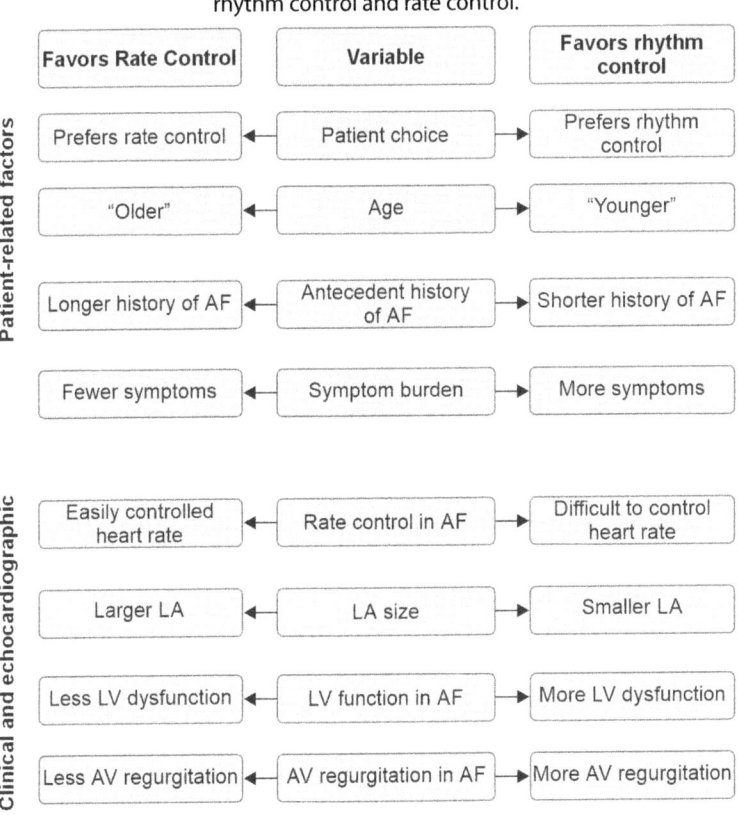

Flowchart 7: Patient and clinical considerations for choosing between rhythm control and rate control.

(AF: atrial fibrillation; AV: atrioventricular; LA: left atrium; LV: left ventricular)

Flowchart 8: Algorithm for treatment choices when required to decrease AF burden (2023 ACC/AHA/ACC/HRS guidelines).

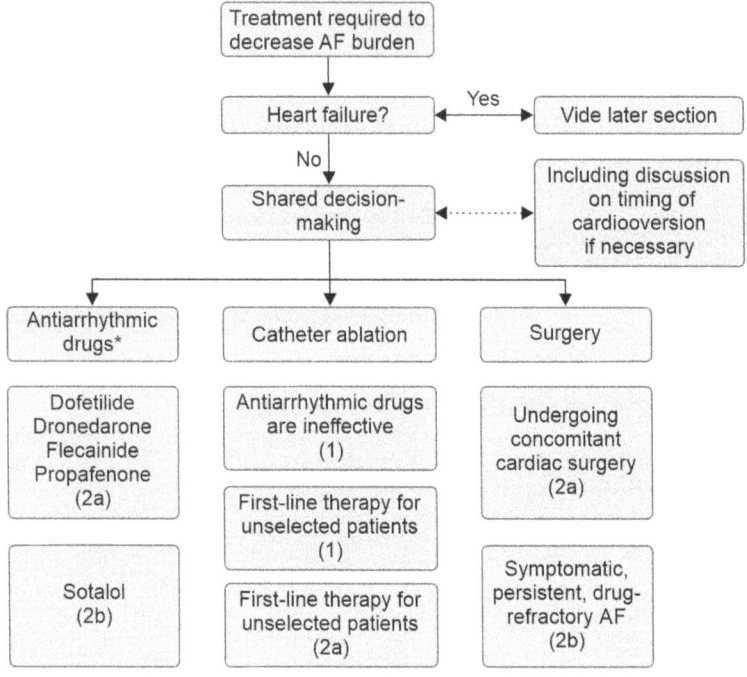

*See later sections

66% of patients in the catheter ablation group were free from recurrent arrhythmia compared to 16% in the antiarrhythmic drug group. Finally, most recently, in the CABANA trial, 80% of patients were on an antiarrhythmic medication and thought to be candidates for AF ablation and were randomized to catheter ablation or continue antiarrhythmic therapy. Catheter ablation was associated with a nearly 50% reduction in recurrent AF (HR 0.52; 95% CI, 0.45–0.60; $p < 0.001$).

- In selected patients with paroxysmal AF, ablation is a suitable first-line option. Several initial RCTs suggested a decrease in recurrent AF or AF burden with catheter ablation when compared with antiarrhythmic drugs. More recent trials have shown a significant reduction in recurrent AF with catheter ablation compared with antiarrhythmic drugs. In a follow-up report

Flowchart 9: Patients with hemodynamically stable AF planned for cardioversion (2023 ACC/AHA/ACC/HRS guidelines).

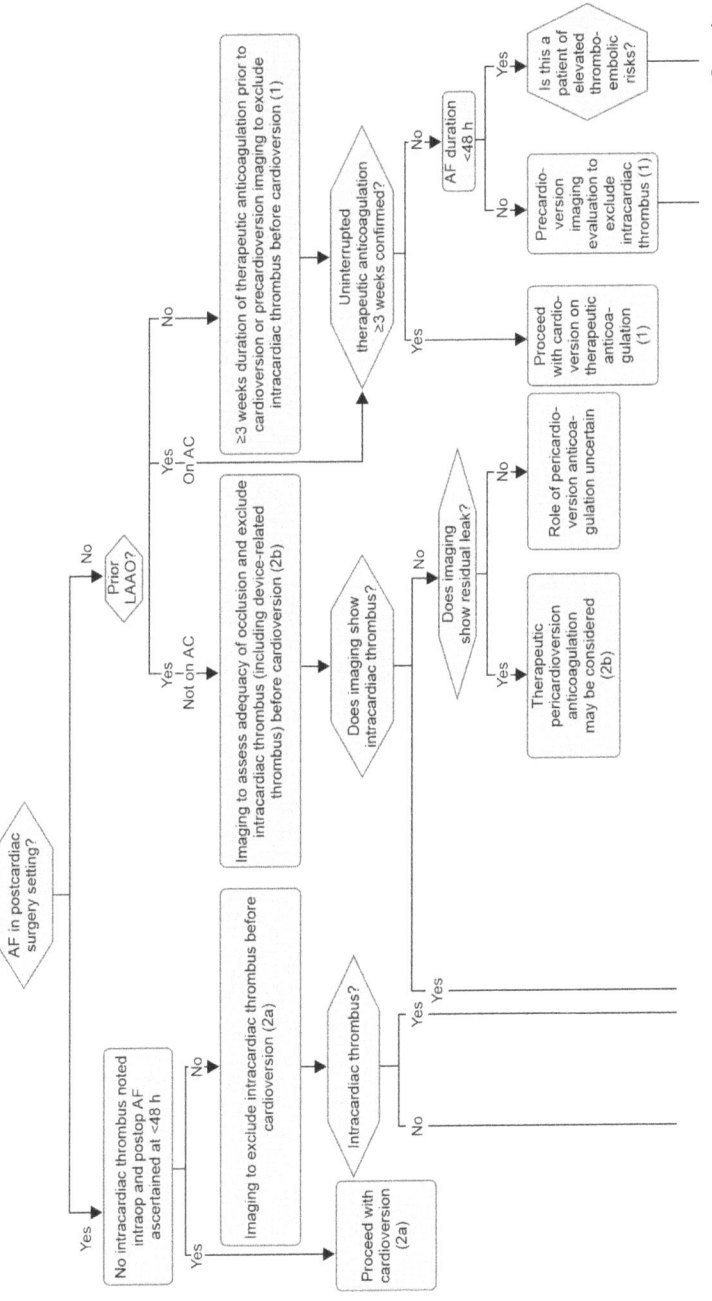

Contd...

Atrial Fibrillation

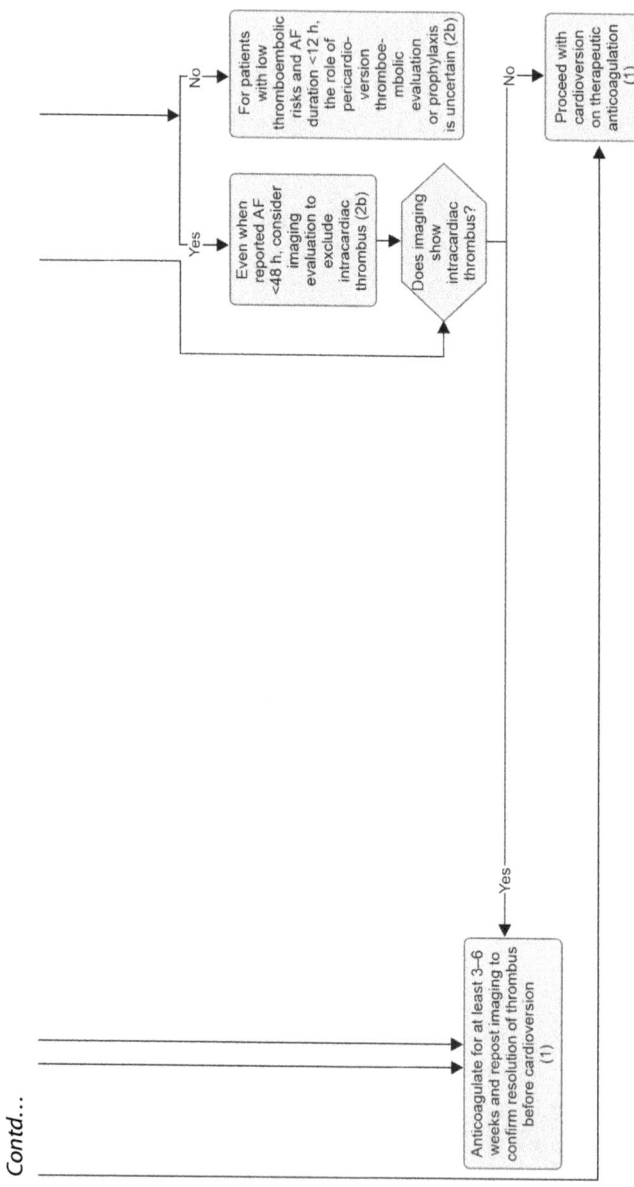

Contd...

TABLE 32: Electrical cardioversion (2023 ACC/AHA/ACC/HRS guidelines) recommendations.

Strength of recommendation	Recommendations
1	In patients with hemodynamic instability attributable to AF, immediate electrical cardioversion should be performed to restore sinus rhythm
1	In patients with AF who are hemodynamically stable, electrical cardioversion can be performed as initial rhythm-control strategy or after unsuccessful pharmacological cardioversion
1	In patients with AF undergoing electrical cardioversion, energy delivery should be confirmed to be synchronized to the QRS to reduce the risk of inducing VF
2a	For patients with AF undergoing elective electrical cardioversion, the use of biphasic of at least 200 J as initial energy can be beneficial to improve success of initial electrical shock
2a	In patients with AF undergoing elective cardioversion, with longer duration AF or unsuccessful initial shock, optimization of electrode vector, use of higher energy, and pretreatment with antiarrhythmic drugs can facilitate success of electrical cardioversion
2b	In patients with obesity and AF, use of manual pressure augmentation and/or further of escalation electrical energy may be beneficial to improve success of electrical cardioversion

TABLE 33: Pharmacological cardioversion (2023 ACC/AHA/ACC/HRS guidelines). Recommendations for pharmacological cardioversion.

Strength of recommendation	Recommendations
2a	For patients with AF, pharmacological cardioversion is reasonable as an alternative to electrical cardioversion for those who are hemodynamically stable or in situations when electrical cardioversion is preferred but cannot be performed
2a	For patients with AF, ibutilide is reasonable for pharmacological cardioversion for those without depressed LV function (LVEF <40%)
2a	For patients with AF, intravenous amiodarone is reasonable for pharmacological cardioversion, although time to conversion is generally longer than with other agents (8–12 hours)
2a	For patients with recurrent AF occurring outside the setting of a hospital, the "pill-in-the-pocket" (PITP) approach with a single oral dose of flecainide or propafenone with a concomitant atrioventricular nodal blocking agent is reasonable for pharmacological cardioversion if previously tested in a monitored setting
2b	For patients with AF, use of intravenous procainamide may be considered for pharmacological cardioversion when other intravenous agents are contraindicated or not preferred

Flowchart 10: Drugs for pharmacological conversion of AF to sinus rhythm (2023 ACC/AHA/ACC/HRS guidelines).

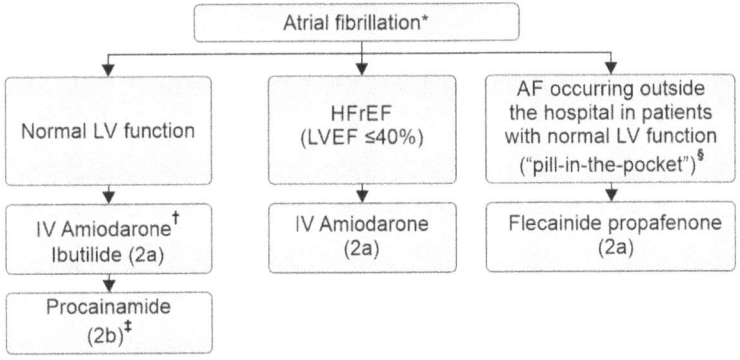

*In the absence of preexcitation.
†First dose administered in a facility that can provide continuous electrocardiographic monitoring and cardiac resuscitation because of the potential for proarrhythmia or postconversion bradycardia.
‡IV amiodarone requires several hours for efficacy; ibutilide is generally effective in 30 to 90 minutes but carries a higher risk of QT interval prolongation and torsades de pointes.
§Recommend avoidance of IV procainamide for patients initially treated with amiodarone or ibutilide to avoid excessive QT interval prolongation and torsades de pointes.

Flowchart 11: Treatment algorithm for drug therapy for maintenance of sinus rhythm (2023 ACC/AHA/ACC/HRS guidelines).

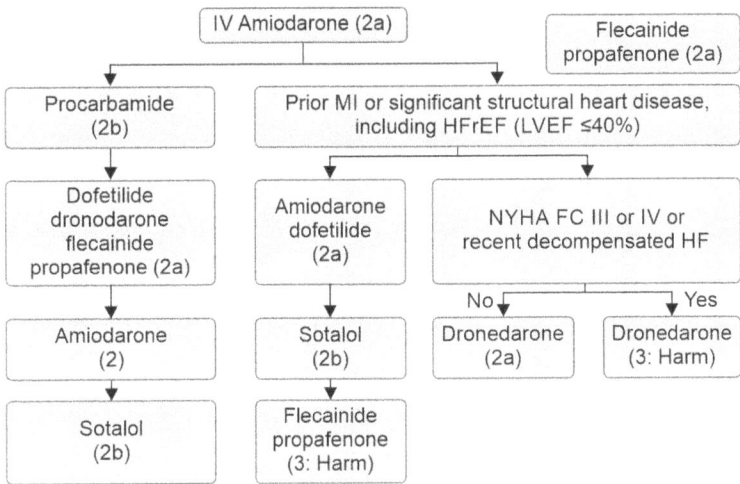

(HFrEF: heart failure with reduced ejection fraction; HF: heart failure; IV: intravenous; LV: left ventricular; LVEF: left ventricular ejection fraction; MI: myocardial infarction; NYHA FC: New York Heart Association functional class)

TABLE 34: Specific drug therapy for maintenance of sinus rhythm in patients with AF.

Drug	Loading dose	Maintenance of dose	Primary Route(s) of elimination	Elimination of half-life	Major adverse effects
Amiodarone	Total loading dose 6–10 g, given 400–800 mg daily in 2–4 divided doses for 1–4 weeks	200 mg once daily	• Liver metabolism • Biliary excretion	14–50 days	AV block, bradycardia, corneal microdeposits, elevation in transaminases, hepatotoxicity, hypothyroidism, nausea, QT prolongation, peripheral neuropathy, photosensitivity, pulmonary fibrosis, skin pigmentation, (blue-gray), TdP
Dofetilide	N/A	CrCl >60 mL/min: 500 µg twice daily; CrCl 40–60 mL/min: 250 µg twice daily; CrCl 20–40 mL/min: contraindicated	Kidney	10 hours	QT prolongation, TdP
Dronedarone	N/A	400 mg twice daily	Liver metabolism	13–19 hours	Abdominal pain, asthenia, bradycardia, diarrhea, nausea and vomiting, QT prolongation, TdP

Contd...

Contd...

Drug	Loading dose	Maintenance of dose	Primary Route(s) of elimination	Elimination of half-life	Major adverse effects
Flecainide	N/A	50–300 mg/d PO divided q 8–12 h	• Liver (70%) • Kidney (30%)	12–27 hours	Atrial flutter, AV block, dizziness, dyspnea, exacerbation of HFrEF, headache, nausea, QT prolongation, VT, and visual disturbances
Propafenone	N/A	150–300 mg	Liver	9 hours	Atrial flutter, bradycardia, AV block, dizziness, dyspnea, exacerbation of HFrEF, nausea, taste disturbance, VT, visual disturbances
Sotalol	CrCl >60 mL/min: 40–80 mg twice daily for 3 days CrCl: 40–60 mL/min; 80 mg once daily for 3 days CrCl <40 mL/min: contraindicated	CrCl >60 mL/min; 80–160 mg twice daily CrCl: 40–60 mL/min; 80–160 mg once daily CrCl <40 mL/min: contraindicated	Kidney	12 hours	AV block, bradycardia, bronchospasm, diarrhea, exacerbation of HFrEF, fatigue, nausea and vomiting, QT prolongation, TdP

(AF: atrial fibrillation; AUC: area under the plasma concentration versus time curve; AV: atrioventricular; CrCl: creatinine clearance; CYP: cytochrome P-450; ER: extended release; HFrEF: heart failure with reduced ejection fraction; IV: intravenous; N/A: not applicable; NAPA: N-acetylprocainamide; p-gp: p-glycoprotein; PO: perorally; TdP: torsades de pointes; VT: ventricular tachycardia)

TABLE 35: Recommended monitoring for patients taking oral amiodarone.

Adverse effect	Baseline testing	Initial follow-up testing	Additional follow-up testing
Hypo- or hyper-thyroidism	TSH (T4 and T3 if TSH is abnormal)	3–6 months	Every 6 months
Hepatotoxicity	AST and ALT	3–6 months	Every 6 months
QT interval prolongation	ECG	Annually	–
Interstitial lung disease	Chest X-ray: Recommended CT chest: Not recommended	Chest X-ray: Unexplained cough or dyspnea or other signs/symptoms suspicious for interstitial lung disease	*CT chest:* As indicated to follow-up ongoing symptoms or chest X-ray findings
Corneal microdeposits (epithelial keratopathy)	Not recommended	Development of visual abnormalities, which may indicate optic neuropathy	–
Dermatological (blue-gray skin discoloration, photosensitivity	Not recommended	Physical examination annually	Development of skin discoloration, severe sunburn
Neurological	Not recommended	Physical examination annually	Development of peripheral neuropathy or other neurological abnormalities

(ALT: alanine transaminase; AST: aspartate transaminase; CT: computed tomography; ECG: electrocardiogram; TdP: torsades de pontes; TSH: thyroid-stimulating hormone)

TABLE 36: AF catheter ablation.

Recommendations for AF catheter ablation (2023 ACC/AHA/ACC/HRS guidelines).

COR	LOE	Recommendations
1	A	In patients with symptomatic AF in whom antiarrhythmic drugs have been ineffective, contraindicated, not tolerated, or not preferred, and continued rhythm control is desired, catheter ablation is useful improve symptoms
1	A	In selected patients (generally younger with few comorbidities) with symptomatic paroxysmal AF in whom rhythm control is desired, catheter ablation is useful as first-line therapy to improve symptoms and reduce progression to persistent AF
1	A	In patients with symptomatic or clinically significant AFL, catheter ablation is useful for improving symptoms
		In patients who are undergoing ablation for AF, ablation of additional clinically significant supraventricular arrhythmias can be useful to reduce the likelihood of future
2a	B-R	In patients (other than younger with few comorbidities) with symptomatic paroxysmal or persistent AF who are being managed with a rhythm-control strategy, catheter ablation as first-line therapy can be useful to improve symptoms
Cost value statement: Intermediate	B-R	Catheter ablation for symptomatic AF provides intermediate economic value compared with antiarrhythmic drug therapy
2b	B-NR	In selected* patients with asymptomatic or minimally symptomatic AF, catheter ablation may be useful for reducing progression of AF and its associated complications

*Younger with few comorbidities and a moderate-to-high burden of AF or persistent AF and AFL.

of 1 study, after 3-year follow-up, catheter ablation continued to be associated with a significant decrease in recurrent atrial tachyarrhythmias when compared with antiarrhythmic drugs. More importantly, episodes of persistent AF developed in only 1.9% of patients randomized to catheter ablation compared with 7.4% of patients in the antiarrhythmic drug arm. All of the studies that have evaluated catheter ablation as an initial strategy for rhythm control in patients with paroxysmal AF, although fairly standard exclusion criteria were used, enrolled relatively young patients (average age approximately 60 years) who had relatively few comorbidities (if present, mainly hypertension).

- AFL is most commonly due to the critical isthmus formed by the inferior vena cava and the tricuspid valve. More rarely, in patients who have not undergone previous ablation procedures, atypical AFL or focal ATs can be observed. Catheter ablation of typical AFL is effective and relatively low risk. In an older meta-analysis of AFL ablation studies, AFL ablation was associated with an acute success rate of 90% and a complication rate of 2.6%. The occurrence of AF after AFL ablation was 34%, with a recurrence rate of 23% in those patients without a history of AF compared with 53% in patients with a history of AF. By 5 years, AF developed in 60–70% of patients regardless of whether the patient had a history of AF before the AFL ablation. Little evidence is available in these studies for the clinical significance of AF after AFL ablation.
- AF can be associated with other atrial arrhythmias, particularly AFL. During ablation for AF, ablation of previously documented or inducible sustained SVT or AFL is useful to reduce the likelihood of recurrent arrhythmias. Although ablation alone for AF in patients with both AF and AFL will reduce the likelihood of AFL, and ablation targeting an inducible SVT in a patient with AF may reduce future AF; in both cases, the likelihood of recurrent arrhythmias is high, although the actual recurrence rate will depend on the specific population. Conversely, prophylactic catheter ablation of the CTI in patients without documented or inducible AFL likely has minimal benefit.
  - Alternatively, in 1 study, cryoballoon PVI as first-line treatment for AFL is equally effective compared with standard

CTI ablation for preventing recurrence of atrial arrhythmia and better at preventing new-onset AF.
- Several randomized trials have compared catheter ablation to AADs as first-line therapy for AF. In the MANTRA- AF study, ablation, and antiarrhythmic drugs as first-line therapy for paroxysmal AF were evaluated. Although no differences in AF were identified during the first 18 months, at 24-month follow-up, ablation was associated with a lower AF burden (ablation 9% vs. antiarrhythmic drugs 18%; $p = 0.004$). Subsequent studies have demonstrated similar results: In the EARLY-AF (Early Aggressive Invasive Intervention for Atrial Fibrillation) study, at 1-year follow-up, recurrent atrial arrhythmias were identified in 43% of the ablation group and 68% of the antiarrhythmic drug group ($p<0.001$), and in the STOP AF First (Cryoballoon Catheter Ablation in an Antiarrhythmic Drug Naive Paroxysmal Atrial Fibrillation) study, recurrent atrial arrhythmias were identified in 25% of the ablation group and 55% of the antiarrhythmic drug group ($p < 0.001$). Procedural complications were observed in 2–5% of patients in all 3 studies. Although AF burden was significantly reduced with ablation compared to antiarrhythmic drug therapy in EARLY-AF, AF burden was low with either strategy (percentage of time in AF: ablation 0.6% vs. antiarrhythmic drugs 3.9%) and in all 3 trials, the average age was ≤60 years. Although these trials enrolled patients with paroxysmal AF, recent studies have consistently found that catheter ablation is more commonly used and also

TABLE 37: Recommendations for techniques and technologies of AF catheter ablation (2023 ACC/AHA/ACC/HRS guidelines).

Strength of recommendation	Recommendations
1	In patients undergoing ablation for AF, PVI is recommended as the primary lesion set for all patients unless a different specific trigger is identified
2b	In patients undergoing ablation for AF, the value of other endpoints beyond PVI such as noninducibility and ablation of additional anatomic ablation targets (e.g., posterior wall sites, low voltage areas, complex fractionated electrograms, and rotors) is uncertain

TABLE 38: Recommendations for management of recurrent AF after catheter ablation (2023 ACC/AHA/ACC/HRS guidelines).

Strength of recommendation	Recommendations
1	In patients with recurrent symptomatic AF after catheter ablation, repeat catheter ablation or antiarrhythmic drug therapy is useful to improve symptoms and get freedom from AF
2a	In some patients who have undergone catheter ablation AF, short-term antiarrhythmic drug therapy after ablation can be useful to reduce early recurrences of atrial arrhythmia and hospitalization

TABLE 39: Recommendations for anticoagulation therapy before and after catheter ablation (2023 ACC/AHA/ACC/HRS guidelines).

Strength of recommendation	Recommendations
1	In patients on warfarin who are undergoing catheter ablation of AF, catheter ablation should be performed on uninterrupted therapeutic anticoagulation with a goal INR of 2.0–3.0
1	In patients on a DOAC who are undergoing catheter ablation of AF, catheter ablation should be performed with either continuous or minimally interrupted oral anticoagulation
1	In patients who have undergone catheter ablation of AF, oral anticoagulation should be continued for at least 3 months after the procedure with a longer duration determined by underlying risk
1	In patients who have undergone catheter ablation of AF, continuation of longer-term oral anticoagulation should be dictated according to the patients' stroke risk (e.g., CHA_2DS_2-VASc score ≥ 2)

effective in patients with persistent AF, particularly if of relatively recent onset (<1 year).

Management of AF in patients with heart failure:
- It can be difficult to determine the extent of the contribution of AF to cardiomyopathy and new onset HFrEF. Allowing AF to

TABLE 40: Complications after AF catheter ablation.

Complication	Frequency of complications	Timing of complicatiosn	Signs and symptoms	Diagnosis	Treatment
LA-esophageal fistula	0.2%	1–4 weeks	Chest pain, pain with swallowing, fever, and stroke symptoms	CT scan of chest	Surgery
Cardiac perforation with tamponade	0.4–1.5%	During procedure	Hypotension	Echocardiography	Pericardiocentesis
CVA/TIA	0.1–1.0%	During procedure and up to 1 week	Neurological findings	MRI or CT scan	Anticoagulate when safe
PV stenosis	0.1–0.8%	Months	Dyspnea and hemoptysis	MRI or CT scan	Stent
Phrenic nerve paralysis	0.2–0.4%	During procedure	Dyspnea	Fluoroscopy	Time
Vascular access complications	1–7%	During procedure and up to 1 month	Pain and swelling at access site	Ultrasound or CT scan	Observation
Vascular access complications requiring surgery	0.1–0.3%	During procedure and up to 1 month	Pain and swelling at access site	Ultrasound or CT scan	Surgery
Death	0.1–0.4%	During procedure			
Pneumonia	0.4–1.0%	Days	Cough and fever	Chest X-ray	Antibiotics

(AF: atrial fibrillation; CT: computed tomography; CVA: cerebrovascular accident; LA: left atrial; MRI: magnetic resonance imaging; PV: pulmonary vein; TIA: transient ischemic attack)

TABLE 41: Recommendations for surgical ablation (2023 ACC/AHA/ACC/HRS guidelines).

Strength of recommendation	Recommendations
2a	For patients with AF who are undergoing cardiac surgery, concomitant surgical ablation can be beneficial to reduce the risk of recurrent AF
2a	In patients undergoing surgical ablation, anticoagulation therapy is reasonable for at least 3 months after the procedure to reduce the risk of stroke or systemic embolism
2b	For patients with symptomatic, persistent AF refractory to antiarrhythmic drug therapy, a hybrid epicardial and endocardial ablation might be reasonable to reduce the risk of recurrent atrial arrhythmia

persist long-term, regardless of reasonable rate control, may result in worsening HF and cardiomyopathy. An early and aggressive approach to rhythm control can reduce AF burden, resulting in favorable ventricular remodeling and halting of any occult arrhythmia-induced cardiomyopathy. In a prespecified subanalysis of 798 HF patients (NYHA class II/ III or LVEF <50%) in EAST-AFNET, early rhythm control significantly improved the composite outcome of death, stroke, or hospitalization for worsening of HF or for ACS (early rhythm control, 94/396; 5.7/100 patient-years) versus usual care (130/402; 7.9/100 patient-years; HR, 0.74; 95% CI 0.56–0.97; $p = 0.03$), and this was not altered by HF status. Safety outcomes in each group were comparable. However, only 17% of the HF population had LVEF <40%. In a post hoc analysis of the CASTLE-AF trial, an AF burden <50% at 6 months postcatheter ablation was associated with significant improvement in the mortality rate and HF hospitalization in patients with AF and HFrEF.

- Multiple RCTs in HFrEF have shown that in patients with symptoms due to AF, ablation improves symptoms and QOL compared with a rate control or an antiarrhythmic drug strategy. In each of 3 meta-analyses, QOL was improved. Although in the past, a trial of antiarrhythmic drugs was advised before pursuing catheter ablation; current data support ablation for AF as first-line therapy even before antiarrhythmic drugs; often patients require both. Data on LVEF, hospitalizations, and mortality rates are less robust, but nearly every larger RCT does show some benefit in these outcomes. Characteristics that may identify patients with a higher likelihood of success or failure with AF catheter ablation have been identified.

- Data for AF catheter ablation are far less robust for HFpEF. The largest analysis for this group of patients was a sub-analysis of the CABANA trial of patients with HF; in this subgroup analysis, patients (35% of the study population) enrolled in the study who had NYHA class II HF experienced improvement in survival, freedom from AF recurrence, and improved QOL compared with the medical therapy group. Most of these had HFpEF. In this subanalysis, catheter ablation was associated with a reduction in the mortality rate and HF. In a meta-analysis on catheter ablation in patients with HFpEF that included 7 studies, patients showed the ablation to be safe and effective and associated with lower hospitalizations and the mortality rates.

ACUTE ISCHEMIC STROKE IN PATIENTS WITH ATRIAL FIBRILLATION

Atrial fibrillation-related ischemic strokes are often fatal or disabling with increased risk of early recurrence within 48 hours to 2 weeks or hemorrhagic transformation, especially in the first days after large cardioembolic lesions and acute recanalization therapy. Notably, ICH is generally associated with higher mortality and morbidity than recurrent ischemic stroke.

Timing of OAC (re)initiation after acute ischemic stroke:
- Early anticoagulation after acute ischemic stroke might cause parenchymal hemorrhage, with potentially serious clinical consequences. Using UFH, LMWH, heparinoids, or VKAs <48 hours after acute ischemic stroke was associated with an increased risk of symptomatic ICH, without significant reduction in recurrent ischemic stroke.

Atrial Fibrillation

Flowchart 12: Management of patients with HF and AF.

Heart failure + AF
- GDMT for HF
- Thromboembolism prophylaxis
- Risk factor modification

Rate control:
- LVEF ≥40% → Beta-blockers or NDCC (1) → Digoxin (2a) → IV Amiodarone* acute rate control (2a)
- LVEF ≤40% → Beta-blockers (1) → Digoxin (2a) → IV Amiodarone* acute rate control (2a)
  - MDCC (Diltiazem, Verapamil) (3: Harm)

Cardioversion if indicated:
- Electrical cardioversion
- Pharmacological cardioversion

Evaluate if appropriate for rhythm control with catheter ablation

Contd...

Atrial Fibrillation

Contd...

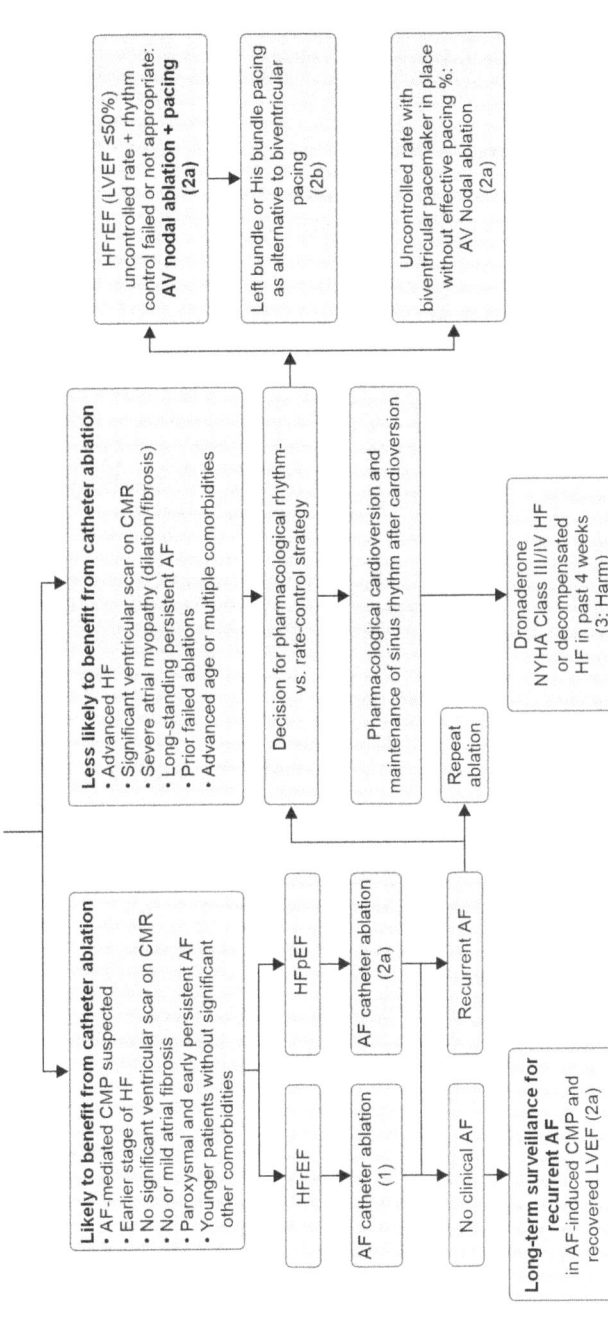

(AF: atrial fibrillation; AV atrioventricular; CMP: cardiomyopathy; CMR: cardiac magnetic resonance; GDMT: guideline-directed medical therapy; HF: heart failure; HFpEF: heart failure with preserved ejection fraction; HFrEF: heart failure with reduced ejection fraction; IV: intravenous; LVEF: left ventricular ejection fraction; NDCC: nonhydropyridine calcium channel blocker; NYHA: New York Heart Association)

TABLE 42: Management of early onset AF, including genetic testing (2023 ACC/AHA/ACC/HRS guidelines).

Strength of recommendation	Recommendations
2b	In patients with an onset of unexplained AF before 30 years of age, electrophysio- logical study to evaluate and treat reentrant supraventricular tachyarrhythmias with a targeted ablation may be reasonable because of the high prevalence of reentrant arrhythmias in this group
2b	In patients with an onset of AF before 45 years of age without obvious risk factors for AF, referral for genetic counseling, genetic testing for rare pathogenic variants, and surveillance for cardiomyopathy or arrhythmia syndromes may be reasonable

TABLE 43: AF with WPW and Preexcitation syndromes (2023 ACC/AHA/ACC/HRS guidelines).

Strength of recommendation	Recommendations
1	Patients with AF with rapid anterograde conduction (preexcited AF) and hemodynamic instability should be treated with electrical cardioversion
1	For patients with AF with rapid anterograde conduction (pre-excited AF), catheter ablation of accessory pathways (Aps) is recommended
1	In patients with AF with rapid anterograde conduction (preexcited AF) and hemodynamic stability, pharmacological cardioversion with intravenous ibutilide or intravenous procainamide is recommended as an alternative to elective cardioversion
3: Harm	For patients with AF with anterograde accessory pathway conduction (preexcited AF), pharmacological agents that block atrioventricular nodal conduction (verapamil, diltiazem, amiodarone, digoxin, adenosine, or beta-blockers) are contraindicated due to risk of precipitating VF or hemodynamic deterioration

TABLE 44: Recommendations for AF with adult congenital heart disease (ACHD) (2023 ACC/AHA/ACC/HRS Guidelines).

Strength of recommendation	Recommendations
1	In adults with congenital heart disease and AF, it is recommended to evaluate for and treat precipitating factors and reversible causes of AF, recognizing that residual hemodynamic sequelae may contribute to the occurrence of the arrhythmia
1	In adults with AF and moderate or complex congenital heart disease, electrophysiological procedures should be performed by operators with expertise in ACHD procedures and in collaboration with an ACHD cardiologist, ideally in specialized centers, when available
1	In adults with congenital heart disease and symptomatic or hemodynamically significant paroxysmal or persistent AF, an initial strategy of rhythm control is recommended regardless of lesion severity as AF in this population is often poorly tolerated
2a	In symptomatic patients with simple congenital heart disease with antiarrhythmic drug-refractory AF, it is reasonable to choose ablation over long-term antiarrhythmic therapies
2b	In adults with congenital heart disease with AF undergoing PVI, it may be reasonable to include an ablative strategy in the right atrium directed at reentrant arrhythmia secondary to atriotomy scars and the CTI
2b	In adults with AF and moderate or severe forms of congenital heart disease, particularly those with low-flow states such as Fontan circulation, blind-ending cardiac chambers, and cyanosis, it may be reasonable to treat with anticoagulation independent of conventional risk score to reduce risk of thromboembolic events

Flowchart 13: Treatment of AF after cardiac surgery (2023 ACC/AHA/ACC/HRS guidelines).

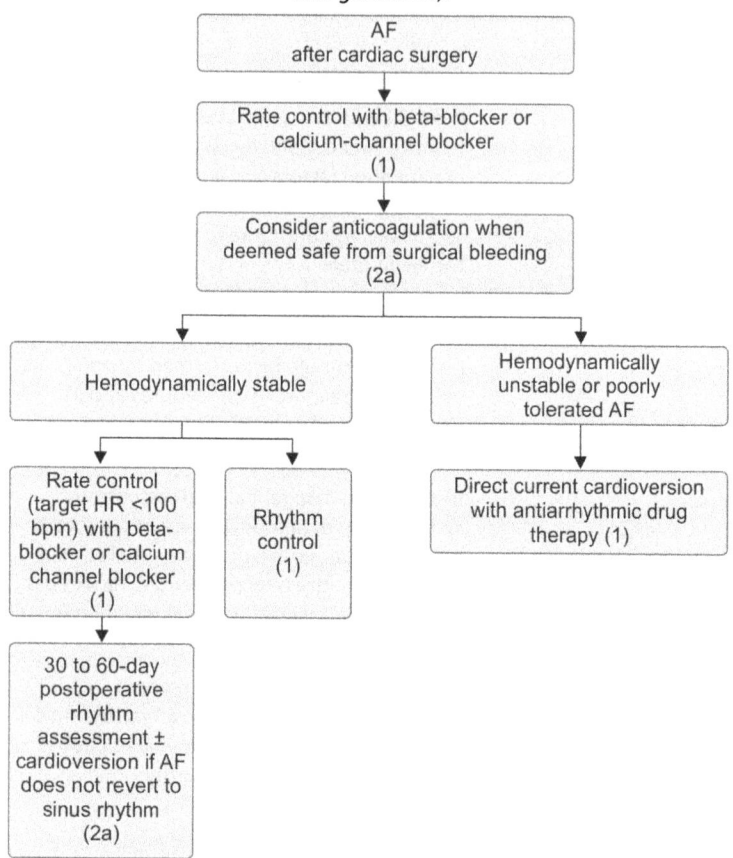

TABLE 45: Recommendations for pulmonary disease (2023 ACC/AHA/ACC/HRS guidelines).

Strength of recommendation	Recommendations
2a	In patients with AF and COPD, it is reasonable to use cardioselective beta-blockers for the rate control of AF, especially where other indications exist (e.g., MI and HF)
2a	In patients with pulmonary hypertension (PH) with pulmonary vascular disease and AF or AFL, a rhythm-control strategy is reasonable to improve functional status and potentially prolong survival

Flowchart 14: Acute medical or surgical illness.

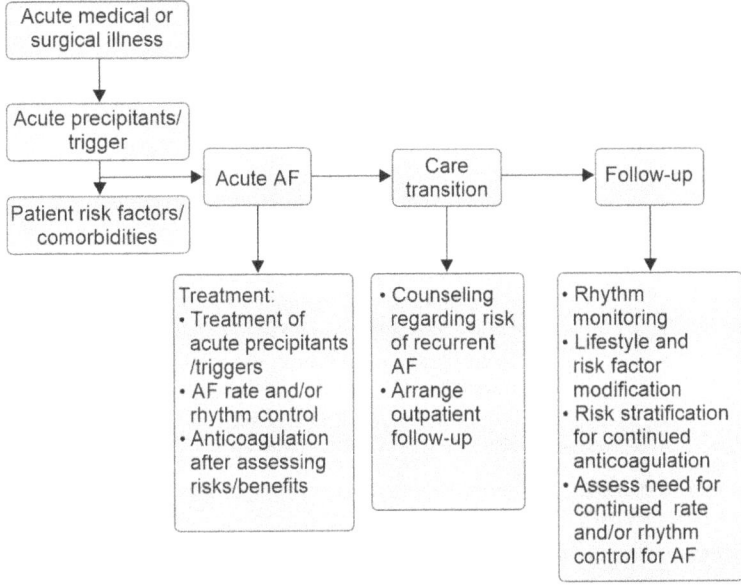

TABLE 46: Recommendations for pregnancy with AF (2023 ACC/AHA/ACC/HRS guidelines).

Strength of recommendation	Recommendations
1	In pregnant patients with AF, DCCV is safe for the patient and fetus and should be performed in the same manner as in patients who are not pregnant
2b	In pregnant individuals with structurally normal hearts and hemodynamically stable AF, pharmacological cardioversion with agents having history of safe use in pregnancy, such as intravenous procainamide, may be considered
2a	In pregnant individuals with AF and without structural heart disease, antiarrhythmic agents with history of safe use in pregnancy (e.g., flecainide and sotalol) are reasonable for maintenance of sinus rhythm

Contd...

Contd...

Strength of recommendation	Recommendations
2a	In pregnant individuals with persistent AF, rate-control agents with a record of safety in pregnancy, such as beta-blockers (e.g., propranolol or metoprolol) and digoxin, either alone or in combination with beta-blockers, are reasonable as first-line agents
2b	Pregnant individuals with AF and elevated risk of stroke may be considered for anticoagulation with the recognition that no anticoagulation strategy is completely safe for both the mother and fetus and an SDM discussion should take place regarding risks of both mother and fetus

TABLE 47: Anticoagulation strategies during pregnancy.

Antenatal options

	Method 1	Method 2	Method 3	Alternative method 4
First trimester	Warfarin ≤5 mg	LMWH	UFH	LMWH
Second trimester	Warfarin	Warfarin	Warfarin	LMWH
Third trimester	Warfarin	Warfarin	Warfarin	LMWH

Delivery planning

	Method 1	Method 2
	Method 1	Method 2
1 week before	Discontinue warfarin → continuous IV UFH	Dose-adjusted LMWH
36 hours before	Continuous IV UFH	Switch to continuous IV UFH
4–6 hours before	Stop IV heparin	Stop IV heparin

- Reportedly, the 90-day risk of recurrent ischemic stroke outweighs the risk of symptomatic ICH in AF patients receiving a NOAC 4–14 days after the acute event (ischemic stroke recurrence rates after mild/moderate ischemic stroke significantly increased with a later NOAC administration, e.g., >14 days). In a small RCT,

Atrial Fibrillation

TABLE 48: Cardio-oncology and anticoagulation considerations (2023 ACC/AHA/ACC/HRS guidelines).

Strength of recommendation	Recommendations
2a	For patients with AF who are at increased risk of systemic thromboembolism and mild or moderate liver disease (Child–Pugh* Class A or B), OAC therapy is reasonable in the absence of clinically significant liver disease-induced coagulopathy of thrombocytopenia
2a	For patients with AF who are at increased risk of systemic thromboembolism and mild or moderate liver disease (Child–Pugh Class A or B) and who are deemed to be candidates for anticoagulation, it is reasonable to prescribe DOACs (Child–Pugh, Class A: any DOAC; Child–Pugh Class B: apixaban, dabigatran, or edoxaban over warfarin)
3: Harm	For patients with AF and moderate liver disease (Child–Pugh Class B) at increased risk of systemic thromboembolism, rivaroxaban is contraindicated due to the potentially increased risk of bleeding

*Child–Pugh scoring is used to assess the severity of liver disease, primarily cirrhosis in patients with diagnosed liver disease.
- *Child–Pugh A (mild):* 5–6 points
- *Child–Pugh B (moderate):* 7–9 points
- *Child–Pugh C (severe):* 10–15 points

The score is based on five variables: Encephalopathy (none = 1 point, grade 2 = 2 points, grade 3 and 4 = 3 points); ascites (none = 1 point, slight = 2 points, moderate = 3 points); total bilirubin (<2 mg/mL = 1 point, 2–3 mg/mL = 2 points, >3 mg/mL = 3 points); albumin (>3.5 mg/mL = 1 point, 2.8–3.5 mg/mL = 2 points, <2.8 mg/mL = 3 points); INR (<1.7 = 1 point, INR 1.7–2.2 = 2 points, INR >2.2 = 3 points).

TABLE 49: Recommendations for cancer with AF and anticoagulation considerations (2023 ACC/AHA/ACC/HRS guidelines).

Strength of recommendation	Recommendations
1	In patients with cancer and AF, multidisciplinary communication including cardiology, oncology and other clinicians, and SDM with the patient is recommended to optimize cancer and AF treatment and to reduce the risk of drug–drug interactions, QTc prolongation, proarrhythmia, bleeding, and thromboembolism

Contd...

Contd...

Strength of recommendation	Recommendations
2a	In patients who are to be initiated on cancer therapies associated with an increased risk of developing AF, increased vigilance for incident AF and treatment of contributing factors are reasonable to decrease morbidity
2a	In most patients with AF and cancer (remote history of receiving active cancer treatment), DOACs are reasonable to choose over VKAs for stroke risk reduction

BOX 1: Thrombotic and bleeding issues in PCI.

Thrombotic risk factors	Bleeding risk factors
• Diabetes mellitus requiring therapy • Prior ACS/recurrent myocardial infarction • Multivessel CAD • Concomitant CAD • Premature CAD (occurring at age of <45 y) or accelerated CAD (new lesion with 2 years) • CKD (eFR <60 mL/min) • Clinical presentation (ACS) • Multivessel stenting • Complex revascularization (left main stenting, bifurcation lesion stenting, chronic total occlusion intervention, and last patient vessel stenting) • Prior stent thrombosis on antiplatelet treatment • Procedural factors (stent expansion), residual dissection, stent length, etc.)	• Hypertension • Abnormal renal or liver function • Stroke or ICH history • Bleeding history or bleeding diathesis (e.g., anemia with hemoglobin <110 g/L) • Labile INR (if on VKA) • Elderly (>65 years) • Drugs (concomitant OAC and antiplatelet therapy, NSAIDs), excessive alcohol consumption *Strategies to reduce bleeding associated with PCI* • Radial artery access • PPIs in patients taking DAPT who are at increased risk of bleeding (e.g., the elderly, dyspepsia, gastroesophageal reflux disease. *Helicobacter pylori* infection and chronic alcohol use) • Nonadministration of unfractionated heparin in patients on VKA with INR >2.5 • Pretreatment with aspirin only, add a P2Y12 inhibitor when coronary anatomy is known if STEMI • GP IIb/IIa inhibitors only for bailout or periprocedural complications • Shorter duration of combined antithrombotic therapy

TABLE 50: Recommendations for patients with AF and ACS, PCI, or CCS (2023 ACC/AHA/ACC/HRS guidelines).

General recommendations for patients with AF and an indication for concomitant antiplatelet therapy	Class
In AF patients eligible for NOACs, it is recommended to use a NOAC in preference to a VKA in combination with antiplatelet therapy	I
In patients at high bleeding risk (HAS-BLED ≥3), rivaroxaban 5 mg OD should be considered in preference to rivaroxaban 20 mg OD for the duration of concomitant single or DAPT to mitigate bleeding risk	IIa
In patients at high bleeding risk (HAS-BLED ≥3), dabigatran 110 mg BID should be considered in preference to dabigatran 150 mg BID for the duration of concomitant single or DAPT to mitigate bleeding risk	IIa
In patients with an indication for a VKA in combination with antiplatelet therapy, the VKA dosing should be carefully regulated with a target INR of 2.0–2.5 and TTR >70%	IIa
Recommendation for AF patients with ACS	
In AF patients with ACS undergoing an uncomplicated PCI, early cessation (≤1 week) of aspirin and continuation of dual therapy with an OAC and a P2Y12 inhibitor (preferably clopidogrel) for up to 12 months is recommended if the risk of stent thrombosis is low or if concerns about bleeding risk prevail over concerns of risk of stent thrombosis, irrespective of the type of stent-used	I
Triple therapy with aspirin, clopidogrel, and an OAC for longer than 1 week after an ACS should be considered when risk of stent, thrombosis outweighs the bleeding risk, with the total duration (≤1 month) decided according to assessment of these risks, and the treatment plan should be clearly specified at hospital discharge	IIa
Recommendations in AF patients with a CCS undergoing PCI	
After uncomplicated PCI, early cessation (≤1 week) of aspirin and continuation of dual therapy with OAC for up to 6 months and clopidogrel is recommended if the risk of stent thrombosis is low or if concerns about bleeding risk prevails over concerns of risk of stent thrombosis irrespective of the type of stent used	I
Triple therapy with aspirin, clopidogrel, and an OAC for longer than 1 week should be considered when risk of stent thrombosis outweighs the bleeding risk, with the total duration (≤1 month) decided according to assessment of these risks, and the treatment plan should be clearly specified at hospital discharge	IIa

rivaroxaban use within 5 days after mild ischemic stroke in AF patients was associated with similar event rates compared with VKA.

As high-quality RCT-derived evidence to inform optimal timing of anticoagulation after acute ischemic stroke is lacking, OAC use in the early post-stroke period is currently based on expert consensus. Several ongoing RCTs [ELAN (NCT03148457), OPTIMAS (EudraCT, 2018- 003859-3), TIMING (NCT02961348), and START (NCT03021928)] are investigating early (<1 week) versus late NOAC initiation in patients with AF-related ischemic stroke.

Long-term secondary stroke prevention:
- There is no evidence that the addition of aspirin to OAC or supratherapeutic INRs would improve outcomes in secondary stroke prevention.
- Compared with VKAs, NOACs were associated with better efficacy in secondary stroke prevention and better safety regarding ICH in a meta-analysis of landmark NOAC AF trial.
- Good adherence to OAC treatment is essential for effective secondary stroke prevention.

There is some evidence to support that strokes can induce AF through neurogenic mechanisms. The first study showed that damage to the insulin increases the odds of AF detection after ischemic stroke and is more prevalent in patients with AF diagnosed after stroke (AFDAS) than among those without AF.

The second study explained the reason why AFDAS detected soon after ischemic stroke is associated with a low risk of ischemic stroke recurrence.

EVIDENCE BASE FOR INTRODUCTION OR REINTRODUCTION OF ANTICOAGULATION AFTER HEMORRHAGIC STROKE

There is inadequate evidence as of date to recommend whether oral anticoagulation should be initiated or reinitiated after ICH to protect against risk of ischemia stroke or other thromboembolic events in these patients. The APACHE-HF trial randomized 101 patients who survived 7–90 days after anticoagulation-associated ICH either to apixaban or no OAC. During a median of 1-9 years of follow-up, there was no difference in nonfatal stroke or vascular death with an annual event rate of 12.6% with apixaban and 11.9% with no OAC ($p = 0.90$). START was an open-label RCT in 203 patients with AF after symptomatic spontaneous ICH. Starting OAC was not noninferior to avoiding long-term OAC (≥1 year) with ICH recurrence in 8% versus 4%. Mortality occurred in 22% patients in the OAC group versus 11% patients where OACs were avoided.

Until additional trial-evidence on this clinical challenge of post-ICH anticoagulation becomes available, an individualized

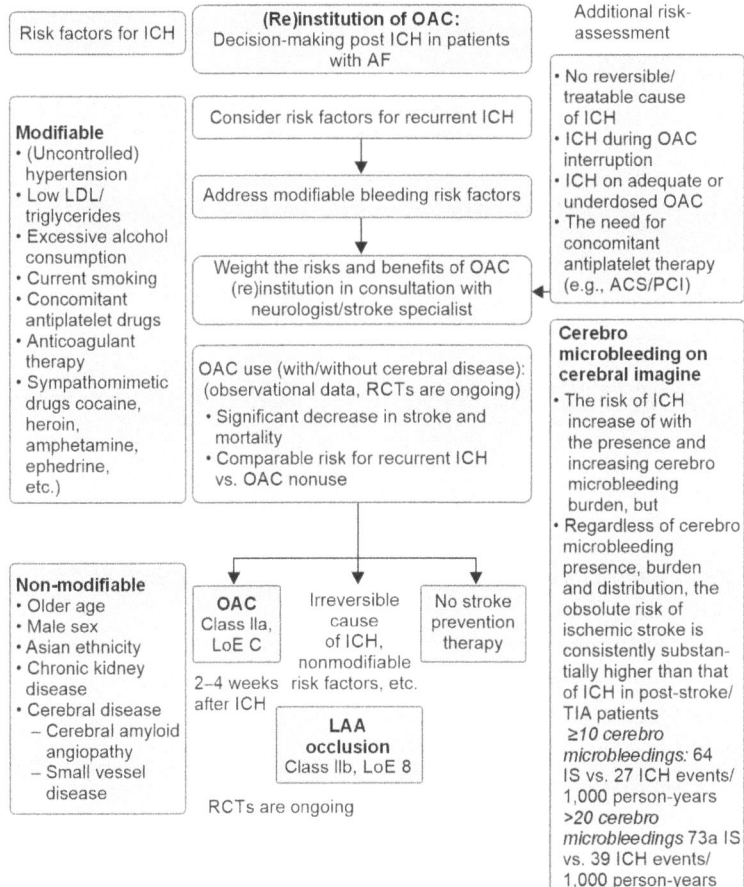

Flowchart 15: Initiation of anticoagulation post-intracranial bleeding.

Flowchart 16: Recommendations for stroke prevention in AF patients after intracranial hemorrhage.

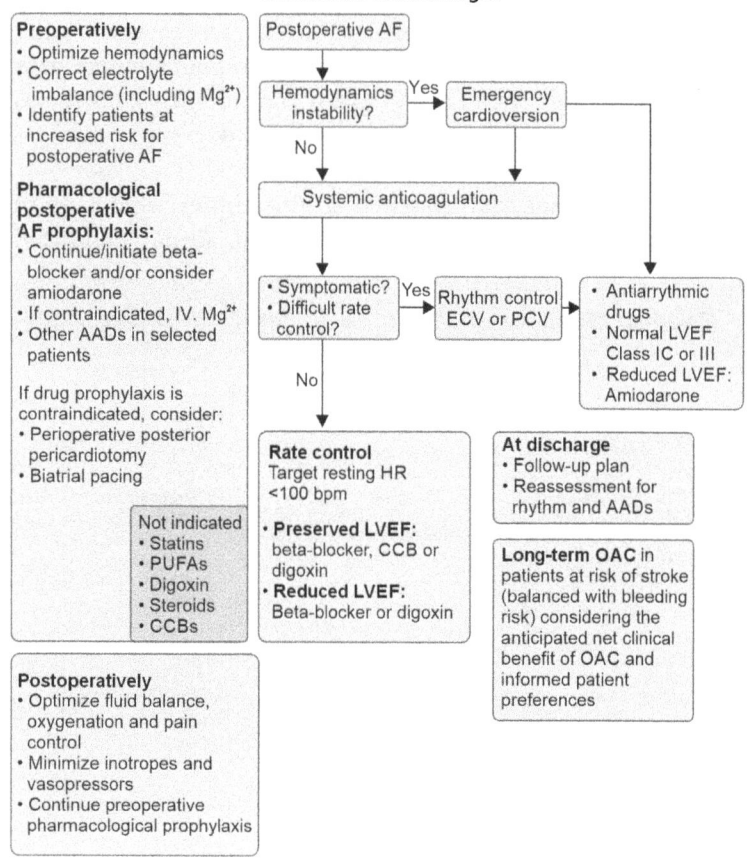

multidisciplinary approach is advised in consultation with an expert team of neurologists.

In AF patients at high-risk of ischemia stroke, reinitiation of OAC with preference for NOACs over VKAs in NOAC-eligible patients should be considered in consultation with a neurologist/stroke specialist after:
- A trauma-related ICH
- Acute spontaneous ICH (which includes subdural, subarachnoid, or intracerebral hemorrhage) after careful consideration of risk and benefits.

SUGGESTED READING

1. Cheung CC, Nattel S, Macle LM, Andrade JG. Management of atrial fibrillation in 2021: An updated comparison of the current CCS/CHRS, ESC and AHA/ACC/HRS Guidelines. Can J Cardiol. 2021;37(10):1607-18.
2. Joglar JA, Chung MK, Armbruster AL, Benjamin EJ, Chyou JY, Cronin EM, et al. 2023 ACC/AHA/ACCP/HRS Guideline for the diagnosis and management of atrial fibrillation: A Report of the American College of Cardiology/American Heart Association Joint Committee on Clinical Practice Guidelines. Circulation. 2024;149(1):e1-e156.
3. Saleh K, Halder S. Arial fibrillation: A contemporary update. Clin Med (Lond). 2023;23(5):437-41.
4. VanGelder IC, Rienstra M, Bunting KV, Casado-Arroyo R, Caso V, Crijns HJGM, et al. 2024 ESC Guidelines for the management of atrial fibrillation developed in collaboration with the European Association for Cardio-Thoracic Surgery (EACTS): Developed by the task force for the management of atrial fibrillation of the European Society of Cardiology (ESC), with the special contribution of the European Heart Rhythm Association (EHRA) of the ESC Endorsed by the European Stroke Organization (ESO). Eur Heart J. 2024;45(36):3314-414.

CHAPTER 7

Tachycardias

Soumitra Kumar

Tachycardias can be broadly classified based on the QRS complex duration into:
- Narrow QRS complex tachycardia when QRS is <120 ms in duration.
- Wide QRS complex tachycardia when QRS is ≥120 ms in duration.

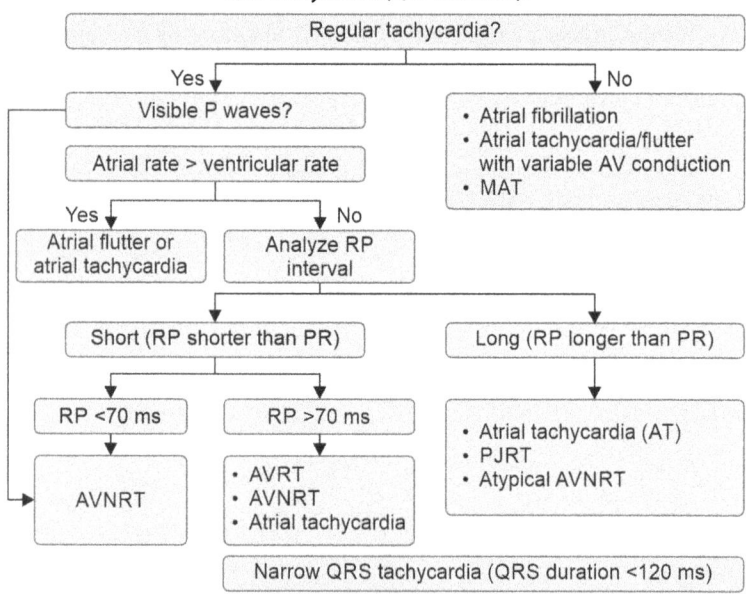

Flowchart 1: Approach to the patient with narrow QRS tachycardia (QRS duration).

*In surface ECG, the onset of QRS wave to the onset of P wave, i.e., RP = 90 ms; as opposed to 70 ms in case of ventriculoatrial interval.
(AT: atrial tachycardia; AV: atrioventricular; AVNRT: AV nodal reentry tachycardia; AVRT: atrioventricular reciprocating tachycardia; MAT: multifocal atrial tachycardia; PJRT: permanent junctional reciprocating tachycardia)

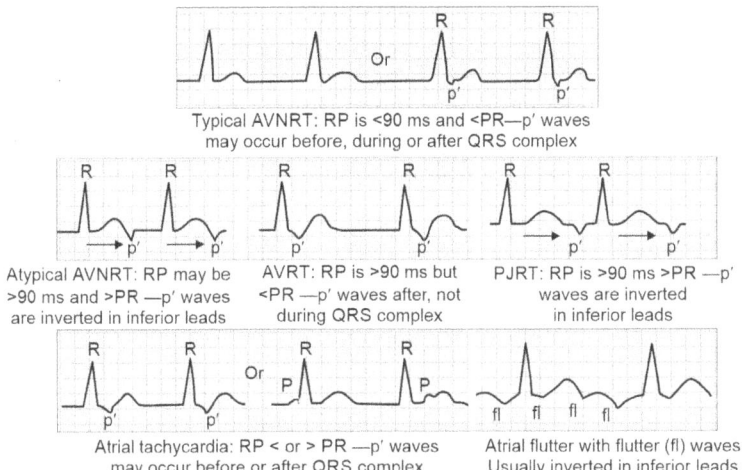

Fig. 1: P wave morphology and its relation with RP and PR Intervals in narrow QRS tachycardia. (AVNRT: AV nodal re-entrant tachycardia. AVRT: AV re-entry tachycardia. PJRT: permanent form of AV junctional reciprocating tachycardia)

P wave morphology and its relationship with RP and PR intervals in narrow QRS tachycardia.

THERAPY OF SINUS TACHYCARDIAS
Focal Atrial Tachycardia

Focal atrial tachycardia (AT) is defined as an organized atrial rhythm ≥100 bpm arising from a discrete origin and disseminating over both atria in a centrifugal pattern. The ventricular rate varies, depending on AV nodal conduction. In asymptomatic young people (<50 years of age), the prevalence of focal AT has been reported to be as low as 0.34% with an increased prevalence of 0.46% in symptomatic arrhythmia patients. Most studies have not reported any gender preferences.

Symptoms may include palpitations, shortness of breath, chest pain, and rarely syncope or presyncope. The arrhythmia may be sustained or incessant. Dynamic, forms with recurrent interruption and reinitiations have also been described.

If patients with pulmonary vein-related (PV) AT, the focus is located at the ostium of the vein (or within 1 cm of the designated ostium) rather than further distally (2-4 cm).

Tachycardias

Flowchart 2: Approach to the patient with narrow QRS complex tachycardia.

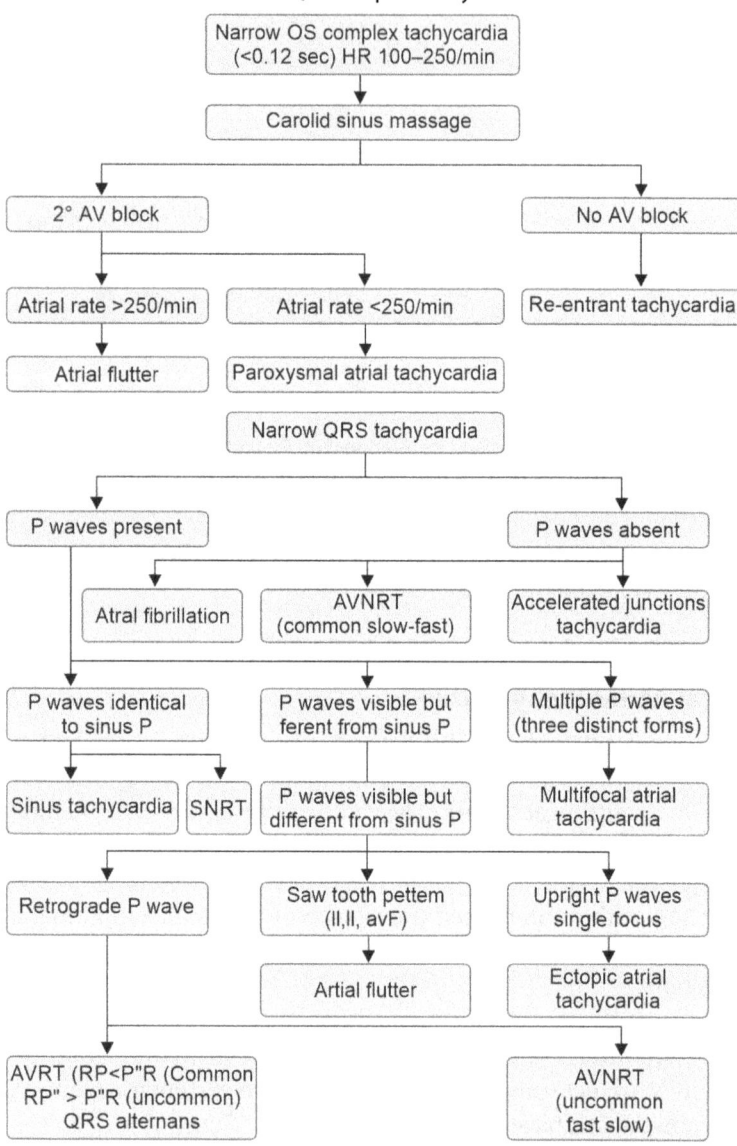

(AVNRT: AV nodal re-entry tachycardia; AVRT: atrioventricular reciprocating tachycardia; SNRT: sinus node recovery time; avF: ateriovenous fistula)

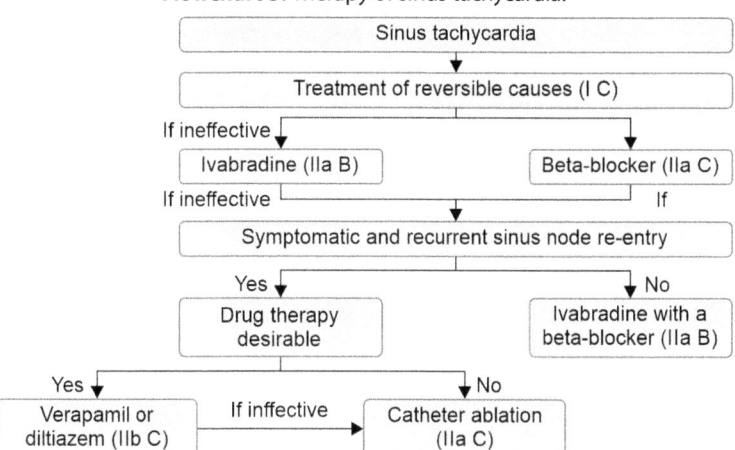

Flowchart 3: Therapy of sinus tachycardia.

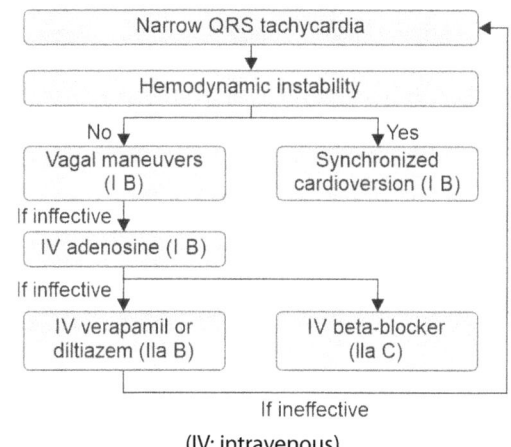

Flowchart 4: Acute therapy of narrow QRS tachycardia in the absence of an established diagnosis.

(IV: intravenous)

Diagnosis

P wave identification from a 12-lead ECG recording during tachycardia is critical. Depending on the AV conduction and AT rate, the P waves may be hidden in the QRS or T waves. The P waves are monographic with stable CL, which helps to rule our organized AF. Adenosine injection can help by slowing the ventricular rate

Flowchart 5: Acute therapy of focal atrial tachycardia.

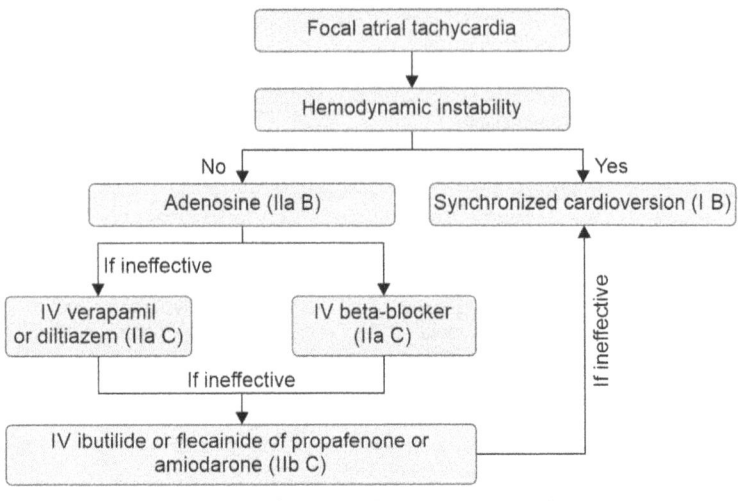

(AT: atrial tachycardia; IV: intravenous)

Flowchart 6: Chronic therapy of focal atrial tachycardia.

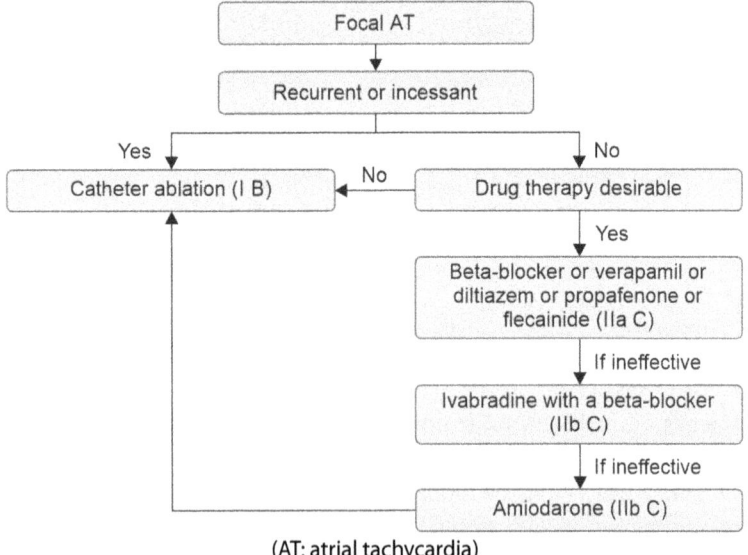

(AT: atrial tachycardia)

TABLE 1: ESC 2019 recommendations for the therapy of multifocal atrial tachycardia.

Recommendations	Class[a]	Level[b]
Acute therapy		
Treatment of an underlying condition is recommended as a first step, If feasible	I	C
IV beta-blockers or IV nondihydropyridine calcium channel blockers (verapamil or diltiazem) should be considered	IIa	B
Chronic therapy		
Oral verapamil or diltiazem should be considered for patients with recurrent symptomatic multifocal AT in the absence of HFrEF	IIa	B
A selective beta-blocker should be considered for patients with recurrent symptomatic multifocal AT	IIa	B
AV nodal ablation followed by pacing (preferable biventricular or His-bundle pacing) should be considered for patients with LV dysfunction due to recurrent multifocal AT refractory to drug therapy	IIa	C

IV = Verapamil and diltiazem are contraindicated in the presence of hypotension or HFrEF
IV = Beta-blockers are contraindicated in the presence of decompensated heart failure
Note:
[a]Class of recommendation
[b]Level of evidence
(AT: atrial tachycardia; HF: heart failure; HFrEF: heart failure with reduced ejection fraction; IV: intravenous; LV: left ventricular)

or less frequently, by terminating focal AT. A discrete P wave with an intervening isoelectric interval suggests a focal AT. However, distinguishing focal from macroreentrant arrhythmias by surface ECG is not always possible. The presence of an isoelectric line does not always rule out a macroreentrant mechanism, particularly in the presence of scar atrial tissue (from structural heart disease or previous extensive ablation/surgery procedures). In a normal heart and in the absence of pervious ablation, the usual ECG localization rules apply.

MACROREENTRANT ATRIAL TACHYCARDIAS

Atrial flutter and focal AT are traditionally defined according to the ECG appearance of continuous regular electrical activity, most commonly a saw-tooth pattern, versus discrete P waves with an isoelectric line in between ECGs with flutter-like appearances are mostly due to macro-co-entrant atrial circuits but microreentry is also possible.

However, MRATs with a significant part of the activation of the circuit in protected areas may display a focal AT pattern, with discrete P waves.

Typical Atrial Flutter: Counter-clockwise and Clockwise

Typical common atrial flutter is the most frequent cavotricuspid isthmus (CTI)-dependent flutter, i.e., a macroreentry circuit around the tricuspid annulus using the CTI as a critical passage at the inferior boundary. Activation goes downward in the RA-free wall, through the CTI, and ascends in the right septum. Activation of the LA is passive. The upper part of the circuit may be anterior or posterior to the superior vena cava. This activation is also known as counter-clockwise (or anticlockwise) when seen from the apex. When the circuit is activated in the opposite direction, i.e., clockwise, it results in different ECG pattern, then called typical reverse flutter.

Diagnosis

In counter-clockwise flutter, the circuit results in regular atrial activation from 250 to 330 bpm with negative saw-tooth waves in inferior leads and positive waves in V1. In clockwise flutter, ECG flutter-waves in inferior leads look positive and broad, and are frequently bimodal negative in V1. Typical atrial flutter has a strong reproducible anatomical dependence, resulting in the morphological reproducibility of the ECG. However, this well-recognized ECG pattern may be significantly altered when atrial activation has been modified, as it is in cardiac surgery involving atrial tissue, after extensive radiofrequency ablation, or in advanced atrial disease. Antiarrhythmic drugs may also modify the typical ECG pattern.

TABLE 2: Recommendations for the therapy of macro-re-entrant atrial arrhythmias (MRATs)/atrial flutter.

Recommendations	Class	Level
Anticoagulation, as in AF, is recommended for patients with atrial flutter and concomitant AV	I	B
Patients with atrial flutter without AF should be considered for anticoagulation, but the threshold for initiation has not been established	IIa	C
Acute therapy		
Hemodynamically unstable patients: Synchronized DC cardioversion is recommended for hemodynamically unstable patients hemodynamically stable patients	I	B
IV ibutilide or IV or oral (in-hospital) dofetilide is recommended for conversion to sinus rhythm	I	B
Low-energy (≤100 biphasic) electrical cardioversion is recommended for conversion to sinus rhythm	I	B
High-rate atrial pacing is recommended for termination of atrial flutter in the presence of an implanted pacemaker or defibrillator	I	B
IV beta-blockers or nondihydropyridine calcium channel blockers (verapamil or diltiazem) (IV) should be considered for control of rapid ventricular rate	IIa	B
Invasive and noninvasive high-rate atrial pacing may be considered for termination of atrial flutter	IIb	B
IV amiodarone may be tried if the above are not available or desirable	IIb	C
Propafenone and flecainide are not recommended for conversion to sinus rhythm	III	B
Chronic therapy		
Catheter ablation should be considered after the first episode of symptomatic typical atrial flutter	IIa	B
Catheter ablation is recommended for symptomatic, recurrent episodes of CTI-dependent flutter	I	A
Catheter ablation is experienced centers is recommended for symptomatic, recurrent episodes of non-CTI-dependent flutter	I	B

Contd...

Contd...

Recommendations	Class	Level
Catheter ablation is recommended in patients with persistent atrial flutter or in the presence of depressed LV systolic function due to TCM	I	B
Beta-blockers or non-dihydropyridine calcium channel blockers (verapamil or diltiazem, in the absence of HFrEF should be considered if ablation is not desirable of feasible	IIa	C
Amiodarone may be considered to maintain sinus rhythm if the above measures fail	IIb	C
AV nodal ablation with subsequent pacing (ablate and pace), either biventricular or His-bundle pacing, should be considered if all the above fail and the patient has symptomatic persistent macroreentrant atrial arrhythmias with fast ventricular rates	IIa	C

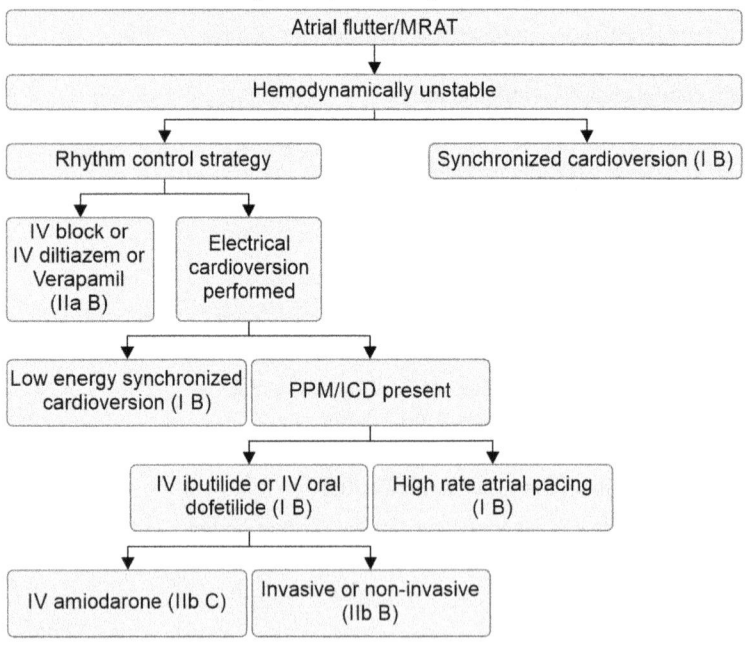

Flowchart 7: Acute therapy of stable atrial flutter or macroreentrant atrial tachycardia (ESC 2019 guidelines).

Flowchart 8: Chronic therapy of atrial flutter/macroreentrant atrial tachycardia (ESC 2019 guidelines).

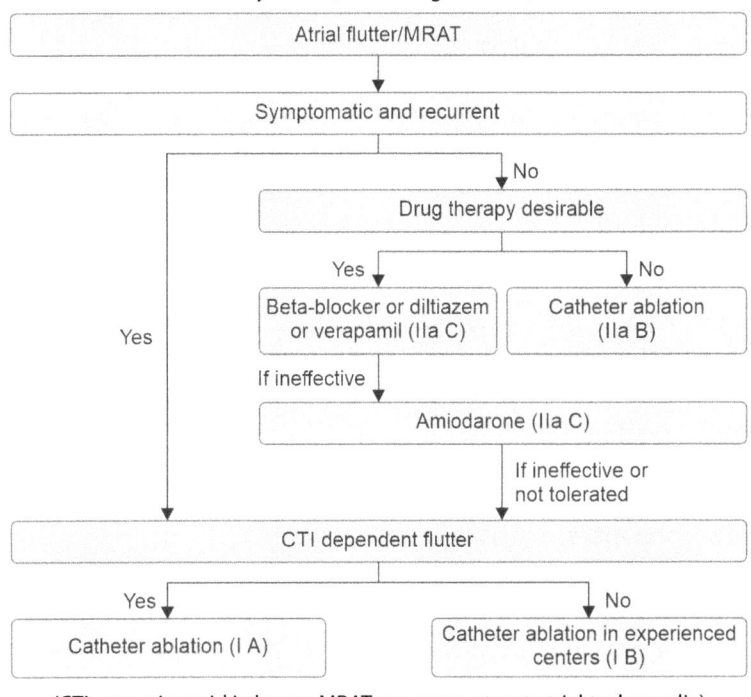

(CTI: cavotricuspid isthmus; MRAT: macroreentrant atrial tachycardia)

In these situations, an atypical ECG does not rule out a circuit of typical flutter using the CTI.

Typical flutter is related to AF in clinical practice, with both being associated with similar clinical settings and coexisting in the same patients. AF may trigger atrial flutter, and after typical flutter ablation AF is frequent. Typical flutter may also frequently occur in patients treated for AF with class IC drugs or amiodarone. In this case, flutter rate may be reduced to <200 bpm facilitating 1:1 AV conduction. The action of antiarrhythmic drugs on ventricular activation may result in wide QRS tachycardia.

Beyond symptoms associated with high-rate and loss of atrial kick, reversible systolic dysfunction, and subsequent DCM are not unusual.

OTHER CAVOTRICUSPID ISTHMUS-DEPENDENT MACROREENTRANT ATRIAL TACHYCARDIA

An atypical ECG pattern may not exclude CTI-dependent MRAT. Lower-loop reentry refers to a circuit rotating around the inferior vena cava instead of around the tricuspid annulus. It may be clockwise or counter-clockwise. when rotating counter-clockwise, it might be considered a variant of typical counter-clockwise flutter with a caudal shift of the cranial turning point posterior to the entry of the superior vena cava, resulting in a similar ECG appearance. Figure-of-eight double-loop reentry may also occur around the inferior vena cava and tricuspid annulus, and mimic typical clockwise atrial flutter. Other circuits using part of the CTI or even restricted inside it are in essence CTI-dependent with a similar ECG appearance to typical common flutter.

Noncavotricuspid Isthmus-dependent Macroreentrant Atrial Tachycardia

The terms non-CTI-dependent MRAT and atypical flutter are used interchangeably, and describe flutter waves in the ECG not suggestive of typical circuits. The pitfall with this use comes from the atypical ECG that may happen when typical circuits develop in diseased atria, most frequently after surgery or extensive ablation, or under the effects of antiarrhythmic drugs. Conversely, upper-loop reentry may mimic a typical flutter ECG pattern without being CTI-dependent. True atypical flutter is actually a posthoc diagnosis when the circuit has been outlined and dependence on CTI has been ruled out.

ATRIOVENTRICULAR JUNCTIONAL ARRHYTHMIAS

Atrioventricular Nodal Reentrant Tachycardia

Atrioventricular nodal reentrant tachycardia (AVNRT) denotes reentry in the area of the atrioventricular node (AVN), but the exact circuit remains elusive. The AVN is a three-dimensional structures with greater variability in the space constraint of tissue, and poor gap junction connectivity due to differential expression of connexin isoforms., conditions that provide an explanation of or dual conduction and nodal reentrant arrhythmogenesis. There has also been considerable histological and electrophysiological evidence that the right and left inferior extensions of the human AVN, and the atrionodal inputs that they facilities may provide the anatomical substrate for the slow pathway. Thus, comprehensive models of the tachycardia circuit for all forms of AVNRT based on the concept of atrionodal inputs have been proposed.

Onset of AVNRT seems to occur bimodally over time. In many patients, attacks indeed manifest early in life. Whereas in a

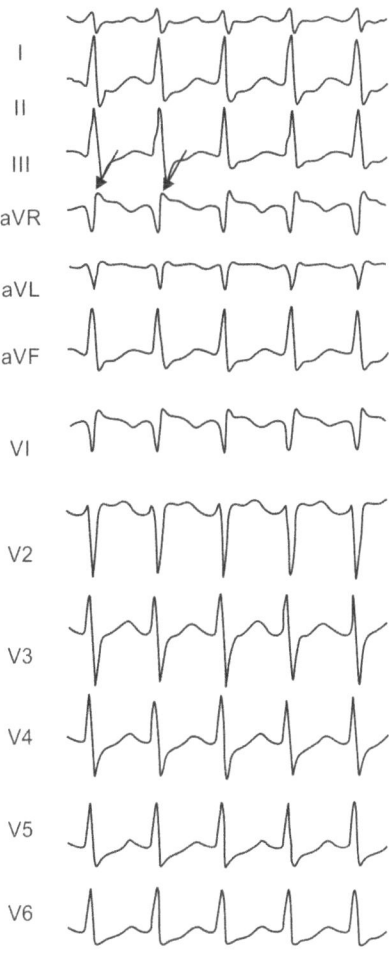

Fig. 2: Typical atrioventricular nodal reentrant tachycardia.

substructural proportion of patients AVNRT starts later, e.g., in the fourth or fifth decade of life. One-half of the patients with minimal symptoms and short-lived, infrequent episodes of tachycardia may become asymptomatic within the next 13 years. AVNRT may result in AF that usually, although not invariably, is eliminated following catheter ablation of AVNRT. Familial AVNRT should be considered.

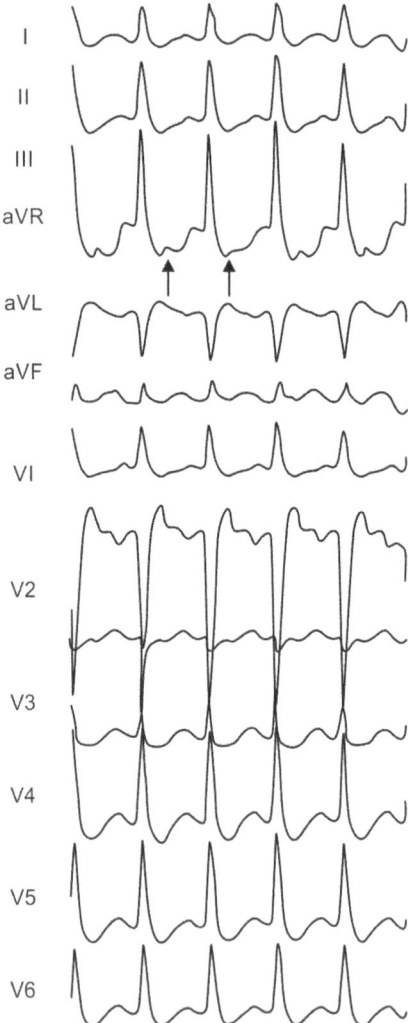

Fig. 3: Atypical atrioventricular nodal reentrant tachycardia.

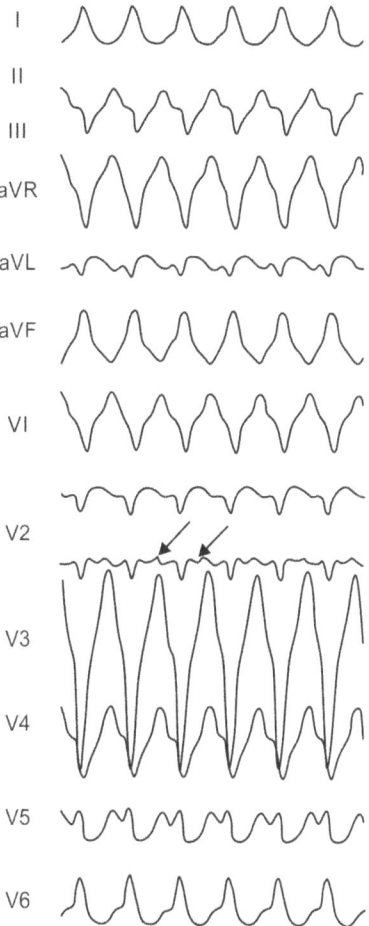

Fig. 4: Atypical AVNRT with (unusual) left bundle branch block aberration.

	HA	VA (His)	AH/HA
TABLE 3: Classification of atrioventricular nodal re-entrant tachycardia types.			
Typical AVNRT	≤70 ms	≥60 ms	>1
Atypical AVNRT	>70 ms	>60 ms	Variable

Flowchart 9: Acute therapy of AVNRT (ESC 2019 Guidelines).

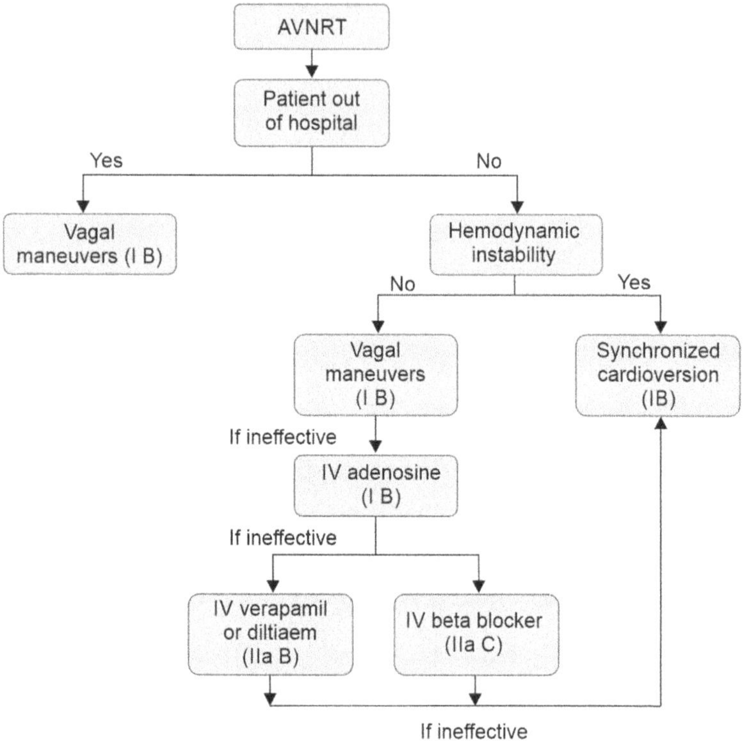

(AVNRT: atrioventricular nodal reentrant tachycardia; IV: intravenous)

Flowchart 10: Chronic therapy atrioventricular nodal re-entrant tachycardia (AVNRT) (ESC 2019 Guidelines).

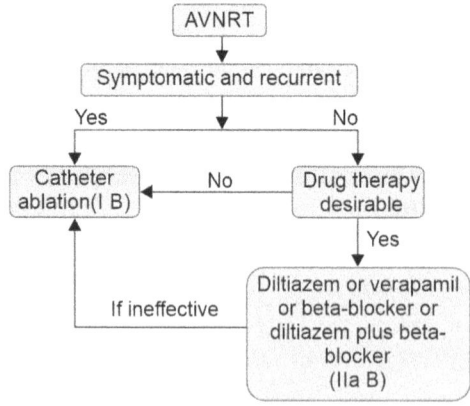

TABLE 4: Recommendations for the management of atrioventricular nodal re-entrant tachycardia (AVNRT) (ESC 2019 Guidelines).

Recommendation	Class	Level
Acute therapy		
Hemodynamically unstable patients: Synchronized DC cardioversion is recommended for hemodynamically unstable patients	I	B
Hemodynamically sable growth: Vagal maneuvers, preferably in the supine position with leg elevation, are recommended	I	B
Adenosine (6–18 mg IV bolus) is recommended if vagal maneuvers fail	I	B
Verapamil or diltiazem IV should be considered if vagal maneuvers and adenosine fail	IIa	B
Beta-blockers (IV esmolol or metoprolol) should be considered if vagal maneuvers and adenosine fail	IIa	C
Synchronized DC cardioversion is recommended when drug therapy fails to convert or control the tachycardia	I	B
Chronic therapy		
Catheter ablation is recommended for symptomatic, recurrent AVNRT	I	B
Diltiazem or verapamil, in patients without HFrEF or beta-blockers should be considered if ablation is not desirable or feasible	IIa	B
Abstinence from therapy should be considered for minimally symptomatic patients with very infrequent, short-lived episodes of tachycardia	IIa	C

WOLF-PARKINSON-WHITE SYNDROME

Wolf-Parkinson-White (WPW) syndrome refers to the presence of an overt (manifest) accessory pathway (AP), thus resulting in the so-called preexcitation, in combination with usually recurrent tachyarrhythmias. During sinus rhythm, a typical pattern in the resting ECG with the following characteristics is present—(1) a short

Flowchart 11: Localization of accessory pathway in WPW syndrome.

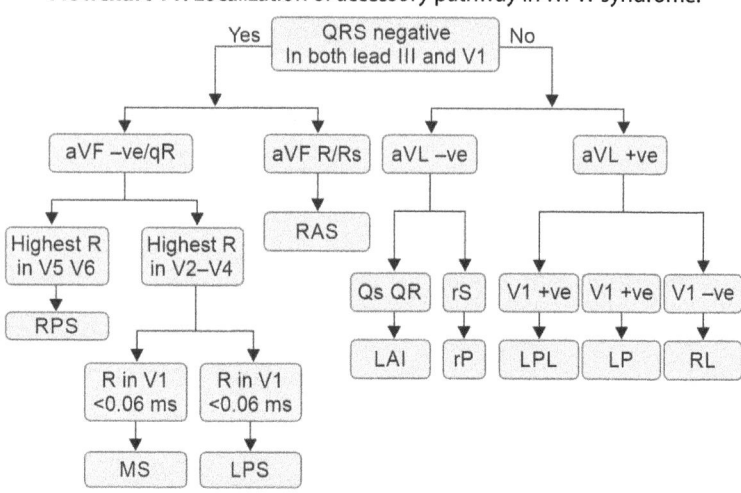

An algorithm for the localization of accessory pathway.
(+ve: QRS complex-positive; –ve: QRS complex-negative, +/–: QRS complex equiphasic; AP: accessory pathway; LAL: left anterolateral; LP: left posterior; LPS: left posteroseptal; MS: mid-septal; RAS: right anteroseptal; RL: right lateral; RP: right posterior; RPS: right posteroseptal; UPL = left posterolateral)

PR interval (≤120 ms); (2) slurred upstroke (or downstroke) of the QRS complex ("delta wave"), and (3) a wide QRS complex (>120 ms). In most cases, APs giving rise to the WPW pattern are seen in structurally normal hearts. Rare, familial forms of preexcitation associated with LV hypertrophy and multisystem disease [mutations in the protein kinase adenosine monophosphate-activated) noncatalytic subunit gamma 2 (*PRKAG2*) gene, Danon and Fabry disease, and others] have also been described.

Several surface ECG algorithms have been developed that can be applied for the localization of APs in the presence of overt preexcitation. Preexcitation on the surface ECG can be intermittent and can even disappear permanently (in ≤35% of cases) over time. Furthermore, various degrees of preexcitation are possible depending on the location of the AP as well as on AV mode conduction properties.

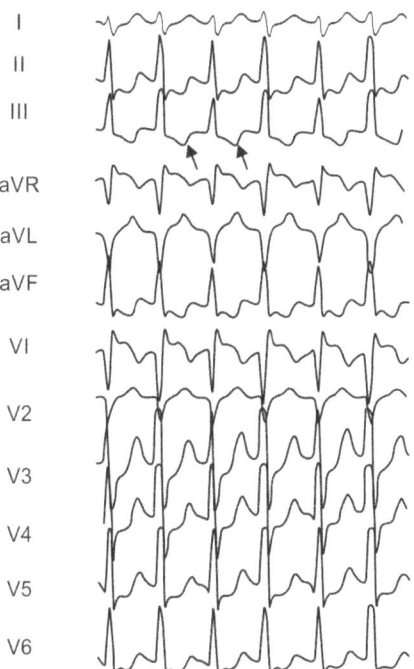

Fig. 5: Atrioventricular re-entrant tachycardia. Orthodromic atrioventricular re-entrant tachycardia (AVRT) due to a concealed posteroseptal accessory pathway. Retrograde P waves are negative during tachycardia in the inferior leads (arrows).

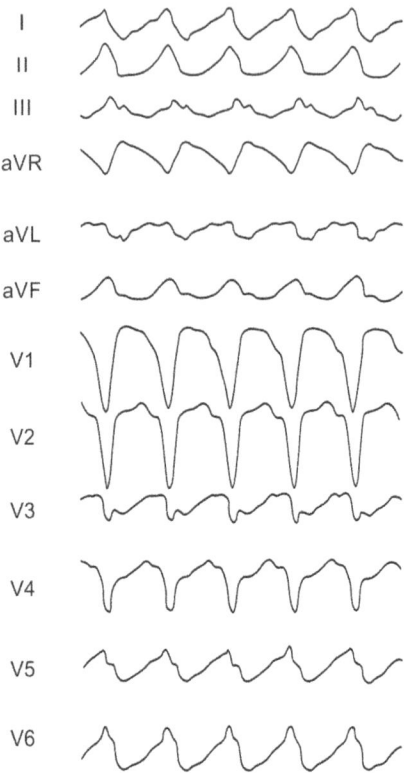

Fig. 6: Antidromic atrioventricular reentrant tachycardia due to an atriofascicular accessory pathway.

TABLE 5: Recommendations for the therapy of atrioventricular reentrant tachycardia due to manifest or concealed accessory pathways (ESC Guidelines 2019).

Recommendation	Class[a]	Level[b]
Acute therapy		
Hemodynamically unstable patients: Synchronized DC cardioversion is recommended for hemodynamically unstable patients	I	B
Hemodynamically stable patients: Vagal maneuver, preferably in the supine position with leg elevation, is recommended	I	B
In orthodromic AVRT, adenosine (6–18 mg IV bolus) is recommended if vagal maneuvers full and the tachycardia is orthodromic	I	B
In orthodromic AVRT, IV verapamil or diltiazem should be considered if vagal maneuvers and adenosine fail	IIa	B
In orthodromic AVRT, IV beta-blockers (esmolol or metoprolol) should be considered in the absence of decompensated HF, if vagal maneuvers and adenosine fail	IIa	C
In antidromic AVRT, IV ibutilide or procainamide or IV flecainide or profanenone or synchronized DC cardioversion should be considered if vagal maneuvers and adenosine fail	IIa	B
In antidromic AVRT, IV amiodarone may be considered in refractory cases	IIb	B
Synchronized DC cardioversion is recommended when drug therapy fails to convert or control the tachycardia	I	B
Clinical therapy		
Catheter ablation of AP(s) is recommended in patients with symptomatic, recurrent AVRT	I	B
Beta-blockers or nondihydropyridine calcium-channel blockers (verapamil or diltiazem in the absence of HFrEF) should be considered if no signs of preexcitation are present on resting ECG, if ablation is Not desirable or feasible	IIa	B
Propafenone or flecainide may be considered in patients with AVRT and without ischemic or structural heart disease, if ablation is not desirable feasible	IIb	B

Contd...

Contd...

Recommendation	Class[a]	Level[b]
Digoxin, beta-blockers, diltiazem, verapamil, and amiodarone are not recommended and are potentially harmful in patients with preexcited AF	III	B

IV = Verapamil and diltiazem are contraindicated in the presence of hypotension or HF-EF
IV = Beta-blockers are contraindicated in the presence of decompensated heart failure
IV = Ibutilide is contraindicated in patients with prolonged QTc interval
IV = Procainamide prolongs the QTc interval but much less than class III agents
IV = flecainide and propafenone are contraindicated in patients with ischemic or structural heart disease. They also prolong the QTc interval but much less than class III agents
IV = Flecainide and propafenone are contraindicated in patients with ischemic or structural heart disease. They are prolong the QTc interval but much less than class III agents
IV = Amiodarone prolongs the QTc but torsades des pointes is rare
[a] Class of recommendation
[b] Level of evidence
(AF: atrial fibrillation; AP: accessory pathway; AVRT: atrioventricular re-entrant tachycardia; DC: direct-current; ECG: electrocardiogram; HFrEF: heart failure with reduced ejection fraction; IV: intravenous)

Flowchart 12: Acute therapy of AVRT.

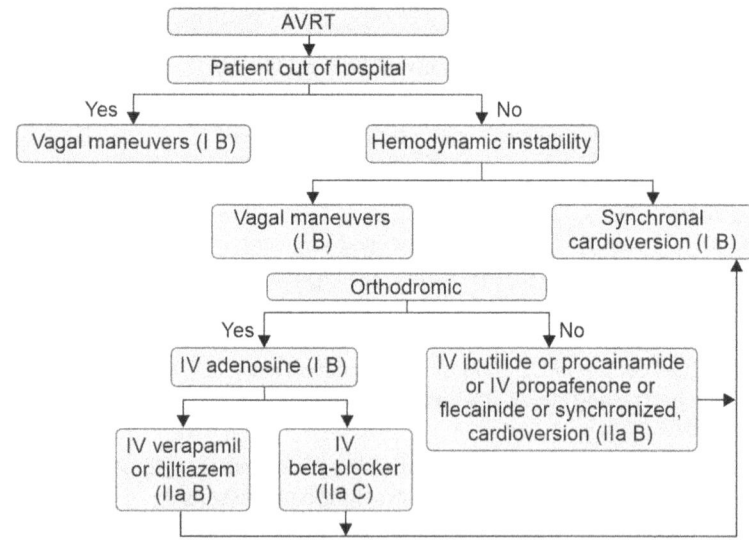

(AVRT: atrioventricular reentrant tachycardia; IV: intravenous)

Flowchart 13: Chronic therapy of AVRT.

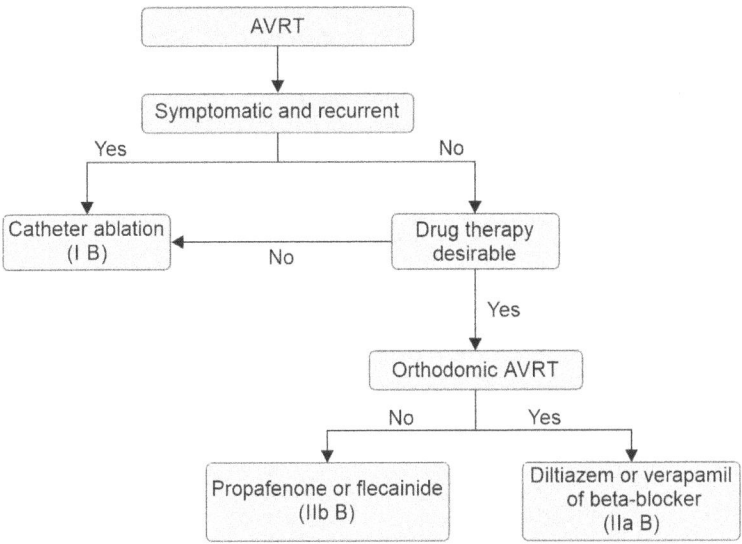

(AVRT: atrioventricular reentrant tachycardia)

Flowchart 14: Acute therapy of preexcited AF (ESC Guidelines 2019).

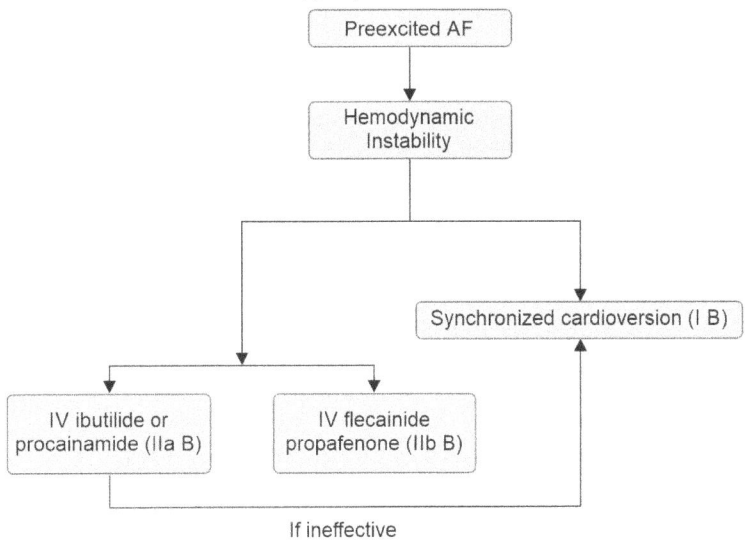

(AF: atrial fibrillation; IV: intravenous)

Flowchart 15: Risk stratification and therapy of patients with asymptomatic preexcitation. High-risk features at electrophysiology study are shortest pre-excited RR interval during atrial fibrillation ≤250 ms, accessory pathway effective refractory period ≤250 ms, multiple accessory pathways, and inducible atrioventricular reentrant tachycardia. Low-risk features at noninvasive risk stratification are induced or intermittent loss of preexcitation on excrete or drug testing, resting electrocardiogram, and ambulatory electrocardiogram monitoring (ESC Guidelines 2019).

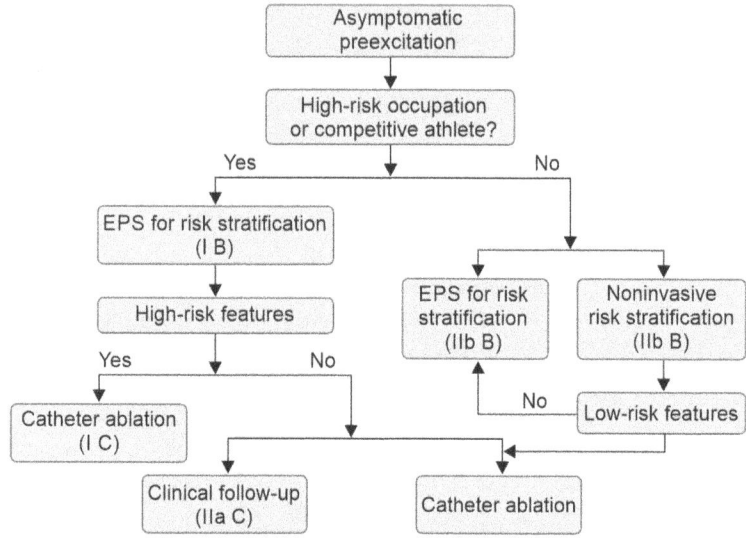

(EPS: electrophysiology study)

TABLE 6: Recommendations for the therapy of supraventricular tachycardia in pregnancy (ESC Guidelines 2019).

Recommendation	Class[a]	Level[b]
Catheter ablation is recommended in symptomatic women with recurrent SVT who plan to become pregnant	I	C
Acute therapy		
Immediate electrical cardioversion is recommended for any tachycardia with hemodynamic instability	I	C
Vagal maneuvers and, if these fail, adenosine are recommended for acute conversion of SVT	I	C
An IV beta-1 selective blocker (except atenolol) should be considered for acute conversion or rate control of SVT	IIa	C
IV digoxin in the latest pocket Gls version should be considered for rate control of AT if beta-blockers fail	IIa	C

Contd...

Contd...

Recommendation	Class[a]	Level[b]
Chronic therapy		
During the first trimester of pregnancy, it is recommended that all antiarrhythmic drugs should be avoided, if possible	I	C
Beta-1 selective (except atenolol) beta-blockers or verapamil, in order of preference, should be considered for prevention of SVT in patients without WPW syndrome	IIa	C
Flecainide or propafenone should be considered for prevention of SVT in patients with WPW syndrome and without ischemic or structural heart disease	IIa	C
Flecainide or propafenone in patients without ischemic or structural heart disease should be considered if AV nodal blocking agents fail to prevent SVT	IIa	C
Digoxin or verapamil should be considered for rate control of AT if beta-blockers fail in patients without WP syndrome	IIa	C
Amiodarone is not recommended in pregnant women	IIa	C
Amiodarone is not recommended in pregnant women	III	C
Fluoroless catheter ablation should be considered in cases of drug-refractory or poorly tolerated SVT, In experienced centers	IIa	C
IV ibutilide is contraindicated in patients with prolonged QTc interval		

[a]Class of recommendation
[b]Level of evidence
(AT: atrial tachycardia; AV: atrioventricular; IV: intravenous; SVT: supraventricular tachycardia; WPW: Wolf–Parkinson–White)

TABLE 7: Recommendations for the therapy of supraventricular tachycardia in patients with suspected or established heart failure due to tachycardiomyopathy (ESC Guidelines 2019).

Recommendation	Class[a]	Level[b]
Catheter ablation is recommended for TCM due to SVT	I	B
Beta-blockers (from the list with proved mortality and morbidity benefits in HFrEF) are recommended, for TCM due to SVT, when catheter ablation fails or is not applicable	I	A
It is recommended that TCM is considered in a patient with reduced LV ejection fraction with an elevated heart rate (>100 bpm)	I	B

Contd...

Contd...

Recommendation	Class[a]	Level[b]
24 hours (or multiday) ambulatory ECG monitoring should be considered for diagnosis of TCM by identifying subclinical or intermittent arrhythmias	IIa	B
AV nodal ablation with subsequent pacing (ablate and pace), either biventricular or His-bundle pacing, is recommended if the tachycardia responsible for the TCM cannot be ablated or controlled by drugs	I	C

[a]Class of recommendation
[b]Level of evidence
(bpm: beats per minute; ECG: electrocardiogram; HFrEF: heart failure with reduced ejection fraction; LV: left ventricular; SVT: supraventricular tachycardia; TCM: tachycardiomyopathy)

TABLE 8: Summary of key electrocardiographic criteria that suggest ventricular tachycardia rather than supraventricular tachycardia in wide complex tachycardia.

AV dissociation	Ventricular rate > atrial rate
Fusion/capture beats	Different QRS morphology from that of tachycardia
Chest lead negative condolence	All precordial chest leads negative
RS in precordial leads	• Absence of RS in precordial leads • RS >100 ms in any lead[a]
QRS complex in aVR	• Initial R wave • Initial R or Q wave >40 ms • Presence of a notch of a predominantly negative complex
QRS axis −90 to ±180°	Both in the presence of RBBB and LBBB morphology
R wave peak time in lead II	R wave peak time ≥50 ms
RBBB morphology	*Lead V1:* Monophasic R, Rsr', biphasic qR complex, broad R (>40 ms), and a double-peaked R wave with the left peak taller than the right (the so-called 'rabbit ear' (sign) *Lead V6:* RS ratio <1 (rS, QS patterns)
LBBB morphology	*Lead V1:* Broad R wave, slurred or notched-down stroke of the S wave *Lead V6:* Q or QS wave

[a]RS: beginning of R to deepest part of S
(AV: atrioventricular; LBBB: left bundle branch block; RBBB: right bundle branch block)

Tachycardias

Flowchart 16: Classic morphology criteria for ventricular tachycardia.

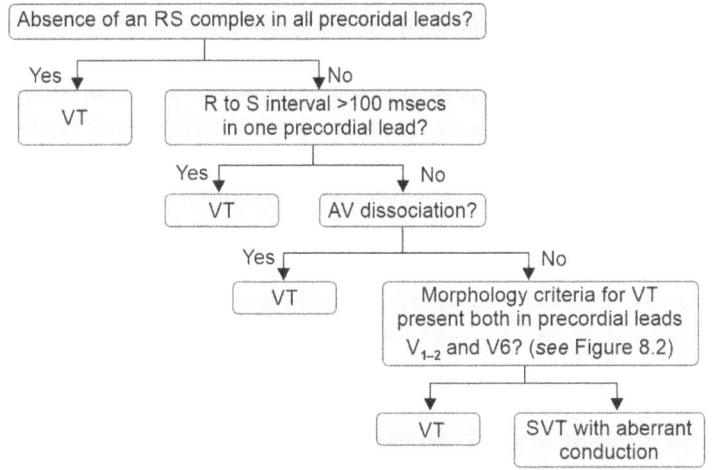

(LBBB: left bundle branch block; RBBB: right bundle branch block; SVT: supraventricular tachycardias; VT: complex tachycardia)

TABLE 9: Brugada criteria for distinguishing ventricular tachycardia from supraventricular tachycardia with aberrancy in wide-complex tachycardias.

	LBBB		RBBB	
	VT	SVT	VT	SVT
Lead V1	In V1, V2 any of: a. r ≥0.04 s b. Notched s downstroke c. Delayed S nadir >0.06 s	In V1, V2 absence of: a. r >0.04 s b. Notched s downstroke c. Delayed S nadir >0.06 s	Taller left peak biphasic RS or QR	Triphasic rsR' or rR'
Lead V6	Monophasic QS		Biphasic rS	Triphasic qRs

(AV: atrioventricular; LBBB: left bundle branch block; RBBB: right bundle branch block)

Flowchart 17: Algorithm of Vereckei.

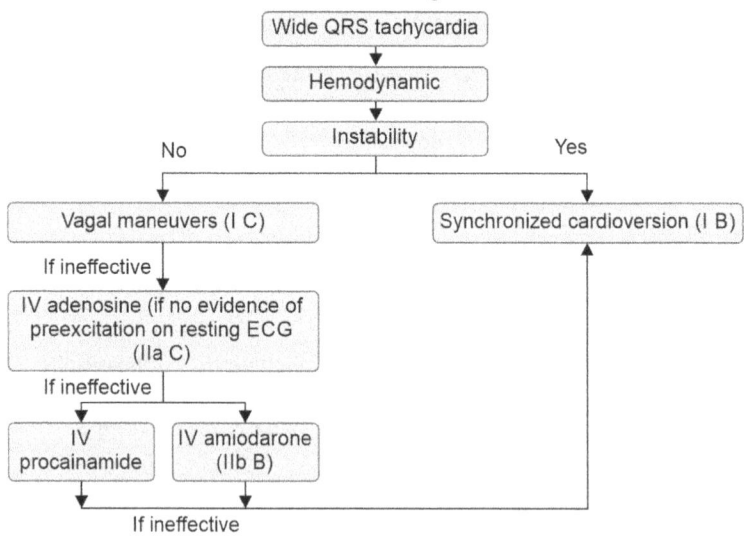

Flowchart 18: Acute therapy of wide complex tachycardia in the absence of an established diagnosis.

(AVRT: atrioventricular re-entrant tachycardia; IV: intravenous)

Flowchart 19: ESC 2019 algorithm for the evaluation of patients presenting with an incidental finding of non-sustained ventricular tachycardia.

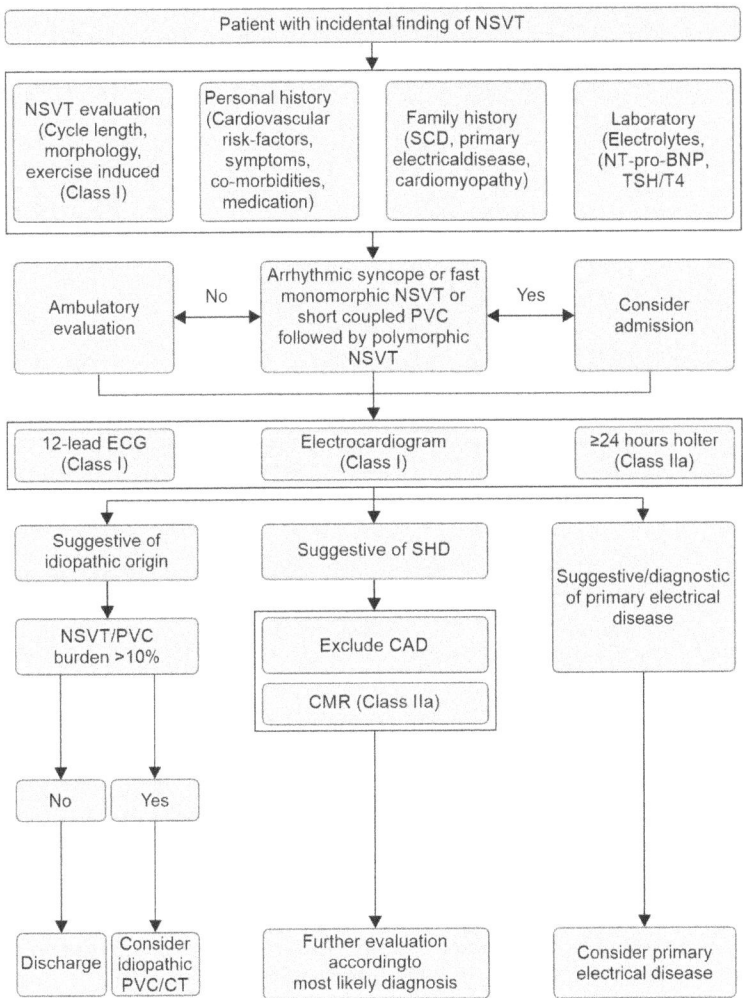

(CAD: coronary disease; CMR: cardiac magnetic resonance; ECG: electrocardiogram; N: no; NSVT: nonsustained ventricular tachycardia; PVC: premature ventricular complex; SCD: sudden cardiac death; SHD: structural heart disease)

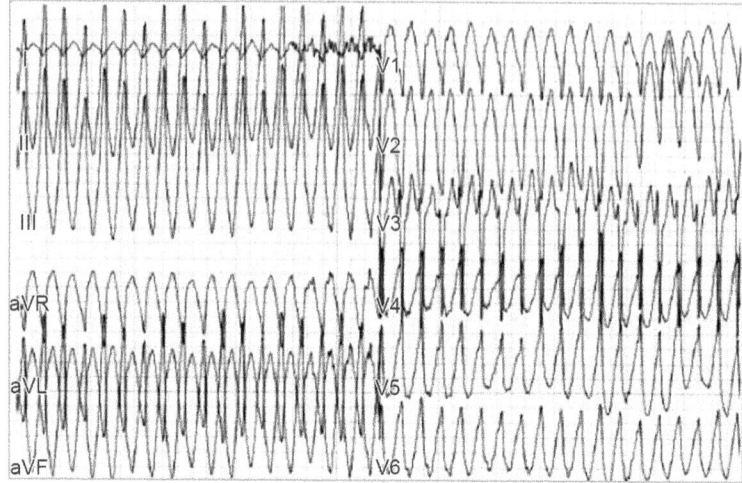
Fig. 7: RVOT VT (LBBB-like, inferior axis, V4 transition).

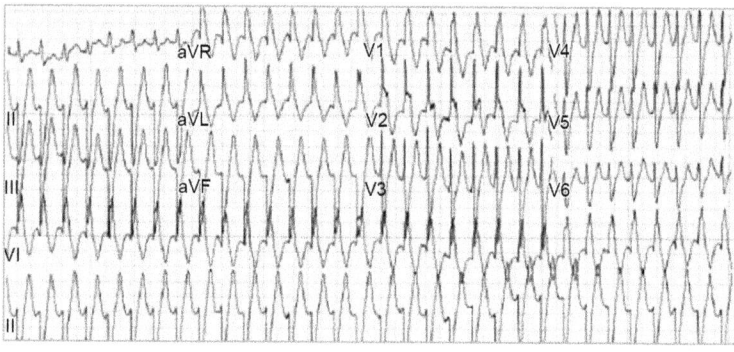
Fig. 8: LV fascicular VT (RBBB like, superior axis, QRS 130 ms).
(ECG pattern of typical idiopathic ventricular tachycardia; LBBB: left bundle branch block; LV: left ventricle; RBBB: right bundle branch block; RVOT: right ventricular outflow tract; VT: ventricular tachycardia)

Flowchart 20: ESC 2019 algorithm for the evaluation of patients presenting with a first sustained monomorphic ventricular tachycardia episode.

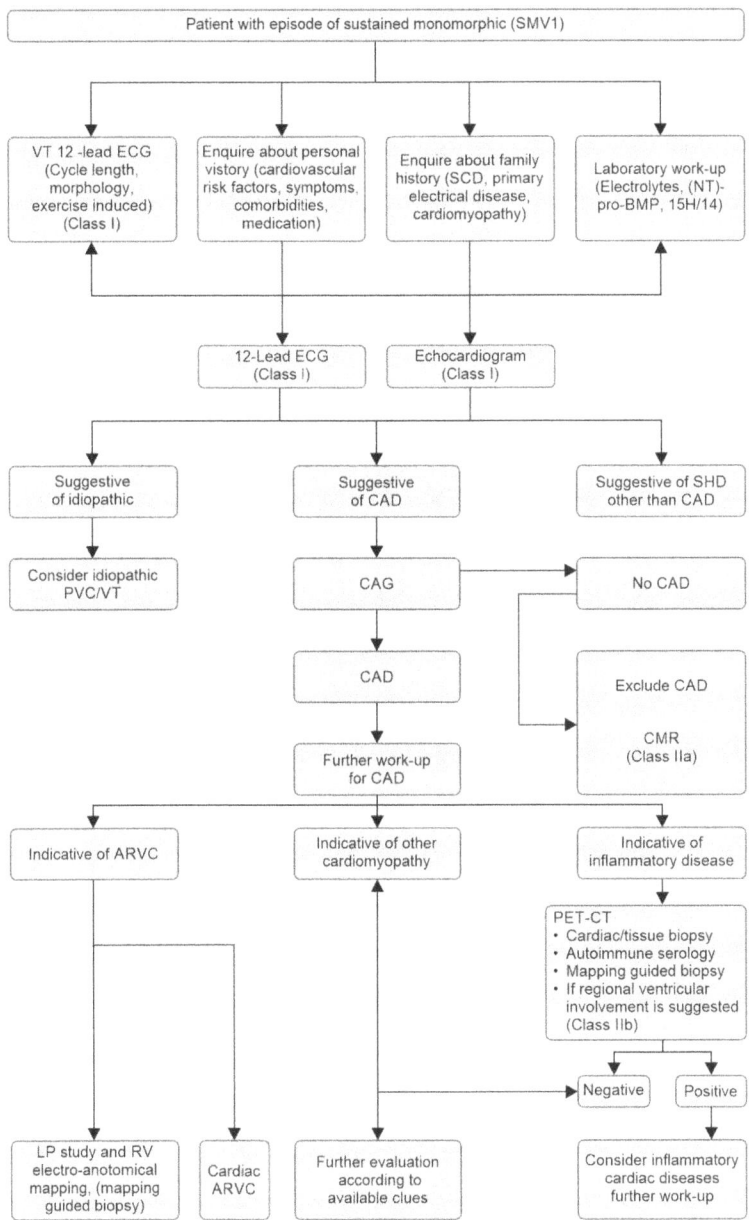

Flowchart 21: Sudden cardiac arrest (SCA).

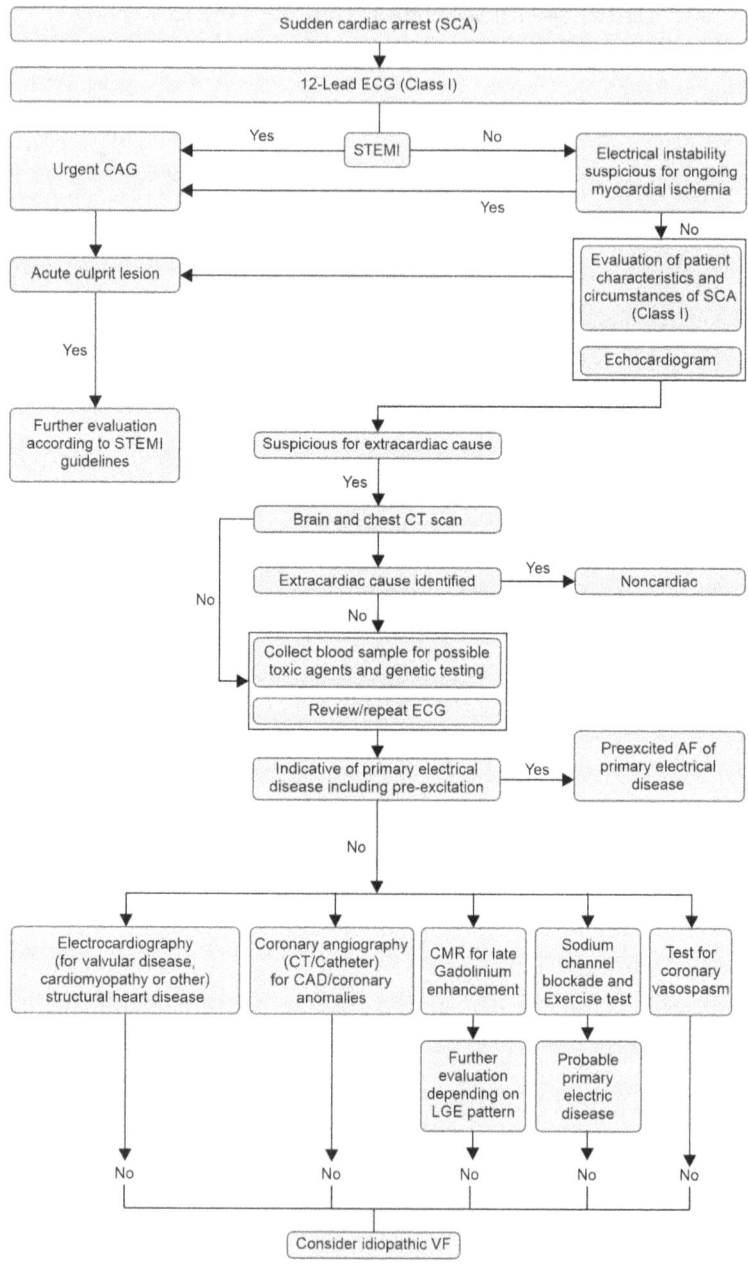

Flowchart 22: Acute management of a patient with regular wide QRS complex tachycardia.

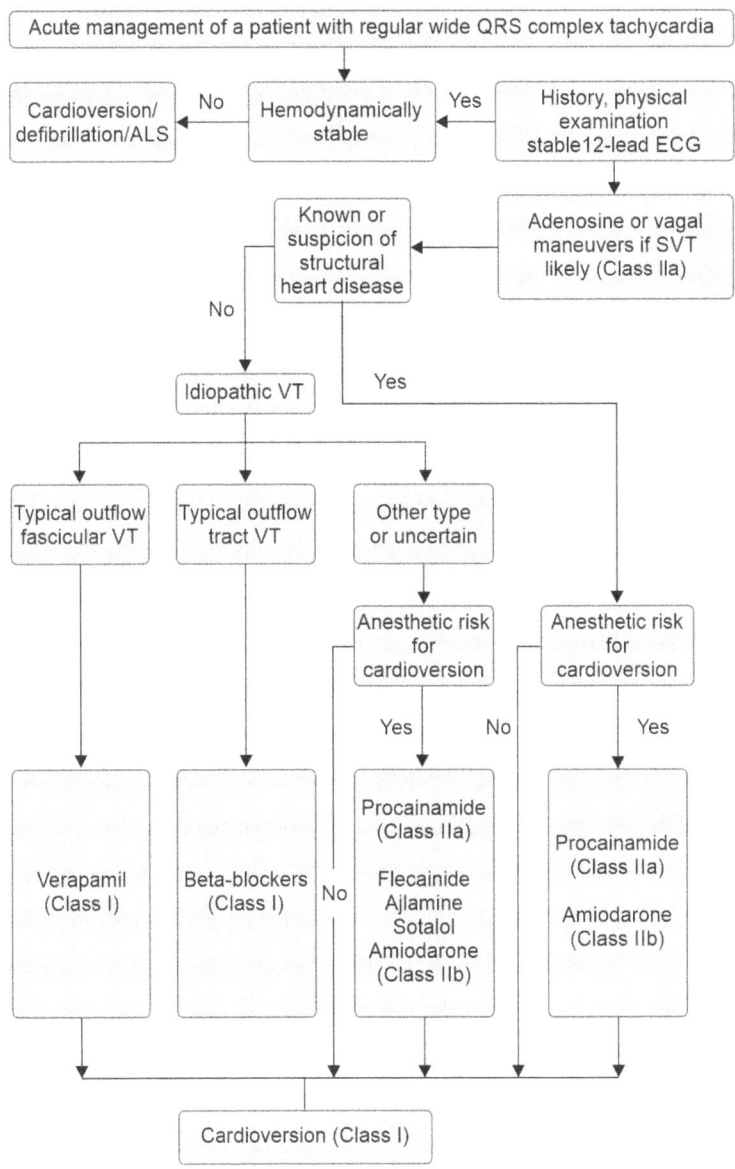

(ALS: advanced life support; ECG: electrocardiogram; SVT: supraventricular tachycardia; VT: ventricular tachycardia)

Tachycardias

Flowchart 23: Patient with electrical storm or repeated ICD discharges.

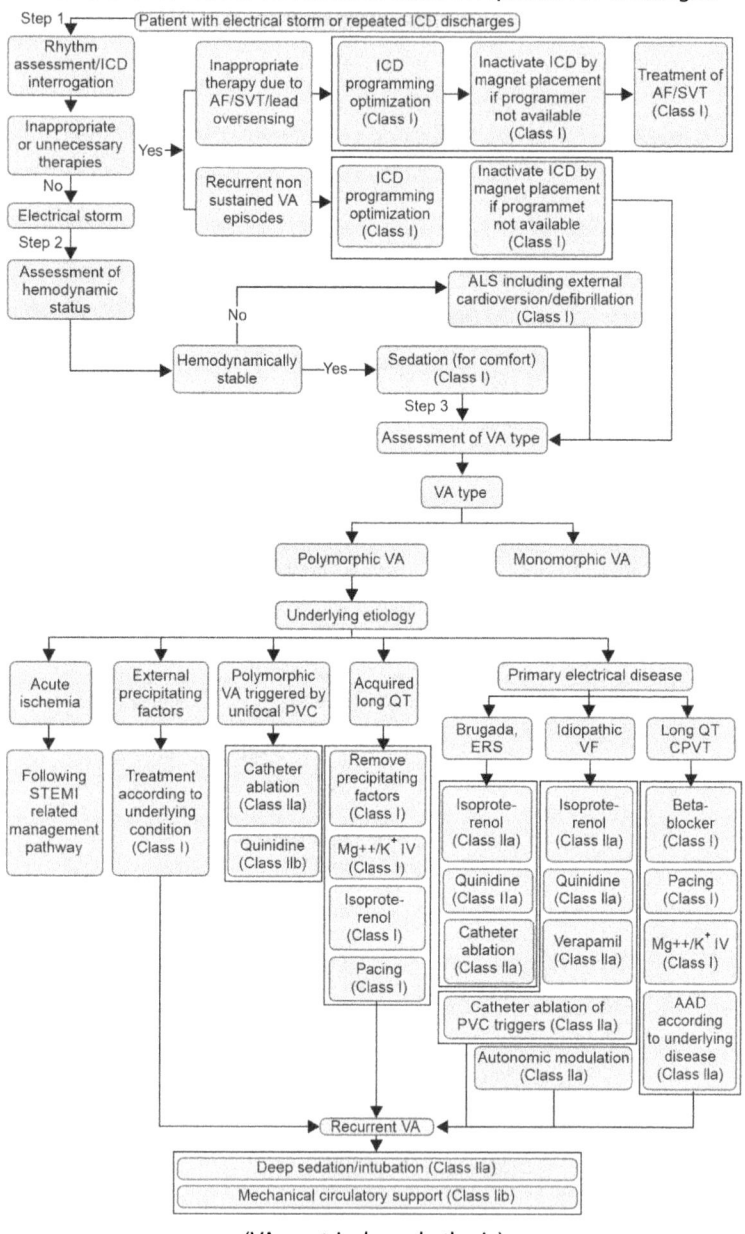

(VA: ventricular arrhythmia)

Flowchart 24: Management of patients with electrical storm or repeated implantable cardioverter defibrillator discharges.

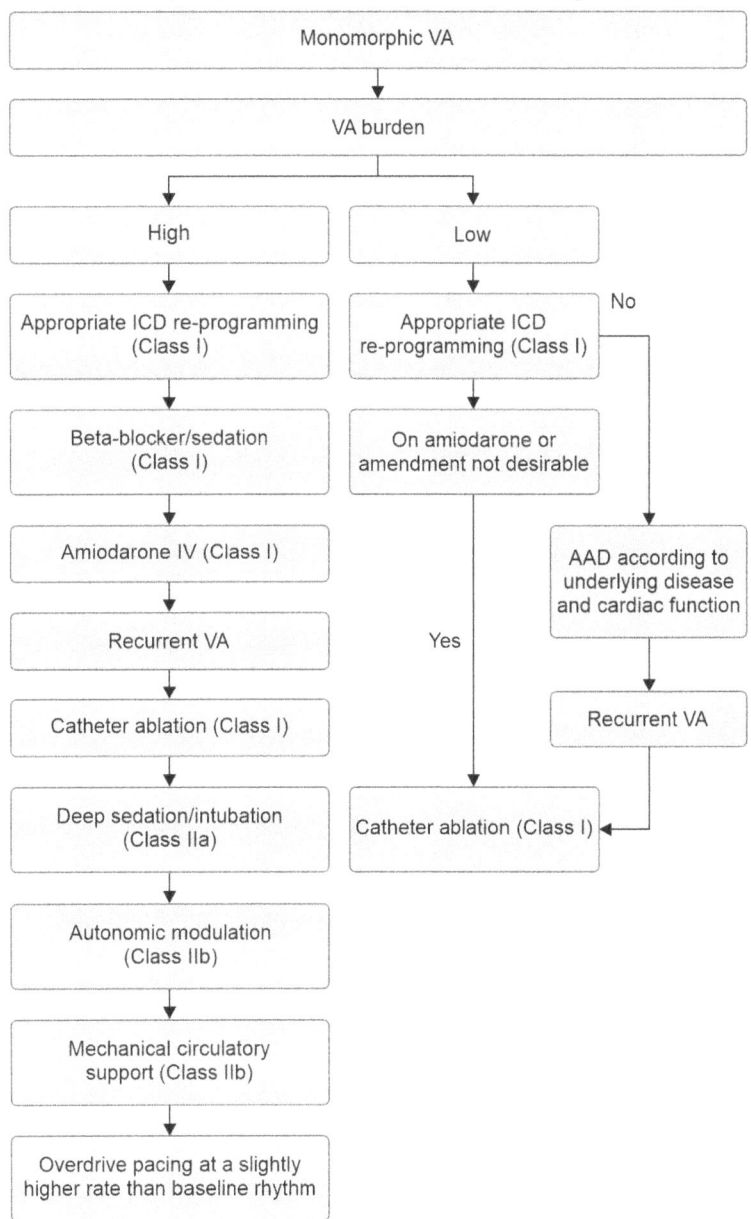

Flowchart 25: ESC 2019 algorithm for the prevention and management of ventricular arrhythmia in ST-elevation myocardial infarction.

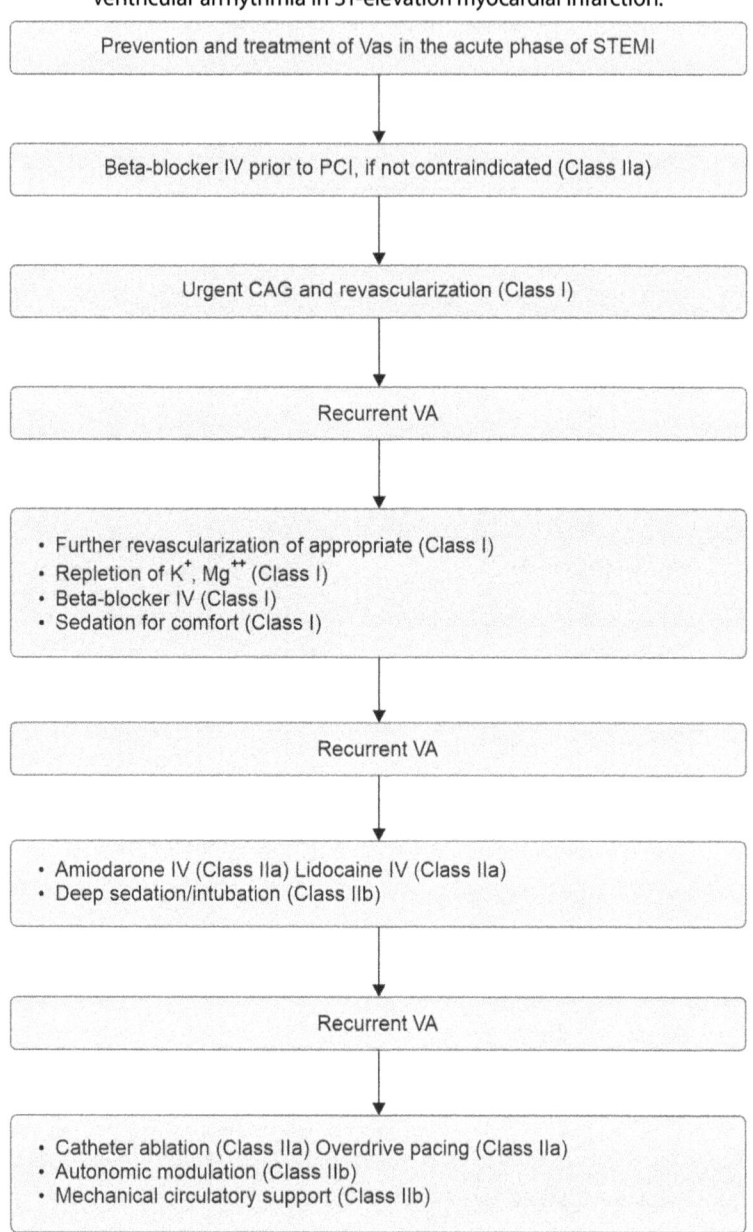

Flowchart 26: Algorithm for risk stratification and primary prevention of sudden cardiac death in patients with chronic coronary artery disease and reduced ejection fraction.

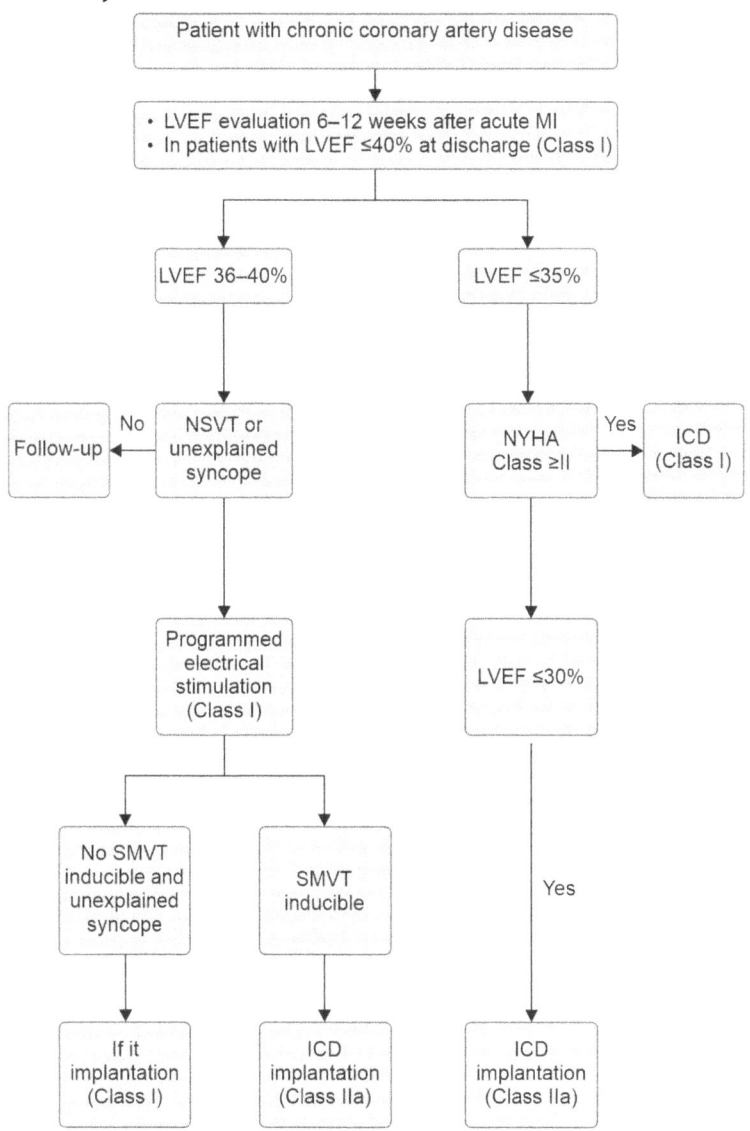

(CAD: coronary artery disease; ICD: implantable cardioverter defibrillation; ILR: implantable loop recorder)

Flowchart 27: Algorithm for the management of sustained monomorphic ventricular tachycardia in patients with chronic coronary artery disease.

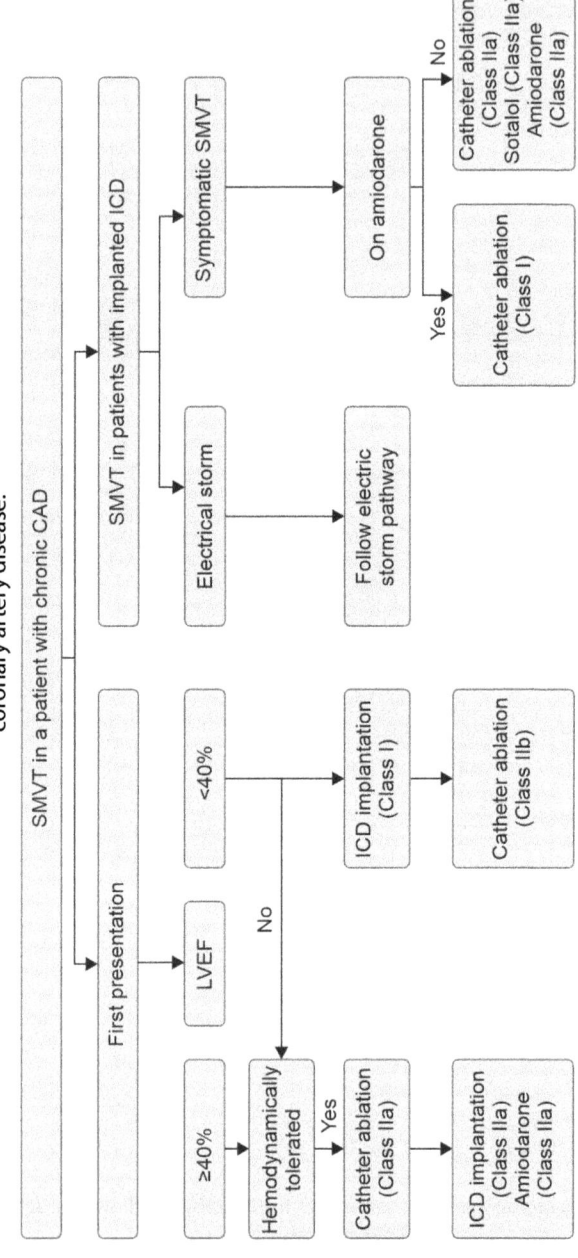

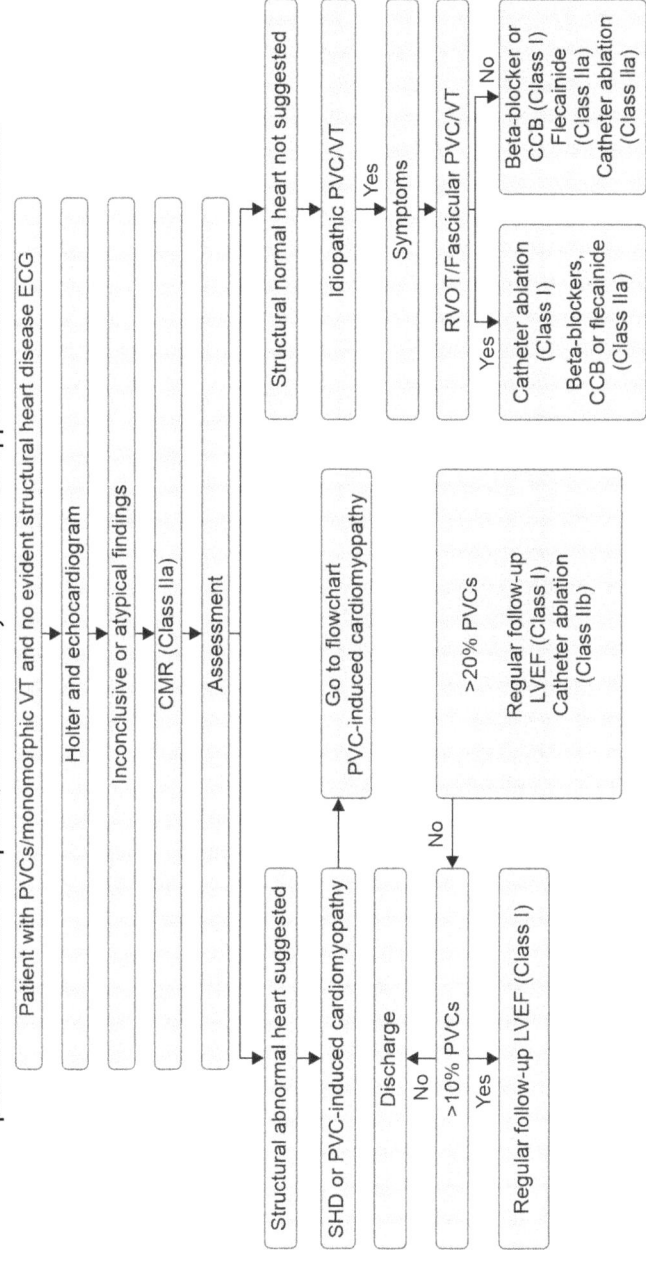

Flowchart 28: Polymorphic ventricular arrhythmia (PVA)—ESC 2019 algorithm for the management of patients with idiopathic premature ventricular complexes/ventricular tachycardia and non-apparent structural heart disease.

TABLE 10: Recommendations for the treatment of patients with frequent idiopathic premature ventricular complexes/ventricular tachycardia or premature ventricular complex-induced cardiomyopathy.

	Ablation	Beta-blocker	CCB	Flecainide	Amiodarone
RVOT/fascicular PVC/VT Symptomatic normal LV function	Class I	Class IIb	Class IIa	Class IIa	Class III
PVC/VT other than RVOT/fascicular Symptomatic normal LV function	Class IIa	Class I	Class I	Class IIa	Class III
RVOT/fascicular PVC/VT LV dysfunction	Class I	Class IIa	Class III	Class IIa	Class IIa
PVC/VT other than RVOT/fascicular LV dysfunction	Class I	Class IIa	Class III	Class IIa	Class IIa
PVC Burden >20%, asymptomatic, normal LV Function	Class IIb				Class III

(CCB: calcium channel blocker; LV: left ventricular; PVC: premature ventricular complex; RVOT: right ventricular outflow tract; VT: ventricular tachycardia)

TABLE 11: ESC 2019 recommendations for the management of patients with premature ventricular complex-induced or premature ventricular complex-aggravated cardiomyopathy.

Recommendation	Class	Level
Diagnostic evaluation		
In patients with an unexplained reduced EF and a PVC burden of at least 10%, PVC-induced cardiomyopathy should be considered	IIa	C
In patients with suspected PVC-induced cardiomyopathy, CMR should be considered PVC-induced cardiomyopathy should be considered	IIa	B
Treatment		
In patients with a cardiomyopathy suspected to be caused by frequent and predominantly monomorphic PVCs, catheter ablation is recommended	I	C
In patients with a cardiomyopathy suspected to be caused by frequent and predominantly monomorphic PVCs treatment with AADs should be considered if catheter ablation is not desired, suspected to be high-risk or unsuccessful	IIa	C
In patients with SHD in whom predominately monomorphic frequent PVCs are suspected to be contributing to the cardiomyopathy, AAD (amiodarone) treatment or catheter ablation should be considered	IIa	B
In nonresponders to CRT with frequent predominantly monomorphic PVCs limiting optimal biventricular pacing despite pharmacological therapy, catheter ablation or AADs should be considered	IIa	C

TABLE 12: ESC 2019 recommendations for diagnostic, risk stratification, sudden cardiac death prevention, and treatment of ventricular arrhythmias in arrhythmogenic right ventricular cardiomyopathy.

Recommendations	Class	Level
Diagnostic evaluation and general recommendations		
In patients with suspected ARVC, CMR is recommended	I	B
In patients with a suspected or definite diagnosis of ARVC, genetic counseling and testing are recommended	I	B

Contd...

Contd...

Recommendations	Class	Level
Avoidance of high-intensity exercise is recommended in patients with a definite diagnosis of ARVC	I	B
Avoidance of high intensity exercise may be considered in carriers of ARVC-related pathogenic mutations and no phenotype	IIb	C
Beta-blocker therapy may be considered in all patients with a definite diagnosis of ARVC	IIB	C
Risk stratification and primary prevention of SCD		
ICD implantation should be considered in patients with definite ARVC and an arrhythmic syncope	IIa	B
ICD implantation should be considered in patients with details ARVC and severe RV or LV systolic Dysfunction	IIa	C
ICD implantation should be considered in symptomatic patients with definite ARVC, moderate right or left ventricular dysfunction, and either NSVT or inducibility of SMVT at PES	IIa	C
In patients with ARVC and symptoms highly suspicious for VA, PES may be considered for risk stratification	IIb	C
Secondary prevention of SCD and treatment of Vas		
ICD implantation is recommended in ARVC patients with hemodynamically not-tolerated VT or VF	I	C
In patients with ARVC and non-sustained or sustained Vas, beta-blocker therapy is recommended	I	C
In patients with ARVC and recurrent, SMVT or ICD shocks for SMVT despite beta-blockers, catheter ablation in specialized centers should be considered	IIa	C
In ARVC patients with indication for ICDs, a device with the capability of ATP programming for SMVT up to high rates should be considered	IIa	B
ICD implantation should be considered in ARVC patients with a hemodynamically tolerated SMVT	IIa	C
In patients with ARVC and recurrent, symptomatic VT despite beta-blockers, AAD treatment should be considered	IIa	C

TABLE 13: ESC 2019 recommendations for risk stratification, sudden cardiac death prevention, and treatment of ventricular arrhythmias in hypertrophic cardiomyopathy.

Recommendations	Class	Level
Risk stratification and primary prevention of SCD		
It is recommended that the 5-year risk of SCD is assessed at first evaluation and at 1–3-year intervals, or when there is a change in clinical status	I	C
ICD implantation should be considered in patients aged 16 years or more with an estimated 5-year risk of SD ≥6%	IIa	B
ICD implantation should be considered in HCM patients aged 16 years or more with an intermediate 5-year risk of SCD (≥4 to <6%) and with (a) significant LE at CMR (usually ≥15% of LV mass) or (b) LVEF <50% or (c) abnormal blood pressure response during exercise test, or (d) LV atypical aneurysm; or (E) presence of sarcomeric pathogenic mutation	IIa	B
In children <16 years of age with HCM and an estimated 5-year risk of SD ≥6% (based on HCM Risk-Kids score) ICD implantation should be considered	IIa	B
ICD implantation may be considered in HCM patients aged 16 years or more with an estimated 5-year risk of SCD of ≥4 to <6%	IIb	B
ICD implantation may be considered in HCM patients aged 16 years or more with a low estimated 5-year risk of SCD (<4%) and with (a) significant LGE at CMR (usually ≥15% of LV mass) or (b) LVEF <50% or (c) LV apical aneurysm	IIb	C
Secondary prevention of SCD and treatment of VAs		
ICD implantation is recommended in HCM patients with hemodynamically not-tolerated VT or VF	I	B
In patients with HCM presenting with hemodynamically tolerated SMVT, ID implantation should be considered	IIa	C
In patients with HCM and recurrent symptomatic VA, or recurrent ICD therapy, AAD treatment should be considered	IIa	C
Catheter ablation in specialized centers may be considered in selected patients with HCM and recurrent symptomatic SMVT or ICD shocks for SMVT, in whom AAD are ineffective, contraindicated, or not tolerated	IIB	C

TABLE 14: ESC 2019 recommendations for implantable cardioverter defibrillator implantation in left ventricular noncompaction.

Recommendations	Class	Level
In patients with LNVC cardiomyopathy phenotype based on CMR or echocardiography, implantation of an ICD for primary prevention of SCD should be considered to follow DCM/HNDCM recommendations	IIa	C

TABLE 15: ESC 2019 recommendations for implantable cardioverter defibrillator implantation in patients with cardiac amyloidosis.

Recommendations	Class	Level
An ICD should be considered in patients with light-chain amyloidosis or transthyretin-associated cardiac amyloidosis and hemodynamically not tolerated-VT	IIa	C

TABLE 16: ESC 2019 recommendations for sudden cardiac death prevention and treatment of ventricular arrhythmias in myocarditis.

Recommendations	Class	Level
Secondary prevention of SCD and treatment of VA		
In patients with hemodynamically not-tolerated SMVT occurring in the chronic phase of myocarditis an ICD implantation is recommended	I	C
In patients with hemodynamically not-tolerated sustained VT or VF during the acute phase of myocarditis, ICD implantation before hospital discharge should be considered	IIa	C
AADs should be considered (preferably amiodarone and beta-blockers) in patients with symptomatic nonsustained or sustained VAs during the acute phase of myocarditis	IIa	C
In postmyocarditis patients with recurrent, symptomatic VT, AAD treatment should be considered	IIa	C
Catheter ablation, performed in specialized centers, should be considered in postmyocarditis patients With recurrent, symptomatic SMVT or ICD shocks for SMVT in whom AADs are ineffective, not tolerated or not desired	IIa	C
In patients with hemodynamically tolerated SMVT occurring in the chronic phase of myocarditis, ICD implantation should be considered	IIa	C

Flowchart 29: Patients with cardiac sarcoidosis.

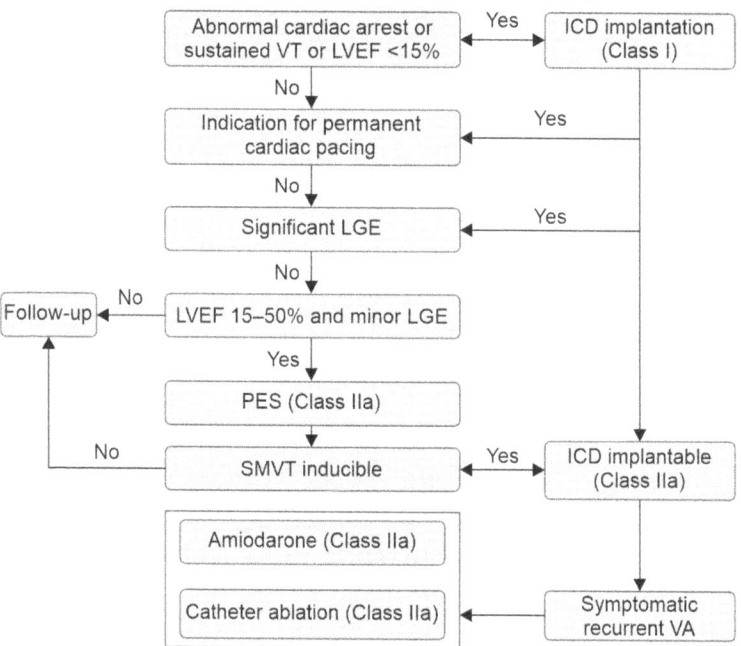

Flowchart 30: ESC 2019 algorithm for the management of patients with for idiopathic ventricular fibrillation.

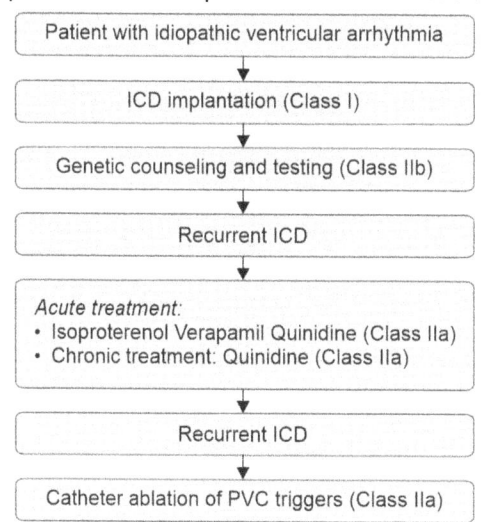

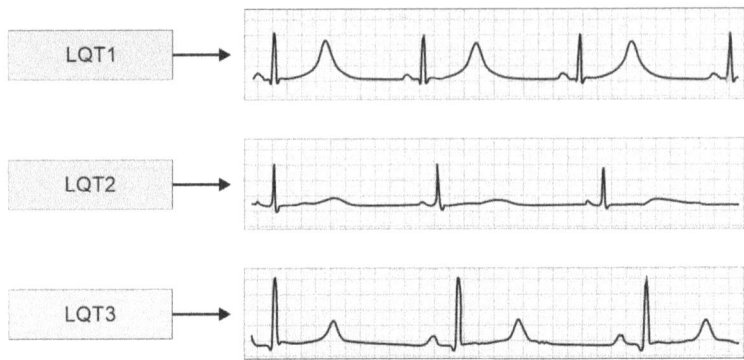

Fig. 9: Modified long QT syndrome diagnostic score.

TABLE 17: ESC 2019 algorithm for the management of patients with long QT syndrome.		
ESC 2019 recommendations for management of patients with Brugada syndrome		
Recommendations	**Class**	**Level**
Diagnosis		
It is recommended that BrS is diagnosed in patients with no other heart disease and a spontaneous type 1 Brugada ECG pattern	I	C
It is recommended that BrS is diagnosed in patients with no other heart disease who have survival a CA due to VF or PVT and exhibit a type 1 Brugada ECG induced by sodium channel Blocker challenge or during fever	I	C
Genetic testing for *SCNSA* gene is recommended for probands with BrS	I	C
BrS should be considered in patients with no other heart disease and induced type 1 Brugada pattern who have at least one of: • Arrhythmic syncope or nocturnal agonal respiration • A family history of BrS • A family history of SD (<45 years old) with a negative autopsy and circumstance suspicious for BrS	IIa	C

Flowchart 31: ECG characteristics in the three major LQTS phenotypes.

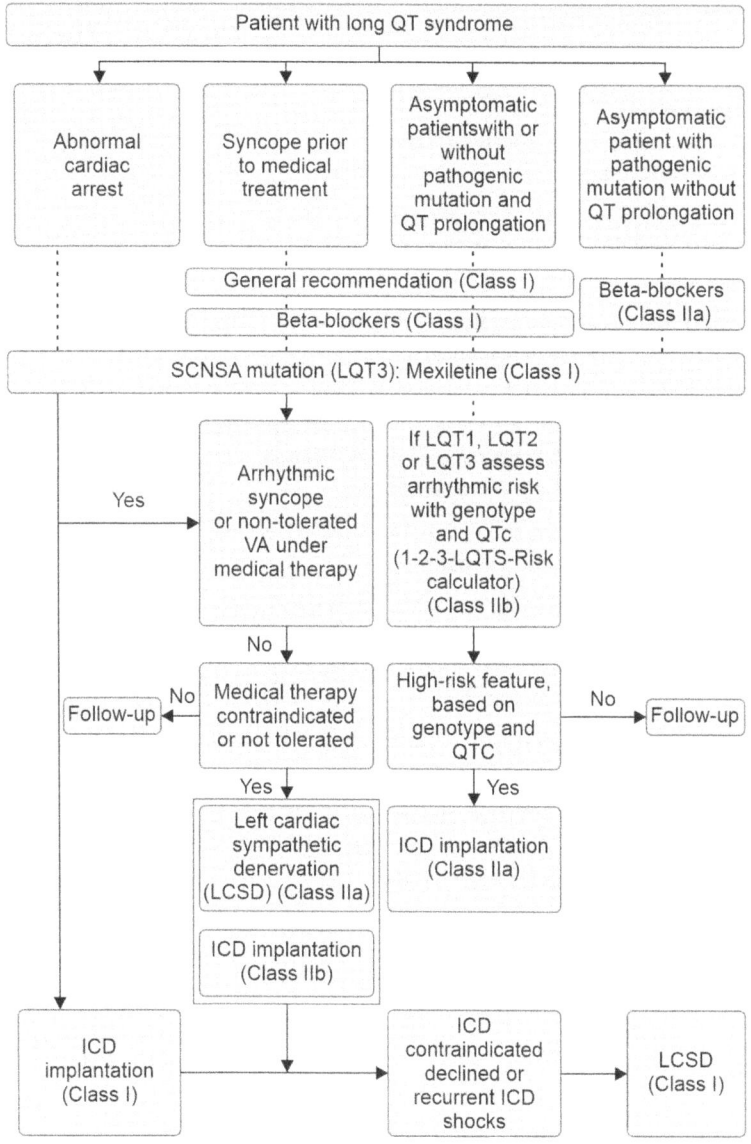

(ICD: implantable cardioverter defibrillator; LCSD: left cardiac sympathetic denervation; LQT: long QT; N: no; VA: ventricular arrhythmia)

TABLE 18: Risk stratification, preservation of SCD, and treatment of VA.

	Class	Level
ICD implantation is recommended in patients with BrS who: • Are survivors of an shorted CA and/or • Have documented spontaneous sustained VT	I	C
ICD implantation should be considered in patients with type 1 Brugada pattern and an arrhythmic syncope	IIa	C
Implantation of a loop recorder should be considered in BrS patient with an unexplained syncope	IIa	C
Quinidine should be considered patients with BrS who qualify for an ICD but have a contraindication, decline, or have recurrent ICD shocks	IIa	C
Isoproterenol infusion should be considered in BrS patients suffering electrical storm	IIa	C
Catheter ablation of triggering PVCs and/or RVOT epicardial substrate should be considered in BrS patients with recurrent appropriate ICD shocks refractory to drug therapy	IIa	C
PES may be considered in asymptomatic patients with a spontaneous type I BrS ECG	IIb	B
ICD implantation may be considered in selected asymptomatic BrS patients with inducible VF during PES using up to 2 extrastimuli	IIb	C
Catheter ablation in asymptomatic BrS patients is not recommended	III	C

TABLE 19: ESC 2019 recommendations for the management of patients with early repolarization pattern/syndrome.

Recommendations	Class	Level
Diagnosis		
It is recommended that the ERP in diagnosed as J-point elevation of ≥1 mm in two adjacent inferior and/or lateral ECG leads	I	C
It is recommended that the ERS is diagnosed in a patient resuscitated from unexplained VF/PVT in the presence of ERP	I	C
In an SCD victim with a negative autopsy and medical chart review, and an ante-mortem ECG demonstrating the ERP, the diagnosis of ERS should be considered	IIa	C
First-degree relatives of ERS patients should be considered for clinical evaluation for ERP with additional high-risk features	IIa	B
Risk stratification, prevention of SCD, and treatment of VA		
ICD implantation is recommended in patients with a diagnosis of ERS who have survived a CA	I	B
Isoproterenol infusion should be considered for ERS patients with electrical storm	I	B
Quinidine in addition to an ICD should be conducted for recurrent VF in ERS patients	IIa	B
ILR should be considered in individuals with ERP and at least one risk feature or arrhythmic syncope	IIa	C
PVC ablation should be considered in ERS patients with recurrent VF episodes triggered by a similar PVC non-responsive to medical treatment	IIa	C
ICD implantation or quinidine may be considered in individuals with ERP arrhythmic syncope and additional risk features	IIa	C
ICD implantation or quinidine may be considered in symptomatic individuals who demonstrates a high-risk	IIa	C
ERP in the presence of a family history unexplained juvenile SD	IIb	C
ICD implantation is not recommended in asymptomatic patients with an isolated ERP	III	C

TABLE 20: ESC 2019 recommendations for the management of patients with catecholaminergic polymorphic ventricular tachycardia.

Recommendations	Class	Level
It is recommended that CPVT is diagnosed in the presence of a structurally normal heart, normal ECG, and exercise or emotion-induced bidirectional or PVT	I	C
It is recommended that CPVT is diagnosed in patients who are carriers of a mutation in disease-causing genes	I	C
Genetic testing and genetic counseling are indicated in patients with clinical suspicion or clinical diagnosis of CPVT	I	C
Epinephrine or isoproterenol challenge may be considered for the diagnosis of CPVT when an exercise test is not possible	IIb	C
Therapeutic interventions		
Beta-blockers ideally nonselective (nadolol or propranolol) are recommended in all patients with a clinical diagnosis of CPVT	I	C
ICD implantation combined with beta-blockers and flecainide is recommended in CPVT patients after aborted CA	I	C
Therapy with beta-blockers should be considered for genetically positive CPVT patients without phenotype	IIa	C
LCSD should be considered in patients with diagnosis of CPVT when the combination of beta-blockers and flecainide at therapeutic dosage are either not effective not tolerated or contraindicated	IIa	C
ICD implantation should be considered in patients with CPVT who experience arrhythmogenic syncope and/or documented bidirectional/PVT while on highest tolerated beta-blocker dose and on flecainide	IIa	C
Flecainide should be considered in patients with CPVT who experience recurrent syncope, polymorphic/bidirectional VT, or persistent exertional PVCs, while on beta-blockers at the highest tolerated dose	IIa	C
PES is not recommended for stratification of SCD risk	III	C

(CA: cardiac arrest; CPVT: catecholaminergic ventricular tachycardia; ECG: electrocardiogram; ICD: implantable cardioverter-defibrillator; LCSD: left cardiac sympathetic denervation; PVT: polymorphic ventricular tachycardia; VT: ventricular tachycardia)

SHORT QT SYNDROME

Short QT syndrome (SQTS) is a rare genetic disorder characterized by a short QT interval premature AF and VF in the context of a structurally normal heart. It has been associated with gain of function mutations in KCNH2, KCNQ1. and loss of function in SLC4A. This panel proposed two QTc cut-off threshold for diagnosis. A QTc ≤320 ms alone or B a QTc ≤360 ms combined with a family history of SQTS, aborted CA in the absence of heart disease or pathogenic mutation. The disease has high mortality in all age groups, including the first months of life. The probability of a first cardiac arrest by the age of 40 years is >40%. While an ICD is used for secondary prevention, primary prevention remains contentious and is based upon prior symptoms and QTc interval. Quinidine is currently the best supported antiarrhythmic drug, but should be monitored for excessive QT prolongation, while isoprenaline may be considered in electrical storm. Drugs that shorten QT interval should be avoided, e.g., nicorandil, loop recorder implantation should be considered in children and young asymptomatic SQTS patients.

TABLE 21: ESC 2019 recommendations for the management of patients with short QT syndrome.

Recommendations	Class	Level
Risk stratification, SCD prevention, and treatment of VA		
ICD implantation is recommended in patients with a diagnosis of SQTS who (a) are survivors of an abnormal CA and/or (b) have documented spontaneous sustained VT	I	C
ILR should be considered in young SQTS patients	IIa	C
ICD implantation should be considered in SQTS patients with arrhythmic syncope	IIa	C
Quinidine may be considered in (a) SQTS patients who qualify for an ICD but present a contraindication to the ICD or refuse it, and (b) asymptomatic SQTS patients and a family history of SCD	IIb	C
Isoproterenol may be considered in SQTS patients with an electrical storm	IIb	C
PES is not recommended for SCD risk stratification in SQTS patients	III	C

SUGGESTED READING

1. Al-Khatib SM, Stevenson WG, Ackerman MJ, Bryant WJ, Callans DJ, Curtis AB, et al. 2017 AHA/ACC/HRS Guideline for Management of Patients with Ventricular Arrhythmias and the Prevention of Sudden Cardiac Death. A report of the American College of Cardiology/American Heart Association Task Force on Clinical Practice Guidelines and the Heart Rhythm Society. Circulation. 2018;13:e272-e391.
2. Brugada J, Katritsis DG, Arbeo E, Arribas F, Bax JJ, Blomström-Lundqvist C, et al; ESC Scientific Document Group 2019 ESC Guidelines for the management of patients with supraventricular tachycardia. The Task Force for the management of patients with supraventricular tachycardia of the European Society of Cardiology (ESC). Eur Heart J. 2020;41(5):655-720.
3. Page RL, Joglar JA, Coldwell MA, Calkins H, Conti JB, Deal BJ, et al; 2015 ACC/AHA/HRS Guideline for the Management of Adult Patients with Supraventricular. Tachycardiac : A Report of the American College of Cardiology/American Heart Association Task Force on Clinical Practice Guidelines and the Heart Rhythm Society. Circulation. 2016;133(14):e506-e574.
4. Zeppenfeld K, T-felt–Hansen J, Riva M, Winkel BG, Behr ER, Blom NA, et al; ESC Scientific Document Group. 2022 ESC Guidelines for the management of patients with ventricular arrhythmias and the prevention of sudden cardiac death. Eur Heart J. 2022;43(40):3997-4126.

8. Cardiopulmonary Resuscitation

Soumitra Kumar

Cardiopulmonary resuscitation (CPR) is a series of lifesaving actions that improve the chance of survival following cardiac arrest.

The newest development in the guidelines of CPR is a change in basic life support (BLS) sequence of steps from airway, breathing, and chest compression (C-A-B) to chest compression, airway, and breathing (C-A-B).

GOALS

- To recognize cardiopulmonary arrest immediately
- To maintain cerebral perfusion until cardiopulmonary function is restored
- To return the patient to baseline neurological function

KEY PRINCIPLES IN RESUSCITATION: STRENGTHENING THE LINKS IN THE CHAIN OF SURVIVAL

- Immediate recognition of cardiac arrest and activation of the emergency response system
- Early CPR with an emphasis on chest compression
- Rapid defibrillation
- Effective advanced life support
- Integrated postcardiac arrest care

ADULT BASIC LIFE SUPPORT

- Make sure the victim, any bystanders and you are safe
  ↓
  Check the victim for a response:
  - Shake his shoulders
  - Ask loudly
  ↓

↓
No response
↓
Shout for help
- Turn the victim on to his back and then open the airway using head tilt and chin lift.
  - Place hand on his forehead and gently tilt his head back
  - Lift chin
  ↓

Flowchart 1: Basic life-support healthcare provider adult cardiac arrest algorithm.

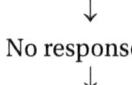

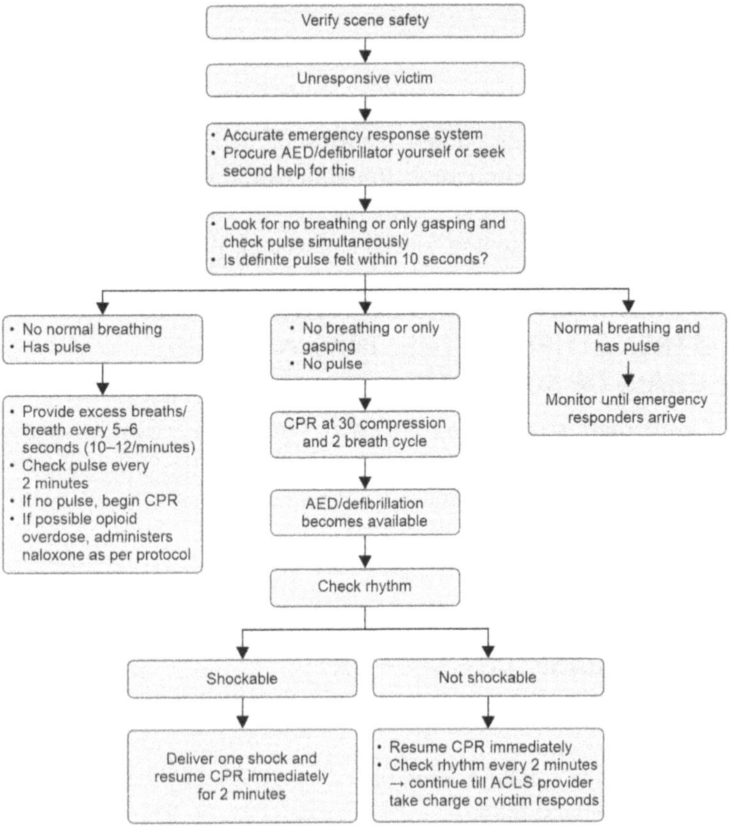

(ACLS: advanced cardiac life-support; AED: automated external defibrillator; CPR: cardiopulmonary resuscitation)

- Keeping airway open; look, listen and feel for normal breathing (take not >10 seconds)
- Look for any chest movements, listen for breath sounds

Flowchart 2: Adult advanced cardiac arrest algorithm.

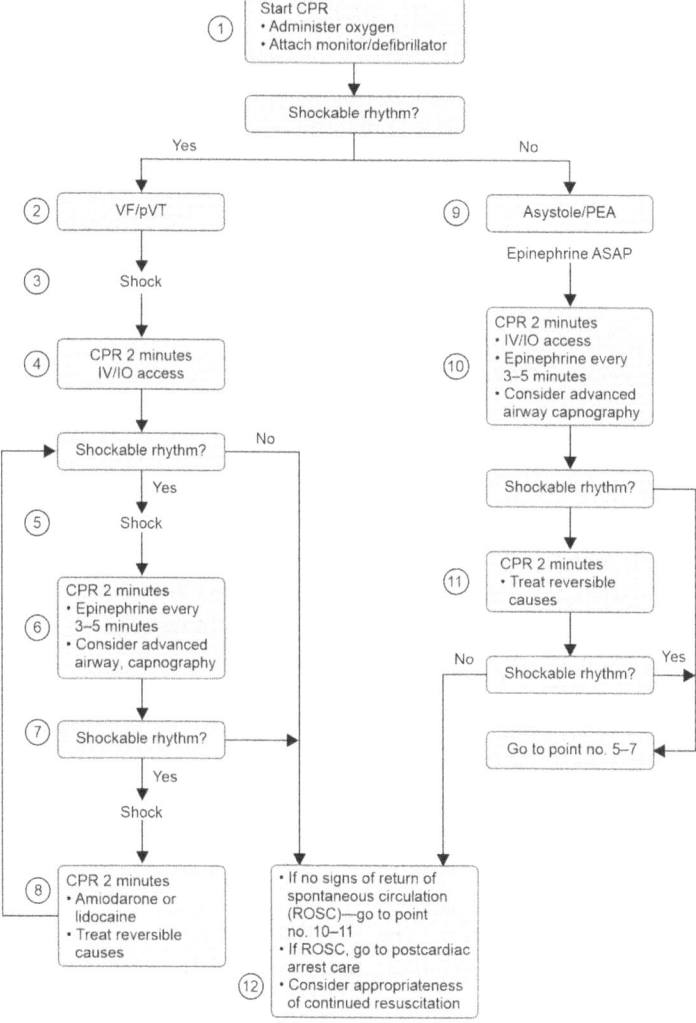

(CPR: cardiopulmonary resuscitation; IO: intraosseous; IV: intravenous)

↓
- Not breathing, alert emergency services, and send someone for automatic external defibrillator
- Kneel by side of victim
- Start chest compression @ 100-120 times/min, (a little <2 compressions for a second)—1″ above xiphoid, depth should be 1½-2″ for adults, 1-1½″ for children, ½-1″ for infants.

↓

- Combined chest compression with rescue breaths:
  - Blow into victim's mouth taking about 1 second to make his chest rise as in normal breathing
  - Continued chest compression rescue breath in a ratio of 30:2

↓

- Stop to check only if he starts breathing normally. Otherwise, do not interrupt resuscitation

↓

- Continue resuscitation until
- Qualified help arrives and takes over

SOME CLARIFICATIONS

- *Shock energy for defibrillation:*
  - *Biphasic:*
    - Manufacturer recommendation (e.g., initial dose of 120-200 J); if unknown, use maximum available.
    - Second and subsequent doses should be equivalent and higher doses may be considered.
  - *Monophasic:* 360 J
- *Drug therapy:*
  - *Epinephrine:* IV/IO dose: 1 mg every 3-5 minutes
  - *Amiodarone:* IV/IO dose:
    - *First dose:* 300 mg/bolus
    - *Second dose:* 150 mg
  - *Lidocaine:* IV/IO dose:
    - *First dose:* 1-1.5 mg/kg
    - *Second dose:* 0.5-0.75 mg/kg
- *Advanced airway:*
  - Endotracheal intubation or supraglottic advanced airway

- Waveform capnography or capnometry to confirm and monitor ET-tube placement
- Once advanced airway is put in place, give 1 breath every 6 seconds (10 breaths/min) with continuous chest compressions (CCCs)
- Return of spontaneous circulation (ROSC):
  - Pulse and blood pressure
  - Abrupt sustained increase in $PETCO_2$ (typically >40 mm Hg)
  - Spontaneous arterial pressure waves with intra-arterial monitoring
- Reversible causes:
  - Hypovolemia
  - Hypoxia
  - Acidosis
  - Hypo/hyperkalemia
  - Hypothermia
  - Tension pneumothorax
  - Cardiac tamponade

Flowchart 3: Opiate-associated emergency algorithm.

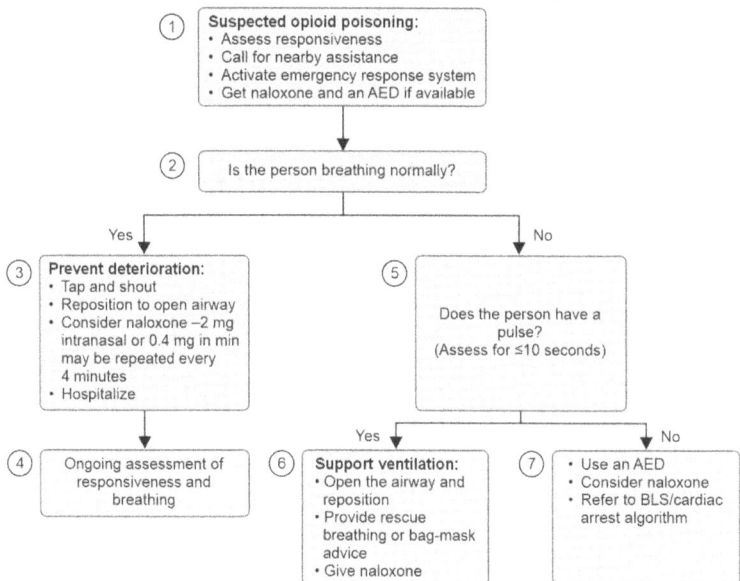

(AED: automated external defibrillator)

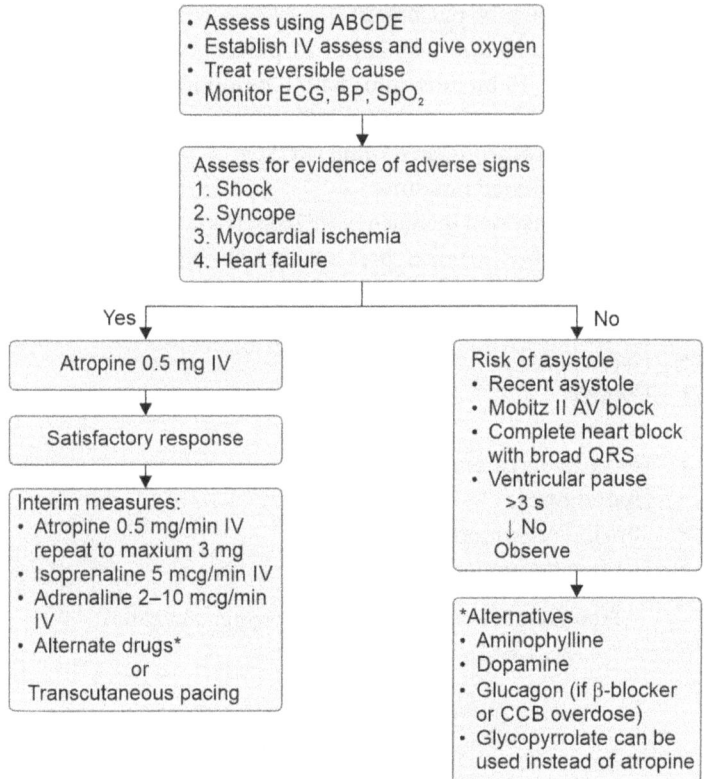

Flowchart 4: Advance cardiac life support bradycardia algorithm.

(ABCDE: airway, breathing, circulation, disability, exposure; BP: blood pressure; CCB: calcium-channel blocker; ECG: electrocardiography; IV: intravenous)

- Toxins
- Pulmonary thrombosis
- Coronary thrombosis

ADVANCED CARDIAC LIFE-SUPPORT

- The victim starts breathing normally
- You become exhausted
- As soon as automated external defibrillator (AED) arrives, switch it on and follow instructions
- Quantitative waveform capnography → if patient end-tidal carbon dioxide ($PETCO_2$—normal values 35–40 mm Hg) is low or decreasing, reassess CPR quality

Cardiopulmonary Resuscitation

Flowchart 5: Tachycardia algorithm.

1. Tachycardia with pulses

2.
- Assess and support ABCs as needed
- Give oxygen
- Monitor ECG (identify rhythm), blood pressure, oximetry
- Identify and treat reversible causes

3. Symptoms persist

Assess for evidence of adverse signs:
- Shock
- Syncope
- Myocardial ischemia
- Heart failure

4. Perform immediate synchronized cardioversion
- Establish IV access and give sedation if patient is conscious; do not delay cardioversion
- Consider expert consultation
- If pulseless arrest develops, see pulseless arrest algorithm

5.
- Establish IV access
- Obtain 12-lead ECG (when available) or rhythm strip. Is QRS narrow?

6. Narrow (<0.12 seconds)
Narrow QRS
Is rhythm regular?

12. Wide (≥0.12 seconds)
Wide QRS
Is rhythm regular?
Expert consultation advised

7. Regular
- Attempt vagal maneuvers
- Give adenosine 6 mg rapid IV push. If no conversion, give 12 mg rapid IV push; may repeat 12 mg dose once

8. Stable
- Does rhythm convert?
  Note: Consider expert consultation

11. Irregular
Irregular narrow-complex tachycardia
Probable atrial fibrillation or possible atrial flutter or multifocal atrial tachycardia
- Consider expert consultation
- Control rate (diltiazem, β-blocker; use β-blockers with caution in pulmonary disease or CHF)
- Consider diagnosis or amiodarone if evidence of heart failure
- Anticoagulate if duration >48 hours

9. Converts
If rhythm converts, probably re-entry Supraventricular tachycardia (SVT)
- Observe for recurrence
- Treat recurrence with adenosine or longer-acting AV nodal blocking agents (such as diltiazem or beta-blockers)

10. Do not convert
If rhythm does not convert, atrial flutter, ectopic atrial tachycardia, or junctional tachycardia
- Control rate (diltiazem, β-blockers; use β-blockers with caution in pulmonary disease of CHF)
- Treat underlying cause
- Consider expert consultation

13. Regular
Amiodarone 300 mg IV over 20–60 minutes

14. Irregular
Magnesium 2 g over 2 minutes

(ABC: airway, breathing, compressions; CHF: congestive heart failure; ECG: electrocardiography)

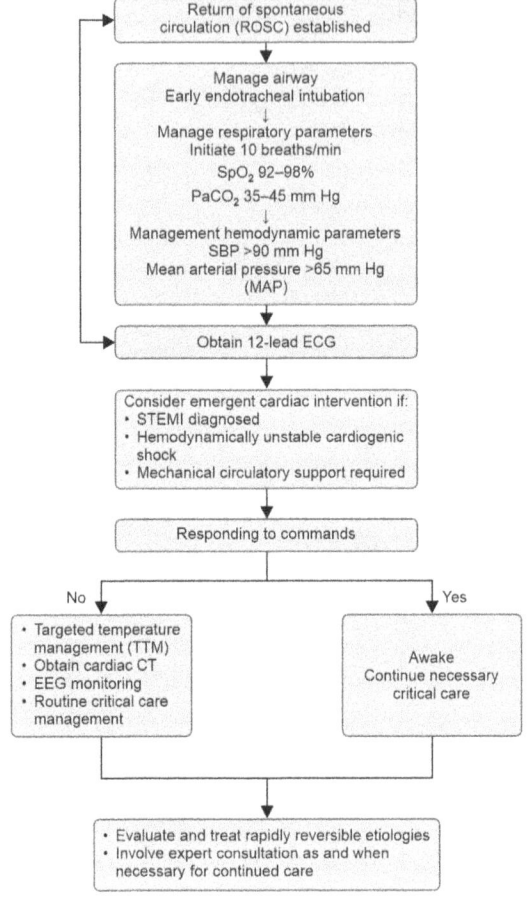

Flowchart 6: Adult postcardiac arrest care algorithm.

CARDIOCEREBRAL RESUSCITATION

The followings are the three pillars of cardiocerebral resuscitation:
1. Compression—only CPR by anyone who witnesses unexpected collapse with abnormal breathing (cardiac arrest)
2. Cardiocerebral resuscitation by emergency medical services (arriving during circulatory phrase of untreated ventricular fibrillation (e.g., > 5 minutes)
    i. *200 CCCs:* Delay intubation, second person applies defibrillation pads and initiates passive oxygen insufflation.

Cardiopulmonary Resuscitation

   ii. Single direct current shock if indicated without postdefibrillation pulse check
   iii. 200 CCCs prior to pulse check or rhythm analysis
   iv. Epinephrine (intravenous or intraosseous) as soon as possible
   v. Repeat (ii) and (iii) three times. Intubate if no ROSC after three cycles
   vi. Continue resuscitation efforts with minimal interruptions of chest compressions until successful or pronounced dead
3. Postresuscitation care to include mild hypothermia (32–34°C) for patients in coma postarrest.

Urgent cardiac catheterization and percutaneous coronary intervention (PCI) unless contraindicated.

The concept of CCC CPR by bystanders came into being with the expectation that eliminating mouth-to-mouth "rescue breathing" will go on a long way toward increasing the incidence of bystander-initiated resuscitation efforts. CCR also changes the approach of those delivering advanced cardiac life-support (ACLS). These changes resulted in dramatic (250–300%) improvement in survival of patients most likely to survive with witnessed cardiac arrest and shockable rhythm. Most aggressive postresuscitation care, including hypothermia and emergent cardiac catheterization and PCI, is required to save even more victims of sudden cardiac arrest.

Initial and late key objectives of postcardiac arrest care include:
- Optimizing cardiopulmonary function and vital organ perfusion after ROSC; anticipate, treat, and prevent multiple organ dysfunction.
- Transportation to an appropriate hospital or critical care unit with a comprehensive postcardiac arrest treatment system of care
- Institute measures to improve long-term neurologically intact survival; temperature control to optimize neurological recovery.
- Identification and intervention for acute coronary syndrome
- Identify causes of arrest and institute measures to prevent recurrence.

Hands only CPR, i.e., chest compressions with no mouth-to-mouth has become especially relevant in the COVID-19 era. The American Heart Association says that for teens and adults experiencing cardiac arrest, lungs, and blood contain enough oxygen to keep vital organ healthy as long as high-quality chest compressions with minimal interruption supplies blood to blood and heart muscle.

PROGNOSTIC FACTORS AFTER CPR

If four of these five predictors are present 24 hours—after CPR a poor prognosis is implied:
1. Absent corneal reflex at 24 hours
2. Absent pupillary reflex at 24 hours
3. Absent withdrawal reflex at 24 hours
4. No motor response at 24 hours and 72 hours
5. EEG more than 24–48 hours provides useful predictive information

TARGETED TEMPERATURE MANAGEMENT POSTCARDIAC ARREST

The concept that hypothermia can provide neuroprotection also has roots in the past where it was observed that infants abandoned and exposed to cold remained alive for prolonged periods. Renewed interest in hypothermia was generated in the 1980s when animal studies provided clues that mild hypothermia (32–35°C) could be beneficial.

Currently available cooling techniques can be divided into three main categories:
  i. Conventional cooling techniques (i.e., cold intravenous fluids)
 ii. Surface cooling systems (i.e., surface blankets or pads)
iii. Intravascular cooling systems (e.g., Thermogard XP system)

Other less known cooling methods include an extracorporeal cooling method using KTEK-3 in Japan, an intranasal cooling system (Rhino Chill) or induction and maintenance of hypothermia through continuous renal replacement therapy (CRRT).

In the CRICS-TRIGGERSEP group trial, moderate therapeutic hypothermia (33°C during the first 24-hour) in comparison to targeted normothermia (37°C) in patients with coma following cardiac arrest secondary to a nonshockable rhythm led to a higher percentage of a favorable neurologic outcome at day 90. The first targeted temperature management (TTM) trial results were somewhat misinterpreted because targeted hypothermia failed to demonstrate and clear benefit and many clinicians gave up this mode of management. The key take-away from TTM-2 trial was that TTM involving pharmacotherapy, device cooling, and timely neurological prognostication is a crucial treatment strategy to improve outcomes in patients who have had a cardiac arrest. The target temperature, at the discretion of the clinician, could be 33°C, 36°C, or 37.5°C or less. In both TTM trials, overall survival at 6 months among patients with out of hospital cardiac arrest was approximately 50%, a significant improvement over historical average of 25%.

The term TTM was coined to cover the deficiencies of the previous term "therapeutic hypothermia" which did not include interventions intended to maintain temperature near 37°C. TTM comprises three district phases:
1. *Induction phase:* When cooling is initiated over 60–80 minutes.
2. *Maintenance phase:* Lasts for 24–28 hours with minimal or no fluctuations in temperature.
3. *Rewarming phase:* It has to be done very slowly at the rate of 0.1–0.2°C per hour to avoid side effects of vasodilatation.

TABLE 1: Side-effects of each phase of TTM.

Phase	Complications	Treatment
1. Induction	• Shivering (≤35.5°C) • Hypovolemia • Hyperglycemia • Electrolyte disturbances • Hypocapnia	• *Drugs*: Fentanyl, tramadol, dexamethasone, and pethidine • *Fluid:* Normal saline/Ringer lactate • Insulin infusion to target blood sugar between 140 and 180 mg/dL • $Na^+/K^+/Mg^{2+}$ values to be checked → supplemented if low decrease minute ventilation
2. Maintenance	Infections	Strict vigilance
3. Rewarming	Hypoglycemia	Strict monitoring of blood sugar and titration of insulin
	• Hyperkalemia • Reperfusion injury	K^+ infusion to be stopped

Flowchart 7: Cardiac arrest in pregnancy in-hospital ACLS algorithm.

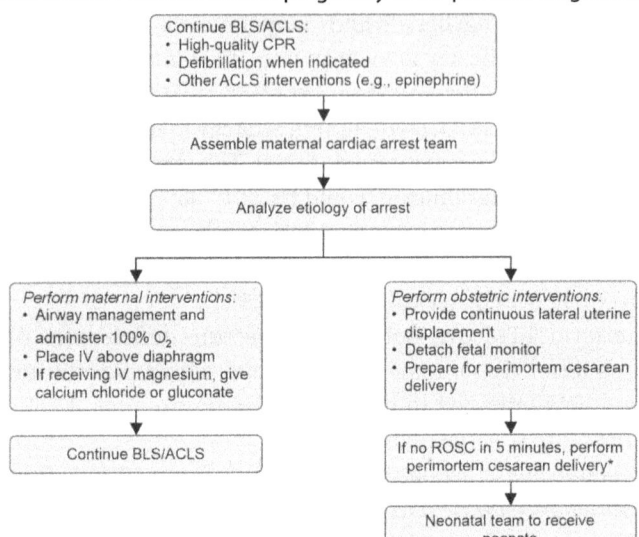

*Ideally, perimortem cesarean section should be performed in 5 minutes, depending on provider resources and skill sets.

COMMON INTERVENTIONS AND MEDICATIONS USED IN ACLS

Interventions

- *Shock—biphasic:* Manufacturer recommendation (e.g., initial dose of 120-200 J); if unknown, use maximum available. Second and subsequent doses should be equivalent and higher doses may be considered.
- *Monophasic*: 360 J synchronized cardioversion: Initial recommended doses:
  - *Narrow regular:* 50-100 J
  - *Narrow irregular:* 120-200 J biphasic or 200 J monophasic
  - *Wide regular:* 100 J
  - *Wide irregular:* Defibrillation dose (not synchronized)
- *Ventilation/oxygenation:* Avoid excessive ventilation. Start at 10-12 breaths/min and titrate to target $PETCO_2$ of 35-40 mm Hg. When feasible, titrate FiO_2 to minimum necessary to achieve $SpO_2 \geq 94\%$.

- *Advanced airway:*
    - Supraglottic advanced airway or endotracheal intubation
    - Waveform capnography to confirm and monitor ET tube placement
    - 8-10 breaths/min with CCCs
- *CPR quality:*
    - Push hard [≥2 inches (5 cm) and fast (≥100/min)] and allow complete chest recoil
    - Minimize interruptions in compressions
    - Avoid excessive ventilation
    - Rotate compressor every 2 minutes
    - If no advanced airway, 30:2 compression: ventilation ratio
    - Quantitative waveform capnography—If $PETCO_2$ <10 mm Hg, attempt to improve CPR quality
    - Intra-arterial pressure—if relaxation phase (diastolic) pressure <20 mm Hg, attempt to improve CPR quality

In intubated patients, failure to achieve an end-tidal carbon dioxide >10 mm Hg by waveform capnography after 20 minutes may be considered as one component of a multimodal approach to decide when to end resuscitation efforts but should not be used in isolation.

Medications

- *Epinephrine:* It is an endogenous catecholamine which acts by stimulating β_1 and α_1 adrenergic receptors. Most commonly used drug during CPR.
    - *Dose:* 10 mL of a 1:10,000 solution repeat after 3-5 minutes; 1 mg IV/IO; for IV QT and wide complex tachycardia of uncertain origin (IIb)
- *Rapid ventricular rate due to accessory pathways:*
    - *Dose:* 5 mg/kg IV infusion as bolus over 20 min-2 hours. In emergency—300 mg slow IV push over 10-60 min ↓ followed by:
        - Infusion of 900 mg over 24 hours
        - Supplementary dose of 150 mg may be repeated every 10 minutes to a maximum of 2 g/24 hours
    - *Side effects:* (1) Hypotension; (2) bradycardia

- *Procainamide:* Blocks open sodium channels and also blocks IKr prolonging action potential duration. It can be used in treating stable monomorphic VT but has been generally replaced by amiodarone for this indication. It can also be used in SVTs, particularly rapidly conducting AF and atrial flutter in WPW syndrome.
  - *Dose:* 20-50 mg/min until arrhythmia suppressed, hypotension ensures, QRS duration increases >50% or maximum dose 17 mg/kg given. Maintenance infusion: 1-4 mg/min. Avoid if prolonged QT or CHF.
- *Sotalol:* It is a class III antiarrhythmic drug with nonselective beta-blocking properties and this combined action makes it effective for a wide range of supraventricular and ventricular arrhythmias.
  - *Dose:* 100 mg (1.5 mg/kg) over 5 minutes. Avoid if prolonged QT.
- *Magnesium indicated in Torsades de pointes:*
  - In VF/pulseless VT—dose is 2 g diluted in 10 mL of D/W IV; push over 10 minutes (IIA). It can be repeated once if necessary.
  - Pulse present—1-2 g in 50-100 mL of D/W IV loading over 5-60 minutes
- *Adenosine:* Endogenous purine nucleotide that depresses AV node and SA node activity.
  - *Indications:*
    - SVT (I)
    - Unstable SVT (IIb)
    - Undefined stable narrow complex SVT
  - *Dose:* 6 mg IV as rapid IV push given over 1-3 seconds through a large vein followed by 20 mL saline flush and elevation of the arm.
    ↓ If not corrected by 2 minutes
    12 mg stat
    ↓ 1-2 minutes 12 mg stat again
    5-10 mg over 15-30 minutes up to total 20 mg

- *Norepinephrine:* It is predominantly an α^{-1} adrenergic stimulant with mild β-receptor agonism and thus is best categorized as a vasopressor.
  - *Dose:* 0.1–0.5 µg/kg/min (in 70 kg adult: 7–35 µg/min)
- *Dopamine:* It evokes most of its effects through activation of adrenergic receptors (β_1, β_2, and α) and also acts via stimulation of dopaminergic receptors (D1 and D2) at low dosage (<4.0 µg/kg/min).
  - *Dose:* 5–10 µg/kg/min as a vasopressor
- *Lignocaine*: It may be considered as an alternative to amiodarone in stable monomorphic VT, polymorphic VT with normal QT and if ventricular function is preserved.
  - *Dose:* Initial 1.0–1.5 mg/kg IV bolus; additional doses of 0.5–0.75 mg/kg IV every 10–15 minutes can be given up to maximum of 3 mg/kg. A maintenance IV infusion of 2–4 mg/min may be acceptable.
  - Side effects include slurred speech, altered sensorium, seizures, bradycardia, and muscle twitching

SUGGESTED READING

1. Calabro L, Bougouin W, Cariou A, De Fazio C, Skrifvars M, Soreide E, et al. Effect of different methods of cooling for targeted temperature management on outcome after cardiac arrest: A systematic review and meta-analysis. Critical Care. 2019;23:285.
2. Ewy GA. Cardiocerebral and Cardiopulmonary Resuscitation—2017 Update. Acute Med Surg. 2017;4(3):227-34.
3. Merchant RM, Topijan AA, Panchal AR, Cheng A, Aziz K, Berg KM, et al; Adult Basic and Advanced Life Support, Pediatric Basic and Advanced Life Support, Neonatal Life Support, Resuscitation Education Science, and Systems of Care Writing Groups. Part 1: Executive summary: 2020 American Heart Association Guideline for Cardiopulmonary Resuscitation and Emergency Cardiovascular Care. Circulation. 2020;142(Suppl.2):S337-S357.

CHAPTER 9

Percutaneous Coronary Intervention in Acute Myocardial Infarction

Shuvanan Ray, Soumitra Kumar

WHY PPCI IS DIFFERENT FROM ELECTIVE PCI, PROTOCOL FOR PPCI?

Acute ST elevation myocardial infarction (STEMI) results from abrupt occlusion of a major epicardial artery which leads to time-dependent myocardial necrosis extending from endocardium to epicardium in a wave front manner. Coronary reperfusion means opening of the artery permitting blood flow uninterruptedly into the microvasculature, and it can be achieved in a timely manner either by primary percutaneous intervention or by fibrinolysis. Reperfusion improves clinical outcomes compared to no reperfusion in nearly all groups of patients presenting with STEMI. A number of mega trials of fibrinolysis established that myocardial salvage and related mortality reduction with fibrinolysis gradually decline with the time passed between the onset of chest pain and introduction of the drug. Initial studies of primary percutaneous coronary intervention (PPCI) did not show this trend and rather stressed a "door to balloon time", i.e., time between the first medical contact and balloon dilatation which if prolonged denied any survival benefit after the procedure. A report from NRMI data, which included a cohort of 29,222 patients with STEMI treated with PCI within 6 hours of presentation. In hospital, mortality was 3%, 4.2%, 5.7%, and 7.4% for door to balloon intervals of 90 minutes or less, 91–120 minutes, 121–150 minutes and >150 minutes respectively ($p < 001$). Nevertheless, the data comparing primary PCI and thrombolysis do not mean that myocardial salvage after primary PCI is not time dependent. They merely indicate that time window for myocardial salvage is wider with primary PCI than thrombolysis. Recent data demonstrated that a shorter door to balloon time (<90 minutes) with a shorter symptom onset to door time (<4 hours) was associated with lowest longer term mortality and short door to balloon time (<90 minutes) are associated with lower mortality in early presenters but not very importantly in late presenters. Based upon the randomized clinical trials, primary PCI is preferred when performed in a timely fashion by an expert operator in patients with ST elevation MI, or an MI with a new or presumably new LBBB or a true posterior MI.

WHY PRIMARY PERCUTANEOUS CORONARY INTERVENTION IS DIFFERENT FROM ELECTIVE PERCUTANEOUS CORONARY INTERVENTION?

Primary PCI involves opening of a thrombus-laden large epicardial artery in a patient with unstable hemodynamics in a time dependent manner to establish free flow through the microcirculation. It requires a sound knowledge base and a technical expertise that is distinctly different from that required to perform elective PCI. The procedure may demand skillful performance at odd hours of the day with relatively a smaller number of supporting personnel.

- *Patients who present in golden hour:* The first 2 hours are very important for salvage of myocardium. If PCI cannot be offering before 120 minutes (even <90 minutes), thrombolysis with fibrin-specific agents should be administered.
- *Between 2 and 12 hours:* In the landmark thrombolysis studies, it is seen that timely thrombolysis is capable for salvaging myocardium. If the patients present within 6 hours of onset of symptoms. After 6 hours thrombolysis becomes less effective, but primary percutaneous coronary intervention (PPCI) is still found useful in these patients but such evidence available on its clinical value remains limited. So, PPCI within this time frame should be offered to patients:
  - Presenting >3-4 hours of symptom onset (short transfer time to PCI capable hospital)
  - With contraindication to thrombolysis
  - With presence of shock or acute heart failure
  - When the diagnosis of STEMI is in doubt
- *Evolved (12-48 hours):* In patients who present late, routine PPCI strategy should be considered. After 48 hours, if the patient is stable without symptomatic of asymptomatic ischemia. PCI is not indicated.

- *Pharmacoinvasive therapy:* PPCI is less capable to achieve microvascular reperfusion in patients who come late. Timely thrombolysis followed by PCI in failed patients or routinely within 3-24 hours (pharmacoinvasive therapy) was tested to different studies, and it is found to be almost equal to timely PPCI in clinical outcomes. Pharmacoinvasive therapy would be the cornerstone of STEMI management in countries where PCI centers are not available everywhere or are not capable to deliver within 90-120 minutes of first medical contact.

Risk stratification for PPCI: Two multivariable models have been devised and validated for patients undergoing PPCI. The Zwolle PPCI risk index and the Cardiac Risk Score. The Zwolle index was based upon a PPCI population in Zwolle, the Netherlands from data on 1,791 patients undergoing PPCI between 1994 and 2001. Controlled abciximab and device investigation to lower late angioplasty complications (CADILLAC) risk score was derived from the 2,082 patients in the CADILLAC trial of abciximab or placebo and stenting or angioplasty in PPCI and then validated using data from the 900 patients in the stent-primary angioplasty in myocardial infarction (STENTPAMI) trial. Seven variables, which are readily available at the time of intervention, were weighted according to their odds ratio for 1 year mortality:

- LVEF <40% - 4 points
- Killip class 2/3 - 3 points
- Renal insufficiency- (estimated CrCl <60 mL/min) - 3 points
- TIMI flow grade after PCI 0-2 - 2 points
- Age >65 years - 2 points
- Anemia (hematocrit - <39% in men, <36% in women) - 2 points
- Triple vessel CAD - 2 points

Patients could be stratified into three risk groups:
- Low risk (score 0-2) - Male 0.1-0.2% at 30 days and 08-0.9% at 1 year
- Intermediate risk (3-5) - Male 1.3-1.9% at 30 days and 4-4.5% at 1 year
- High risk (>6) - Male 6.6-8.1% at 30 days and 12.4-13.2% in 1 year

PROTOCOL FOR PRIMARY PERCUTANEOUS CORONARY INTERVENTION

Preprocedural Protocol

At Home

- Chew aspirin 325 mg (not enteric coated)
- Call emergency service
- Prehospital ECG (if available immediately)

At Hospital

- Establish a PPCI orientation program
- All patients with confirmed or suspected AMI undergo emergency angiography; thrombolysis withheld. Referring physicians (e.g., physicians, internists, and noninvasive cardiologists) and catheterization laboratory staff members are educated about invasive treatment.
- Percutaneous transluminal coronary angioplasty (PTCA) should be performed as rapidly as possible.
- Catheterization laboratory team is called in as soon as intimation is received that a patient of myocardial infarction is being transported or has arrived at the ER.
- An abbreviated history is taken, and a physical examination is performed in the ER; laboratory samples are drawn, and medications are given. If ECG has been done, patient may be taken directly to the Coronary Care Unit by passing the ER.

Adjunctive Pharmacology

Antiplatelet Therapy

Recommendations:
- In patients undergoing PCI, a loading dose of aspirin, followed by daily dosing, is recommended to reduce ischemic events (Class 1 recommendation).
- In patients with acute coronary syndrome (ACS) undergoing PCI, a loading dose of P2Y12 inhibitor, (clopidogrel, ticagrelor, and prasugrel) followed by daily dosing, is recommended to reduce ischemic events (Class 1 recommendation).

- In patients with ACS undergoing PCI, it is reasonable to use ticagrelor or prasugrel in preference to clopidogrel to reduce ischemic events, including stent thrombosis (Class 2a recommendation).
- In patients undergoing PCI within 24 hours after fibrinolytic therapy, a loading dose of 300 mg of clopidogrel followed by daily dosing is recommended to reduce ischemic events (Class 1 recommendation)
- In patients <75 years of age undergoing PCI within 24 hours after fibrinolytic therapy, ticagrelor may be a reasonable alternative to clopidogrel to reduce ischemic events (Class 2b recommendation).
- In patients undergoing PCI who have a history of stroke or transient ischemic attack, prasugrel should not be administered (Class 3 recommendation).
- In patients undergoing PCI who are P2Y12 inhibitor naïve, intravenous cangrelor may be reasonable to reduce periprocedural ischemic events (Class 2b recommendation).
- In patients with ACS undergoing PCI with large thrombus burden, and resultant no reflow or slow flow, intravenous glycoprotein IIb/IIIa inhibitor agents are reasonable to improve procedural success (Class 2a recommendation).

Scientific evidence base for the recommendations: In the early days of PCI, aspirin was found to be effective at decreasing coronary thrombosis with balloon angioplasty. Contemporary oral P2Y12 inhibitors used in PCI include clopidogrel, ticagrelor, and prasugrel. A loading dose of 600 mg of clopidogrel is associated with a shorter time to platelet inhibition and therefore is the preferred dose. TRITON-TIMI 38 trial with prasugrel and PLATO trial with ticagrelor in ACS patients reduced the rate of composite endpoint of death from vascular causes, MI, or stroke in comparison to clopidogrel. These agents were also associated with a lower rate of stent thrombosis. These more potent agents should be used with caution in other patients because of increased bleeding risk. One trial (POPULAR AGE) albeit with open-label design tested use of clopidogrel versus ticagrelor or prasugrel in patients aged 70 years or older in non-STEMI patients suggested that with similar outcomes, clopidogrel may be a reasonable alternative for older patients with ACS. Further studies in this regard are indicated.

In the CLARITY trial, clopidogrel pretreatment in conjunction with fibrinolytic therapy resulted in a 46% reduction in the rate of cardiovascular death or recurrent MI or stroke at 30 days among patients referred for PCI. Major and minor bleeding was similar between the groups. A loading dose of 600 mg may be used for most patients, whereas lower 300 mg loading dose is generally reserved for older patients or those at higher risk of bleeding. In more recent times, the TREAT trial was designed to study the safety of ticagrelor in patients treated with fibrinolytic therapy for STEMI. In this study, ticagrelor was found to be non-inferior to clopidogrel in rates of TIMI major bleeding, fatal bleeding, and intracranial bleeding.

Cangrelor is a potent, direct, reversible, short-acting intravenous P2Y12 inhibitor with rapid onset of platelet inhibition, and restoration of platelet function within 1 hour of discontinuation. The CHAMPION program (CHAMPION PLATFORM, CHAMPION PCI, and CHAMPION PHOENIX) compared cangrelor with a loading dose of clopidogrel given at the time of PCI in three large scale clinical trials, cangrelor resulted in lower rates of prespecified secondary outcomes of stent thrombosis and death. There was a reduction in periprocedural MI and intraprocedural stent thrombosis.

Many of the trials of glycoprotein IIb/IIIa in the setting of ACS were conducted in the period before the use of potent P2Y12 inhibitors or before routine testing or when time to coronary angiography was often prolonged. In contemporary practice, with shortening of revascularization times and use of potent DAPT, benefit of GPIIb/IIIa receptor inhibitor agents is diminished. Its use is now generally reserved for patients with a large thrombus burden or no-reflow or slow-flow that is believed to be attributable to distal embolization of thrombus.

Anticoagulant Therapy

Recommendations:
- In patients undergoing PCI, administration of intravenous unfractionated heparin (UFH) is useful to reduce ischemic events (Class I recommendation).

[*Dose:* 70-100 u/kg initial bolus to achieve a target ACT of 250-300 seconds; additional UFH as needed (e.g., 2000-5000 u) to achieve ACT of 250-300 seconds].

- In patients with heparin-induced thrombocytopenia undergoing PCI, bivalirudin or argatroban should be used to replace UFH to avoid thrombotic complications (*Class I recommendation:* 2b).
  [*Dose:* In patients who are anticoagulant naïve, bivalirudin 0.75 mg/k, and IV bolus followed by 1.75 mg/kg/hour IV infusion to be administered].
- In patients undergoing PCI for ACS, bivalirudin may be a reasonable alternative to UFH to reduced bleeding (*Class of recommendation:* 2b) [*Dose:* In patients who are anticoagulant naïve, bivalirudin 0.75 mg/kg bolus, and 1.75 mg/kg/hour IV infusion to be administered].
- In patients on therapeutic subcutaneous enoxaparin, in whom last dose was administered within 12 hours of PCI, UFH should not be used for PCI and may increase bleeding (*Class of recommendation:* 3).
- Use of intravenous enoxaparin may be considered at the time of PCI to reduce ischemic events, only if upstream subcutaneous enoxaparin has been used to treat patients with unstable angina or NSTE-ACS (*Class of recommendation:* 2b).

Scientific evidence base for the recommendations: Based on the finding of HEAT-PPCI and MATRIX trials, UFH is recommended in addition to ticagrelor or prasugrel without a GIIb/IIIa inhibitor rather than bivalirudin or UFH plus routine GPIIb/IIIa inhibitor use. This is based on a lower rate of definite stent thrombosis and lower cost. For patients who receive clopidogrel rather than either prasugrel or ticagrelor, either heparin or bivalirudin is a reasonable choice. In patient who are at an increased bleeding risk, including women, those with renal dysfunction or those who undergo femoral access, bivalirudin is a reasonable choice. Fondaparinux is not recommended for primary PCI because of a higher incidence of guide catheter-related thrombosis.

Procedural Protocol

Arterial access: Radial and Femoral Approaches for Percutaneous Coronary Intervention

Recommendations: In patients with ACS undergoing PCI, a radial approach is indicated in preference to a femoral approach to reduce the risk of death, vascular complications, or bleeding (*Class of recommendation:* 1).

Scientific evidence base for the recommendation: Over the past decade, proportion of patients undergoing radial artery catheterization and PCI has increased exponentially. The MATRIX trial demonstrated a significantly lower rate of the coprimary endpoint of net adverse clinical events (30-day death, nonfatal infarction and stroke, and non-CABG major bleeding) among patients with ACS randomized to transradial approach than among those randomized to the transfemoral approach. The difference was driven by a lower rate of bleeding events and a lower 30-day mortality rate. A pre-specified subgroup analysis of patients with STEMI enrolled in RIVAL trial demonstrated a lower mortality rate at 30 days with transradial access. This was supported by a meta-analysis of RCTs. Although the SAFARI-STEMI trial failed to show any difference in 30-day mortality rate between radial and femoral access, this trial was stopped early for futility and enrolled less than half the sample size that was planned. In patients, who have a high likelihood of future CABG, radial access of the dominant artery will allow preservation of the non-dominant radial artery for use as a bypass graft.

Choice of Stent Type

Recommendations: In patients undergoing PCI, DES should be used in preference to BMS to prevent restenosis, MI, or acute stent thrombosis (*Class of recommendation:* 1).

Scientific evidence base for the recommendation: Earlier studies comparing outcomes with first generation DES and BMS reported an increase in late stent thrombosis and increased mortality rate with DES. There has been a notable improvement in DES technology, including optimization of drug polymer and stent design which has ensured the safety and efficacy. Several meta-analyses suggest that stents can be ranked from more to less safe as follows—durable-polymer DES ≥ biodegradable-polymer DES > BMS. Newer generation DES were defined as any DES released after the original sirolimus-eluting and paclitaxel-eluting DES. For this reason, there are limited roles for the use of BMS except for unusual circumstances, such as lack of DES availability or when patient is not in a position to receive DAPT for >1 month. The COMFORTABLE AMI clinical trial compared patients of STEMI randomized to receive a BMS or a biodegradable polymer biolimus-eluting group. The EXAMINATION clinical trial in STEMI patients showed that in patients who received a second-generation everolimus-eluting stent (EES) had significantly lower rate of definitive thrombosis compared to those receiving a BMS.

Also, all-cause mortality at 5 years was also significantly lower in favor of the EES arm. In the BVS EXAMINATION clinical trial comparing fully reasonable vascular scaffolds (BVS) to EES, no difference was found in device-oriented composite endpoints between the two groups. However, at the 2-year follow-up, rate of definitive thrombosis was often higher in the BVS group compared to EES group. It should be mentioned in this regard that long-term results of RCTs have proved a significantly higher rate of BVS thrombosis and that was the reason of their withdrawal from the market.

Thrombectomy

Recommendations: In patients with STEMI, routine aspiration thrombectomy before primary PCI is not useful (*Class of recommendation:* 3, i.e., no benefit).

Scientific evidence supporting the recommendation: Initial studies (TAPAS and EXPIRA) of aspiration thrombectomy in STEMI demonstrated an improvement in myocardial blush grades and rates of ST-segment-elevation resolution. Patient enrolled in contemporary trials of thrombectomy (thrombus aspiration) (Frobert et al., Jolly et al., Lagerqvist et al.) did not derive a benefit of reduction in infarct size or improvement in death, reinfarction, stent thrombosis or target-lesion revascularization at 30 days or 1 year or cardiovascular death, recurrent MI, cardiogenic shock or NYHA Class IV heart failure at 3 months or 1 year. INFUSE-AMI trial which combined use of intracoronary abciximab with thrombus aspiration also did not yield any benefit. In the TOTAL trial those patients who were assigned to thrombus aspiration arm were found to have a small but statistically significant increased risk of stroke. A patient-level meta-analysis also demonstrated a trend toward a higher rate of stroke. In the subgroup of patients with high thrombus burden, although thrombus aspiration was associated with a small but statistically significant reduced rate of cardiovascular death and a small but statistically significant increased rate of stroke. A sub-analysis of the EXAMINATION trial confirmed that the use of thrombectomy was associated with a higher rate of direct-stenting, lower rate of post-dilatation and a smaller number of stents implanted with a larger stent size. However, optimized angiographic result did not impact the long-term outcomes since no difference at 2 years in terms of clinical endpoints were found. Hence, clearly additional selective studies in patients with high thrombus burden are needed. mechanical (rheolytic) thrombectomy (JETSTENT trial) also did not result in benefit for the patients.

Revascularization of the Infarct related artery with ST elevation myocardial infarction

Recommendations:
- In patients with STEMI and ischemic symptoms for <12 hours, PCI should be performed to improve survival (*Class of recommendation:* 1).
- In patients with STEMI and cardiogenic shock or hemodynamic instability, PCI, or CABG (when PCI is not feasible) is indicated to improve survival irrespective of the time delay from MI onset (*Class of recommendation:* 1).
- In patients with STEMI who have mechanical complications (e.g., ventricular septal rupture, mitral valve insufficiency because of papillary muscle infarction or rupture, or free wall rupture or free wall rupture). CABG is recommended at the time of surgery, with the goal of improving survival (*Class of recommendation:* 1).
- In patients with STEMI and evidence of failed reperfusion after fibrinolytic therapy, rescue PCI of the infarct artery

should be performed to improve clinical outcomes (*Class of recommendation*: 1).

- In patients with STEMI who are treated with fibrinolytic therapy, angiography within 3-24 hours with the intent to perform PCI is reasonable to improve clinical outcomes (*Class of recommendation:* 2a). (Pharmacoinvasive therapy).
- In patients with STEMI who are stable and presenting 12-24 hours after symptom onset, PCI is reasonable to improve clinical outcomes (*Class of recommendation:* 2a).

Scientific evidence base for the recommendations: Multiple RCTs and meta-analyses (Keeley et al., Zijlstra et al., GUSTO IIb, Andersen et al., Grines et al.) have shown that primary PCI reduces death, MI, stroke, and major bleeding as compared with fibrinolysis, especially when treatment delays are minimized. The benefit is observed even if patients are transferred from non-PCI hospitals provided transfer times are reasonable and total ischemic time after presentation is <120 minutes.

Revascularization strategies in cardiogenic shock are discussed in the relevant chapter of this treatise: Emergency CABG along with surgical management of mechanical complications of STEMI continues to be high. Currently, only a few medical or percutaneous treatment modalities to effectively treat ventricular rupture, papillary muscle rupture leading to severe mitral regurgitation or ischemic ventricular septal rupture. No RCT has investigated whether adding CABG to emergent surgical repair of the mechanical complications is beneficial or not. Neither has any RCT examined whether emergent cardiac surgery is beneficial over initial medical stabilization and delayed surgery. Placement of a mechanical support device may be useful in temporizing a patient affected with mechanical complication of STEMI.

Revascularization strategies with regard to "Rescue PCI" and "Pharmacoinvasive therapy" (Routine early angiography with the intent to perform PCI following fibrinolytic therapy) are discussed in the chapter on "STEMI".

Percutaneous coronary intervention in patients of ST elevation myocardial infarction presenting after 12 hours of symptom onset:

This is not well studied in asymptomatic patients. BRAVE-2 was a small trial in asymptomatic STEMI patients with symptom onset >12 hours but <48 hours before presentation. Invasive strategy had a reduction in left ventricular infarct size (primary endpoint) compared with a conservative strategy. This also was a reduction in adjusted 4-year mortality rate in the invasive arm. This was supported by the observational data from Prospective National Observational Study in terms of lower adjusted 1-year mortality rate. This evidence should be weighed against potential for harm when PCI of a totally occluded artery is performed >24 hours after symptom onset. Hence, as evidence suggests delayed PCI of an infarct-related artery beyond 24-hours should be considered only in patients with a patient artery. Followed by the smaller DECOPI trial which enrolled patients presenting 2–15 days after symptom onset, the OAT trial also demonstrated that PCI of a totally occluded vessel did not reduce cardiovascular events at 4 years of follow-up and there was a trend toward a higher rate of recurrent infarction in the group assigned to PCI. It should be noted that patients who demonstrated severe ischemia on noninvasive stress testing were not enrolled in this trial. There have been no RCTs which have examined the benefit of PCI in patients with STEMI presenting >12 hours but who have clinical evidence of ongoing ischemia, acute severe heart failure or life-threatening arrhythmias. A strategy of delay reperfusion by PCI appears justified in these patient sub-groups with an expectation to improve outcomes.

In situations in which PCI is not possible for anatomic reasons or because of presence of severe left main or multivessel disease or in cases where PCI is unsuccessful, CABG can be an effective primary reperfusion strategy, particularly if a large area of myocardium is at risk. However, in cases of no-reflow following PCI, since CABG is unlikely to improve perfusion to the subtended myocardium, it may be actually harmful in this setting. As per European Society of Cardiology (ESC) 2017 STEMI Guidelines, three categories have been described:

- Patients who are still early in the course of STEMI I (12–48 hours) should undergo PCI.

- Those beyond 48 hours with evidence of silent ischemia or viability should also undergo PCI.
- Patients who are truly stable and asymptomatic beyond 48 hours from onset of symptoms, with no evidence of silent ischemia or viability, can safely be treated with medical therapy.

Revascularization of the non-infarct related artery in patients with ST elevation myocardial infarction: Around 50% of patients with STEMI show multivessel coronary artery disease. Multiple clinical trials have examined the best revascularization strategy, i.e., treat the culprit lesion (>70% diameter stenosis with ≥2 mm vessel size) only versus complete revascularization. Initial trials like PRAMI and CULPRIT showed that complete revascularization was superior to the PCI of infarct-related lesion only, in the terms of composite endpoint of death, reinfarction, heart failure, and refractory angina/repeat revascularization.

Measuring the fractional flow reserve (FFR) of coronary flow to guide the need for non-culprit lesion revascularization has been suggested. The DANAMI-3 PRAMI CULPRIT and COMPARE-ACUTE trials demonstrated that FFR-guided complete revascularization significantly reduced the risk of future CV events compared to the conventional angiographic approach. Similar results have been replicated by the Compare-Acute trial.

The COMPLETE clinical trial randomized 4,041 patients to complete revascularization versus culprit lesion therapy who were followed up for up to 3 years. Complete revascularization was superior to culprit-only approach to reduce the risk of cardiovascular death or myocardial death, myocardial infarction or ischemia-induced revascularization. In a systemic review of 10 randomized trials that included 7,030 patients with STEMI and MVD, complete revascularization was associated with reduced CV mortality compared with infarct-related artery (IRA)-only PCI. All-cause mortality was comparable in both groups. Complete revascularization was also associated with a reduced composite of CV death or new MI, supporting complete revascularization in patients with STEMI and MVD. Currently, the BioVasc trial is exploring the best time to perform complete revascularization, whether immediate or delayed. Both American (ACC/AHA/SCAI) and ESC guidelines currently recommend complete revascularization of the on-culprit lesions of

Flowchart 1: Algorithm for revascularization of non-infarct coronary artery lesion in patients with ST elevation myocardial infarction (STEMI).

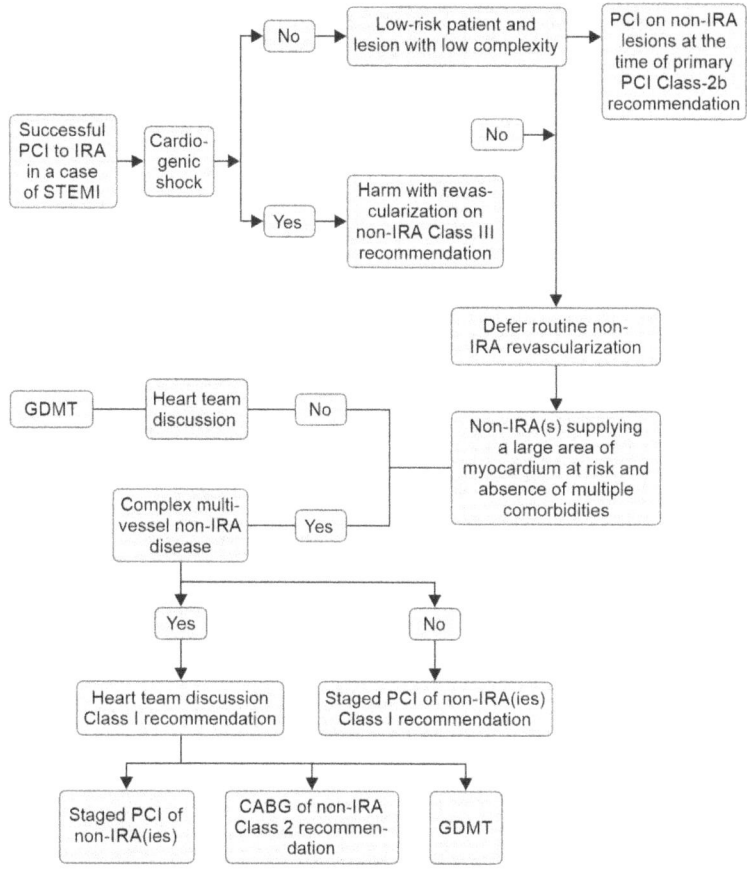

(GDMT: guideline-directed medical therapy; IRA: infarct-related artery)

patients with STEMI and multivessel disease during hospitalization and before hospital discharge.

It should, however, be noted that in the aforementioned trials, only one-third had triple-vessel disease and most of these trials excluded patients with left main disease, chronic total occlusion (CTO) of the non-infarct artery or complex non-infarct artery disease. Revascularization of non-infarct arteries includes those with a large area of myocardium at risk and those without significant comorbidities that would enhance the risk of revascularization.

Flowchart 2: Patients with ACS undergoing PCI of IRA with an angiographically significant stenosis of ≥1 non-IRA.

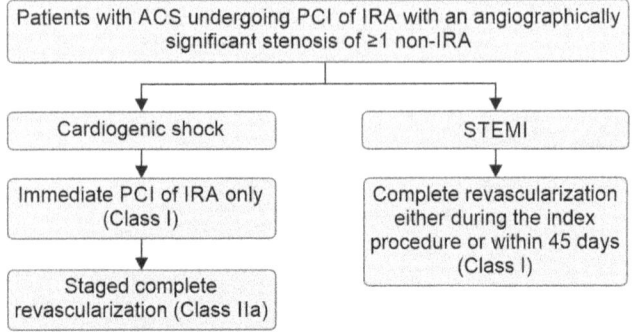

Flowchart 3: Pathophysiology of no-reflow.

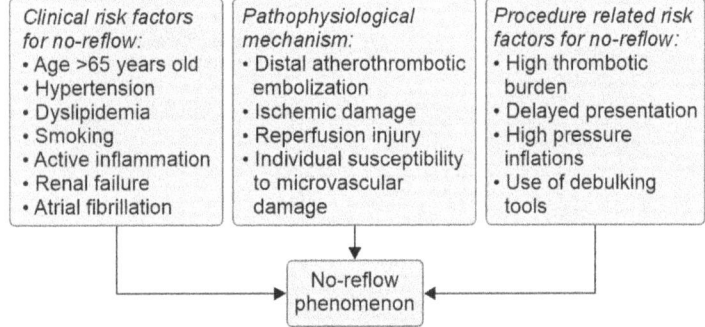

NO REFLOW: PREVENTION AND TREATMENT

No reflow is defined as thrombolysis in myocardial infarction (TIMI) flow grade <3 and myocardial blush grade <3 as manifestations of abnormal epicardial blood flow despite relief of coronary obstruction. It is a challenging complication of PCI occurring mainly in STEMI-related PCI and saphenous vein graft (SVG) PCI but can occur during elective PCI. Clinically, patient can experience hemodynamic instability, ischemic symptoms, and ST-elevation.

MAIN DIAGNOSTIC METHODS FOR ASSESSING NO-REFLOW

- *Coronary angiography:* TIMI flow grade and "Myocardial Blush Grade" (MBG) are two parameters that have been the mainstay

of diagnosis of non-reflow. Interobserver and intraobserver variabilities associated with subjective angiographic assessment are their limitations.
- *Coronary flow reserve (CFR) and microvascular resistance index (IMR):* CFR value ≥2.0 is considered normal. An IMR >40 is a multivariable associate of left ventricular and clinical outcomes after STEMI regardless of infarct size. Complimentary assessment of microcirculation by the IMR and CFR may be useful to evaluate myocardial viability and predict the long-term prognosis of STEMI patients.
- *Myocardial contrast echocardiography (MCE):* Among patients with TIMI 3 flow, microvascular obstruction (MVO) extension, as detected and quantified by MCE, is the most powerful independent predictor of LV remodeling after STEMI compared with persistent ST-segment elevation on ECG and degree of MBG.

Cardiac magnetic resonance (CMR) and position emission tomography (PET) are also extremely valuable for viability assessment but are expensive and not widely available.

Cardiac magnetic resonance (CMR) and PET are also very informative tools in assessment of microvascular obstruction (MVO) but are expensive and not widely available.

MANAGEMENT OF NO-REFLOW
Pharmacotherapy
- *Adenosine:* Intravenous 70 µg/kg/min infusion
  Intracoronary 100–200 µg bolus
- *Side effects:* Bradycardia, hypotension, chest pain, and dyspnea
- *Sodium nitroprusside:* Intracoronary—60–100 µg bolus
  Side effects: Bradycardia and hypotension
- *Verapamil:* Intracoronary—100–500 µg bolus (maximum 1 mg)
  Side effects: Bradycardia and transient heart block
- *Diltiazem:* Intracoronary—400 mg bolus (maximum 5 mg)
  Side effects: Bradycardia and hypotension
- *Nicardipine:* Intracoronary—200 µg (maximum 1 mg)
  Side effects: Bradycardia and hypotension
- *Epinephrine:* Intracoronary—80–100 µg bolus
  Side effects: Malignant arrhythmias

- *Nicorandil:* 500 µg (maximum 5 mg)
  Side effects: Malignant arrhythmias
- *Streptokinase:* 250 kU over 3 min
  Side effect: Bleeding
- *Tenecteplase:* 5 mg (maximum 25 mg)
  Side effect: Bleeding
- *Tissue plasminogen activator (tPA):* 0.025–5 mg/kg/hour
  Side effect: Bleeding
- *Abciximab:* 0.25 mg/kg bolus, then 0.125 mg/kg/min (maximum 10 µg/min) infusion for 12 hours
  Side effect: Bleeding
- *Eptifibatide:* 180 µg/kg bolus, then further 180 µg/kg bolus 10 minutes later, then 2 µg/kg/min infusion for up to 18 hours. If creatinine clearance <50 mL/min, reduce infusion by 50%.
  Side effect: Bleeding
- *Tirofiban:* 25 µg/kg over 3 min, then 0.15 µg/kg/min infusion for up to 18 hours. If creatinine clearance <30 mL/min reduce infusion by 50%
  Side effect: Bleeding

Nonpharmacological Treatment

- *Ischemic conditioning:* Ischemic preconditioning is the most powerful endogenous mechanism capable of reducing the extent of myocardial infarction by cycles of coronary balloon occlusion and reperfusion. Although ischemic preconditioning

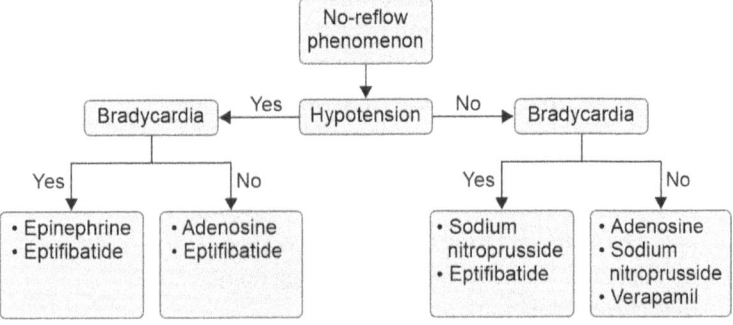

Flowchart 4: Use of pharmacotherapy on the basis of underlying hemodynamic parameters.

has been shown to reduce no reflow in small studies, larger randomized trials of POST, DANAMI-3, Impost, POSTEMI, and LIPSIA CONDITIONING have not supported its choice in clinical practice.
- *Thrombus aspiration:* Despite early positive results, it is neither indicated in routine primary PCI nor in situations of no reflow.

Another mechanical approach is to reduce distal embolization during STEMI consists of placement of filters, devices placed before stent deployment, which however, have never documented an effective improvement in microvascular flow, infarct extension, or clinical outcomes.

Pressure-controlled intermittent coronary sinus occlusion (PICSO) is a device which by increasing cardiac venous pressure and thus improves perfusion of the microcirculation. The Ox-AMI–PICSO study demonstrated less extension of infarction at 6 months in patients treated with PICSO compared with control group.

FUTURE PERSPECTIVE

- Therapeutic hypothermia which has shown favorable results in animals, but results are controversial in humans.
- Another technique is hyperoxemic reperfusion, evaluated in AMIHOT 1 and AMIHOT II studies, documented a reduction in final infarct size in spite of an increase in bleeding. It has been recently approved by FDA.
- A "tailored" anti-inflammatory approach in patients with evidence of myocardial oedema at CMR could be another therapeutic target.

ANTIPLATELET THERAPY AFTER PRIMARY PERCUTANEOUS CORONARY INTERVENTION

Risk Assessment to Guide Antiplatelet Therapy after Percutaneous Coronary Intervention

Bleeding Risk
- *Clinical variables:*
  - Previous major bleeding
  - Anemia

- Reduced platelet count
- Prior stroke
- Severe liver disease
- Malignancy
- Fragility
- *Procedural features:*
- Non-radial access
- Periprocedural use of GPIIb/IIIa inhibitors
- Use of thrombolytic agents
- Antiplatelets or anticoagulants before PCI
  - *Scores:* ARC-HBR, Blee MACS, CREDO-Kyoto, PRECISE-DAPT, PARIS, DAPT, and REACH

Antiplatelet Responsiveness

- *Platelet function testing*:
  - High platelet reactivity (HPR)
  - Optimal platelet reactivity (OPR)
  - Low platelet reactivity (LPR)
- *Genetic testing*:
  - Ultra-rapid (UR), rapid (RM), and normal (NM)
  - Intermediate (IM) or poor metabolizer (PM)

Ischemic Risk

- *Clinical variables:*
  - Acute coronary syndrome
  - Diabetes
  - Age >75 years
  - Chronic kidney disease
  - History of recurrent MI or stent thrombosis
  - BMI >30
  - Polyvascular atherosclerotic disease
- *Procedural features:*
  - Multivessel disease
  - Lesion length (>60 mm)
  - Number of stents implanted (≥3)
  - PCI of last patent vessel
  - Bifurcation or CTO

- Sub-optimal result (i.e., malapposition, under expansion, and periprocedural injury)
- *Scores:* ESC thrombotic definition
  - SYNTAX II
  - GRACE
  - TIMI
  - CADILLAC
  - PAMI
  - EPICOR
  - DAPT
  - GUSTO
- *Strategies focusing on ischemic events*
  - Use of prasugrel or ticagrelor over clopidogrel
  - Prolonging DAPT duration
  - Guided escalation
- *Strategies focusing on bleeding events*
  - Shortening DAPT
  - Guided de-escalation
  - Unguided de-escalation
  - Aspirin-free

CURRENT GUIDELINES OF EUROPEAN SOCIETY OF CARDIOLOGY 2023 ACUTE CORONARY SYNDROME GUIDELINES OF USE OF ANTIPLATELET THERAPY IN ACUTE CORONARY SYNDROME

ST-Elevation Myocardial Infarction

- *Before percutaneous coronary intervention:*
  - Aspirin (*Recommendation:* IA)
  - Routine P2Y12 inhibitor (*Recommendation:* IIb)
- *During percutaneous coronary intervention:*
  - Prasugrel (*Recommendation:* IA)
  - Ticagrelor (*Recommendation:* IA)
  - Clopidogrel (*Recommendation:* IA)
  - Prasugrel over ticagrelor (*Recommendation:* IIa B)
- *After percutaneous coronary intervention:*
  - DAPT for 12 months (*Recommendation:* IA)

TABLE 1: Randomized controlled trials (RCTs) testing antiplatelet strategies aiming at reducing ischemic events among patients undergoing PCI for ACS.

Primary endpoint met?	Study name	Year of publication	Treatment arms and population
Yes	TRITON TIMI 38	2007	Prasugrel vs. clopidogrel among ACS
Yes	PALTO	2008	Ticagrelor vs. clopidogrel among ACS
No	PHILO	2015	Ticagrelor vs. clopidogrel among ACS
No	PRAGTUE 18	2016	Ticagrelor vs. prasugrel among STEMI patients
No	ELDERLY ACS 2	2018	Reduced dose of prasugrel 5 mg vs. clopidogrel among ACS
Yes	TICAKOREA	2019	Ticagrelor vs. clopidogrel among ACS
Yes	ISAR-REACTS 5	2019	Ticagrelor vs. prasugrel among ACS
No	Popular Age	2020	Ticagrelor vs. clopidogrel among elderly (>70 years ACS
RCTs with prolonged DAPT duration			
No	DES-LATE	2010	12 months vs. 24 months DAPT
No	PRODIGY	2012	6 months vs. 24 months DAPT 30 days after PCI
Yes	DAPT	2014	12 months vs. 30 months DAP
No	ARCTIC interruption	2014	12 months vs. 18 months DAPT
No	ITALIC	2015	6 months vs. 24 months DAPT
Yes	PEGASUS-TIMI 54	2015	Ticagrelor 90 mg or ticagrelor 60 mg vs. Placebo 1–3 years after MI
No	OPTIDUAL	2016	12 months vs. 48 months DAPT
RCTs with platelet function testing (PFT)			
No	GRAVITAS	2011	High dose 150 mg vs. standard dose clopidogrel 75 g daily among clopidogrel non-responders defined by PFT

Contd...

Contd...

Primary endpoint met?	Study name	Year of publication	Treatment arms and population
No	ARCTIC	2012	High dose 150 mg clopidogrel vs. standard dose clopidogrel 75 mg daily among clopidogrel non-responders by PFT
No	TRIGGER-PCI	2012	Prasugrel vs. clopidogrel among clopidogrel non-responders defined by PFT
Yes	PHARMCLO	2018	Prasugrel or ticagrelor among clopidogrel non-responders defined by genetic testing vs. standard therapy
Yes	PATH-PCI	2019	Ticagrelor among clopidogrel non-responders defined by PFT vs. standard therapy
No	TAILOR-PCI	2020	Prasugrel or ticagrelor among clopidogrel non-responders defined by genetic testing vs. standard therapy
RCTs with shortening DAPT			
Yes	EXCELLENT	2012	6 vs. 12 months DAPT
Yes	RESET	2012	3 vs. 12 months DAPT
Yes	OPTIMIZE	2013	3 vs. 12 months DAPT
Yes	SECURITY	2014	6 vs. 12 months DAPT
Yes	ISAR-SAFE	2015	6 vs. 12 months DAPT
Yes	I-LOVE IT2	2016	3 vs. 12 months DAPT
Yes	NIPPON	2017	6 vs. 12 months DAPT
Yes	DAPT-STEMI	2018	6 vs. 12 months DAPT
Yes	SMART-DATE	2018	6 vs. 12 months DAPT
Yes	OPTIMA-C	2018	6 vs. 12 months DAPT

Contd...

Contd...

Primary endpoint met?	Study name	Year of publication	Treatment arms and population
Yes	One-month DAPT	2021	1 vs. 6–12 months DAPT in non-complex PCI
Yes	MASTER-DAPT	2021	1 vs. 5 months DAPT among high bleeding risk patients
RCTs with P2Y12 monotherapy			
Yes	GLOBAL-LEADERS	2018	Ticagrelor monotherapy for 23 months vs. DAPT with Ticagrelor for 12 months
Yes	TWILIGHT	2019	Ticagrelor monotherapy after 3 months of DAPT vs. standard DAPT in uneventful patients with high risk PCI
Yes	SMART-CHOICE	2019	P2Y12 inhibitor monotherapy after 3 months of DAPT vs. standard DAPT
Yes	STOPDAPT-2	2019	Clopidogrel monotherapy after 1 month of DAPT vs. standard DAPT
Yes	TICO	2020	Ticagrelor monotherapy after 3 months of DAPT vs. standard DAPT
No	STOP DAPT-2 ACS	2021	Clopidogrel monotherapy after 1 month of DAPT vs. standard DAPT among ACS
RCTs with unguided de-escalation			
Yes	TOPIC	2017	Clopidogrel-based DAPT vs. standard DAPT
Yes	• HOST-REDUCE • POLYTHEC-ACS	2020	Prasugrel 5 mg based DAPT vs. prasugrel 10 mg based DAPT
Yes	TALOS-MI	2021	Clopidogrel based DAPT vs. ticagrelor based DAPT

(Yes: Primary endpoint met; No: Primary endpoint not met)

TABLE 2: Overlapping of PEGASUS TIMI 54 and COMPASS trials.

ASA + Ticagrelor 60 mg bid		ASA + Rivaroxaban 2.5 mg bid
No history of ischemic stroke	CAD	Previous ischemic stroke (except last month)
No risk of bradycardia	High ischemic risk outweighing bleeding risk	No chronic heart failure (NYHA III/IV class or EF <30%)
No recent CABG	• >12 months post-PCI • Good tolerance of DAPT • Diabetes mellitus • Non end-stage CKD • No indication for P2Y12	Polyvascular disease

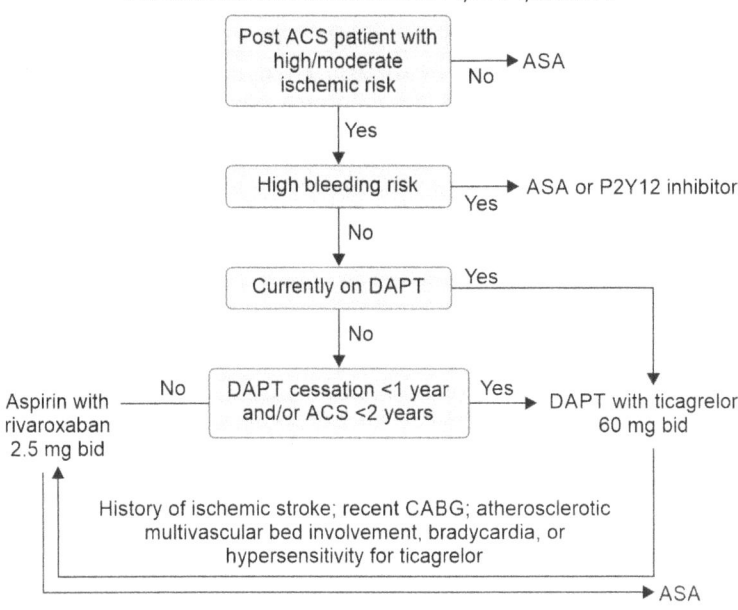

Flowchart 5: Choice between SAPT, DAPT, and DPI.

- Extended DAPT or DPI (high ischemic risk) (*Recommendation:* IIa A)
- 1-month DAPT → Clopidogrel (very high bleeding risk) (*Recommendation:* IIa B)
- 3-month DAPT → Aspirin (high bleeding risk) (*Recommendation:* IIa B)
- 3-month DAPT with ticagrelor → ticagrelor (*Recommendation:* IIa B)
- Extended DAPT or DPI (moderate ischemic risk) (*Recommendation:* IIb A)
- Guided de-escalation (*Recommendation:* IIb A)

RECOMMENDATIONS FOR ANTIPLATELET THERAPY IN PATIENTS WITH ATRIAL FIBRILLATION OF ANTICOAGULATION AFTER PERCUTANEOUS CORONARY INTERVENTION

- It is recommended to discontinue aspirin treatment after 1–4 weeks while maintaining P2Y12 inhibitors in addition to a non-vitamin K oral anticoagulant (rivaroxaban, dabigatran, apixaban, or edoxaban) or warfarin to reduce the risk of bleeding (*Recommendation:* 1BR).
- In patients with atrial fibrillation who are undergoing PCI are taking oral anticoagulant therapy and are treated with DAPT or a P2Y12 inhibitor monotherapy, it is reasonable to choose a non-vitamin K oral anticoagulant over warfarin to reduce the risk of bleeding (*Recommendation:* Class 2a BR).

SUGGESTED READING

1. Angiolillo DJ, Galli M, Phillipe-Collet J, Kastrati A, O'Donoghue ML. Antiplatelet therapy after Percutaneous Coronary Intervention. EuroIntervention. 2022;17(17):e1371-96.
2. Annibali G, Serocca J, Aranzulla TC, Meliga E, Maiellaro F, Musumeci G, et al. No Reflow Phenomenon: A Contemporary Review. J Clin Med. 2022;11(8):2233.
3. Byrne RA, Rossello X, Coughlan JJ, Barbato E, Berry C, Chieffo A, et al. 2023 ESC Guidelines for the management of acute coronary syndromes. Eur Heart J. 2023;44(38):3720-3826.

4. Kubica J, Adamski P, Niezgoda P, Alexopoulos D, Badarienė J, Budaj A, et al. Prolonged antithrombotic therapy in patients after acute coronary syndrome: A critical appraisal of current European Society of Cardiology guidelines. Cardiol J. 2020;27(6):661-76.
5. Lawton JS, Tamis-Holland JE, Bangalore S, Bates ER, Beckie TM, Bischoff JM, et al. 2021 ACC/AHA/SCAI Guideline for Coronary Artery Revascularization: A Report of the American College of Cardiology/American Heart Association Committee on Clinical Practice Guidelines. J Am Coll Cardiol. 2022;79(2):e21-e129.
6. Ortega-Paz L, Brugaletta S, Sabate M. State-of-the art and future perspective of percutaneous interventions for the management of STEMI. REC Interv Cardiol. 2021;3:204-212.
7. Sanchez JS, Stefanini GG, Timing and Completeness of revascularization in acute coronary syndrome. Heart. 2021;0:1-9.

CHAPTER 10

Acute Pulmonary Embolism

Soumitra Kumar

PREDISPOSING FACTORS FOR VENOUS THROMBOEMBOLISM

Strong Risk Factors

- Fracture of lower limb
- Hospitalization for heart failure or atrial fibrillation/flutter (within previous 3 months)
- Hip or knee replacement
- Major trauma
- Myocardial infarction (within previous 3 months)
- Previous VTE
- Spinal cord injury

Moderate Risk Factors

- Arthroscopic knee surgery
- Autoimmune diseases
- Blood transfusion
- Central venous lines
- Intravenous catheters and leads
- Chemotherapy
- Congestive heart failure or respiratory failure
- Erythropoiesis-stimulating agents
- Hormone replacement therapy (depends on formulation)
- In vitro fertilization
- Oral contraceptive therapy
- Post-partum period
- Infection (specifically pneumonia, urinary tract infection, and HIV)
- Inflammatory bowel disease
- Cancer (highest risk in metastatic disease)

- Paralytic stroke
- Superficial vein thrombosis
- Thrombophilia

Weak Risk Factors

- Bed rest >3 days
- Diabetes mellitus
- Arterial hypertension
- Immobility due to sitting (e.g., prolonged car or air travel)
- Increasing age
- Laparoscopic surgery (e.g., cholecystectomy)
- Obesity
- Pregnancy
- Varicose veins

TREATMENT IN THE ACUTE PHASE

Hemodynamic and Respiratory Support

Oxygen Therapy and Ventilation

Hypoxemia is one of the features of severe PE, and is mostly due to the mismatch between ventilation and perfusion. Administration of supplemental oxygen is indicated in patients with PE and SaO_2

TABLE 1: Recommendation for diagnosis.

Recommendations	Class[a]	Level[b]
Suspected PE with hemodynamic instability		
In suspected high-risk PE, as indicated by the presence of hemodynamic instability, bedside echocardiography or emergency CTPA (depending on availability and clinical circumstances) is recommended for diagnosis	I	C
It is recommended that IV anticoagulation with UFH, including a weight-adjusted bolus injection, be initiated without delay in patients with suspected high-risk PE	I	C
Suspected PE without hemodynamic instability		
The use of validated criteria for diagnosis PE is recommended	I	B

Contd...

Contd…

Recommendations	Class[a]	Level[b]
Initiation of anticoagulation is recommended without delay in patients with high or intermediate clinical probability of PE while diagnostic workup is in progress	I	C
Clinical evaluation		
It is recommended that the diagnostic strategy be based on clinical probability, assessed either by clinical probability of PE while diagnostic workup is in progress	I	A
D-dimer		
Plasma D-dimer measurement, preferably using a highly sensitive assay, is recommended in outpatients/emergency department patients with low or intermediate clinical probability, or those that are PE-unlikely, to reduce the need for unnecessary imaging and irradiation	I	A
As an alternative to the fixed D-dimer cut-off, a negative D-dimer test using an age-adjusted cut-off (age × 10 μg/L, in patients aged >50 years) should be considered for excluding PE in patients with low or intermediate clinical probability, or those that are PE-unlikely	IIa	B
As an alternative to the fixed or age-adjusted D-dimer cut-off, D-dimer levels adapted to clinical probability[c] should be considered to exclude PE	IIa	B
D-dimer measurement is not recommended in patients with high clinical probability, as a normal result does not safely exclude PE, even when using a highly sensitive assay	III	A
CTPA		
It is recommended to reject the diagnosis of PE (without further testing) if CTA is normal in a patient with low or intermediate clinical probability, or who is PE unlikely	I	A
It is recommended to accept the diagnosis of PE (without further testing) if CTPA shows a segmental or more proximal filing defect in a patient with intermediate or high clinical probability	I	B
It should be considered to reject the diagnosis of PE (without further testing) if CTPA is normal in a patient with high clinical probability or who is PE likely	IIa	B

Contd…

Contd...

Recommendations	Class[a]	Level[b]
Further imaging tests to confirm PE may be considered in cases of isolated subsegmental filling defects	IIb	C
CT venography is not recommended as an adjunct to CTPA	III	B
V/Q scintigraphy		
It is recommended to reject the diagnosis of PE (without further testing) if the perfusion lung scan is normal	I	A
It should be considered to accept that the diagnosis of PE (without further testing) if the V/Q scan yields high probability for PE	IIa	B
V/Q SPECT		
V/Q SPECT may be considered for PE diagnosis	IIb	B
Lower-limb CUS		
It is recommended to accept the diagnosis of VTE (and PE), if a CUS shows a proximal DVT in a patient with clinical suspicion of PE	I	A
If CUS shows only a distal DVT, further testing should be considered to confirm PE	IIa	B
If a positive proximal CUS us used to confirm PE, assessment of PE severity should be considered to permit risk-adjusted management	IIa	C
MRA		
MRA is not recommended for ruling out PE	III	A

[a]Class of recommendation
[b]Level of evidence
[c]D-dimer cut-off levels adapted to clinical probability according to the YEAS model (signs of DVT hemoptysis and whether an alternative diagnosis is less likely than PE) may be used. According to this model. PE is excluded in patients without clinical items and D-dimer levels <1,000 μg/L or in patients with one or more clinical items and D-dimer levels <500 μg/L.
(CT: computed tomography; CTPA: computed tomography pulmonary angiography/angiogram; CUS: compression ultrasonography; DVT: deep vein thrombosis; IV: intravenous; MRA: magnetic resonance angiography; PE: pulmonary embolism; SPECT: single-photon emission computed tomography; UFH: unfractionated; V/Q: ventilation/perfusion (lung scintigraphy); VTE: venous thromboembolism)

> **BOX 1:** Transthoracic echocardiographic parameters in the assessment of right ventricular pressure overload.
> - Enlarged right ventricle, parasternal long axis view
> - Dilated RV with basal RV/LV ratio >1.0, and McConnell sign (arrow), four-chamber view
> - Flattened intraventricular septum (arrows) parasternal short axis view
> - Distended inferior vena cava with diminished inspiratory collapsibility, subcostal view
> - *60/60 sign:* Coexistence of acceleration time of pulmonary ejection <60 ms and midsystolic "notch" with mildly elevated (<60 mm Hg) peak systolic gradient at the tricuspid valve
> - Right heart mobile thrombus detected in right heart cavities (arrow)
> - Decreased tricuspid annular plane systolic excursion (TAPSE) measured with M-Mode (<16 mm)
> - Decreased peak systolic (S') velocity of tricuspid annulus (<9.5 cm/s)

<90%. Severe hypoxemia/respiratory failure that is refractory to conventional oxygen supplementation could be explained by right-to-left shunt through a patent foramen ovale or atrial septal defect. Further oxygenation techniques should also be considered, including high-flow oxygen (i.e., a high-flow nasal cannula)and mechanical ventilation (noninvasive or invasive) in cases of extreme instability (i.e., cardiac arrest), taking into consideration that correction of hypoxemia will not be possible without simultaneous pulmonary reperfusion. Patients with RV failure are frequently hypotensive or are highly susceptible to the development of severe hypotension during induction of anesthesia, intubation, and positive-pressure ventilation.

Consequently, intubation should be performed only if the patient is unable to tolerate or cope with noninvasive ventilation. When feasible, noninvasive ventilation or oxygenation through a high-flow nasal cannula should be preferred; if mechanical ventilation is used, care should be taken to limit its adverse hemodynamic effects. In particular, positive intrathoracic pressure induced by mechanical ventilation may reduce venous return and worsen low CO due to RV failure in patients with high-risk PE; therefore, positive end-expiratory pressure should be applied with caution. Tidal volumes of approximately 6 mL/kg lean body weight should be used in an

TABLE 2: Classification of pulmonary embolism severity and the risk of early (in-hospital or 30 day) death.

Early mortality risk		Hemo-dynamic instability	Indicators of risk		
			Clinical parameters of PE severity and/or comorbidity: PESI class III – V or sPESI ≥1[a]	RV dysfunction on TTE or CTPA	Elevated cardiac troponin levels[b]
High		+	(+)	+	(+)
Intermediate	Intermediate-high	–	+	+	+
	Intermediate-low	–	+	One (or none) positive	
Low		–	–	–	Assessment optional; If assessed, negative

[a]Original and simplified Pulmonary Embolism Severity Index (PESI)

Parameter	Original PESI	Simplified PESI (sPESI)
Age	Age in years	1 point (if age >80 years)
Male sex	+ 10 points	–
Cancer	+ 30 points	1 point
Chronic heart failure	+ 10 points	–
Chronic pulmonary disease	+ 10 points	1 point
Pulse rate ≥110 bpm	+ 20 points	1 point
Systolic BP <100 mm Hg	+ 30 points	1 point
Respiratory rate >30 breaths per min	+ 20 points	–
Temperature <36 °C	+ 20 points	–
Altered mental status	+ 60 points	–
Arterial oxyhemoglobin saturation	+ 20 points	1 point

PESI: Class I: ≤65 points; Class II: 66–85 points; Class III: 86–106 points; Class IV: 106–125 points; Class V: >125 points

[b]NT-proBNP ≥600 ng/L, H-FABP ≥6 ng/mL or copeptin ≥24 pmol/L may provide additional prognostic information

(BP: blood pressure; CTPA: computed tomography pulmonary angiography; H-FABP: heart-type fatty acid-binding protein; NT-proBNP: N-terminal pro B-type natriuretic peptide; PE: pulmonary embolism; PESI: pulmonary embolism severity index; RV: right ventricular; sPESI: simplified pulmonary embolism severity index; TTE: transthoracic echocardiogram)

TABLE 3: Recommendations for prognostic assessment.

Recommendations	Class[a]	Level[b]
Initial risk stratification of suspected or confirmed PE, based on the presence of hemodynamic Instability, is recommended to identify patients at high risk of early mortality	I	B
In patients without hemodynamic instability, further stratification of patients with acute PE into intermediate and low-risk categories is recommended	I	B
In patients without hemodynamic instability, use of clinical prediction rules integrating PE severity and comorbidity, preferably the PESI or sPESI, should be considered for risk assessment in the acute phase of PE	IIa	B
Assessment of the RV by imaging methods[c] or laboratory biomarkers[d] should be considered, even in the presence of a low PESI or a negative sPESI		
In patients without hemodynamic instability, use of validated scores combining clinical imaging, and laboratory PE-related prognostic factors may be considered to further stratify the severity of he acute PE episode	IIb	C

[a]Class of recommendation
[b]Level of evidence
[c]Transthoracic echocardiography or computed tomography pulmonary angiography
[d]Cardiac troponins or natriuretic peptides
(PE: pulmonary embolism; PESI: pulmonary embolism severity index; RV: right ventricle; sPESI: simplified pulmonary embolism severity index)

attempt to keep the end-inspiratory plateau pressure <30 cmH$_2$O. If intubation is needed, anesthetic drugs more prone to cause hypotension should be avoided for induction.

Mechanical Circulatory Support and Oxygenation

The temporary use of mechanical cardiopulmonary support, mostly with venoarterial extracorporeal membrane oxygenation (ECMO), may be helpful in patients with high risk PE, and circulatory collapse or cardiac arrest. Survival of critically ill patients has been described in a number of case series, but no RCTs testing the efficacy and

Flowchart 1: Suspected PE in a patient with hemodynamic instability.

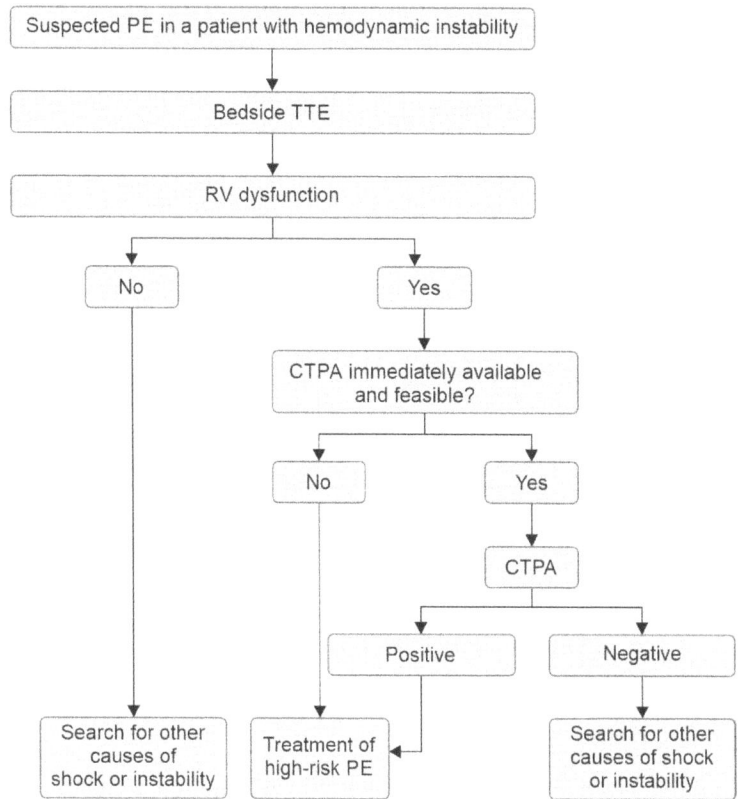

safety of these devices in the setting of high-risk PE have been conducted date. Use of ECMO is associated with a high incidence of complications, even when used for short periods, and the results depend on the experience of the center as well as patient selection. The increased risk of bleeding related to the need for vascular access should be considered, particularly in patients undergoing thrombolysis. At present, the use of ECMO as a stand-alone technique with anticoagulation is controversial and additional therapies, such as surgical embolectomy, have to be considered.

A few cases suggesting good outcomes with use of the Impella catheter in patients in shock caused by acute PE have been reported.

Flowchart 2: Suspected PE in a patient without hemodynamic instability.

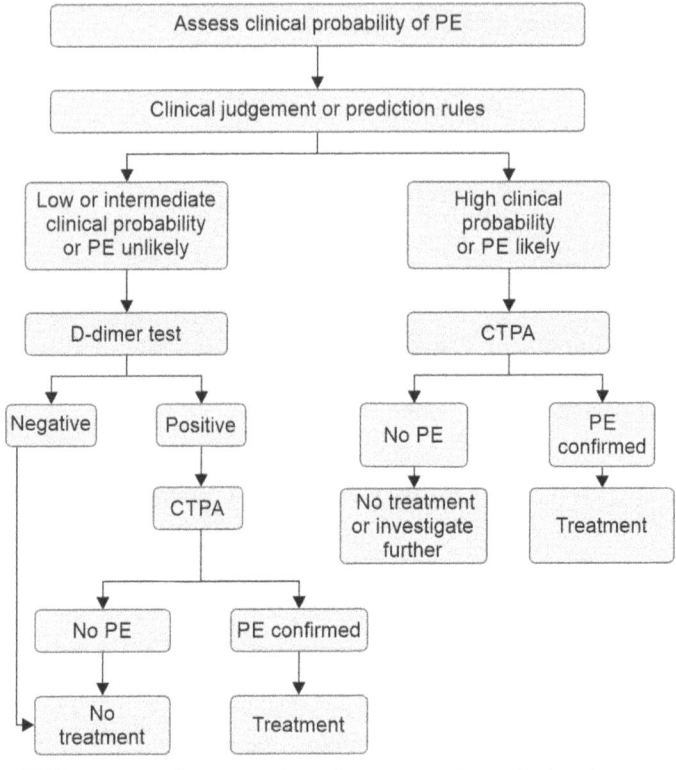

(CTPA: computed tomography pulmonary angiography/angiogram; PE: pulmonary embolism)

INITIAL ANTICOAGULATION

Parenteral Anticoagulation

In patients with high or intermediate clinical probability of PE, anticoagulation should be initiated while awaiting the results of diagnostic tests. This is usually done with subcutaneous weight-adjusted low-molecular weight heparin (LMWH) or fondaparinux, or IV unfractionated heparin (UFH). Based on pharmacokinetic data, an equally rapid anticoagulant effect can also be achieved with a nonvitamin K antagonist oral anticoagulant (NOAC), and phase III clinical trials have demonstrated the non-inferior efficacy

TABLE 4: Treatment of right ventricular failure in acute high-risk pulmonary embolism.

Strategy	Properties and use	Caveats
Volume optimization		
Cautious volume loading, saline, or Ringer's Lactate, ≤500 mL over 15–30 minutes	Consider in patients with normal—low central venous pressure (due, for example, to concomitant hypovolemia)	Volume loading can over-distend the RV, worsen ventricular interdependence and reduce CO
Vasopressors and inotropes		
Norepinephrine, 0.2–1.0 µg/kg/min[a]	Increases RV inotropy and systemic BP, promotes positive ventricular interactions, and restores coronary perfusion gradient	Excessive vasoconstriction may worsen tissue perfusion
Dobutamine, 2–20 µ/kg/min	Increases RV inotropy, lowers filling pressures	May aggregate arterial hypotension if used alone, without a vasopressor, may trigger or aggregate arrhythmias
Mechanical circulatory support		
Venoarterial ECMO/ extracorporeal life support	Rapid short-term support combined with oxygenator	Complications with use over longer periods (>5–10 days), including bleeding and infections; no clinical benefit unless combined with surgical embolectomy, requires an experienced team

[a]Epinephrine is used in cardiac arrest.
(CO: cardiac output; BP: blood pressure; ECMO: extracorporeal membrane oxygenation; RV: right ventricle/ventricular)

of a single-oral drug anticoagulation strategy using higher doses of adoption for 7 days or rivaroxaban for 3 weeks.

The LMWH and fondaparinux are preferred over UFH for initial anticoagulation in PE, as they carry a lower risk of inducing major bleeding and heparin-induced thrombocytopenia. Neither

LMWH nor fondaparinux needs routine monitoring of anti-Xa levels. Use of UFH is now-a-days largely restricted to patients with overt hemodynamic instability or imminent hemodynamic decompression in whom primary reperfusion treatment will be necessary. UFH is also recommended for patients with serious renal impairment [creatinine clearance (CrCl) ≤30 mL/min] or severe obesity. If LMWH is prescribed in patients with CrCl 15–30 mL/min, an adapted dosing scheme should be used. The dosing of UGH is adjusted based on the activated partial thromboplastin.

Nonvitamin K Antagonist Oral Anticoagulants

The NOACs are small molecules that directly inhibit one activated coagulation factor, which is thrombin for dabigatran and factor Xa for apixaban, edoxaban, and rivaroxaban.

Phase III trials on the treatment of acute VTE (supplementary as well as those on extended treatment beyond the first 6 months, demonstrated the noninferiority of NOACs compared with the combination of LMWH with VKA for the prevention of symptomatic or lethal VTE recurrence, along with significantly reduced rates of major bleeding. The different drug regimens tested in these trials are displayed. In a meta-analysis, the incidence rate of the primary efficacy outcome was 2.0% for NOAC-treated patients and 2.2% for VKA-treated patients [relative risk (RR) 0.88, 95% CI 0.74–1.05]. Major bleeding occurred in 1.1% of NOAC-treated patients and 1.7% of VKA-treated patients for an RR of 0.60 (95% CI 0.41–0.88). Compared with VKA-treated patients, critical site major bleeding occurred less frequently in NOAC-treated patients (RR 0.38, 95% CI 0.23–0.62); in particular, there was a significant reduction in intracranial bleeding (RR 0.37, 95% CI 0.21–0.68) and in fatal bleeding (RR 0.36, 95% CI 0.15–0.87) with NOACs compared with VKAs.

Vitamin K Antagonists

The VKAs have been the gold standard in oral anticoagulation for >50 years. When VKAs are used, anticoagulation with UFH, LMWH, or fondaparinux should be continued in parallel with the oral anticoagulant for ≥5 days and until the international normalized ratio (INR) value has been 2.0–3.0 for 2 consecutive days. Warfarin may be started at a dose of 10 mg in younger (e.g., aged <60 years) otherwise healthy patients and at a dose ≤5 mg in older patients. The daily dose is adjusted according to the INR over the next 5-7 days, aiming for an INR level of 2.0-3.0. Pharmacogenetic testing may increase the precision of warfarin dosing. When used in addition to clinical parameters, pharmacogenetic testing improves anticoagulation control and may be associated with a reduced risk of bleeding but does not reduce the risk of thromboembolic events or mortality.

REPERFUSION TREATMENT

Systemic Thrombolysis

Thrombolytic therapy leads to faster improvements in pulmonary obstruction, PAP, and PVR in patients with PE, compared with UFH alone; these improvements are accompanied by a reduction in RV dilation on echocardiography. The greatest benefit is observed when treatment is initiated within 48 hours of symptom onset, but thrombolysis can still be useful in patients who have had symptoms for 6-14 days. Unsuccessful thrombolysis, as judged by persistent clinical instability and unchanged RV dysfunction on echocardiography after 36 hours, has been reported in 8% of high-risk PE patients.

A meta-analysis of thrombolysis trials that included (but were not confined to) patients with high-risk PE, defined mainly as the presence of cardiogenic shock, indicated a significant reduction in the combined outcome of mortality and recurrent PE. This was achieved with a 9.9% rate of severe bleeding and a 1.7% rate of intracranial hemorrhage.

In normotensive patients with intermediate-risk PE, defined as the presence of RV dysfunction and elevated troponin levels, the impact of thrombolytic treatment was investigated in the Pulmonary Embolism Thrombolysis (PEITHO) trial. Thrombolytic therapy was associated with a significant reduction in the risk of hemodynamic decompensation or collapse, but this was paralleled by an increased risk of severe extracranial and intracranial bleeding. In the PEITHO trial, 30-day death rates were low in both treatment groups, although meta-analyses have suggested a reduction in PE related and overall mortality of as much as 50-60% following thrombolytic treatment in the intermediate-risk category.

Accelerated IV administration of recombinant tissue type plasminogen activator (rtPA; 100 mg over 2 hours) is preferable to prolonged infusions of first-generation thrombolytic agents (streptokinase and urokinase). Preliminary reports on the efficacy and safety of reduced-dose rtPA need confirmation by solid evidence before any recommendations can be made in this regard. UFH may be administered during continuous infusion of alteplase, but should be discontinued during infusion of streptokinase or urokinase. Reteplase, desmoteplase, or tenecteplase have also been investigated; at present, none of these agents are approved for use in acute PE.

It remains unclear whether early thrombolysis for (intermediate or high-risk) acute PE has an impact on clinical symptoms, functional limitation, or CTEPH at long-term follow-up. A small randomized trial of 83 patients suggested that thrombolysis might improve functional capacity at 3 months compared with anticoagulation alone. In the PEITHO trial, mild persisting symptoms, mainly dyspnea, were present in 33% of the patients at long-term (at 41.6 ± 15.7 months) clinical follow-up. However, the majority of patients (85% in the tenecteplase arm and 96% in the placebo arm) had a low or intermediate probability based on the ESC guidelines definition of persisting or new-onset PH at echocardiographic follow-up. Consequently, the findings of this study do not support a role for thrombolysis with the aim of preventing long-term sequelae after intermediate-risk PE, although they are limited by the fact that clinical follow-up was available for only 62% of the study population.

Percutaneous Catheter-directed Treatment

Mechanical reperfusion is based on the insertion of a catheter into the pulmonary arteries via the femoral route. Different types of catheters are used for mechanical fragmentation, thrombus aspiration, or more commonly a pharmacomechanical approach combining mechanical or ultrasound fragmentation of the thrombus with in situ reduced-dose thrombolysis.

Most knowledge about catheter-based embolectomy is derived from registries and pooled results from case series. The overall procedural success rates (defined as hemodynamic stabilization,

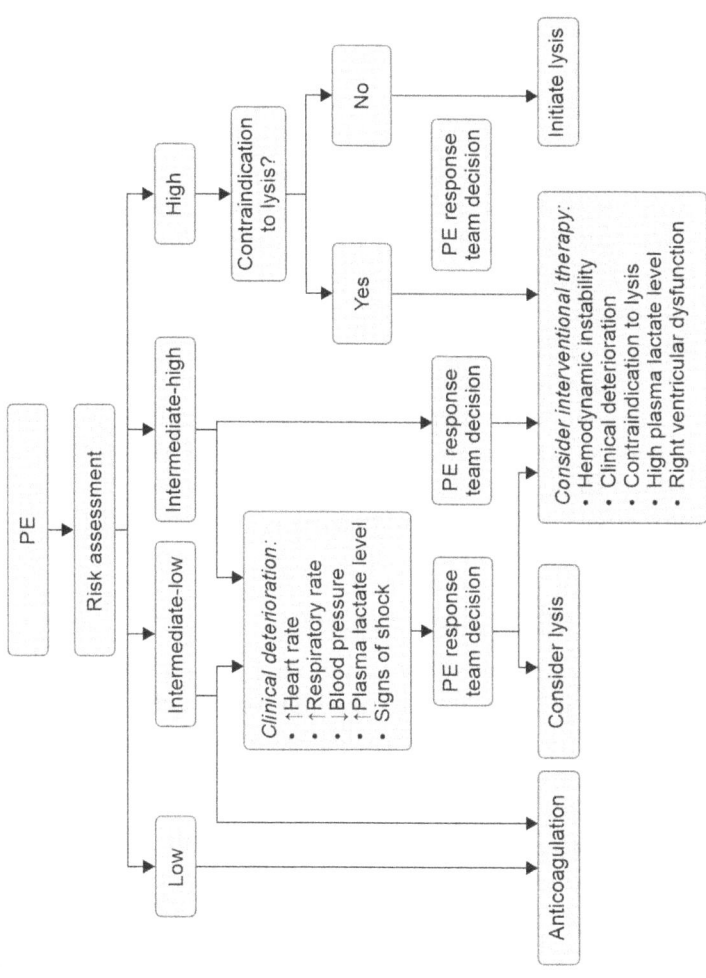

Flowchart 3: Treatment algorithm for pulmonary embolism (PE). Interventional therapies can be considered in patients with high-risk PE and contraindications to systemic thrombolysis and in patients with intermediate-risk and low-risk PE if their condition deteriorates despite anticoagulation.

correction of hypoxia, and survival to hospital discharge) of percutaneous catheter-based therapies reported in these studies have reached 87%; however, these results may be subject to publication bias. One RCT compared conventional heparin-based treatment and a catheter-based therapy combining ultrasound-based clot fragmentation with low-dose in situ thrombolysis in 59 patients with intermediate-risk PE. In that study, ultrasound-assisted thrombolysis was associated with a larger decrease in the RV/LV diameter ratio at 24 hours, without an increased risk of bleeding. Data from two prospective cohort studies and a registry, with a total of 352 patients, support the improvement in RV function, lung perfusion, and PAP in patients with intermediate- or high-risk PE using this technique. Intracranial hemorrhage was rare, although the rate of Global Utilization of Streptokinase and Tissue Plasminogen Activator for Occluded Coronary Arteries (GUSTO) severe and moderate bleeding complications was 10% in one of these cohorts. These results should be interpreted with caution, considering the relatively small numbers of patients treated, the lack of studies directly comparing catheter directed with systemic thrombolytic therapy, and the lack of data from RCTs on clinical efficacy outcomes.

SURGICAL EMBOLECTOMY

Surgical embolectomy in acute PE is usually carried out with cardiopulmonary bypass, without aortic cross-clamping and cardioplegic cardiac arrest, followed by incision of the two main pulmonary arteries with the removal or suction of fresh clots. Recent reports have indicated favorable surgical results in high-risk PE, with or without cardiac arrest, and in selected cases of intermediate-risk PE. Among 174–322 patients hospitalized between 1999 and 2013 with a diagnosis of PE in New York state, survival and recurrence rates were compared between patients who underwent thrombolysis (n = 1,854) or surgical embolectomy (n = 257) as first-line therapy. Overall, there was no difference between the two types of reperfusion treatment regarding 30-day mortality (15 and 13%, respectively), but thrombolysis was associated with a higher risk of stroke and reintervention at 30 days. No difference was found

TABLE 5: Recommendations for acute phase treatment of high-risk pulmonary embolism.[a]

Recommendations	Class[b]	Level[c]
It is recommended that anticoagulation with UFH, including a weight-adjusted bolus injection, be initiated without delay in patients with high-risk PE	I	C
Systemic thrombolytic therapy is recommended for high-risk PE	I	B
Surgical pulmonary embolectomy is recommended for patients with high-risk PE in whom thrombolysis is contraindicated or has failed	I	C
Percutaneous catheter-directed treatment should be considered for patients with high-risk PE, in whom thrombolysis is contraindicated or has failed[d]	IIa	C
Norepinephrine and/or dobutamine should be considered in patients with high-risk PE	IIa	C
ECMO may be considered, in combination with surgical embolectomy or catheter-directed treatment, in patients with PE and refractory circulatory collapse or cardiac arrest	IIb	C

[a] See **Table 3** for definition of high-risk PE. After hemodynamic stabilization of the patient, continue with anticoagulation treatment as in intermediate or low-risk PE
[b] Class of recommendation
[c] Level of evidence
[d] If appropriate expertise and resources are available on-site
(ECMO: extracorporeal membrane oxygenation; PE: pulmonary embolism; UFH: unfractionated heparin)

in terms of 5-year actuarial survival, but thrombolytic therapy was associated with a higher rate of recurrent PE requiring readmission compared with surgery (7.9 vs. 2.8%). However, the two treatments were not randomly allocated in this observational retrospective study, and the patients referred for surgery may have been selected. An analysis of the Society of Thoracic Surgery Database with multicenter data collection, including 214 patients submitted for surgical embolectomy for high- ($n = 38$) or intermediate-risk ($n = 176$) PE, revealed an in-hospital mortality rate of 12%, with the worst outcome (32%) in the group experiencing preoperative cardiac arrest.

Recent experience appears to support combining ECMO with surgical embolectomy, particularly in patients with high-risk PE with or without the need for cardiopulmonary resuscitation. Among patients who presented with intermediate-risk PE ($n = 28$), high-risk PE without cardiac arrest ($n = 18$), and PE with cardiac arrest ($n = 9$), the in-hospital and 1 year survival rates were 93 and 91%, respectively.

SUGGESTED READING

1. Hobohm L, Keller K, Konstantinides S. Pulmonary Embolism. Inn Med (Heidelb). 2023;64(01):40-9.
2. Keller K, Hobohm L, Ebner M, Kresoja KP, Münzel T, Konstantinides SV, et al. Trends in thrombolytic treatment and outcomes of acute pulmonary embolism in Germany. Eur Heart J. 2020;41(04):522-9.
3. Konstantinides SV, Meyer G, Becattini C, Bueno H, Geersing GJ, Harjola VP, et al; ESC Scientific Document Group. 2019 ESC Guidelines for the diagnosis and management of acute pulmonary embolism developed in collaboration with the European Respiratory Society (ERS). Eur Heart J. 2020;41(04):543-603.
4. Opitz CF, Meyer FJ. Pulmonary embolism: An update based on the revised AWMF-S2K Guideline. Hamostaseologie. 2024;44:111-8.

CHAPTER 11

Acute Cardiac Care in Pediatric Practice

Soumitra Kumar, Achyut Sarkar

There are varied types of cardiac emergencies in neonates, infants, and children. While some of these may ultimately require treatment at a center staffed with specialists in pediatric cardiology and pediatric cardiovascular surgery, the initial recognition of the emergency, stabilization, and management do devolve on the emergency physician when a child presents to the emergency room.

The incidence of congenital heart disease (CHD) in the general population is approximately 1% of live births. In the past few decades, advances have been made in the medical and surgical management of the more severe forms of CHD. As a result of this, there are now more survivors with severe forms of CHD. These patients may frequent the emergency rooms, and their distinctive physiology requires comprehension by the caregivers so as to provide adequate and appropriate therapy. Importantly, they may have emergencies related not only to the cardiovascular system, but also neurological, gastrointestinal, infections, and other problems.

Commonly encountered pediatric cardiac emergencies:
- Cardiopulmonary arrest
- Shock
- Arrhythmias
- Hypercyanotic ("Tet") spells
- Cyanosis in the newborn
- Congestive heart failure
- Cardiac emergencies in the patient with a functional single ventricle
- Cerebrovascular accidents
- Brain abscess

ARRHYTHMIAS

Several types of arrhythmias are seen in pediatric patients; however, supraventricular tachycardia (SVT) is the most frequently encountered arrhythmia both in the neonatal period and childhood and will be discussed in this chapter. SVT is the most common arrhythmia of the pediatric age group requiring medical treatment. Although patients with CHD may develop SVT, it is more commonly seen in children with structurally normal hearts. The heart rate in SVT frequently exceeds 250 beats per minute in the neonates, above 220 beats per minute in infants, and over 150 beats per minute in older children. It is usually characterized by a narrow QRS complex unless there is aberrant ventricular conduction. Approximately 70% of SVTs are reentrant in type, involving an accessory pathway [Wolff-Parkinson-White syndrome (WPW)]; if the pathway manifests antegrade conduction of the impulse from the atria to the ventricle, a short PR interval and a delta wave are seen on a surface electrocardiogram; however, it should be pointed out that WPW pattern is not seen while the child is in SVT. It is seen only after conversion to sinus rhythm. If the preexcitation is not present on ECG, the pathway may be concealed or there is an alternate mechanism.

MANAGEMENT OF SUPRAVENTRICULAR TACHYCARDIA

- Child is hemodynamically stable
  - Vagal maneuvers (ice-to-face, Valsalva)
  - Adenosine 100 µg/kg rapid IV push; may be increased to 200 µg/kg in 50 µg increments until there is a response
  - Esmolol at bolus dose of 200-400 µg/kg over 10 minutes, followed by 75 µg/kg/min infusion
  - Amiodarone (bolus infusion of 5 mg/kg infused over a 20-60 minutes followed by continuous infusion of 10-15 mg/kg/day)
  - Procainamide (loading dose of 7-15 mg/kg given over a 30-45 minutes followed by a maintenance dose of 40-50 µg/kg/minute)
  - Verapamil* 0.1 mg/kg slow IV push; may increase to 0.2 mg/kg in 15 minutes if no response (maximum dose 5 mg)

---

*Verapamil should not be used in patients under 1 year of age, those taking beta-blockers, or signs of congestive heart failure (CHF).

- Child is hemodynamically unstable
  - Immediate synchronized DC cardioversion at 0.5–2 Joules/kg
  - Transesophageal pacing (if a cardiologist experienced enough to do the procedure is available)

Treatment of Supraventricular Tachycardia with Pulse
See **Table 1**.

Treatment of Wide Complex Tachycardia with a Pulse
See **Table 2**.

TABLE 1: AHA 2020 recommendations for treatment of supraventricular tachycardia with a pulse.

Class of recommendation	Recommendations
1	• If IV/IO access is readily available, adenosine is recommended for the treatment of SVT • For hemodynamically stable patients whose SVT is unresponsive to vagal maneuvers and/or IV adenosine, expert consultation is recommended
2a	It is reasonable to attempt vagal stimulation first unless the patient is hemodynamically unstable or it will delay chemical or electric synchronized cardioversion
2a	If the patient with SVT is hemodynamically unstable with evidence of cardiovascular compromise (i.e., altered mental status, signs of shock, and hypotension), it is reasonable to perform electric synchronize cardioversion starting with a dose of 0.5–1.0 Joules/kg, if unsuccessful increase the dose of 2.0 Joules/kg
2b	• For a patient with unstable SVT unresponsive to vagal maneuvers, IV adenosine, electric synchronized • Cardioversion, and for whom expert consultation is not available, it may be reasonable to consider either procainamide or amiodarone

TABLE 2: AHA 2020 recommendations for treatment of wide-complex tachycardia with a pulse.

Class of recommendation	Recommendations
1	If the patient with a wide-complex tachycardia is hemodynamically stable, expert consultation is recommended prior to administration of antiarrhythmic agents
2a	If the patient with a wide-complex tachycardia is hemodynamically unstable with evidence of cardiovascular compromise (i.e., altered mental status, signs of shock, and hypotension), it is reasonable to perform electric synchronized cardioversion starting with a dose of 0.5–1.0 Joules/kg. If unsuccessful, increase the dose to 2.0 Joules/kg

MANAGEMENT OF VENTRICULAR FIBRILLATION/ PULSELESS VENTRICULAR TACHYCARDIA

The risk of ventricular fibrillation/pulseless ventricular tachycardia (VF/pVT) steadily increases throughout childhood and adolescence but remains less frequent than in adults. Cardiac arrest due to an initial rhythm of VF/pVT has better rates of survival to hospital discharge with favorable neurological function than cardiac arrests due to an initial nonshockable rhythm. Shockable rhythms may be the initial rhythm of the cardiac arrest (primary VF/pVT) or may develop during the resuscitation (secondary VF/pVT). Defibrillation is the definitive treatment for VF/pVT. The shorter the duration of VF/pVT, the more likely the shock will result in a perfusing rhythm **(Tables 3 and 4)**.

Defibrillator Paddle Size, Type, and Position
See **Tables 5**.

Type of Defibrillator
See **Tables 6**.

Flowchart 1: Approach to palpable pulse with poor perfusion.

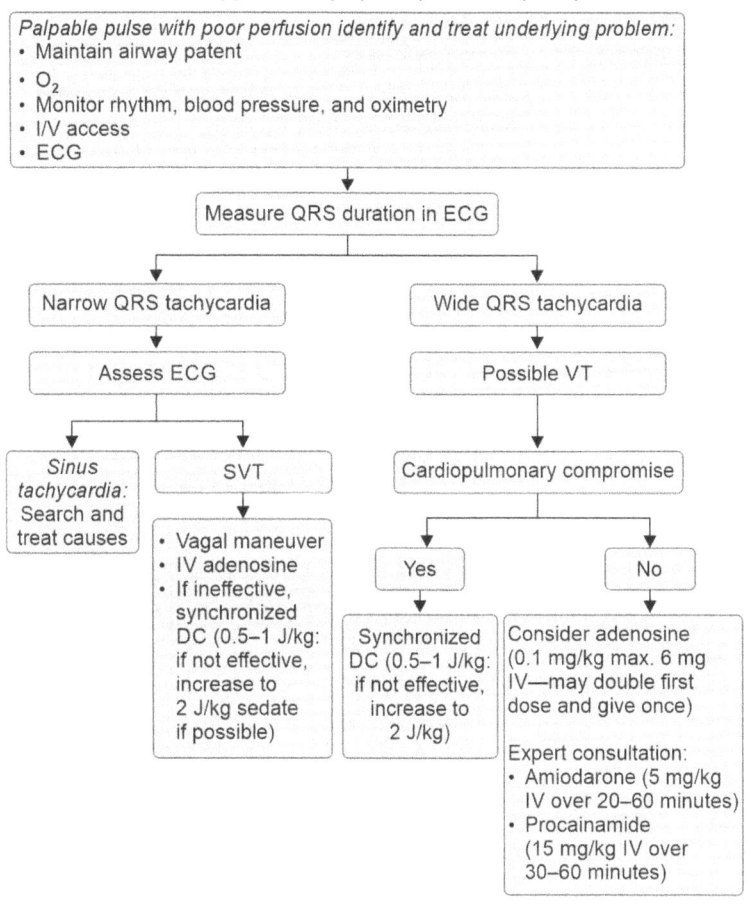

(DC: direct current; ECG: electrocardiogram; IV: intravenous; SVT: supraventricular tachycardia; VT: ventricular tachycardia)

TABLE 3: AHA 2020 recommendations for energy dose for treatment of VF/pVT.	
Class of recommendations	Recommendations
2a	It is reasonable to use an initial dose of 2–4 J/kg of monophasic or biphasic energy for defibrillation but for ease of teaching, an initial dose of 2 J/kg may be considered

Contd...

Contd...

Class of recommendations	Recommendations
2b	• For refractory VF, it may be reasonable to increase the defibrillation dose of 4 J/kg • For subsequent energy levels, a dose of 4 J/kg may be reasonable, and higher energy levels may be considered, though not to exceed. 10 J/kg or the adult maximum dose

TABLE 4: AHA 2020 recommendations for coordination of shock and CPR.

Class of recommendations	Recommendations
1	Perform CPR until the device is ready to deliver a shock
1	A single shock followed by immediate chest compressions is recommended for children with VF/pVT
1	Minimize interruptions of chest compressions

TABLE 5: AHA 2020 recommendations for defibrillator paddle size, type and position.

Class of recommendations	Recommendations
1	Use the largest paddles or self-adhering electrodes that will fit on the child's chest while still maintaining good separation between the pads/paddles
2b	When affixing self-adhering pads, either anterior-lateral placement or anterior-posterior placement may be reasonable
2b	Paddles and self-adhering pads may be considered equally effective in delivering electricity

TABLE 6: AHA 2020 recommendations for type of defibrillator.

Class of recommendations	Recommendations
1	When using an AED on infants and children <8 years old, use of a pediatric attenuator is recommended
2	For infants under the care of a trained healthcare provider, a manual defibrillator is recommended when a shockable rhythm is identified

Contd...

Contd...

Class of recommendations	Recommendations
2b	If neither a manual defibrillator nor an AED equipped with a pediatric attenuator is available, an AED without a dose attenuator may be used

Flowchart 2: Pediatric bradycardia with a pulse algorithm.

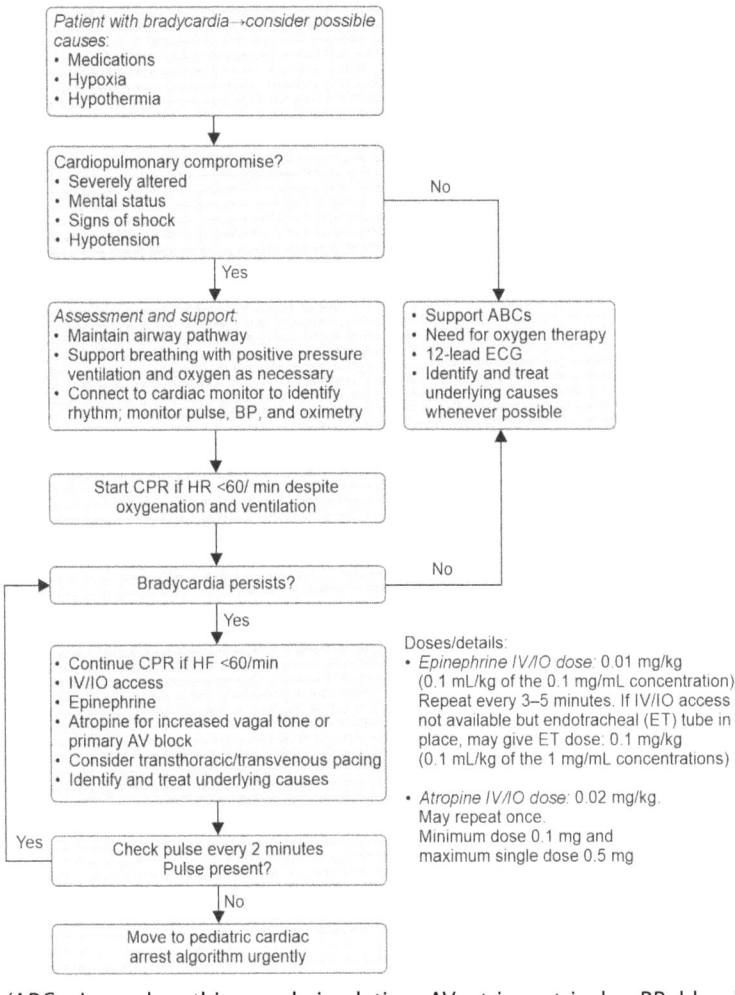

(ABC: airway, breathing, and circulation; AV: atrioventricular; BP: blood pressure; CPR: cardiopulmonary resuscitation; ECG: electrocardiogram; HR: heart ate; IO: intraosseous; IV: intravenous)

PEDIATRIC BASIC LIFE SUPPORT FOR LAY RESCUERS

See **Flowcharts 3 and 4** below.

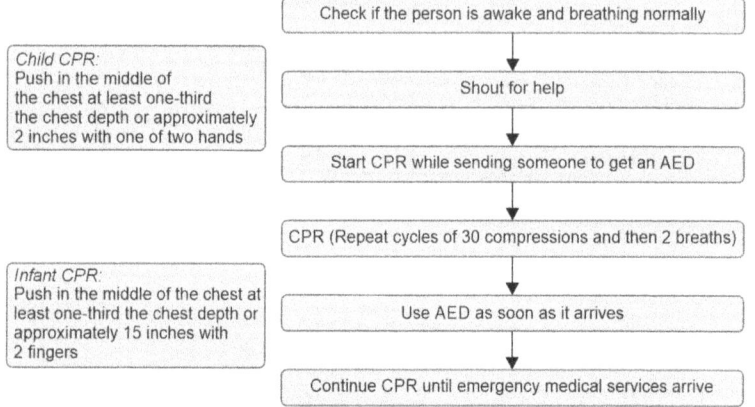

Flowchart 3: Pediatric basic life support (BLS) for lay rescuers.

(AED: automated external defibrillator; BLS: basic life support; CPR: cardiopulmonary resuscitation)

HYPERCYANOTIC (TET) SPELL

Hypercyanotic or "Tet" spells may happen in infants and children with unrepaired tetralogy of Fallot and other cardiac anomalies with large interventricular communication and pulmonary outflow tract obstruction. The spell is manifested by increase in rate and depth of respiration (hyperpnea) and cyanosis and may worsen to limpness and syncope; however, the babies usually recover subsequently. These spells are usually self-limited but may rarely lead to grave complications such as syncope, seizure-like episodes, cerebrovascular accidents, or even death. The spell may last for a few minutes to a few hours. These spells are most usually observed between the ages of 1 and 12 months, with a highest frequency between the ages of 2 and 3 months. The spells may occur at any time of the day but are most frequent in the morning after waking from sleep; defecation, crying, and feeding are usual precipitating

Acute Cardiac Care in Pediatric Practice

Flowchart 4: Pediatric basic life support algorithm for healthcare providers—single rescuer.

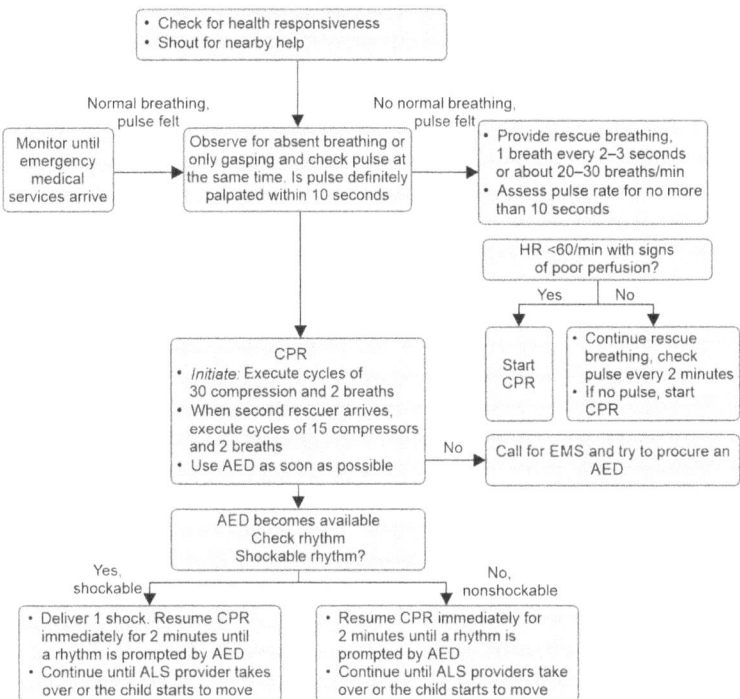

factors. Examination reveals an agitated and cyanotic infant, and a previously heard cardiac murmur of right ventricular outflow obstruction is either absent or markedly obtunded in intensity during the spell.

Management of hypercyanotic spells:
- Knee-to-chest position
- Oxygen via face mask (discontinue if it causes further agitation in the patient)
- Morphine 0.1 mg/kg intramuscular or intravenous
- Normal saline bolus 10 mL/kg intravenous
- Esmolol loading dose of 500 μg/kg/dose followed by an infusion of 50–100 μg/kg/min

Flowchart 5: Pediatric cardiac arrest algorithm.

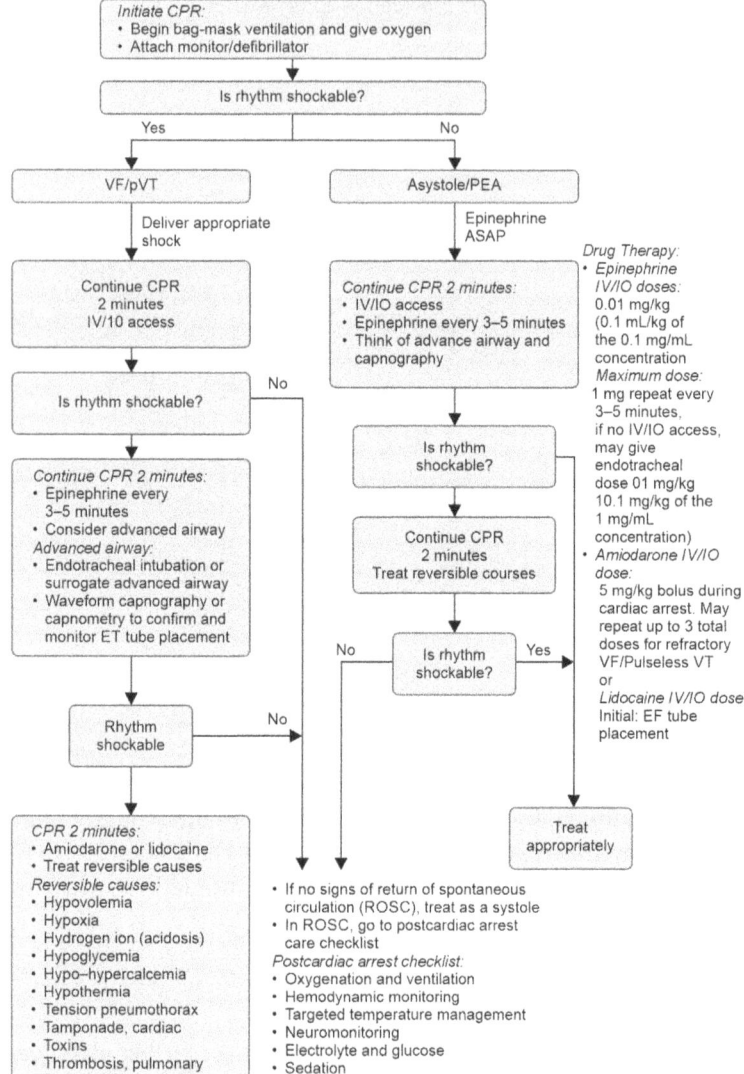

(ASAP: as soon as possible; CPR: cardiopulmonary resuscitation; ET: endotracheal; IO: intraosseous; IV: intravenous; PEA: pulseless electrical activity; VF/pVT: ventricular fibrillation/pulseless ventricular tachycardia)

- Phenylephrine 5-10 µg/kg intravenous (maximum dose 5 mg) or norepinephrine as a continuous infusion of 0.05-0.5 µg/kg/min (the rate of infusion should be titrated to increase the systolic blood pressure by 15-20% of the control value)
- Correct any acidosis with sodium bicarbonate 1-2 mEq/kg intravenous.
- Correct any electrolyte imbalance.
- Persistent or refractory spells may require emergency Blalock-Taussig shunt (B-T shunt) or ECMO.

CONGESTIVE HEART FAILURE

There are numerous conditions that may precipitate CHF in children; the most common are large left-to-right shunts, such as VSD, patent ductus arteriosus, single ventricle lesions without pulmonary stenosis, among others. Other causes are primary myocardial dysfunction, as seen in myocarditis or cardiomyopathy and ductal-dependent lesions such as hypoplastic left heart syndrome, severe coarctation of the aorta, or interruption of the aortic arch. The child in CHF usually demonstrates tachypnea, retractions of chest wall, poor feeding, diaphoresis particularly with exertion or feeding, and failure to thrive. Examination may reveal tachypnea, tachycardia, cardiomegaly, hepatomegaly, and poor perfusion reflected by cool extremities and retarded distal capillary refill. Cardiac murmurs indicative of the basic cardiac lesion may be present in some patients. For a child with a large left-to-right shunt, the initial presentation with signs of CHF may be at 6-8 weeks of age. It is at this time that the pulmonary vascular resistance naturally drops and, consequently, the left-to-right shunt increases. In addition, any intercurrent respiratory or gastrointestinal illness (usually viral) may precipitate CHF. A child with myocarditis or cardiomyopathy may present at any age. Ductal-dependent lesions usually present within the first few days to weeks after discharge from birth admission.

Management of acute CHF:
- Furosemide 1 mg/kg/dose; may be repeated up to every 6 hours
- Respiratory support as needed
- Correct acidosis or metabolic derangements.

- Milrinone 0.25–0.75 µg/kg/min if not hypotensive
- Dopamine 5–10 µg/kg/min
- Prostaglandin E1 (PGE1) for babies with ductal-dependent systemic perfusion (0.05–0.1 µg/kg/min; reduce to 0.025 µg/kg/min once the baby is stabilized)

CARDIAC EMERGENCIES IN PATIENT WITH FUNCTIONAL SINGLE VENTRICLE

In-depth understanding of the precise physiology of patients born with complex congenital heart lesions with single-functioning ventricle is required to adequately address their care. There are several types of cardiac defects that have single functioning ventricle, and these include hypoplastic left heart syndrome, tricuspid atresia, single ventricle, unbalanced atrioventricular canal defects, and others. The common finding among these defects is that the heart has only one functioning ventricle and this ventricle pumps blood to both the body and lungs. Treatment of these defects requires a three-staged surgical approach, starting in the neonatal period and are completed between 2 and 4 years of age.

Stage I

Single ventricle physiology patients born with obstruction of pulmonary blood flow receive an aortic-to-pulmonary artery shunt, usually a modified B-T shunt. This shunt (GORE-TEX graft) is typically placed from the subclavian artery to the ipsilateral pulmonary artery. In patients who have single ventricle physiology with unrestricted pulmonary blood flow, the blood will preferentially flow to the lungs since the pulmonary vascular resistance is lower than the systemic vascular resistance. This results in severe CHF and decreased systemic perfusion. These patients receive a pulmonary artery band as a temporizing measure.

Stage II

Irrespective of the surgery done for palliation in the neonatal period, all patients will undergo a bidirectional Glenn procedure This consists of anastomosing the superior vena cava to the right pulmonary artery, end-to-side. The previously created B-T shunt is ligated.

Stage III

These patients eventually undergo Fontan procedure, usually 1 year following the bidirectional Glenn procedure. The Fontan, as performed at the current time, consists of connecting the inferior vena cava to the pulmonary artery via an extracardiac conduit; the superior vena cava has previously been connected to the pulmonary artery during stage II, bidirectional Glenn. After the Fontan procedure, the single functioning ventricle pumps blood only to the body and the blood flow to the lungs is directly from the systemic veins, completely passive, and the two circulations are finally separated. Most patients receive a fenestration between the extracardiac conduit and the atrial mass, the so-called fenestrated Fontan.

The most feared, and most fatal, complication in patients with aortopulmonary shunts (e.g., B-T shunt) is an occlusive thrombus within the GORE-TEX graft. Since the shunt is the only source of pulmonary blood flow, rapid evaluation, diagnosis, and management are essential to ensure a successful outcome. Any patient with fever, vomiting, diarrhea, or decreased oral intake should be monitored closely until the fever has resolved for at least 24 hours. Supplemental intravenous fluids should also be provided as long as fever, vomiting, or diarrhea persists, or until oral intake improves.

A patient with a severely obstructed shunt will present with severe cyanosis and respiratory distress. If the diagnosis is not made readily, rapid hemodynamic deterioration leading to cardiac arrest may occur. A continuous murmur of the shunt should normally be heard on auscultation. If the shunt is obstructed, the murmur disappears or is severely obtunded in intensity. Management of an acutely obstructed shunt involves first the airway, breathing, and circulation as initial assessment and basic life support. Intubation is indicated as is cardiopulmonary resuscitation. In the case of suspected shunt obstruction, heparin may be given to prevent the progression of the thrombus. A pediatric cardiac and cardiovascular surgical consultation should be sought immediately in the case of suspected shunt occlusion. Emergency transcatheter opening of the shunt by interventional pediatric cardiologist or shunt revision or placing the infant on ECMO by pediatric cardiovascular surgeon is urgently warranted. Unfortunately, even with the best of care, this condition carries a high mortality rate. Patients with shunts are on platelet antagonist aspirin routinely in an effort to prevent this complication.

NEUROLOGICAL EVENTS

Cerebrovascular accidents (CVAs) and brain abscess are potential complications with cyanotic CHD; this is presumed to be due to intracardiac right-to-left shunt in the uncorrected or palliated cyanotic CHD patients. CVA used to be seen in older times in association with relative anemia in infants and children <2 years old, but is not as commonly seen in the current day and this is probably related to early surgery for the cyanotic CHD. Similarly, the CVA seen in older children with severe polycythemia has also become rare and is again related to early surgical intervention in cyanotic CHD. These days effective surgical palliation of complex cyanotic CHD patients leaves many infants and children on the contrary at risk for development of CVA prior to complete separation of the systemic and pulmonary circuits either by complete biventricular repair or by single ventricular, Fontan type of palliation. Another group of patients with severe primary myocardial disease may have CVAs due to dislodgement of left ventricular thrombi.

Recognition of stroke in the pediatric population calls for a high index of suspicion. While adolescents and young adults may present with more typical symptoms such as hemiparesis or dysarthria, the diagnosis can be missed or delayed in the young patient presenting with nonspecific symptoms. Atypical signs and symptoms of stroke in children may be as nonspecific as headache or seizures.

The management of acute stroke in children is similar to that currently in practice for adults. Combined use of reperfusion and neuroprotection should be considered after a pediatric neurology/ stroke team consultation, especially when the time horizons are satisfied. Once considered ineligible for thrombolytic therapy, the treatment is mostly symptomatic and includes adequate hydration, correction of anemia or polycythemia, anticonvulsants (if seizures are present), and physiotherapy. A detailed discussion of treatment of pediatric stroke is beyond the scope of this chapter; and those interested, are advised to refer to recent reviews on the subject.

SUGGESTED READING

1. Cashen K, Gupta P, Lieh-Lai M, Mastropietro C. Infants with single ventricle physiology in the emergency department are physicians prepared? J Pediatr. 2011;159(2):273-7.
2. Rao PS. Cardiac emergencies in pediatric practice. Physician's Digest. 2008;17:30-6.
3. Rao PS. Neonatal cardiac emergencies: Management strategies. Neonatology Today. 2008;3:1-5.
4. Topjian AA, Raymond TT, Atkins D, Chan M, Duff JP, Joyner BL Jr, et al.; Pediatric Basic and Advanced Life Support Collaborators. Part 4: Pediatric Basic and Advanced Life Support: 2020 American Heart Association Guidelines for cardiopulmonary resuscitation and emergency cardiovascular care. Circulation. 2020;142(16_suppl_2):S469523.
5. Yates MC, Rao S. Pediatric cardiac emergencies. Emergency Med. 2013;3(6).

12. Hypertensive Emergencies

Soumitra Kumar

DEFINITIONS

Physicians in emergency departments frequently triage patients with "hypertensive crises" which is actually an acute, severe rise in blood pressure (BP) presenting with a broad profile ranging from asymptomatic patients to patients with life-threatening target organ damage. "Hypertensive emergencies" are situations where very high BP values (often ≥220/120 mm Hg) are associated with acute hypertension-mediated organ damage involving heart, retina, brain, kidneys, and large arteries. The type of organ damage is the key determinant of choice of treatment, target BP, and timeframe over which BP should be reduced.

Malignant hypertension is a hypertensive emergency with severe BP rise (≥229/120 mm Hg) and advanced retinopathy, defined as presence of bilateral retinal flame-shaped hemorrhages, cotton wool spots, or papilledema.

Hypertensive encephalopathy is another hypertensive emergency characterized by severe hypertension and one or more of the following features: Seizures, lethargy, cortical blindness, and coma, which cannot be explained alternatively.

Thrombotic microangiopathy (TMA) is another situation of severe BP elevation marked by Coomb's negative hemolysis (indicated by raised lactate dehydrogenase, unmeasurable haptoglobin, or schistocytes) and thrombocytopenia in the absence of another plausible cause and amelioration with BP-lowering treatment.

Other examples of hypertensive emergencies are severe hypertension associated with (1) intracranial hemorrhage and resultant acute stroke, (2) acute coronary syndrome, (3) cardiogenic pulmonary edema, (4) acute aortic disease, and (5) preeclampsia and eclampsia or HELLP syndrome.

The term *"hypertensive urgencies"* refers to situations where patients present with very high BP values, usually >180/110 mm Hg but without any manifestation of acute hypertension-mediated target organ damage. Since cardiovascular risk of these patients is not particularly high in short term, it should not be viewed differently from *severe asymptomatic uncontrolled hypertension*. So, hypertensive crisis should only include "hypertensive emergencies" where immediate treatment is warranted, and the term "hypertensive crisis", which incorporates urgency and emergency, has thus become obsolete.

Epidemiology: Across the continents, 1 in every 200 patients at the emergency department (ED) presents with a suspected hypertensive emergency. Heart failure, stroke, and myocardial infarction represent the largest proportion of all hypertensive emergencies, followed by intracranial hemorrhage and aortic dissociation. Advanced improvements with the availability of effective therapy are:
- *1-year survival:* 90%
- *5-year survival:* 80%
- Death beyond 5 years is usually due to coronary artery disease (CAD)

There is insufficient data from RCTs to suggest that any individual drug is superior to another in improving morbidity and mortality in these situations.

PATHOPHYSIOLOGY

Majority of patients presenting with malignant hypertension to the ED have undetected or uncontrolled essential hypertension. However, 20–40% are shown to have secondary hypertension, most commonly renal parenchymal disease and renal artery stenosis. Endocrine hypertension is rare.

Initiating events for sudden escalation of BP is yet to be deciphered. In experimental models, development of acute hypertensive microcoagulopathy is preceded by an accentuation of renal vasoconstriction and microvascular damage that in turn leads to marked activation of renin–angiotensin system. Pressure-induced natriuresis is another factor that leads to activation of renin–angiotensin system through contraction of blood

Flowchart 1: Pathophysiology of acute severe hypertensive-mediated organ damage in malignant hypertension.

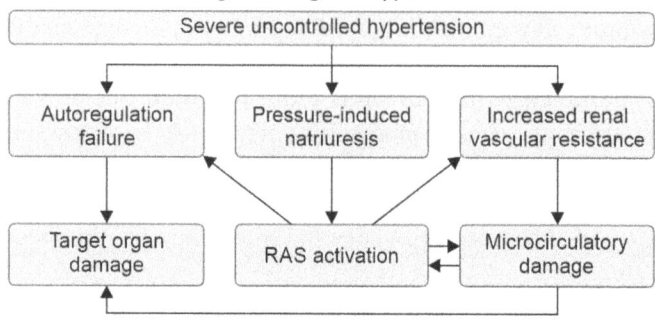

(RAS: renin–angiotensin system)

volume. Microvascular damage and failure of auto-regulatory systems constitute the foundation of target-organ damage in malignant hypertension and explain the occurrence of thrombotic microangiopathy (TMA), encephalopathy, and retinopathy.

CLINICAL PRESENTATIONS

There is no specific BP threshold that can be incriminated with hypertension-mediated target organ damage. Rate of BP increase appears to be more important than the absolute BP value in the causation of target-organ damage and hypertensive emergencies.

A quick medical history-taking is very important:
- Non-adherence to antihypertensive drugs or drug-withdrawal
- Use of specific drugs (e.g., steroids, NSAIDs, cyclosporine, sympathomimetics, cocaine, and antiangiogenic therapy)
- Secondary cause of hypertension (e.g., renoparenchymal disease and renal vascular disease)

Symptoms suggestive of "Hypertensive emergencies" are: Headache, visual disturbances, chest pain, dyspnea, focal or general neurological symptoms, dizziness (resulting from cerebral autoregulation), gastrointestinal manifestations (abdominal pain, nausea, and anorexia), somnolence, tonic–clonic seizures, cortical blindness proceeding at times to loss of consciousness.

Physical examination should include measurement of BP in both arms appropriately following the current guidelines and measurement should be repeated over time because, in a significant proportion of patients, BP will fall even without antihypertensive medication. Measurement of lower-limb BP is helpful in detecting aortic dissection. Fundoscopy is mandatory to detect retinal changes.

Proposed diagnostic studies in hypertensive emergencies are as follows:
- Hemoglobin and platelet count
- Creatinine, sodium, potassium, lactic dehydrogenase (LDH), and haptoglobin
- Urine
  - Quantitative protein loss
  - Sediment for RBCs, leukocytes, cylinders, and casts
- ECG
- Troponin-T, CK, and CK-MB*
- Peripheral blood smear (if indicated, to detect schistocytes)*
- Chest X-ray (in suspected pulmonary edema)*
- Transthoracic echocardiography including long ultrasound (if pulmonary edema is suspected)*
- CT (or MRI) brain (to rule out intracranial hemorrhage)*
- CT-angiography of thorax and abdomen (if acute aortic disease is suspected)*
- Renal ultrasound (postrenal obstructions, kidney size, and left-to-right difference in size)*

APPROACH TO MANAGEMENT OF HYPERTENSIVE EMERGENCIES DEPENDING ON TARGET ORGAN DAMAGE IN QUESTION

- Malignant hypertension and hypertensive encephalopathy
  - In this situation, large reductions in BP [>50% decrease in mean arterial pressure (MAP)] may lead to ischemic stroke and death.
  - Sodium nitroprusside, labetalol, nicardipine, and urapidil all appear to be safe and effective options in this situation. Labetalol is preferred to sodium nitroprusside since it spares cerebral blood flow for a given BP reduction and does not increase intracranial pressure.

---
*Tests to be carried out on appropriate indication

- Fendolopam, a short-acting selective dopamine-1 agonist, and clevidipine, an ultra-short-acting calcium channel blocker both administered intravenously are additional options but are not widely available.
- BP lowering response to renin–angiotensin system blockers is unpredictable in malignant hypertension. Some teams use oral ACB-inhibitors and if effective, they cause sudden decrease in BP, especially if the patient is volume depleted because of pressure-natriuresis. Intravenous (IV) saline infusion can be useful in such settings in order to preserve cerebral blood flow.

- Acute stroke (Ischemic and Hemorrhagic)
  - Ischemic stroke
    - If thrombolytic therapy is indicated, lowering BP <185/110 mm Hg is recommended before thrombolytic therapy is initiated. Same BP criteria have been used in recent trials that investigated the effect of thrombectomy with or without prior thrombolysis.
    - Overall, in ischemic stroke, acute BP reduction within first 5–7 days is associated with adverse neurological outcome. Unless there is another pressing reason like acute coronary event, acute heart failure, aortic dissection, it is probably safe to lower MAP by 15% in the first 24 hours. In concomitant situations mentioned earlier, faster reduction is advisable.
  - Hemorrhagic stroke
    - The Intensive BP reduction in Acute Cerebral Hemorrhage Trial (INTERACT)-2 showed that treatment to systolic BP <140 mm Hg in patients with intracerebral hemorrhage reduced intracranial hematoma and had a borderline significant effect in improving functional outcome. On the other hand, the more recent Antihypertensive Treatment of Acute Cerebral Hemorrhage II (ATACH-2) trial failed to show any benefit of acute BP lowering treatment. In the two trials, despite having same BP target, there were large discrepancies in the BP target and achieved BP target. This factor may have mitigated any positive effect.

- If acute BP reduction is intended, labetalol is the preferred choice but nicardipine and sodium nitroprusside are useful alternatives.
- Acute coronary syndrome
  - In case of acute coronary syndrome with severe hypertension, afterload needs to be reduced without an increase in heart rate and preserving adequate diastolic filling time so as to decrease myocardial oxygen demand.
  - Both nitroglycerine and labetalol have been used to lower BP in this situation. If nitroglycerine is used, additional beta-blockade may be indicated if tachycardia is present.
  - Sodium nitroprusside is best avoided in acute myocardial infarction since it decreases regional coronary blood flow in patients with coronary abnormalities.
  - Urapidil may be a good alternative for the management of hypertension in patients with myocardial ischemia.
- Acute cardiogenic pulmonary edema
  - In hypertensive heart failure, i.e., acute pulmonary edema caused by severe hypertension, both nitroglycerine and sodium nitroprusside can be used as they optimize preload and decrease afterload. Nitroprusside is preferred as it acutely decreases both pre- and afterload. High dose of nitroglycerine (>200 mg/min) may be required to attain targeted BP-lowering effect.
  - Urapidil, in comparison to nitroglycerine, achieves better BP control without precipitating reflex tachycardia.
  - Noninvasive continuous positive airway pressure may be of adjunctive benefit as it acutely reduces both pulmonary edema and venous return.
  - Concomitant use of loop diuretics decreases volume overload and may also reduce BP.
- *Acute aortic disease:* Reduction of aortic wall stress and disease progression is most important in patients with acute aortic disease of rupture, and hence reduction of systolic BP to 120 mm Hg and heart rate to 60 bpm or less is vitally important. Beta-blockers are therefore considered first-line treatment. Esmolol can be used along with ultra-short-acting vasodilator

drugs such as nitroprusside or clevidipine. In case these agents are not available, longer-acting agents like metoprolol or labetalol bolus can be used. However, these agents are associated with the disadvantage that prolonged hypotension may be precipitated. Even in absence of systemic hypertension, BP should be reduced. After control of BP, angiography or transesophageal echocardiography or both should be performed. The need for surgical intervention is determined based on involvement of the ascending aorta.

- *Hypertensive retinopathy in malignant hypertension:* Typical features are flame-shaped hemorrhages and cotton wool spots (grade III) with or without presence of papilledema (Grade IV) detected in both eyes. Grade III and Grade IV retinopathy have the same background and are associated with similar prognosis. Presence of hypertensive retinopathy in suspected hypertensive emergency denotes severe activation of renin–angiotensin system and more pronounced hypertension-mediated organ damage.
- *TMA in malignant hypertension:* Detachment of the endothelium is one of the pathological hallmarks of hypertensive microangiopathy. High-shear forces in severe (malignant) hypertension are responsible for this. Following detachment of subendothelium, exposure of blood to subendothelium leads to coagulation cascade activation, platelet activation, and formation of a fibrin network. This in turn has two ramifications that are as follows: (1) Formation of platelet-rich thrombi resulting in obliteration of the microcirculation, (2) platelet consumption and intravascular hemolysis as a consequence of trapping and destruction of erythrocytes within the fibrin network.
  - Thrombotic thrombocytopenic purpura (TTP) and hemolytic uremic syndrome (HUS) are close differential diagnosis of TMA. However, only moderate thrombocytopenia and fewer schistocytes are seen in TMA compared to more severe manifestations in two other afore-mentioned conditions. Presence of severe hypertension and advanced retinopathy supports the diagnosis of hypertensive emergency leading to TMA. Measurement of activity of von Willebrand factor

cleaving proteinase, ADAMTS13, which is normal or slightly reduced in hypertension-induced TMA, helps to distinguish from TTP where its activity is very low. BP-lowering treatment will usually improve TMA associated with severe hypertension within 24-48 hours; in contrast, specific other treatments are required for TTP or HUS.

ECLAMPSIA AND SEVERE PREECLAMPSIA

Preeclampsia is gestational hypertension accompanied by ≥1 of the following new-onset conditions at or after 20 weeks gestation:
- Proteinuria
- Other maternal organ dysfunction, including:
  - AKI (creatinine ≥90 μmol/L or 1 mg/dL
  - Liver involvement (elevated transaminases >40 u/L) with or without right upper quadrant or epigastric abdominal pain
  - Neurological complications like eclampsia, altered mental status, blindness, stroke, clonus, severe headaches, and persistent visual scotomata.
  - Hematological complications (thrombocytopenia, disseminated intravascular coagulation, and hemolysis).
  - Uteroplacental dysfunction such as fetal growth retardation, abnormal umbilical artery doppler waveform analysis, or stillbirth.

Distinction between early and late-onset and mild and severe preeclampsia may be useful for research purposes. However, for practical clinical purposes, all cases of preeclampsia should be considered as one that at any time is capable of becoming severe and life-threatening for mother and baby. Level of BP itself is not a dependable parameter to stratify immediate risk in preeclampsia because some women may develop significant organ malfunction such as renal impairment or neurological complications even at mild levels of hypertension. BP at or >160/110 mm Hg is thought to be only surrogate markers for the risk of stroke as well as a reflection of increased severity of the overall condition of preeclampsia.

The consensus is to lower systolic and diastolic BP <160/105 mm Hg to prevent acute hypertensive complications in the mother. Both labetalol and nicardipine have been shown to be safe and effective for treatment of severe preeclampsia and IV BP lowering therapy is deemed essential. Fetal heart rate monitoring becomes necessary for both the drugs. Otherwise, timely initiation of oral antihypertensive (e.g., methyldopa or long-acting nifedipine) may help in BP control in preeclampsia and prevent maternal or fetal complications. Hydralazine (associated with adverse perinatal complications) or nitroprusside (associated with fetal cyanide toxicity) are not indicated anymore.

Urgent delivery in preeclampsia is necessitated when ≥1 of the following indications emerge:
- Inability to control maternal BP despite using ≥3 classes of antihypertensives in appropriate doses.
- Maternal oxygen saturation is <90%.
- Progressive worsening of liver function, creatinine, hemolysis, or platelet count.
- Emerging neurological features, such as severe intractable headache, repeated visual scotomata, or eclampsia
- Abruptio placenta
- Reversed end-diastolic flow in the upper abdominal doppler velocimetry, a nonreassuring cardiotocograph or stillbirth

Prevention of Eclampsia in Women with Preeclampsia

In the landmark MAGPIE trial, women with preeclampsia were given magnesium sulfate ($MgSO_4$) if they had severe hypertension and at least 3+ of proteinuria or slightly lower measurements (150/100 mm Hg and at least 2+ of proteinuria) in the presence of at least two signs or symptoms of imminent eclampsia (likely symptoms are headache, visual symptoms, or clonus) $MgSO_4$ was given either intravenously or intramuscularly (IM). Loading dose was 4 g $MgSO_4$ IV. IV infusion dose used for maintenance was 1 g $MgSO_4$ per hour and for intramuscular maintenance regimen following the IV loading dose, 10 g $MgSO_4$ is given IM, followed by 5 mg $MgSO_4$ IM every 4 hours. The International Society for the Study of Hypertension in Pregnancy (ISSHP) recommends that because the cost-benefit is greatest, all preeclamptic women in low-and-middle-income countries should receive $MgSO_4$. It also recommends that each unit should have a consistent policy on their use of $MgSO_4$ that incorporates appropriate monitoring, identifying the risks of $MgSO_4$ infusion, and assessment of maternal and fetal outcomes. The dosing regimens used in MAGPIE trial should be used.

Management of Eclampsia

Comprehensive protocols for the management of eclampsia (and severe hypertension) should be available in all appropriate areas.

There are four main aspects to care for the woman who sustains eclampsia.
1. Resuscitation
2. Prevention of further seizures:
   a. Treatment should be commenced with magnesium sulfate (4 g//IV over 10-15 minutes) followed by an IV infusion (1-2 g/h) for 24-48 h. There is no need to measure serum magnesium levels provided renal function is normal.
   b. In the event of a further seizure, a further 2-4 g of magnesium sulfate is given IV over 10 minutes.
   c. Intravenous diazepam (2 mg/min) may be given while the magnesium sulfate is being prepared if the seizure is prolonged.
   d. Magnesium infusion should not be used for >12 hours in women with oliguria or renal impairment and serum magnesium levels should be monitored during this time.
3. Control of hypertension:
   a. Control of severe hypertension to levels below 160/100 mm Hg by parenteral therapy is essential.
   b. First-line drugs are IV labetalol and IV hydralazine.
   c. Tablet nifedipine may be used (maximum dose 50 mg).
   d. IV nicardipine or labetalol infusion can be tried if IV/PO shots are ineffective.
   e. Close monitoring of BP for at least 4 hours is advised even after successful control of BP.
   f. Short IV nitroprusside should be reserved only in extreme emergency.

4. Delivery:
   a. Arrangements for delivery should be decided once the women's condition is stable.
   b. In the meantime, close fetal monitoring should be maintained.

MANAGEMENT OF SEVERE HYPERTENSION IN SPECIAL SITUATIONS

- *Hypertensive crisis after coronary artery bypass surgery:* Paroxysmal hypertension in the immediate postoperative period is a frequent and serious complication of cardiac surgery. Paroxysmal hypertension is the most frequent complication of coronary artery bypass surgery, occurring in 30–50% of patients. It occurs just as in normotensive patients as it does in those with a history of chronic hypertension.

Flowchart 2: Perioperative management of hypertension with pheochromocytoma.

| Malignant hypertension or Inadequate preoperative blood pressure control (diastolic BP >110 mm Hg) or Mild-to-moderate hypertension In patients with history of ischemia during cerebrovascular accident, myocardial ischemia, heart failure, or renal insufficiency | → | Postpone elective surgery until blood pressure is adequately controlled for 2–3 weeks |

↓

- Administer blood pressure and antianginal medications on the morning of surgery
- Continuation of beta-blockers within few hours of surgery decreases risk of dysrhythmia and myocardial ischemia during surgery
- *Adequate hypovolemia:* Diuretics should be withheld for 1–2 days preoperatively except in patients with overt heart failure or fluid overload

↓

Manage postoperative hypertension with nitroprusside or nitroglycerin in patients with complications or labetalol in patients without complications

↓

Carefully institute oral antihypertensive at low dose and titrate based on orthostatic blood pressure measurements

The initial management of post-bypass surgery hypertension should focus on attempts to ameliorate reversible causes of sympathetic activation, including patient agitation on recovery from anesthesia, tracheal or nasopharyngeal irritation from the endotracheal tube, pain, hypothermia with shivering ventilator asynchrony, hypoxia, hypercarbia, and volume depletion. If these general measures fail to lower BP, further therapy should be guided by measurement of systemic hemodynamics. Intravenous nitroglycerin or nitroprusside is the drug of choice to provide a controlled decrease in systemic vascular resistance (SVR) and BP. Nitroglycerin may be the preferred drug because it dilates intracoronary collateral arteries.

- *Pheochromocytoma:* In most patients, pheochromocytoma causes sustained hypertension that sometimes becomes malignant as evidenced by the presence of hypertensive neuroretinopathy.

  Prompt control of BP is mandatory to prevent life-threatening complications. Although the nonselective alpha-blocker phentolamine often is cited as therapy of choice for pheochromocytoma-related hypertensive crisis, sodium nitroprusside is equally effective and easier to administer. After adequate alpha-blockade is achieved, based on the presence of moderate orthostatic hypotension, oral beta-blocker therapy can be initiated as needed to control tachycardia.

- *Poorly controlled hypertension in surgical patients:* Although adequate preoperative control of BP is imperative, aggressive parenteral therapy to do so can lead to precipitous fall of BP, which carries the risk of significant complications such as hypovolemia, electrolyte abnormalities, and marked intraoperative BP liability. General anesthesia is accompanied by a 30% decrease in cardiac output. In normotensive persons and patients with adequately treated hypertension, anesthesia is not associated with a decrease in SBP. Therefore, decrease in MAP is modest (25-30%). However, in patients with inadequate preoperative BP control, anesthesia is associated with a concomitant decrease in SVR of approximately 27%. The combined decrease in cardiac output and SVR leads to a

TABLE 1: Summary of hypertensive emergencies requiring immediate BP lowering.

Clinical presentation	Timeline and target BP	First-line treatment	Alternative
Malignant hypertension with or without TMA or acute renal failure	Several hours, MAP −20% to −25%	• Labetalol • Nicardipine	• Nitroprusside • Urapidil
Hypertensive encephalopathy	Immediate, MAP −20% to −25%	• Labetalol • Nicardipine	Nitroprusside
Acute ischemic stroke and BP >220 mm Hg systolic or >120 mm Hg diastolic	1 h, MAP −15%	• Labetalol • Nicardipine	Nitroprusside
Acute ischemic stroke with indication for thrombolytic therapy and BP >185 mm Hg systolic or >110 mm Hg diastolic	1 h, MAP −15%	• Labetalol • Nicardipine	Nitroprusside
Acute hemorrhagic stroke and systolic BP >180 mm Hg	Immediate, systolic BP <130 mm Hg	• Labetalol • Nicardipine	Urapidil
Acute coronary event	Immediate, systolic BP <140 mm Hg	• Nitroglycerine • Labetalol	Urapidil
Acute cardiogenic pulmonary edema	Immediate, systolic BP <140 mm Hg	Nitroprusside or Nitroglycerine (with loop diuretic)	Urapidil (with loop diuretic)
Acute aortic disease	Immediate, systolic BP <120 mm Hg and heart rate <60 bpm	Esmolol and nitroprusside or nitroglycerine or nicardipine	Labetalol or Metoprolol
Eclampsia and severe preeclampsia/HELLP	Immediate, systolic BP < 160 mm Hg and diastolic BP <105 mm Hg	Labetalol or nicardipine and magnesium sulfate	

(BP: blood pressure; HELLP: hemolysis, elevated liver enzymes and low platelets; TMA: thrombotic microangiopathy)

TABLE 2: Intravenous drugs for the treatment of hypertensive emergencies.

Drug	Onset of action	Duration of action	Dose	Contraindications	Adverse effects
Esmolol	1–2 minutes	10–30 minutes	0.5–1 mg/kg as bolus; 50–300 mg/kg/min as continuous infusion	History of second or third-degree AV block (and in the absence of rhythm support), systolic heart failure, asthma, and bradycardia	Bradycardia
Metoprolol	1–2 minutes	5–8 hours	15 mg intravenous (IV), usually given as 5 mg, and repeated at 5 minutes intervals as needed	History of second or third-degree AV block, systolic heart failure, asthma, and bradycardia	Bradycardia
Labetalol	5–10 minutes	3–6 hours	0.25–0.5 mg/kg; 2–4 mg/min until goal BP is reached, thereafter 5–20 mg/h	History of second or third-degree AV block, systolic heart failure, asthma, and bradycardia	Bronchoconstriction and fetal bradycardia
Fenoldopam	5–15 minutes	30–60 minutes	0.1 µg/kg/min, increase every 15 minutes until goal BP is reached		
Clevidipine	2–3 minutes	5–15 minutes	2 mg/h, increase every 2 min with 2 mg/h until goal BP		Headache and reflex tachycardia

Contd...

Contd...

Drug	Onset of action	Duration of action	Dose	Contraindications	Adverse effects
Nicardipine	5–15 minutes	30–40 minutes	5–15 mg/h as continuous infusion, starting dose 5 mg/h. Increase every 15–30 minutes with 25 mg until goal BP; thereafter, decrease to 3 mg/h	Liver failure	Headache and reflex tachycardia
Nitroglycerine	1–5 minutes	3–5 minutes	5–200 mg/min, 5 mg/min increase every 5 min		Headache and reflex tachycardia
Nitroprusside	Immediate	1–2 minutes	0.3–10 mg/kg/min, increase by 0.5 mg/kg/min every 5 minutes until goal BP	Liver/kidney failure (relative)	Cyanide intoxication
Enalaprilat	5–15 minutes	4–6 hours	0.62–1.25 mg IV	History of angioedema	
Urapidil	3–5 minutes	4–6 hours	12.5–25 mg as bolus injection, 5–40 mg/h as continuous infusion		
Clonidine	30 minutes	4–6 hours	150–300 µg IV in 5–10 minutes		Sedation and rebound hypertension
Phentolamine	1–2 minutes	10–30 minutes	0.5–1 mg/kg bolus injections OR 50–300 µg/kg/min as continuous infusion		Tachyarrhythmias and chest pain

profound MAP (45%) during anesthesia. This intraoperative hypotension predisposes to myocardial ischemia, cerebrovascular accidents, and acute renal failure. Hence, more gradual and sustained adequate preoperative BP control should be the goal in all hypertensive patients.

- In patients with autonomic hyperactivity, resulting from suspected methamphetamine or cocaine intoxication, initial treatment with benzodiazepines is indicated in first place. For additional BP lowering, intravenous phentolamine, nicardipine, or nitroprusside are indicated. Alternatively, clonidine can be used. However, if coronary ischemia is suspected, treatment with nitroglycerin and aspirin should be administered next to benzodiazepines, and as a next line, in non-ST-segment elevation myocardial infarction, percutaneous coronary intervention (PCI) should be considered. Beta-blockers (including labetalol) should be avoided since they do not seem to relieve coronary vasoconstriction. Rather, nondihydropyridine calcium channel blockers, like verapamil and diltiazem, can be used to treat tachyarrhythmias under close ECG monitoring.

PROGNOSIS AND FOLLOW-UP

In patients admitted to coronary care unit (CCU) with hypertensive emergency, mortality has been detected to be significantly higher (4.6%) when compared with hypertensive patients without a hypertensive emergency (9.8%).

Few studies have been conducted with regard to optimal follow-up in patients with previous hypertensive emergency. In absence of such data, extrapolated guidelines for severe hypertension in general should be applied. Improving adherence is of paramount importance. In-depth etiological work-up and monitoring of hypertension-indicated organ damage are indispensable. Simplification of therapy like use of frontline fixed combination therapy including diuretics or other antihypertensive therapy and reinforcing dietary sodium restriction are vital steps in preventing recurrent hospitalization for hypertensive emergencies.

SUGGESTED READING

1. Brown MA, Magee LA, Kenny LC, Karumanchi SA, McCarthy FP, Saito S, et al. Hypertensive disorders of pregnancy. ISSHP classification, diagnosis, and management recommendations for international practice. Hypertension. 2018;72(1):24-43.
2. Cremer A, Amraour F, Lip GY, Morales E, Rubin S, Segura J, et al. From malignant hypertension to hypertension-MOD: A modern definition for an old but still dangerous emergency. J Hum Hypertens. 2016;30:463-6.
3. Miller J, McNaughton C, Joyce K, Binz S, Levy P. Hypertension management in emergency departments. Am J Hypertens. 2020;33(10):927-4.
4. Muiesan ML, Salvetti M, Amadoro V, di Somma S, Perlini S, Semplicini A, et al. An update on hypertensive emergencies and urgencies. J Cardiovasc Med (Hagerstown). 2014;16(5):372-82.
5. Van den Born BH, Lip GYH, Brguljan-Hitij J, Cremer A, Segura J, Morales E, et al. ESC Council on hypertensive position document on the management of hypertensive emergencies. Eur Heart J Cardiovasc Pharmacother. 2019;5(1):37-46.

13 Acid-base Disturbance

CHAPTER

Sujata Majumder, Amitava Mazumdar

The objective is to detect acid-base disorder from arterial blood gas (ABG) analysis and correlate with clinical and other laboratory findings to reach at a definite diagnosis. Sometimes multiple acid-base disorders are present due to presence of either multiple diseases at a time or multiple components of a disease at a time. Body tries to maintain pH in physiologic range (7.35–7.45) to maintain all the enzymes to remain active.

Whenever any disease process makes the pH to any extreme then body tries by compensatory means to bring the pH toward physiology range. In extreme pH, people cannot survive.

TYPES OF ACID-BASE DISORDER

- *Metabolic acidosis:* pH low, HCO_3^- low
- *Metabolic alkalosis:* pH high, HCO_3^- high

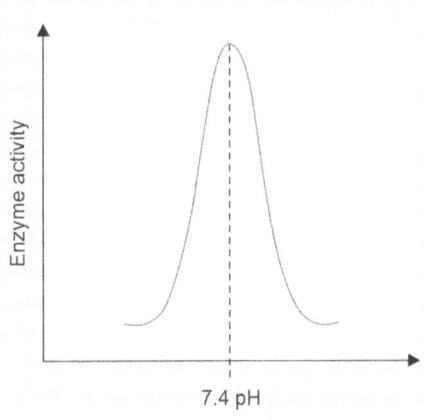

Fig. 1: Curve showing relationship between enzyme activity and pH.

- *Respiratory acidosis:* pH low, $PaCO_2$ high
- *Respiratory alkalosis:* pH high, $PaCO_2$ low

NORMAL VALUES

- pH = 7.35–7.45
- $PaCO_2$ = 35–45 mm Hg
- HCO_3 = 22–26 mmol/L
- BE = +2 to –2

APPROACH TO DIAGNOSE MIXED ACID-BASE DISORDERS

- *CO_2 bicarbonate (Boston) approach:* Check pH → check $PaCO_2$ and HCO_3^- → determine primary acid based order from the table, a measure compensation from second column of the table → look for overshoot changes → that will be the second disorder.
- *Anion gap (AG) approach:* Measure AG (Na^+ - Cl^- - HCO_3^-) → measure corrected AG = AG –2.5 (reduction in albumin from 4.5 g/dL) → if >10 then high AG acidosis is present → measure delta AG (AG-10) and delta 24 –HCO_3^- → measure their ratio.
- *Stewart's approach:* There are three independent variables, namely $PaCO_2$, strong ion difference (SID), ATOT. In respiratory disorders, there is change in $PaCO_2$. Metabolic disorders are addressed with SID and ATOT. In metabolic alkalosis, SID is increased and in metabolic acidosis, SID is decreased.

$$SID = [Na^+] + [K^+] + [Ca^{+2}] + [Mg^{+2}] - [Cl^-] - [lactate^-] - [other\ strong\ ions] = [HCO_3^-] + [A^-]$$

Under normal conditions, concentration of lactate and other strong ions is very low and can be ignored. The formula could therefore be simplified to:

$$SID = [Na^+] + [K^+] + [Ca^{+2}] + [Mg^{+2}] - [Cl^-] = [HCO_3^-] + [A^-]$$

The SID, therefore, can be calculated as the difference between fully dissociated cations and anions or sum of bicarbonate and $[A^-]$, where $[A^-]$ represents total charges contributed by all nonbicarbonate buffers, primarily albumin, phosphate, and, in whole blood, hemoglobin.

Strong ion gap (SIG) = apparent SID (SID_a) - effective SID (SID_e)
$$SID = [Na^+] + [K^+] + [Ca^{+2}] + [Mg^{+2}] - [Cl^-].$$
$$SID = [HCO_3^-] + [A^-]$$

TABLE 1: Compensatory changes.

Acid-base disorder	Method of compensation	Prediction of compensation	PH	$PaCO_2$	HCO_3^-
Met acidosis	Hyperventilation	↓$PaCO_2$ 1.25 mm Hg per mmol/L in [HCO_3^-]	↓	↓	↓
Met alkalosis	Hypoventilation	↑$PaCO_2$ 0.75 mm Hg per mmol/L in [HCO_3^-]	↑	↑	↑
Acute respiratory acidosis	*1, 2, 3	[HCO_3^-] 0.1 mmol/L per mm Hg in $PaCO_2$	↓	↑	↑
Chronic respiratory acidosis	*1, 2, 3	↑[HCO_3^-] 0.4 mmol/L per mm Hg in $PaCO_2$	↓	↑	↑
Acute respiratory alkalosis	*Opposite of 1,2,3	↓[HCO_3^-] 0.2 mmol/L per mm Hg in $PaCO_2$	↑	↓	↓
Chronic respiratory alkalosis	*Opposite of 1,2,3	↓[HCO_3^-] 0.4 mmol/L per mm Hg in $PaCO_2$	↑	↓	↓

*The kidneys regulate plasma [HCO_3^-] through three main processes: (1) "Reabsorption" of filtered HCO_3^-, (2) formation of titratable acid, and (3) excretion of NH_4^+ in the urine.

Flowchart 1: Approach to diagnosis of metabolic pH abnormalities.

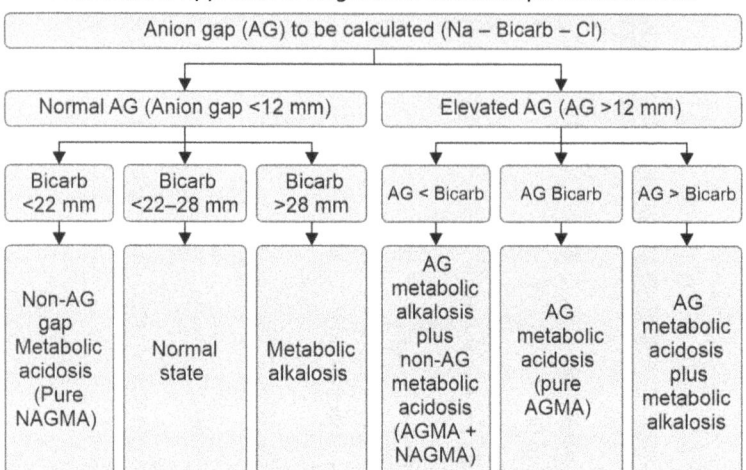

TABLE 2: Base deficit/excess (Copenhagen) approach.	
Disturbance	**BDE vs. PaCO₃**
Acute respiratory acidosis	$\Delta BDE = 0$
Acute respiratory alkalosis	$BDE = 0$
Chronic respiratory acidosis	$BDE = 0.4, \Delta PaCO_2$
Metabolic acidosis	$\Delta PaCO_2 = \Delta BDE$
Metabolic alkalosis	$\Delta PaCO_2 = 0.6, \Delta BDE$
BDE = Base deficit/excess	
Change of $PaCO_2$ more/less than above equation will indicate mixed disorder	

ATOT: Total concentration of weak acids = *[HA + A⁻] (all nonbicarbonate buffer pairs)* contributed primarily by serum proteins with phosphate and other buffers playing a minor role. An increase in serum protein would result in metabolic acidosis and a decrease, metabolic alkalosis.

RESPIRATORY ACIDOSIS

Chronic respiratory acidosis management: Therapeutic measures are guided by the presence or absence of severe hypercapnic encephalopathy or hemodynamic instability. An aggressive

Acid-base Disturbance

TABLE 3: Classification of primary acid-base disturbances.

Parameter	Acidosis	Alkalosis
Respiratory	↑$PaCO_2$	↓$PaCO_2$
Nonrespiratory (metabolic)		
• Abnormal SID		
– Water excess/deficit	↓SID, ↓[Na]	↑SID, ↑[Na]
– Imbalance of strong anions		
- Chloride excess/deficit	↓SID, ↑[Cl]	↑SID, ↓[Cl]
- Unidentified anion excess	↓SID, ↑[XA]	
• Nonvolatile weak acids		
– Serum albumin	↑[Alb]	↓[Alb]
– Inorganic phosphate	↑[Pi]	↓[P>]

(Alb: albumin concentration; Pi: inorganic phosphate concentration; XA: concentration of unidentified strong anion)

Metabolic acidosis—high AG and normal Ag

Normal

	A⁻ 10	HCO₃⁻
Na⁺ 140	Cl⁻ 106	24

Metabolic acidosis

Normal anion gap (hyperchloremic)

	A⁻ 10	HCO₃⁻
Na⁺ 140	Cl⁻ 126	4

Causes
Renal acidification defects
• Proximal renal tubular acidosis
• Classic distal tubular acidosis
• Hyperkalemic distal tubular acidosis
• Early renal failure
Gastrointestinal loss of bicarbonate
• Diarrhea
• Small bowel losses
• Ureteral diversion
• Anion exchange resins
• Ingestion of $CaCl_2$
Acid infusion
• HCl
• Arginine HCl
• Lysine HCl

High anion gap (normochloremic)

	A⁻ 30	HCO₃⁻
Na⁺ 140	Cl⁻ 106	4

Causes
Endogenous acid load
• Ketoacidosis
  – Diabetes mellitus
  – Alcoholism
  – Starvation
• Uremia
• Lactic acidosis
Exogenous toxins
• Osmolar gap present
  – Methanol
  – Ethylene glycol
Osmolar gap absent
• Salicylate
• Paraldehyde

Fig. 2: Individual acid-base disorders.

TABLE 4: Signs and symptoms of metabolic acidosis.

Respiratory system	Cardiovascular system	Metabolism	Central nervous system	Skeleton
• Hyperventilation • Respiratory distress and dyspnea • Decreased strength of respiratory muscles and promotion of muscle fatigue	• Impairment of cardiac contractility, venoconstriction, and centralization of blood volume • Reductions in cardiac output, arterial blood pressure, and hepatic and renal blood flow • Sensitization to reentrant arrhythmias and reduction in threshold for ventricular fibrillation • Increased sympathetic discharge but attenuation of cardiovascular responsiveness to catecholamines cardiovascular responsiveness to catecholamines	• Increased metabolic demands • Insulin resistance • Inhibition of anaerobic glycolysis • Reduction in adenosine triphosphate synthesis • Hyperkalemia increased protein degradation	• Impaired metabolism • Inhibition of cell volume regulation • Progressive obtundation • Coma	Osteomalacia fractures

TABLE 5: Approach to diagnosis and treatment of high AG acidosis.

High AG acidosis	Diagnostic clue	Treatment plan
Lactic acidosis L-lactate → (type A) poor tissue perfusion, (type B) aerobic disorders, D-lactate → ↑formation by gut bacteria	Serum lactate >5 mmol/L	• Underlying condition correction • Tissue perfusion restoration • Vasoconstrictors should be avoided • Alkali therapy when pH <7.15, to make pH 7.2 over 30–40 minutes • Cautious fluid administration after correction risk of overshoot alkalosis (lactate will convert to HCO_3^-)
Keto-acidosis Diabetic K Alcoholic K	• Blood sugar high, history of missed insulin, pancreatitis, AMI, sepsis, pain abdomen • History of alcoholism/alcohol withdrawal, poor nutrition, vomiting	• IV fluid • Insulin in DKA • Underlying condition correction in DKA • Electrolytes correction • Dextrose when needed
Starvation renal failure	• High serum creatinine, low urine output, sometimes combined high and normal AG acidosis	• Alkali supplement • Hemodialysis, if needed • General measures • Fomepizole hemodialysis
Ethylene glycol	• Associated osmolar gap (measured osmolality—calculated osmolality >15–20 mmol/L), oxalate crystal in urine	
Methanol Salicylate	• Associated osmolar gap • Associated respiratory alkalosis	• Gastric lavage, activated charcoal • Alkali replacement (if noalkalemia) • Acetazolamide (if alkalemia) • Treat hypokalemia, hypoglycemia • Hemodialysis (bicarbonate dialysate)

(AMI: acute myocardial infarction; DKA: diabetic ketoacidosis; IV: intravenous)

TABLE 6: Metabolic alkalosis.

	Signs and symptoms of metabolic alkalosis				
Central nervous system	Cardiovascular system	Respiratory system	Neuromuscular system	Metabolic effects	Renal (associated potassium depletion)
Headache	Supraventricular and ventricular arrhythmias	Hypoventilation with attendant hypercapnia and hypoxemia	Chvostek's sign	Increased organic acid and ammonia production	Polyuria
Lethargy	Potentiation of digitalis toxicity		Trousseau's sign	Hypokalemia	Polydipsia
Stupor	Positive inotropic ventricular effect		Weakness (severity depends on degree of potassium depletion)	Hypocalcemia	Urinary concentration defect
Delirium				Hypomagnesemia	
Tetany				Hypophosphatemia	
Seizures					
Potentiation of hepatic encephalopathy					

Flowchart 2: Causes of metabolic alkalosis.

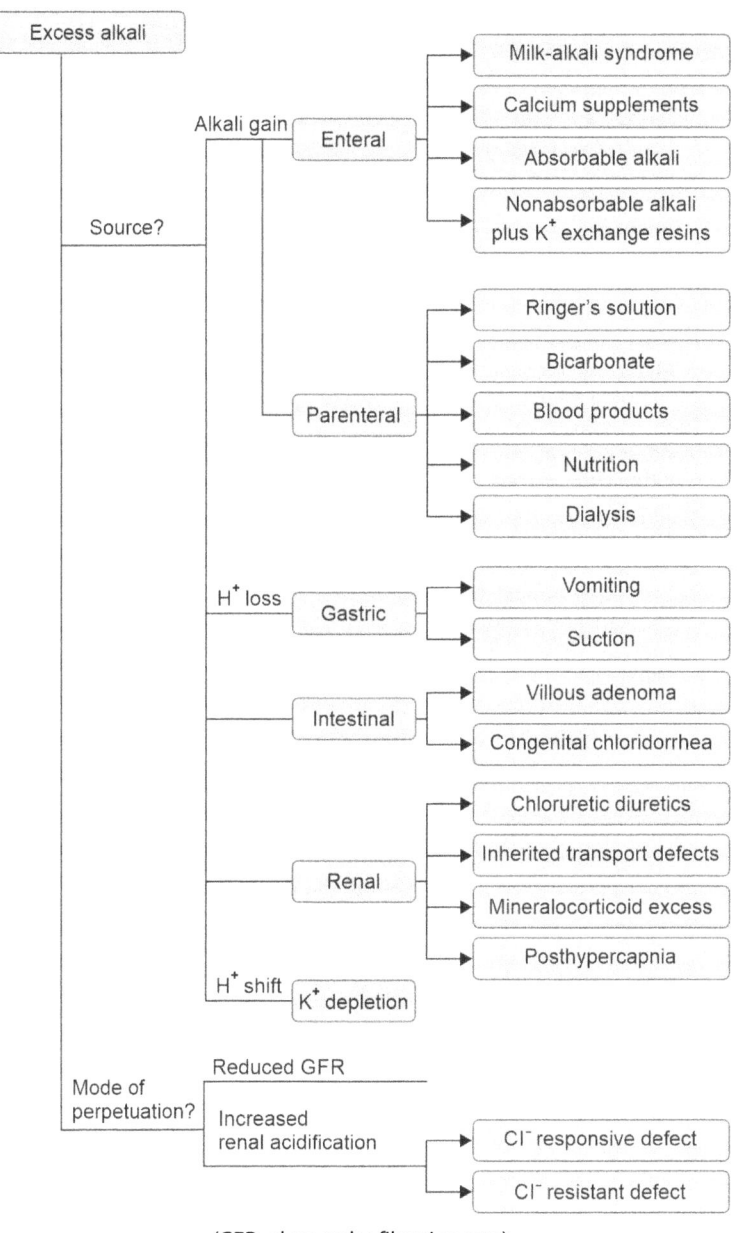

(GFR: glomerular filtration rate)

TABLE 7: Signs and symptoms of respiratory acidosis.

Central nervous system	Respiratory system	Cardiovascular system

• Mild-to-moderate hypercapnia
  – Cerebral vasodilation
  – Increased intracranial pressure
  – Headache
  – Confusion
  – Combativeness
  – Hallucinations
  – Transient psychosis
  – Myoclonic jerks
  – Flapping tremor
• Severe hypercapnia
• Manifestations of pseudotumor cerebri
• Stupor
• Coma
• Constricted pupils
• Depressed tendon reflexes
• Extensor plantar response
• Seizures
• Papilledema
	• Breathlessness
	• Central and peripheral cyanosis (especially when breathing room air)
	• Pulmonary hypertension
		• Mild-to-moderate hypercapnia
		  – Warm and flushed skin
		  – Bounding pulse
		  – Well-maintained cardiac output and blood pressure
		  – Diaphoresis
		• Severe hypercapnia
		  – Cor pulmonale
		  – Decreased cardiac output
		  – Systemic hypotension
		  – Cardiac arrhythmias
		  – Prerenal azotemia
		  – Peripheral edema tumor

Flowchart 3: Diagnostic clue of metabolic alkalosis.

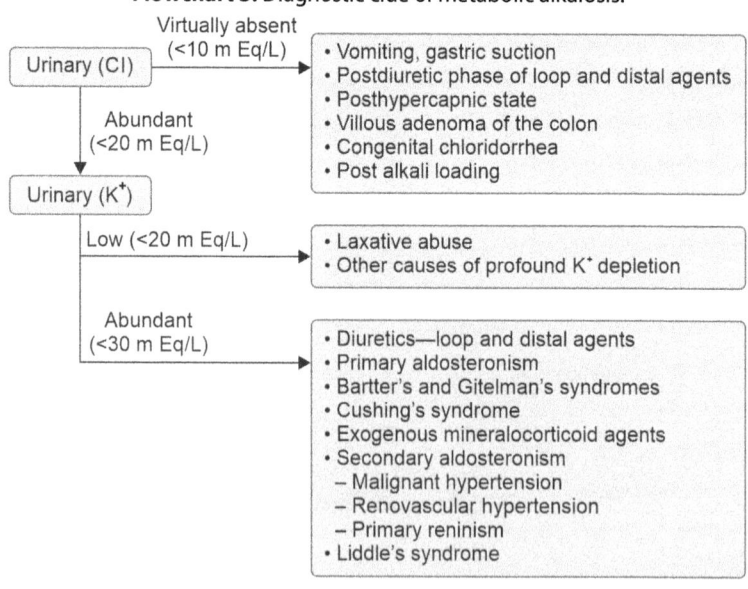

Flowchart 4: Management of metabolic alkalosis.

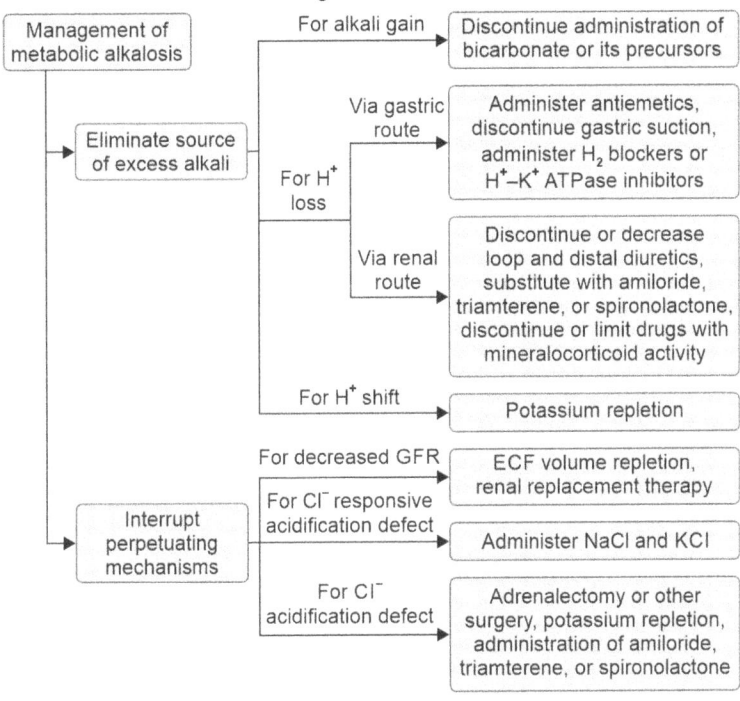

(GFR: glomerular filtration rate; ECF: extracellular fluid; KCl: Kyoto circling)

TABLE 8: Respiratory alkalosis.		
Signs and symptoms of respiratory alkalosis		
Central nervous system	**Cardiovascular system**	**Neuromuscular system**

• Cerebral vasoconstriction
• Reduction in intracranial pressure
• Light-headedness
• Confusion
• Increased deep tendon reflexes
• Generalized seizures
	• Chest oppression
	• Angina pectoris
	• Ischemic electrocardiographic changes
	• Normal or decreased blood pressure
	• Cardiac arrhythmias
	• Peripheral vasoconstriction
		• Numbness and paresthesias of the extremities
		• Circumoral numbness
		• Laryngeal spasm
		• Manifestations of tetany
		  – Muscle cramps
		  – Carpopedal spasm
		  – Trousseau's sign
		  – Chvostek's sign

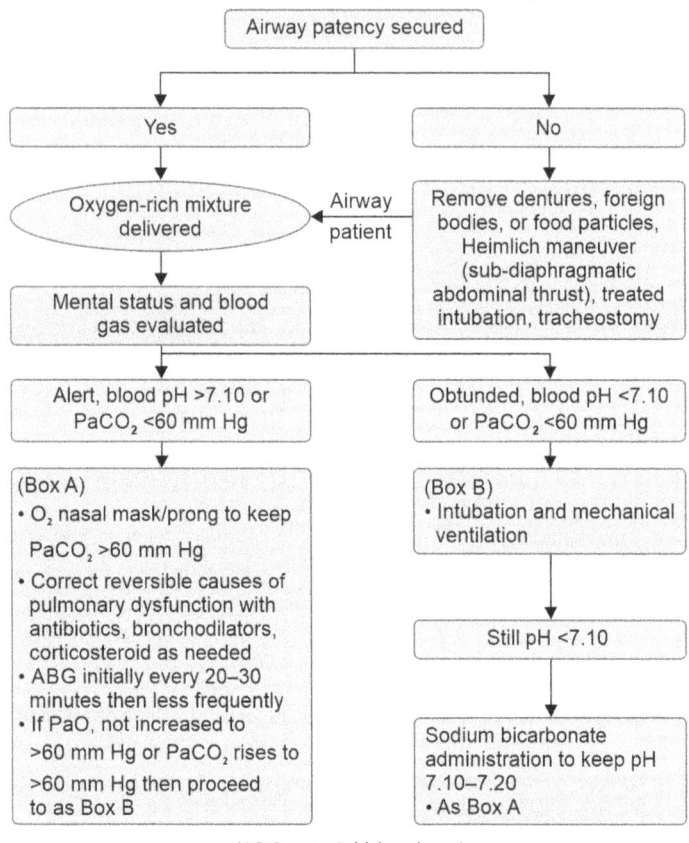

Flowchart 5: Acute respiratory acidosis management.

(ABG: arterial blood gas)

approach that favors the early use of ventilator assistance is most appropriate for patients with acute respiratory acidosis. In contrast, a more conservative approach is advisable in patients with chronic hypercapnia because of the great difficulty often encountered in weaning these patients from ventilators. As a rule, the lowest possible inspired fraction of oxygen that achieves adequate oxygenation (PaO_2 on the order of 60 mm Hg) is used. Unlike acute respiratory acidosis, the underlying cause of chronic respiratory acidosis only rarely can be resolved.

Role of dialysis in acid-base disorders: In ethyl glycol poisoning, when the arterial pH is <7.3 or the osmolar gap exceeds 20 mOsm/kg.

TABLE 9: Causes of respiratory alkaloids.

Hypoxemia or tissue hypoxia	Central nervous system stimulation	Drugs or hormones	Stimulation of chest receptors	Miscellaneous
• Decreased inspired oxygen tension • High attitude • Bacterial or viral pneumonia • Aspiration of food, foreign object, or vomitus • Laryngospasm • Drowning • Cyanotic heart disease • Severe anemia • Left shift deviation of oxyhemoglobin curve • Hypotension • Severe circulatory failure • Pulmonary edema	• Voluntary pain • Anxiety syndrome hyperventilation syndrome • Psychosis • Fever • Subarachnoid hemorrhage • Cerebrovascular accident • Meningoencephalitis • Tumor • Trauma	• Analeptics • Doxapram • Xanthines • Salicylates • Catecholamines • Angiotensin II • Vasopressor agents • Progesterone • Medroxyprogesterone • Dinitrophenol • Nicotine	• Pneumonia • Asthma • Pneumothorax • Hemothorax • Flail chest • Acute respiratory distress syndrome • Cardiogenic and noncardiogenic pulmonary edema • Pulmonary embolism • Pulmonary fibrosis	• Pregnancy • Early sepsis • Hepatic failure • Mechanical hyper-ventilation • Heat exposure • Recovery from metabolic acidosis

Flowchart 6: Management of respiratory alkaloids.

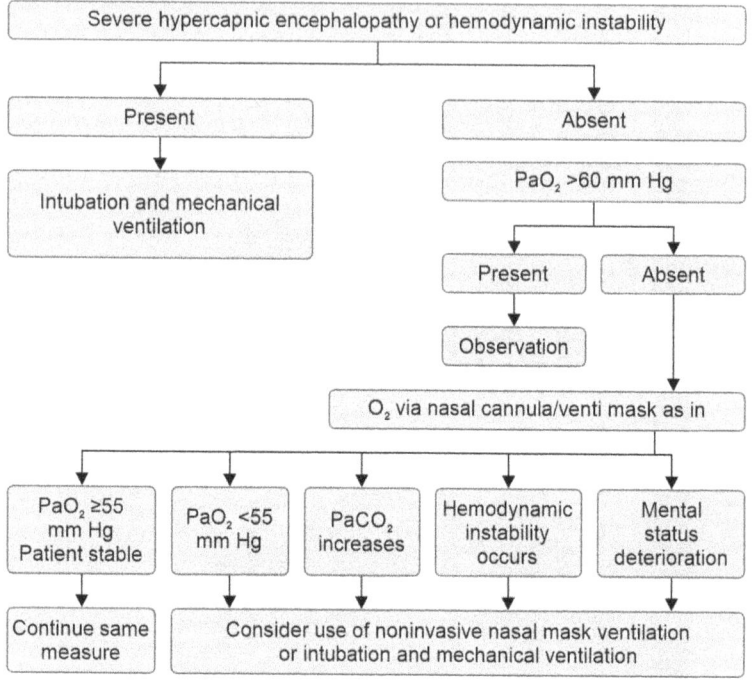

Flowchart 7: Management of respiratory alkalosis.

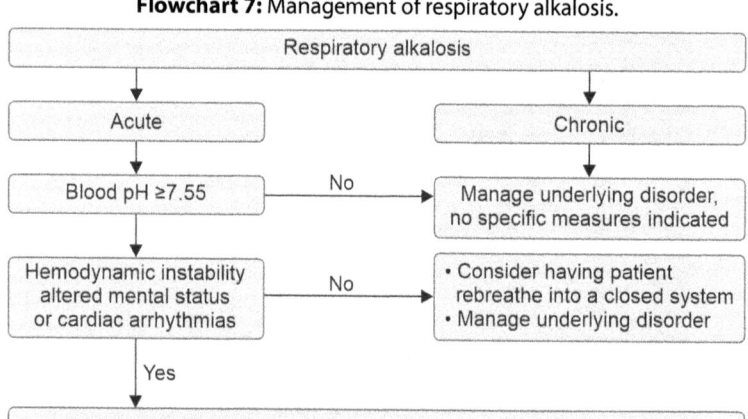

PSEUDORESPIRATORY ALKALOSIS

Presence of arterial hypocapnia in patients with profound circulatory shock has been termed as "pseudorespiratory alkalosis". This situation arises when alveolar ventilation is supported but the circulation is grossly inadequate. Mixed venous PCO_2 is significantly elevated but the arterial PCO_2 is normal or even decreased consequent to decrease CO_2 delivery to the lungs and increased pulmonary transit time. Overall, there is marked tissue acidosis, unusually involving both metabolic (resulting from tissue hypoperfusion and hyperlactatemia) and respiratory (resulting from markedly depressed CO_2 clearance) components. Arterial oxygen saturation also may appear to be adequate despite tissue hypoxemia. This condition becomes quickly fatal unless cardiac output is rapidly corrected.

SUGGESTED READING

1. Adrogué HJ, Madias NE. Management of life-threatening acid-base disorders (Part I). N Engl J Med. 1998;338:26-34.
2. Al-Jaghbeer M, Kellum JA. Acid-base disturbances in intensive care patients: etiology, pathophysiology and treatment. Nephrol Dial Transplant. 2015;30:1104-11.
3. Bruno CM, Valenti M. Acid-base disorders in patients with chronic obstructive pulmonary disease: a pathophysiological review. J Biomed Biotechnol. 2012;2012:915150.
4. Hood VL, Tannen RL. Protection of acid-base balance by pH regulation of acid production. N Engl J Med. 1998;339(12):819-26.

14 Electrolyte Imbalance

CHAPTER

Amitava Mazumdar, Sujata Majumder

HYPONATREMIA

Hyponatremia is categorized as acute or chronic hyponatremia on the basis of its duration being less or more than 48 hours. However, 48 hours' cut off is not essentially a strict one; it is the average time taken by the cells to adapt a hypotonic extracellular fluid. Hyponatremia is usually hypotonic, i.e., defined by reduced effective plasma osmolality and if of acute onset, it is this variety that leads to cerebral edema if hyponatremia is severe (serum sodium <125 mmol/L). Non-hypotonic causes also exist which do not associated with risk of cerebral edema. The ground for treatment of acute hyponatremia is to reduce brain cellular swelling by infusing hypertonic saline.

On the contrary, in chronic hyponatremia, brain cells have time to adjust to their hypotonic environment through the release of intracellular osmoles. In this state of adjustment, brain cells become sensitive to rapid correction of hyponatremia, and this may precipitate in osmotic demyelination.

These severe complications, i.e., cerebral edema and osmotic demyelination are fortunately rare in hyponatremia. However, they need to be treated or avoided whenever possible and treated as necessary.

Since the onset of hyponatremia often cannot be ascertained, rather than classifying hyponatremia into acute or chronic, it is preferred by some to classify it into symptomatic or asymptomatic. Another controversial issue is whether chronic hyponatremia requires treatment. Although chronic hyponatremia is associated with reduced survival, it is not clear if this is directly related to hyponatremia or to the severity of the underlying disorder causing hyponatremia. One meta-analysis suggested that correction of hyponatremia may provide a survival benefit, but this analysis was limited by the retrospective and observational nature of the studies that were included. A correct reasoning for treatment in chronic hyponatremia is a situation where patients exhibit neuromuscular or neurological symptoms. Further decrease in serum sodium can occur in cases of "acute on chronic hyponatremia" which generally produces symptoms and requires treatment. Treatment of chronic hyponatremia is etiology directed (e.g., treatment of underlying disease or interruption of a causative drug). However, chronic hyponatremia is also referred to as euvolemic hyponatremia [syndrome of inappropriate antidiuretic hormone (SIADH) secretion] and hypervolemic hyponatremia (liver cirrhosis and heart failure). Treatment usually relies on fluid restriction or stimulation of renal water excretion by loop diuretics, urea, or vasopressin-receptor antagonists (VRAs).

Hyponatremia: Plasma (Na^+) <135 mmol/L.

Clinical features: Primarily neurologic due to cerebral edema and depends on acuity and magnitude of fall in plasma Na^+.

Diagnostic approach:
Serum Na^+ <135 mmol/L
↓

(Rule out pseudohyponatremia vide later)
Calculate plasma osmolality = 2 Na^+ (mmol/L) + BUN (mg/dL)/2.8 + glucose (mg/dL)/18
↓

High (>275-290 mmol/L)—exclude hyperglycemia
Normal—exclude hyperlipidemia, hyperproteinemia, and bladder irrigation with glycine in TURP patient
↓

True hyponatremia
↓

Assess volume status and urinary Na^+
↓

- *Hypovolemic patient:*
  - U_{Na^+} *>20 mmol/L:* Renal losses, diuretic excess, osmotic dieresis, mineralocorticoid deficiency, salt losing deficiency, and cerebral salt wasting, etc.
  - U_{Na^+} *<20 mmol/L:* Extrarenal losses, vomiting, diarrhea, third spacing of fluids, burns, trauma, and pancreatitis, etc.

- *Hypervolemic patient:*
  - U_{Na^+} >20 mmol/L: Acute or chronic renal failure.
  - U_{Na^+} <20 mmol/L: Nephrotic syndrome, cirrhosis, and cardiac failure, etc.
- *Euvolemic patient:*
  - U_{Na^+} >20 mmol/L: Glucocorticoid deficiency, hypothyroidism, stress, drugs [e.g., SSRIs, TCAs, antipsychotic drugs, non-steroidal anti-inflammatory drugs (NSAIDs), carbamazepine, vincristine, cyclophosphamide, iphosphomide, nicotine, narcotics, clofibrate, MDMA, desmopressin, oxytocin, and vasopressin, etc.] and SIADH

Clinical Approach

Asymptomatic or nausea, malaise, headache, lethargy, confusion, obtundation, stupor, seizures, coma → excess mortality in hospitalized patients.

Adaptive mechanism in chronic hyponatremia minimizes symptoms.

What is Pseudohyponatremia?

Serum osmolality is governed by contributions from all molecules in the body that cannot easily move between the intracellular and extracellular space. Sodium is the most abundant electrolyte, but glucose, urea, plasma proteins, and lipids are also important. A patient with diabetic ketoacidosis may have hyponatremia, but normal osmolality, due to hyperglycemia, hypertriglyceridemia, and ketonemia. Patients with acute renal failure may have hyponatremia due to uremia. If a patient has hyponatremia, with low measured and calculated serum osmolality, we call this hypotonic hypernatremia. If serum osmolality is normal or high, this is isotonic or hypertonic hyponatremia-pseudohyponatremia.

Hyponatremia: Treatment

Goals

- To increase plasma Na^+ concentration by decreasing water intake and promoting water loss
- To correct the underlying disorder

Individual Situations

- Mild, asymptomatic case → no treatment
- Mild, asymptomatic cases with extracellular fluid (ECF) volume contraction → Na^+ repletion with isotonic saline (raise plasma Na^+ by 0.5-1 mmol/L/hour and <10-12 mmol/L/24 hours).
- Mild, asymptomatic cases with edematous states → restriction of Na^+ and water intake, correction of hypokalemia, loss of free water in excess of Na^+ using loop diuretics.
- Hyponatremia with renal failure, SIADH, and primary polydipsia → dietary water restriction to less than urine output.

Severe symptomatic acute (<2 days) hyponatremia (plasma Na^+ 110-115 mEq/L) suffers from altered mental status and seizure. In this case, correction is indicated with hypertonic normal saline IV over 2-4 hours. The principle of treatment is to raise serum Na^+ concentration 1 mEq/L for first 3-4 hours and not >10-12 mEq/L in 24 hours.

Repleting the Sodium Deficit

Four steps:
1. Find the patient's normal body weight.
2. Calculate the serum sodium deficit, divide by half to find how much you will replace—from this calculate the total body sodium deficit [serum deficit × total body water (TBW)].
3. Calculate the rate of replacement (ROR) (replace the serum deficit at 0.5 mEq/hour).
4. Calculate how much of your chosen fluid is required.

If you are going to use hypertonic saline, you must calculate the sodium deficit—it is conventional only to correct half of the deficit. The normal serum sodium is 140 mEq/L.

Step 1: Find out the patient's weight in kilograms prior to illness.

Step 2: Calculate the sodium deficit.

It is usual to correct only half the sodium deficit (NaD)—(hence the deficit/2).

Sodium deficit (NaD) = desired sodium - patient's sodium/2

If the patient's weight is 70 kg, and the serum sodium is 120, then the desired change is 10 mEq/L.

Total body deficit of sodium is the sodium deficit × TBW. NaD × (weight in kg × 0.6) = total deficit (TD)

Using the formula: 10 × (70 × 0.6) = 420 mEq.

Step 3: Calculate the ROR.

Most physicians replace the deficit at no >0.5 mEq/hour. The patient has a deficit of 10 mEq, so at this rate, it will be replaced over 20 hours (10/0.5).

ROR in hours = NaD/0.5

Step 4: Replace the sodium deficit with the fluid of your choice.

So, TD/(Na fluid/mL) ROR = per hour fluid replacement.

If we are using 3% saline in this 70 kg male patient with a serum sodium of 120 (420/0.513)/20 = 41 mL/hour.

That is after 20 hours, assuming no other fluids are given, the patient's serum sodium will rise to 130 mEq/L. If 0.9% saline is given: (420/0.13)/20 = 160 mL/hour.

In case of chronic hyponatremia serum Na^+ concentration is to be increased more slowly 5-8 mEq/L in 24 hours. Osmotic demyelination syndrome (ODS) develops on rapid correction of hyponatremia.

Uses of Vasopressin Receptor Antagonists (Vaptans)

Vasopressin receptor V_2 antagonists (V_2RAs) have become a mainstay of treatment of *euvolemic* (i.e., *SIADH*, postoperative *hyponatremia*) and *hypervolemic hyponatremia* (i.e., *CHF* and *cirrhosis*). V_2RAs predictably cause *aquaresis* leading to increased [Na^+] in majority

TABLE 1: The amount of fluid required depends on the sodium content of that fluid.

Fluid (infusate)	Na content mEq/L	Sodium concentration mEq/mL
Lactated ringers	130	0.13
0.9% NaCl	154	0.154
1.8%	308	0.38
3% NaCl	513	0.513
5% NaCl	855	0.855

of patients with hyponatremia due to SIADH, CHF, and cirrhosis. The optimum use of VRAs has not yet been determined, but some predictions can be made with reasonable certainty. For hyponatremia in hospitalized patients who are unable to take medication orally or for those in whom a more rapid correction of hyponatremia is desired, *conivaptan* (V_1/V_2RA) will likely be the preferred agent. Selective V_2RAs such as *tolvaptan, lixivaptan*, etc., will likely be useful in patients for whom oral therapy is suitable and for more chronic forms of hyponatremia. Tolvaptan is the one most commonly used and available in India. Start with 15 mg PO/day and do not exceed 30 mg PO/day or 30 days of treatment to avoid liver injury. Not studied in patients with creatinine clearance <10 mL/minutes. Avoid use of tolvaptan in patients with underlying liver disease.

HYPERNATREMIA—PLASMA (NA^+) >145 MMOL
Hypernatremia

Introduction: Hypernatremia is seen in patients who do not have ready access to water. This includes infants, incapacitated patients (with hypodipsia) and patients with severe illness, and multiple comorbidities.

Flowchart 1: Etiology of hypernatremia.

```
                    Etiology of hypernatremia
                              │
                ┌─────────────┴─────────────┐
                ▼                           ▼
```

Dehydration (water loss)	Sodium gain
• Osmotic diarrhea (loss of water exceeds less of solutes) • Loop diuretics (furosemide, bumetanide, and torsemide) • Central and nephrogenic diabetic insipidus, e.g., with lithium, amphotericin B, ofloxacin, clozapine, demeclocycline, and orlistat, etc. • Drug-induced nephrogenic diabetes insipidus, e.g., with lithium, amphotericin B, ofloxacin, clozapine, demeclocycline, and orlistat, etc. • Osmotic diuretics (e.g., hyperglycemia or mannitol) • Enteral feeding if free water administration is deficient • Hypothalamic lesions affecting thirst (rare)	• Administration of hypertonic intravenous solutions (sodium bicarbonate or sodium chloride) to infants or patients in the ICU • Acute salt poisoning—accidental or due to attempted suicide • Hypertonic feeding solutions

Clinical Features
Severity depends on acuity—magnitude of rise in plasma Na^+. Neurologic—altered mental status, weakness, neuromuscular irritability, focal neurologic deficits, coma, or seizures, increased risk of SAH, or ICH.

Others—polyuria, thirst, signs, and symptoms of volume depletion.

Clinical Approach
Example
For a 60 kg man with Na = 160 mEq/L, K = 3.0 mEq/L ideal fluid is 5% dextrose or half NS with 20 mEq/L KCl.

$$\text{Change in Na} = \frac{\text{Na infused} + \text{K infused} - \text{Sodium Na}}{\text{TBW} + 1}$$

$$= \frac{0 + 20 - 160}{(60 \times 0.5) + 1} = \frac{140}{31}$$

$$= 4.5 \text{ mEq/L}$$

So, 2.66 L of 5% D reduce 12 mEq/L that means 2.66L/24 hours or 110 mL/hour of 5% dextrose reduces sodium at 0.5 mEq/L/hour.

However, not included in this equation is insensible loss of 10 mL/kg. GI loss should be included every day in addition to calculated total fluid intake.

HYPERKALEMIA
Introduction
Certain patient populations have an increased risk of hyperkalemia-associated morbidity and mortality, including patients with advanced stages of chronic kidney disease (CKD), heart failure, resistant hypertension, diabetes, myocardial infarction, and/or combination of these conditions. Additive risks factors include renin-angiotensin-aldosterone system (RAAS) inhibitors usage, advanced age, and drugs such as heparin, B-blockers, NSAIDs, calcineurin inhibitors,

Flowchart 2: Approach to diagnosis of hyponatremia.

```
History – Thirst, diaphoresis, diarrhea, polyuria, medications list
                    (current and recent)
                            ↓
Physical examination – Mental status, neurologic assessment, hydration
                            ↓
                       ECF volume
              ↓                            ↓
          Increased                   Not increased
              ↓                            ↓
      Administration of           Measure urine volume
   hypertonic NaCl/NaHCO₃             and osmolality
    (primary Na⁺ excess in       ↓                    ↓
           urine)           Polyuria with      Minimum volume (500 mL/day)
      (Na⁺) >100 mmol/L     submaximal         of maximally concentrated
                            urine osmolality   urine (>800 mosm/kg)
                                  ↓                    ↓
                       Calculate urine osmolality  Insensible water loss, GI
                       excretion rate (urine vol. × water loss, remote renal
                       urine osmolality)            water loss
                            ↓                            ↓
              Urine osmolality <250            >750 mosm/day
                   mosm/kg                         ↓
                            ↓                Diuretics, osmotic diuresis
              Renal response to 10 mg        (confirm by measuring urine
              intranasal desmopressin              glucose/urea)
              after careful water restriction
                ↓                    ↓
      Urine osmolality ↑≥50%   Urine osmolality ±
                ↓                    ↓
               CDI                  NDI
```

(CDI: central diabetes insipidus; ECF: extracellular fluid; NDI: nephrogenic diabetes insipidus)

trimethoprim, pentamidine, and K⁺ sparing diuretics. Generally, risk of hypokalemia progressively increases as the estimated glomerular filtration rate (eGFR) decreases particularly with levels <15 mL/min/1.73 m²; patients receiving RAAS inhibitors therapy with eGFR <60 mL/min per 1.73 m² have been increased risk of hyperkalemia which increases further as eGFR declines.

Acute hyperkalemia management decides by on magnitude or severity of increase in K^+ concentration and its manifestations such as ECG changes and severe muscle weakness. The REVEAL-ED (Real World Evidence for Treatment of Hyperkalemia in the Emerging Department) study demonstrated that there are several deficiencies associated with current management of acute hyperkalemia. Intravenous calcium, inhaled β_2 agonists, oral sodium polystyrene sulfonate (SPS), intravenous sodium bicarbonate, dialysis, and intravenous diuretics are various treatment options that have been utilized. Most commonly utilized option (64%) was insulin/glucose infusion in the first 4 hours. However, the treatment option most likely to attain normokalemia within 4 hours is dialysis.

Chronic hyperkalemia is often asymptomatic and is likely to be identified in patients with regular and frequent testing. Current recommendations for management include use of loop or thiazide diuretics, modification of RAAS-inhibitor dose, and removal of other hyperkalemia – inducing medications (NSAIDs, herbal drugs, etc.). Recently, internationally approved K^+ binding agents may provide benefits for management of chronic hyperkalemia.

Plasma [K⁺] >5.0 mEq/L

Clinical Features

Impaired membrane excitability → weakness of muscles, flaccid paralysis, hypoventilation → metabolic acidosis.

Cardiac toxicity → ECG changes of increased T wave amplitude, increased PR interval and QRS duration, loss of P waves, sine-wave pattern, VF, or a systole.

Clinical Approach

Treatment

It depends on severity (>7.5 mmol/L—potentially fatal):
- Exogenous K^+ intake and antikaliuretic drugs discontinued.
  - Membrane excitability by IV calcium-gluconate—10 mL of a 10% solution over 2–3 minutes → repeat if no ECG change after 5–10 minutes.

Flowchart 3: Approach to diagnosis of hyperkalemia.

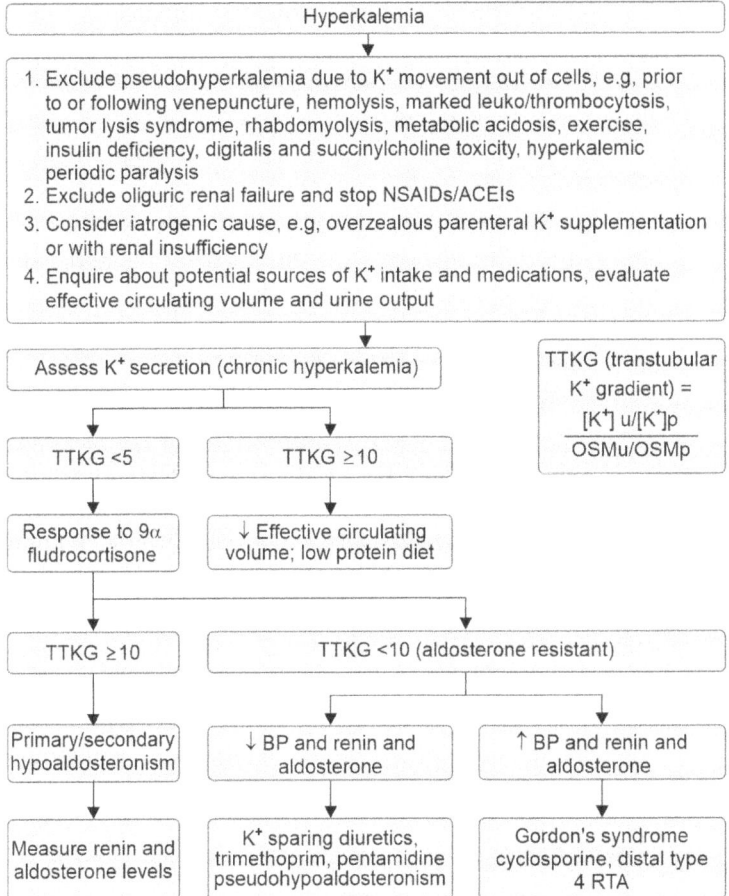

(ACEI: angiotensin-converting enzyme inhibitors; NSAIDs: nonsteroidal anti-inflammatory drugs; TTKG: trans-tubular potassium gradient)

- Shifting K^+ into cells by insulin—10 U of regular insulin in 100 mL of 25% dextrose → effect within 15–30 minutes and lasts for several hours.
- IV $NaHCO_3$ (alkali therapy) in cases of severe hyperkalemia with metabolic acidosis—isotonic solution of 3 amp per liter (134 mmol/L).

- β_2 adrenergic agonists ↑ cellular uptake of K^+ either parenterally or in nebulized form → onset of action in 30 minutes and effect lasts for 2-4 hours.
- Loop and thiazide diuretics, often in combination, ↑ K^+ excretion if renal function is adequate.
- Sodium polystyrene sulfonate (kayexalate/K—bind powder)—a cation exchange resin which promotes exchange of Na^+ for K^+ in GIT → by mouth, usual dose is 25-50 g mixed with 100 mL of 20% sorbitol to prevent constipation → effect within 1-2 hours and lasts for 4-6 hours → retention enema also available.
- Recent clinical studies suggest that newer K^+ binders, Patiromer sorbitex calcium (supported by PEARL-HF, AMETHYST-DN, AMBER, OPAL-HK trials) and sodium zirconium cyclosilicate (supported by ENERGIZE, HARMONIZE, HARMONIZE-OLE, HARMONIZE-GLOBAL, and DIALIZE trials) have given the scope to optimize the long-term management of chronic hyperkalemia. The characteristics of old and newer K^+ binding agents are compared in the table below.
- Hemodialysis is the most rapid and effective way → reserved for patients with renal failure and those with severe life-threatening hyperkalemia unresponsive to conservative measures.
- Treatment of underlying cause by either dietary modification, volume expansion, correction of acidosis, or exogenous mineralocorticoid.

HYPOKALEMIA

Hypokalemia (K^+ <3.5 mEq/L)

Introduction

Severe and life-threatening hypokalemia is defined when potassium levels are <2.5 mEq/L. In hospitalized patients, as many as 20% of hospitalized patients are detected to have hypokalemia but only in 4-5%, this is clinically significant. More than 50% of clinically significant hypokalemia have concomitant magnesium deficiency and in practice, most frequently observed in patients receiving loop or thiazide diuretic therapy, Hypokalemia associated with magnesium deficiency is often refractory to treatment with K^+.

TABLE 2: Comparison of new potassium binders.

Characteristic	Sodium polystyrene sulfonate (SPS)	Patiromer	Sodium zirconium cyclosilicate (SZS)
Approval date	1958	US 2015 Eu 2017	US 2018 Eu 2018
Mechanism of action	K^+ binding in exchange for Na^+ in GI tract for Ca^{2+} (↑ fecal excretion)	K^+ binding in exchange in GS tract (↑ fecal excretion)	K^+ binding in exchange for H^+ and Na^+ in GI tract (↑ fecal excretion)
Site of action	Colon	Colon	Small and large intestines
Onset of action	Variable (several hours)	7 hours	1 hour
Dosing	15 g 1–4 times (oral) 30–50 g 1–2 times (rectal)	8.4 g QD (oral) titrate up to 16.8 or 25.2 g QD	10 g TID (oral) for initial correction of hyperkalemia (for ≤48 hours) then 5 g QOD to 15 g QD for maintenance
Serious adverse effects	Cases of fatal GI injury reported	None reported	None reported
Common side effects	GI disorders (constipation diarrhea, nausea vomiting, gastric irritation), hypomagnesemia, and systemic alkalosis	GI disorders, abdominal discomfort, constipation, diarrhea, nausea, flatulence, and hypomagnesemia	GI disorders (constipation, diarrhea, nausea, and vomiting), mild-to-moderate edema

Causes of Hypokalemia

- *Gastrointestinal loss:* Chronic diarrhea, villous adenoma of colon, and clay (bentonite) ingestion
- *Intracellular shift:* Gluconeogenesis during total parenteral nutrition or enteral hyperalimention, β2 agonist stimulation, e.g., albuterol
  Familial periodic paralysis
  Hypokalemic thyrotoxic periodic paralysis
- *Renal potassium loss:* Cushing's syndrome
  Primary hyperaldosteronism
  Glucocorticoid-remediable congenital adrenal hyperplasia
  Bartter syndrome
  Gitelman syndrome
  Liddle syndrome
  Renal tuberculosis
  Fanconi syndrome
  Hypomagnesemia
- *Drugs:* Thiazides
  Loop diuretics
  Osmotic diuretics
  Laxatives
  Amphoterium B
  Penicillins in high doses
  Theophylline

Clinical Features

- *Mild-to-moderate hypokalemia:* Asymptomatic or with mild symptomatology especially in elderly people or in people suffering from heart or kidney disease
- *Severe hypokalemia:* *Renal features:* Metabolic acidosis, rhabdomyolysis, and nephrogenic diabetes insipidus
- *Nervous system:* Leg cramps, weakness and paresis, and ascending paresis

- *Gastrointestinal system:* Constipation or intestinal paralysis
- *Respiratory failure:* Respiratory failure
- *Cardiovascular system:* ECG changes (U waves, T-wave flattening, and ST-segment changes)
  Cardiac arrhythmias
  Heart failure

Treatment

To Correct K^+ Deficit and Decreased Ongoing Losses

Oral correction for mild-to-moderate hypokalemia (serum potassium 3.0–3.5 mEq/L) is suggested. When the average deficit of potassium is about 200–400 mEq, 50–100 mEq/day of potassium correction is recommended. Aver-age oral dose is 60–80 mEq/day. 10 mEq potassium salt are given for each.

0.1 mEq/L reduction in serum potassium.

IV replacement: IV potassium administered in case of severe hypokalemia, i.e., serum K^+ <3 mEq/L. The maximum concentration of administered K^+ should be 40 mEq/L via peripheral vein and 100 mEq/L via central vein. The rate of infusion should not be >20 mEq/h. Average rise of K level 0.25 mEq/L occurs when 20 mEq/L is given within 1 hour. Treat judiciously and under close observation of ECG and neuromuscular examination.

HYPERMAGNESEMIA

Etiology—renal failure, therapy with Mg containing antacids and laxatives and during treatment of preeclampsia with IV Mg.

Clinical Features

Only if >4 mEq/L.

Neuromuscular, e.g., areflexia, lethargy, weakness, paralysis, respiratory failure; cardiac, e.g., hypotension, bradycardia, prolonged PR, QRS and QT intervals, complete heart block, and asystole.

Flowchart 4: Approach to diagnosis of hypokalemia.

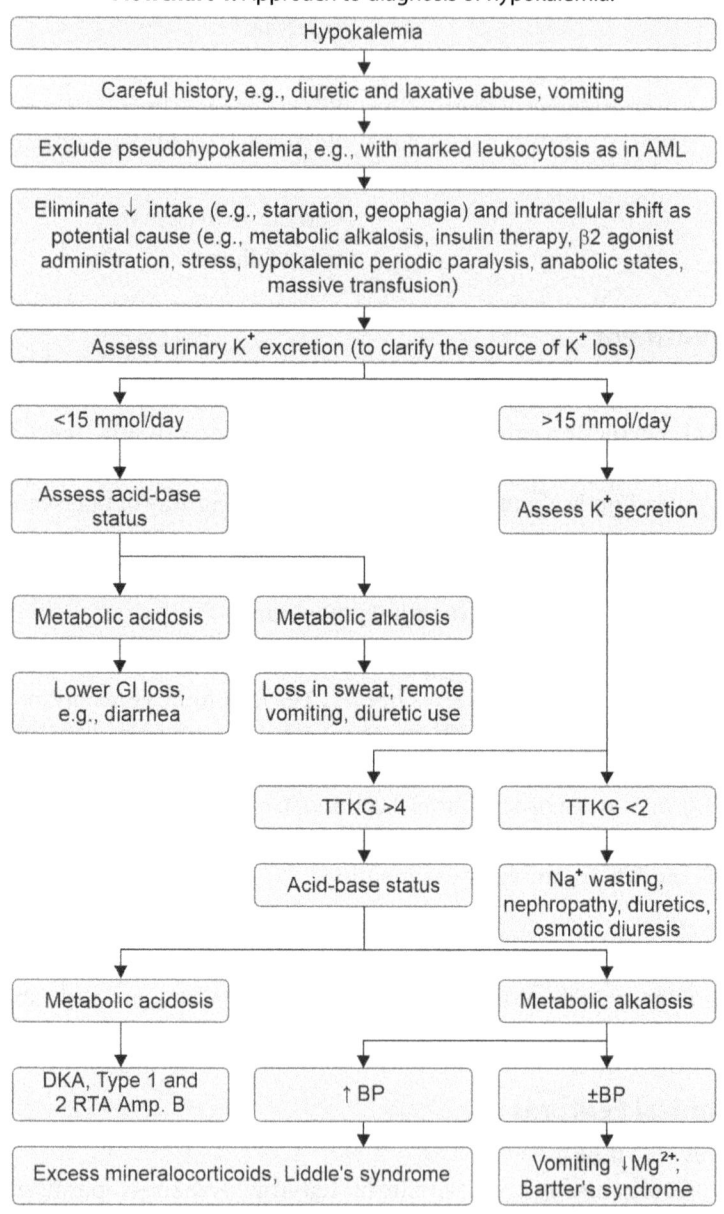

(AML: acute myelogenous leukemia; DKA: diabetic ketoacidosis; GI: gastrointestinal; RTA: renal tubular acidosis; TTKG: trans-tubular potassium gradient)

Electrolyte Imbalance 383

Therapy

Just withdrawal of Mg preparation suffices if asymptomatic. In case of severe symptomatic hypermagnesemia symptomatic 10% calcium-gluconate, 10–20 mL IV over 10 minutes to be administered. If renal function is normal IV frusemide after rehydration with NS will increase renal clearance of magnesium. Mechanical ventilation, temporary pacing, and hemodialysis may be required.

HYPOMAGNESEMIA

Etiology

Decreased intestinal absorption, e.g., malnutrition, malabsorption, chronic diarrhea, nasogastric aspiration; increased renal excretion, e.g., hypercalcemia, osmotic diuresis, drugs, alcoholism, and alcohol withdrawal.

Clinical Features

Neurologic, e.g., lethargy, confusion, tremor, fasciculations, ataxia, nystagmus, tetany, seizures; ECG, e.g., prolonged PR and QT interval, atrial, and ventricular arrhythmias.

Therapy

Mild hypomagnesemia (serum Mg 1.5 mEq/L) 240 mg elemental Mg required in 24 hours.

While more severe hypomagnesemia (K^+ serum level 1.2–1.5 mEq/L), 720 mg elemental Mg required in 24 hours. In severe hypomagnesemia (<1.2 mEq/L of serum Mg)—1–2 g $MgSO_4$ IV slowly over 15 minutes followed by 1 mEq/kg body weight in 24 hours. After first day, the dose 0.5 mEq/kg/day for three consecutive days to correct intracellular deficit.

1 amp = 2 mL of the 50% solution = 1 g = 8.12 mEq of magnesium ≅8 mEq Mg^{++}

Deep tendon reflex should be examined frequently, and ideal serum magnesium level is <2.5 mEq/L.

HYPERCALCEMIA

A serum calcium >11 mg/dL with normal serum albumin or an ionized calcium >5.2 mg/dL defines hypercalcemia.

Causes of Hypercalcemia

- Primary hyperparathyroidism
- Secondary hyperparathyroidism (CKD)
- Malignancy (lung, breast, and multiple myeloma)
- Sarcoidosis
- Vitamin D intoxication and milk alkali syndrome
- Familial hypocalciuric hypercalcemia
- Drug such as lithium thiazide
- Thyrotoxicosis

Clinical Features

Anorexia, vomiting, constipation, abdominal pain, polyuria, nephrolithiasis, weakness, depression, and confusion.

Diagnosis

PTH↑, PO_4↓ in hyperparathyroidism, serum Cl: HCO_3 = 33:1 suggestive of primary hyperparathyroidism.

BUN↑, Cl↑, HCO_3↑ in milk alkali syndrome. PTH↓, ↑PO_4, ↑1.25 $(OH)_2$, D_3 in vitamin D intoxication and chronic granulomatous disease.

ECG: Shortened QT interval.

Treatment

Isotonic saline (0.9% NS) for correction of dehydration and excretion of calcium. Maintenance fluid adjusted if urine as produced at 100–150 mL/hour. Fluid to be cautiously used in elderly patients.

Frusemide: It is used after volume correction. IV bisphosphonate
   Calcitonin
   Steroid
   Oral phosphate by increasing Ca^{2+} deposition

HYPOCALCEMIA

A serum calcium <8.4 mg/dL with normal sodium albumin or an ionized calcium <1.2 mg/dL is called hypocalcemia.

Causes of Hypocalcemia
- Hypoalbuminemia
- Hypoparathyroidism due to postsurgical hungry bone syndrome
- Hypomagnesemia
- Liver disease and kidney disease
- Nutritional deficiency of vitamin D_3. Lack of sun-exposure
- Respiratory and metabolic alkalosis
- Severe acute hyperphosphatemia, i.e., conditions such as tumor lysis syndrome, rhabdomyolysis, and acute renal failure
- Invasive blood transfusion and anticonvulsant drug

Clinical Features
Paresthesia, muscle spasm, irritability, depression, and psychosis. Chvostek's syndrome, Trousseau's sign, lethargy, laryngeal spasm, and seizure. ECG—prolonged QT interval.

Treatment
Before correcting hypocalcemia, first hypomagnesemia and hyperphosphatemia should be corrected.

Mild hypocalcemia treated with 1 amp of 10 mL 10% calcium-gluconate (containing 90 mg elemental calcium slowly over 10 minutes). Severe hypocalcemia treated with 6 amp of calcium-gluconate (60 mL) dissolved in 500 mL of 5% dextrose. Now 1 mL of solution contains 1 mg calcium. Then, infusion rate is 0.5-2 mg/kg/hour.

Chronic Treatment
- Salt (1-2 g elemental calcium) TDS
- 6 weeks of ergocalciferol 50,000 IV weekly in CKD patient
- Calcitriol to be taken as it increases phosphate absorption.

HYPOPHOSPHATEMIA
A serum phosphate <2.8 mg/dL defines hypophosphatemia. Causes are:
- *Increased renal excretion:* Hypoparathyroidism, ECF volume expansion with dieresis, proximal tubular transport defect (e.g.,

Fanconi's syndrome), cancer-induced hypophosphatemia, and familial hypophosphatemic rickets.
- *Inadequate intake or absorption:* Malabsorption, chronic diarrhea, malnutrition, phosphate-binding antacids, vitamin D deficiency, or resistance.
- *Redistribution into cells:* Refeeding after starvation, treatment for diabetic ketoacidosis, and respiratory alkalosis.

Clinical Features
Proximal muscle weakness, impaired diaphragmatic function, confusion, par esthesia, dysarthria, seizure, coma, heart failure, and hypoxia (due to decreased concentration of 2, 3 DPG).

Investigation
Renal excretion of >100 mg by 24 hours urine collection, serum 25 (OH) D3↓, PTH↑.

Treatment
Management involves administering oral phosphate supplements and high-protein/high-dairy dietary supplements which are rich in naturally occurring phosphate. In severe hypophosphatemia (<1 mg/dL) intravenous treatment with sodium or potassium phosphate 0.08–0.16 mmol/kg in 0.45% saline administered over 6 hours is indicated. However, intravenous phosphate administration is associated with the risk of precipitating hypocalcemia and metastatic calcification.

HYPERPHOSPHATEMIA
A serum phosphate level >5 mg/dL defines hyperphosphatemia.
- Acute and chronic renal failure
- Tumor lysis syndrome and rhabdomyolysis, crush injury
- Hypoparathyroidism
- Acromegaly
- Thyrotoxicosis
- Vitamin D intoxication
- Metabolic acidosis

Clinical Features
Relate to hypocalcemia and metastatic calcification, particularly in chronic renal failure with tertiary hyperparathyroidism.

Treatment
Phosphate binders are calcium acetate and calcium carbonate. Aluminum hydroxide may be used with caution in chronic kidney disease patients. Management also involves volume expansion with intravenous normal saline and dialysis in extreme cases.

SUGGESTED READING
1. Adrogue HJ, Madias NE. Hypernatremia. N Engl J Med. 2000;342(20):1493-9.
2. Kardalas E, Paschou SA, Anagnostis P, Muscogiuri G, Siasos G, Vryonidou A. Hypokalemia: a clinical update. Endocr Connect. 2018; 7(4):R135-46.
3. Kovesdy CP, Appel LJ, Grams ME, Gutekunst L, McCullough PA, Palmer BF, et al. Potassium homeostasis in health and disease: a scientific workshop cosponsored by the National Kidney Foundation and American Society of Hypertension. Am J Kidney Dis. 2017;70:844-58.
4. Spasovski G, Vanholder R, Allolio B, Annane D, Ball S, Bichet D, et al. Clinical practice guideline on diagnosis and treatment of hyponatremia. Nephrol Dial Transplant. 2014;Suppl 2:i1-i39.
5. Sterns RH. Treatment of severe hyponatremia. Clin J Am Soc Nephrol. 2018;13:641-9.
6. Vesbalis JG, Goldsmith SR, Greenberg A, Korzelius C, Schrier RW, Sterns RH, et al. Diagnosis, evaluation and treatment of hyponatremia: expert panel recommendations. Am J Med. 2013;126:s1-s42.
7. Weisinger JR, Bellorin-Font E. Magnesium and phosphorus. Lancet. 1998;352(9125):391-6.

CHAPTER 15

Management of Adult Severe Acute Asthma

Sumit Sen Gupta

DEFINITION OF SEVERE ASTHMA

Acute severe asthma (previously termed status asthmaticus) is an acute exacerbation of asthma that does not respond to standard treatments of inhaled bronchodilators and steroids.

Definition of acute severe asthma as given in International ERS/ATS Guidelines 2013 is as following:

Asthma which requires treatment with high dose inhaled corticosteroids (CS) and second controller (LABA or leukotriene modifier/theophylline) for the previous year or systemic CS for ≥50% of the previous year to prevent it from becoming "uncontrolled" or which remains "uncontrolled" despite this therapy.

- *Uncontrolled* asthma is defined as at least one of the following:
  - *Poor symptom control:* Asthma control questionnaire (ACQ0 consistently >1.5, asthma control test (ACT) ≤19
  - *Frequent severe exacerbations:* Two or more bursts of systemic CSs (>3 days each) in the previous year
  - *Serious exacerbations:* At least one hospitalization, ICU stay or mechanical ventilation in the previous year
  - *Airflow limitation:* After appropriate bronchodilator withhold FEV1 <80% predicted (in the face of reduced FEV_1/FVC defined as less than the lower limit of normal).
- *Controlled* asthma that worsens on tapering of these high doses of inhaled CS or systemic CS (or additional biologics).

Asthma Control Questionnaire

Scores range from 0 to 6 (higher is worse). A score of 0.0-0.75 is classified as well-controlled asthma; 0.75-1.5 as a "grey zone"; and >1.5 as poorly controlled asthma. The ACQ score is calculated as the average of 5, 6, or 7 items—all versions of the ACQ include five symptom questions. The minimum clinically important difference is 0.5.

Asthma Control Test

Scores range from 5 to 25 (higher is better). Scores of 20-25 are classified as well-controlled asthma; 16-20 as not well-controlled; and 5-15 as very poorly controlled asthma. The ACT includes four symptom/reliever questions plus a patient self-assessed level of control. The minimum clinically important difference is 3 points.

Despite the rising prevalence, there seems to be some improvement in the hospital admissions associated with life-threatening asthma. The ICU admission rate for hospitalized asthma patients ranges from 1 to 10% from various studies. In a comprehensive analysis of almost two million hospitalizations for asthma in the United States, the healthcare utilization patterns were examined and compared between 2000 and 2008. The findings revealed that the proportion of cases requiring invasive mechanical ventilation (IMV) decreased from 1.40% in 2000 to 0.73% in 2008. However, this was seen in the cost of five-fold increase in the utilization of noninvasive ventilation

DIFFERENTIAL DIAGNOSIS OF ACUTE ASTHMA

12-39 years

- Vocal cord dysfunction
- Hyperventilation
- Bronchiectasis
- Congenital heart disease
- Inhaled foreign body

40+ years

- Chronic obstructive pulmonary disease (COPD)
- Vocal cord dysfunction
- Hyperventilation
- Bronchiectasis
- Cardiac failure
- Parenchymal lung disease
- Pulmonary embolism/hypertension
- Central airway obstruction

ASSESSMENT OF ACUTE ASTHMA
Moderate Acute Asthma
- Increasing symptoms
- Peak expiratory flow (PEF) >50–75% of best or predicted
- Prefers sitting to lying, not agitated
- Accessory muscles not working
- No features of acute severe asthma
- SpO_2 90–95% (on room air)

Acute Severe Asthma
Any one of the following:
- Peak expiratory flow (PEF) 33–50% of best or predicted
- Cannot complete sentences in one breath
- Respiratory rate ≥25 breaths/min
- Pulse rate ≥110/min
- Sits hunched forwards, agitated
- Accessory muscles in use

Life-threatening Asthma
Any one of the following:
- PEF <33% of best or predicted
- SpO_2 <92%
- Silent chest, cyanosis or feeble respiratory effort
- Bradycardia, arrhythmia, or hypotension
- Exhaustion, confusion, or coma

Patients with severe attacks may not be distressed and may not have all these abnormalities. The presence of any should alert the healthcare team.

MANAGEMENT OF ACUTE ASTHMA EXACERBATION
Oxygen Therapy and Targets
Although asthma is primarily a large airways disease, some patients with acute asthma exacerbation may ongoing present with hypoxemia of varying severity, and targeted oxygen therapy is recommended. The BTS debate guidelines currently recommend an

Management of Adult Severe Acute Asthma

Flowchart 1: Management of asthma exacerbations in primary care.

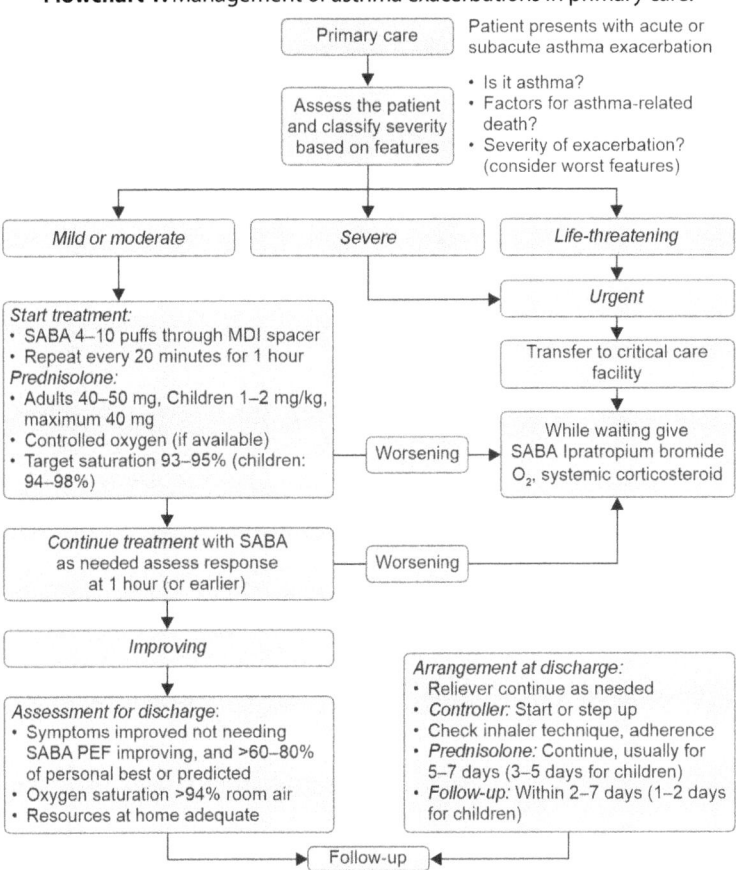

Review symptoms and signs: Is the exacerbation resolving? Should steroid be continued? *Reliever:* Reduce to as essential; *Controller:* Continue higher dose for short term (1–2 weeks) or long-term (months), depending on background to exacerbation; *Adults/adolescents:* ICS-formoterol formulation is advisable. *Risk factors:* To be assessed and corrected whenever they are modifiable.

[ICS: inhaled corticosteroid; SABA: short-acting beta-2-agonist (doses are for salbutamol)]

oxygen saturation of 94–98% However, there is concerning the level at which oxygen targets should be set for critically ill patients, with concern regarding the effects of hypoxemia on adverse outcomes. A randomized controlled trial (RCT) of 106 patients presenting to the ED with acute severe asthma concluded that routine high-concentration oxygen therapy (8 L/min via a medium-concentration

Flowchart 2: Advanced therapeutic options for acute moderate to near fatal asthma.

```
                    IV magnesium sulphate
                              ↓
              Target oxygen saturations 94–98%
                              ↓
   Increasing frequency of nebuliszed bronchodilators with worsening severity
                              ↓
                 Steroids (oral/intravenous)
                              ↓
```

Acute moderate:	Acute severe:	Life threatening:
• Worsening symptoms	• Inability to complete sentences	Altered consciousness, exhaustion arrythmia, hypotension cyanosis, silent chest, oxygen saturation <92% PaO$_2$ <8 kPa, "normal" PaCO$_2$
• Respiratory rate <25	• Respiratory rate >25	
• Heart rate <110	• Geart rate >110	

```
                    ECMO/ECCO$_2$R
                         ↓
                    IV salbutamol
                         ↓
                   IV aminophylline
                         ↓
                      Mucolytics
                         ↓
                      NIV/HFNO
                         ↓
              Invasive mechanical ventilation
                         ↓
         IV ketamine/inhalational anesthetic agents
```

Hudson facemask) significantly increases PaCO$_2$ and recommended a titrated regime where oxygen is only administered to patients suffering from hypoxemia with an oxygen saturation of ≤92%.

Nebulized Bronchodilators

Nebulized β$_2$ adrenoceptor agonists (salbutamol/albuterol) are essential components in the treatment of acute asthma exacerbations of all severity as well as for day-to-day maintenance. β_2 adrenoceptors are G-protein-coupled transmembrane receptors that are found mainly in airway smooth muscle cells. They activate the enzyme adenylyl cyclase, which produces cyclic adenosine monophosphate (cAMP) that in turns activates protein kinase A and modification of intracellular calcium concentrations. Differences in the activity of β_2 agonists mediate the dynamics of how airway smooth muscle responds. Salbutamol directly activates the adrenoceptor, while salmeterol interacts with a receptor-specific auxiliary binding site. The first-line therapy for rapid bronchodilation requires the use of high-dose nebulized β_2 agonists driven by either oxygen or air depending on the degree of hypoxemia. Patients with minimal response to the initial dose may require continuous or "back-to-back" nebulization. Intravenous β_2 agonists are reserved for those patients in whom the nebulized therapy cannot be used reliably or in those who require additional bronchodilation during extreme states. Adverse effects of β_2 agonist they primarily include tachycardia and tremor but also have effects on serum potassium and glucose. Although quite effective to tide over acute exacerbations, long-term use leads to development of tolerance.

Systemic Corticosteroids

The beneficial effects of corticosteroids in the management of acute asthma are well-established have long been known. A 2001 Cochrane review including 12 studies and 863 patients concluded that corticosteroids given within the first hour of presentation to the ED significantly reduced the rate of hospital admission in patients presenting with acute asthma. Corticosteroids reduce mortality, asthma relapses, subsequent hospitalization, and requirement for β_2 agonist therapy. Since they take time to work, the earlier they are administered in the acute attack, the better should be the outcome. The BTS guidelines advise giving steroids in adequate doses to all patients with acute asthma exacerbation. Regarding the route by which steroids are given, studies have shown that the efficacy between oral, intravenous, and intramuscular routes is similar. Furthermore, there appears to be little difference in efficacy between different formulations of corticosteroids—for example, prednisolone, dexamethasone, and methylprednisolone. A standard dose of 40–50 mg of prednisolone or 400 mg of hydrocortisone (100 mg four times a day) for a minimum duration of 5 days is currently recommended. Although there are several acute side effects from systemic corticosteroids use in ICUs, including hyperglycemia, hypernatremia, water retention, delirium, and weakness, the benefits of short-term modest doses of systemic corticosteroids clearly outweigh these adverse events.

Magnesium Sulphate

Intravenous (IV) and nebulized magnesium sulphate ($MgSO_4$) has long been proposed as a treatment for severe acute asthma.

The mechanism of action of $MgSO_4$ is incompletely partially understood but is thought to comprise the following:

Inhibition of the cellular uptake of calcium via activation of Na^+ Ca^{2+} pumps, muscle relaxation via inhibition of myosin and calcium interaction and calcium-dependent acetylcholine release at motor neuron terminals, and inhibition of prostacyclin and nitric oxide synthesis.

A Cochrane review and meta-analysis of 13 studies including 2,313 patients concluded that "a single infusion of 1.2 g or 2 g IV $MgSO_4$ over 15–30 minutes reduces hospital admissions and improves lung function in adults with acute asthma who have not responded sufficiently to oxygen, nebulized short-acting $β_2$ agonists and IV corticosteroids". However, the effect of $MgSO_4$ on patients with life-threatening or near-fatal asthma in negating the need for mechanical ventilation and mortality of mechanically ventilated ICU patients is yet to be known. Currently, magnesium sulphate is recommended for those who have continue to refractory symptoms in spite of standard preliminary management.

Intravenous Aminophylline

Methylxanthines can cause bronchial smooth muscle relaxation through multiple mechanisms and are one of the most commonly prescribed drugs for asthma worldwide. The effect of methylxanthines is due to a combination of inhibition of phosphodiesterase enzymes, translocation of calcium, adenosine receptor blockade, and modulation of GABA receptors, resulting in the accumulation of cyclic adenosine monophosphate and subsequent bronchodilation.

However, intravenous aminophylline has a narrow therapeutic index and should only be used with caution, as it requires monitoring of plasma concentrations to avoid adverse index.

Hence, the guidelines currently do not recommend the routine use of intravenous aminophylline; however, it continues to be used in patients with severe asthma as a salvage therapy to provide additional bronchodilation.

Intravenous Salbutamol

There are studies going back to the mid-1970s exploring the effect of IV β_2 agonists for the treatment of acute asthma. However, it is unclear if IV β_2 agonists offer additional bronchodilation beyond the use of regular nebulization that leads to better outcomes.

Currently, there is no evidence to support the use of IV β_2 agonists in patients with severe asthma in the ICU. However, it is available as an additional bronchodilator treatment in those with severe airflow obstruction, and it continues to be used as a rescue therapy in ICU patients.

ADVANCED MANAGEMENT IN THE ICU FOR ACUTE LIFE-THREATENING ASTHMA

Patients with acute life-threatening and near-fatal asthma should be admitted to the ICU for close supervision and to initiate additional measures to optimize bronchodilation and ventilation. However, subsequent management of such patients is generally not addressed by current guidelines due to a lack of high-quality evidence. In this section, the use of noninvasive respiratory support measures, ventilation strategies, and other advanced measures available to optimize patient care in the ICU will be discussed.

High-Flow Nasal Oxygen

Asthma patients admitted to the ICU are frequently hypoxic, and supplemental oxygen therapy is one of the most common first-line treatments provided either via low-flow nasal cannula (LFNC) or via facemask. LFNC can deliver supplemental oxygen at a maximum rate of 4–6 liters (L) per minute, while a standard reservoir mask can deliver a maximum rate of 15 L per minute.

A meta-analysis of four randomized controlled trials comprising of 175 patients demonstrated that although HFNO appeared to significantly lower dyspnea score, there was no significant impact on gas exchange, rate of intubation, or length of hospital stay. Although a trial of high-flow nasal oxygen (HFNO) is worthy of consideration for improvement of dyspnea in certain patients, it should not be looked upon as an alternative to mechanical ventilation.

Noninvasive Ventilation

Noninvasive ventilation (NIV) has the physiological impact of reducing the work of breathing and further alveolar recruitment, thereby improving dynamic lung compliance. Acute respiratory failure from asthma is associated with significant morbidity. While NIV is an established practice for hypercapnic respiratory failure for COPD patients, the use of NIV during acute asthma exacerbations remains a questionable issue. Patients with acute severe asthma often present with hypoxemic respiratory failure rather than hypercapnic respiratory failure, and the primary aim is to optimize oxygenation while alleviating airway symptoms with bronchodilator therapy. However, patients with later stage life-threatening or near-fatal asthma may develop hypercapnic respiratory failure, often necessitating endotracheal intubation and mechanical ventilation.

In a large multicenter retrospective cohort study in ICUs, 25% of patients received NIV for acute asthma exacerbation, and for those who received IMV (27%), 21% received NIV before IMV initiation.

Large randomized controlled trials are required to evaluate the clinical efficacy of NIV in acute asthma exacerbations for preventing IMV and the effect on mortality. While NIV is not an alternative to IMV, the use of NIV should be limited to safe situations where IMV can be utilized rapidly, and at-risk patients can be monitored very closely.

INTUBATION

Approximately 2% of all acute severe asthma patients will worsen to require intubation and mechanical ventilation. Among ICU patients, nearly 36–46% may require invasive mechanical ventilation within

24 hours of admission. The decision to intubate is a clinical one, albeit considering other investigations and the projected deterioration of the patient's condition. Although variable depending on a combination of factors, the clinical indications for intubation in acute severe asthma are detailed below:

Relative and Immediate Indications for Intubation

Immediate Indications

- Cardiac arrest
- PaO_2 <60 mm Hg (8.0 kPa) and/or $PaCO_2$ >46.5 mm Hg (6.5 kPa)
- Severe obtundation or coma
- Impending respiratory failure with gasping or inability to speak
- Respiratory arrest

Relative Indications

- Progressive exhaustion
- Increasing use of accessory muscles or change in rate/depth of respiration
- Change in posture or speech
- Failure to reverse severe respiratory acidosis despite intensive therapy
- Altered sensorium
- Severe hypoxemia with maximal oxygen delivery
- Silent chest

Intubation in the context of these relative indications can be challenging. The induction agents commonly used are propofol and ketamine in combination with opiates and a paralyzing agent. There are several potential complications that may occur during endotracheal intubation. Some are specific to asthma patients. These include worsening of bronchospasm and significant air trapping during and after intubation. Cardiovascular collapse may result from depleted intravascular volume status, vasodilation from anesthetic medications, and increased intrathoracic pressure leading to impaired cardiac output need to be anticipated and managed successfully to prevent cardiac arrest.

Potential Complications Arising from Endotracheal Intubation in an Asthmatic Patient
- Laryngospasm
- Worsening bronchospasm
- Significant air trapping

Potential Complications during Intubation
- Aspiration
- Barotrauma/volutrauma
- Cardiovascular collapse
- Cardiac arrhythmias
- Cardiac arrest

Mechanical Ventilation

Although life-threatening asthma is rare, a small proportion of patients may require IMV. While IMV is not a specific therapy for asthma, it is to be viewed upon as a last resort while allowing time for bronchodilator therapy to take effect. Patients with life-threatening asthma may end up with severe respiratory distress, hypoxemia, arrhythmias, and pulse paradoxus due to air trapping with cardiovascular instability or, at later stages, hypercapnia, and respiratory arrest. High airway pressures and dynamic hyperinflation may be complicated by air trapping, barotrauma, the development of pneumothorax, and hemodynamic instability. Emphasis of mechanical ventilation in asthma should be avoiding dynamic hyperinflation. The ventilation mode can be volume-assisted or controlled pressure-cycled ventilation with a tidal volume of 6–8 mL/kg body weight as a starting point. Minute ventilation should be adjusted to allow adequate time for the expiratory phase. Higher inspiratory to expiratory ratio (I:E) time is often required at 1:3 or 1:4 with a low respiratory rate (e.g., 12–14/min). Despite this, in the event of continued breath stacking, disconnecting the ventilator circuit followed by manual decompression is required to improve the dynamic hyperinflation.

Establishing optimal positive end-expiratory pressure (PEEP) during mechanical ventilation for patients with asthma is a contentious issue. In practice, most advocate an applied PEEP of zero or reduced levels of PEEP below the intrinsic PEEP to minimize hyperinflation. Permissive hypercapnia is often adopted with deep sedation and neuromuscular paralysis at early stages to prevent patient-ventilator desynchrony. Standard ideal ventilator settings following mechanical ventilation are detailed below:

Proposed Ventilator Settings

- *Fraction inspired O_2:* Titrate to achieve oxygen saturations 94–98%
- *Respiratory rate:* 12–14 breath/minute
- *Mode:* Volume-assisted or controlled pressure-cycled
- *Tidal volume:* 6–8 mL/kg IBW
- *Inspiratory:* Expiratory ratio—1:3–1:4
- *For air trapping:* Consider disconnecting the ventilator circuit followed by manual decompression to improve the dynamic hyperinflation

Anesthetic Agents

Ketamine

Despite some bronchodilator effects demonstrated by ketamine and some anecdotal data to suggest few benefits when used as an anesthetic agent in asthma, scientific literature thus far does not support its use.

Inhalational anesthetic agents: Inhalational anesthetic agents such as isoflurane, sevoflurane, enflurane, and halothane with the exception of desflurane are known to induce bronchodilation.

It must be noted that use of inhalational anesthetic agents in the ICU may only be performed with the support presence of appropriate gas-scavenging equipment along with specialized delivery devices which are designed to conserve inhalational anesthetics.

While its use as an additional rescue therapy continues, further studies are needed to evaluate the clinical impact of such devices on robust patient outcomes.

Extracorporeal CO_2 removal: Extracorporeal carbon dioxide removal ($ECCO_2R$) provides a means of fast and effective treatment of CO_2

removal in acute hypercapnic respiratory failure; however, in comparison to extracorporeal membrane oxygenation (ECMO), the blood is not oxygenated before returning to the body. Given the solubility and diffusion characteristics of carbon dioxide compared to oxygen, $ECCO_2R$ requires much lower blood flow rates. Utilizing this system, the deleterious effects of IMV can be lessened. Application of $ECCO_2R$ in hypoxemic respiratory failure in acute asthma remains unestablished.

Extracorporeal membrane oxygenation: Extracorporeal membrane oxygenation is not a standard feature of asthma guidelines and use of ECMO in near fatal asthma is a rarity. However, in asthma refractory to standard intensive therapy (near-fatal asthma or status asthmaticus), ECMO may help to improve gas exchange without the expense of aggressive IMV.

FOLLOW-UP AFTER AN EXACERBATION

All patients must be followed up regularly by a healthcare provider until symptoms and lung function return to normal and the goal should be reverting an exacerbation again. Each exacerbation should be viewed upon as a possible failure in chronic asthma care.

MEDICATIONS FOR MAINTENANCE TREATMENT

Inhaled Corticosteroids

Beclometasone, budesonide, ciclesonide, fluticasone propionate, fluticasone furoate, mometasone, triamcinolone.

Devices: DPIs (dry powder inhalers) or pMDIs (pressurized method dose inhalers).

Inhaled corticosteroids (ICS)-containing medications are the most effective anti-inflammatory medications for asthma. ICS reduce symptoms, increase lung function, reduce airway hyperresponsiveness, improve quality of life, and reduce the risk of exacerbations, asthma-related hospitalizations, and death adherence with ICS alone (i.e. not in combination with a bronchodilator) is usually very poor.

Inhaled Corticosteroids in Combination with a Long-acting Beta-2-Agonist Bronchodilator

Beclometasone-formoterol, budesonide-formoterol, fluticasone furoate- vilanterol, fluticasone propionate formoterol, fluticasone propionate-salmeterol, mometasone-formoterol and mometasone-indacaterol.

Devices: pMDIs or DPIs.

When a low-dose of ICS alone fails to achieve good control of asthma, the addition of long-acting beta-2-agonist (LABA) to maintenance ICS improves symptoms, lung function, and reduces exacerbations in more patients, more rapidly, than doubling the dose of ICS.

Leukotriene Modifiers (Leukotriene Receptor Antagonists)

Tablets: For example, montelukast, pranlukast, zafirlukast, and zileuton.

Target one part of the inflammatory pathway in asthma. Sometimes used as an option for maintenance therapy, mainly only in children.

When used alone: Less effective than low-dose ICS.

When added to ICS: Less effective than ICS-LABA.

Add-on Maintenance Medications

Long-acting Muscarinic Antagonists

Tiotropium, ≥6 years, by mist inhaler, added to ICS-LABA.

Combination ICS-LABA-LAMA inhalers for adults ≥18 years: Beclometasone-formoterol-glycopyrronium; fluticasone furoate-vilanterol-umeclidinium; mometasone-indacaterol-glycopyrronium.

Devices: pMDIs or DPIs or mist inhalers.

An add-on option at Step 5 in combination or separate inhalers for patients with uncontrolled asthma despite ICS-LABA. Modestly improves lung function but not symptoms or quality of life; small reduction in exacerbations. For patients with exacerbations, ensure that ICS is increased to at least medium dose before considering need for add-on LAMA.

Anti-immunoglobulin E (Check Your Local Eligibility Criteria)

Omalizumab, ≥6 years, subcutaneous (SC) injection

An add-on option for patients with severe allergic asthma uncontrolled on high-dose ICS-LABA. May also be indicated for nasal polyps and chronic spontaneous (idiopathic) urticaria. Self-administration may be an option.

Anti-IL5 and Anti-IL5R

Anti-IL5: Mepolizumab (≥6 years, SC injection) or reslizumab (≥18 years, intravenous infusion). Anti-IL5 receptor benralizumab (≥12 years, SC injection).

Add-on options for patients with severe eosinophilic asthma uncontrolled on high-dose ICS-LABA. Maintenance OCS dose can be significantly reduced with benralizumab and mepolizumab. Mepolizumab may also be indicated for eosinophilic granulomatosis with polyangiitis (EGPA), hypereosinophilic syndrome or chronic rhinosinusitis with nasal polyposis. For mepolizumab and benralizumab, self-administration may be an option.

Adverse effects: Headache and reactions at injection sites are common but minor.

Anti-IL4R

Medications: Anti-interleukin 4 receptor alpha: Dupilumab, ≥6 years, SC injection.

An add-on option for patients with severe eosinophilic or type 2 asthma uncontrolled on high-dose ICS-LABA, or patients requiring maintenance OCS. Not advised for patients with current or historical blood eosinophils ≥1,500/μL. May also be indicated for treatment of skin conditions including moderate-severe atopic dermatitis, chronic rhinosinusitis with nasal polyps, and eosinophilic esophagitis. Self-administration may be an option.

Anti-thymic Stromal Lymphopoietin

Tezepelumab, SC injection, ≥12 years.

An add-on option for patients with severe asthma uncontrolled on high-dose ICS-LABA. In patients taking maintenance OCS, no significant reduction in OCS dose compared with placebo.

Systemic Corticosteroids

These include prednisone, prednisolone, methylprednisolone, hydrocortisone tablets, and dexamethasone. Given by tablets or suspension or by IM or IV injection.

Short-term treatment (usually 5-7 days in adults) is important in the treatment of severe acute exacerbations, with main effects seen after 4-6 hours. For acute severe exacerbations, OCS therapy is preferred to IM or IV therapy and is effective in preventing short-term relapse. Tapering is required if OCS given for >2 weeks. Patients should be reviewed after any exacerbation, to optimize their inhaled therapy in order to reduce the risk of future exacerbations. As a last resort, long-term treatment with OCS may be required for some patients with severe asthma, but side-effects are problematic. Patients for whom this is considered should be referred for specialist review if available, to have treatment optimized and phenotype assessed.

Anti-inflammatory Reliever Medications

Low-dose Combination Inhaled Corticosteroid-formoterol

Beclometasone-formoterol or budesonide-formoterol pMDIs or DPIs.

Low-dose ICS-formoterol can be taken before exercise to reduce exercise-induced bronchoconstriction, and it can be taken before or during allergen exposure to reduce allergic responses.

Recommended maximum doses in any day. The maximum total dose recommended in a single day (maintenance plus reliever doses) for beclometasone-formoterol is 48 µg formoterol (delivered dose 36 µg), and for budesonide-formoterol 72 µg).

Short-acting Bronchodilator Reliever Medications

Short-acting Inhaled Beta-2-Agonist Bronchodilators

For example, salbutamol (albuterol and terbutaline). Administered by pMDIs, DPIs and rarely, as solution for nebulization or injection.

Inhaled short-acting inhaled beta-2-agonists (SABAs) provide quick relief of asthma symptoms and bronchoconstriction, and for pretreatment before exercise. SABAs should be used only as needed (not regularly) and at the lowest dose and frequency required. SABA-only treatment is not recommended because of the risk of severe exacerbations and asthma-related death. Currently, inhaled SABAs are the most commonly used bronchodilator for acute exacerbations requiring urgent primary care visit or ED presentation.

Short Anticholinergics

For example, ipratropium bromide and oxitropium bromide. May be in combination with SABAs. pMDIs or DPIs.

As noted use: Ipratropium is a less effective reliever medication than SABAs, with slower onset of action. Short-term use in severe acute asthma, where adding ipratropium to SABA reduces the risk of hospital admission.

SUGGESTED READING

1. Global initiative for Asthma. (2024). Global Strategy for Asthma Management and Prevention. Available from www.ginasthma.org. [Last accessed March, 2025].
2. Lin SY, Azar A, Suarez-Cuervo C, Diette GB, Brigham E, Rice J, et al. The role of immunotherapy in the treatment of asthma. Rockville (MD): Agency for Healthcare Research and Quality (US); 2018. (AHRQ Comparative Effectiveness Reviews, No. 196.)
3. Mortimer K, Reddel HK, Pitrez PM, Bateman ED. Asthma management in low and middle-income countries: case for change. Eur Respir J. 2022;60(3):2103179
4. Reddel HK, Brusselle G, Lamarca R, Gustafson P, Anderson GP, Jorup C. Safety and effectiveness of as-needed formoterol in asthma patients taking inhaled corticosteroid (ICS) – formoterol or ICS-salmeterol maintenance therapy. J Allergy Clin Immunol Pract. 2023; 11(7);2104-14.E3.

Management of Acute Exacerbation of Chronic Obstructive Pulmonary Disease

Sumit Sen Gupta

DEFINITION

Chronic obstructive pulmonary disease (COPD) is a heterogeneous lung condition characterized by chronic respiratory symptoms (dyspnea, cough, sputum production, and/or exacerbations) due to abnormalities of the airways (bronchitis and bronchiolitis) and/or alveoli (emphysema) that cause persistent, often progressive, airflow obstruction.

CAUSES AND RISK FACTORS

Chronic obstructive pulmonary disease results from interactions of gene (G) with the environment (E) occurring over the lifetime (T) of the individual (GETomics) that damage the lungs and/or influence normal development/aging processes.

The major environment related exposures leading to COPD are tobacco smoking and the inhalation of toxic particles and gases from household indoor and outdoor air pollution, but there are other environmental and host-related factors (including abnormal lung development and accelerated lung aging) that can also contribute.

The most relevant genetic risk factor identified till dates for COPD are mutations in the *SERPINA1* gene that lead to α-1 antitrypsin deficiency. A number of other less deformed genetic variants have also been associated with reduced lung function and risk of COPD, but the extent of other individual contribution size is rather limited.

DIAGNOSTIC CRITERIA

In the appropriate clinical context (see "Definition" and "Causes and Risk Factors" above), the presence of partially reversible airflow obstruction (i.e., $FEV_1/FVC < 0.7$ postbronchodilation) measured by spirometry confirms the diagnosis of COPD.

TABLE 1: Clinical indicators for considering a diagnosis of COPD.

Dyspnea that is	• Progressive over time • Worsen with exercise • Persistent • Recurrent wheeze
Chronic cough	May be intermittent and may be nonproductive
Recurrent lower respiratory tract infections	
History of risk factors	• Tobacco smoke (including popular local preparations) • Smoke from home cooking and heating fuels • Occupational dusts, vapors, fumes, gases, and other chemicals • Host factors (e.g., genetic factors, developmental abnormalities low birth weight, prematurity, childhood, respiratory infections, etc.)

Few individuals can have respiratory symptoms and/or structural lung lesions (e.g., emphysema) and/or physiological abnormalities (including low FEV_1, gas trapping, hyperinflation, reduced lung diffusing capacity, and/or rapid FEV_1 decline) in absence of airflow obstruction ($FEV_1/FVC \geq 0.7$ postbronchodilation). These subjects may be labelled "Pre-COPD". The term "PRISm" (Preserved Ratio Impaired Spirometry) has been proposed to identify those with normal ratio but abnormal spirometry. Subjects with Pre-COPD or PRISm are at risk of developing airflow obstruction over time, but not all of them do.

INITIAL ASSESSMENT

Once the diagnosis of COPD has been established by spirometry, in order to guide therapy COPD assessment must focus on considering the following five basic aspects:
- Severity of airflow obstruction
- Nature and magnitude of current symptoms
- Previous history of moderate and severe exacerbations
- Blood eosinophil count
- Presence and type of other diseases (multimorbidity).

TABLE 2: Differential diagnosis of COPD.

Diagnosis	Suggestive features
COPD	• Symptoms slowly progressive • History of tobacco smoking or other risk factors (e.g., indoor/outdoor pollution)
Asthma	• Variable airflow obstruction • Symptoms vary widely from day to day • Symptoms worse at night/early morning • Allergy, rhinitis, and/or eczema are often present • Often involves children • Family history often present
Congestive heart failure	• Chest X-ray shows dilated heart pulmonary edema • Pulmonary function tests indicate volume restriction, not airflow obstruction
Bronchiectasis	• Large volumes of purulent sputum • Commonly associated with bacterial infection • Chest X-ray/HRCT shows bronchial dilation
Tuberculosis	• Onset at all ages • Chest X-ray shows lung infiltrate • Microbiological confirmation • High local prevalence of tuberculosis
Obliterative bronchiolitis	• Generally involves children • Seen after lung or bone marrow transplantation • HRCT on expiration shows hypodense areas
Diffuse panbronchiolitis	• Predominantly seen in patients of Asian descent • Most patients are male and nonsmokers • Almost all have chronic sinusitis • Chest X-ray and HRCT show diffuse small centrilobular nodular opacities and hyperinflation

These features tend to be characteristic of the respective diseases, but are not mandatory. For example, a person who has never smoked may develop COPD (especially in LMICs, where other risk factors may be more important than cigarette smoking)
(HRCT: high-resolution computed tomography)

BOX 1: Global Initiative for Chronic Obstructive Lung Disease (GOLD) grades and severity of airflow obstruction in COPD (based on postbronchodilator FEV_1).

In COPD patients ($FEV_1/FVC <0.7$):
- *GOLD 1:* Mild $FEV_1 \geq 80\%$ predicted
- *GOLD 2:* Moderate $50\% \leq FEV_1 <80\%$ predicted
- *GOLD 3:* Severe $30\% \leq FEV_1 <50\%$ predicted
- *GOLD 4:* Very severe $FEV_1 <30\%$ predicted

DEFINITION OF ACUTE EXACERBATION OF CHRONIC OBSTRUCTIVE PULMONARY DISEASE

An acute exacerbation of chronic obstructive pulmonary disease (AECOPD) is defined as an event characterized by increased dyspnea and/or cough and sputum that worsens in <14 days, which may be accompanied by tachypnea and/or tachycardia and is often associated with increased local and systemic inflammation caused by infection, pollution, or other insult to the airways.

DIAGNOSIS AND ASSESSMENT

- Perform a comprehensive clinical assessment for evidence of COPD and potential respiratory and nonrespiratory concomitant diseases, including consideration of alternative causes for the patient's symptoms and signs, primarily pneumonia, heart failure, and pulmonary embolism
- *Evaluate:*
  - Extent of severity of dyspnea that can be determined by using a visual analog scale (VAS), and documentation of the presence of cough
  - Signs (tachypnea and tachycardia), sputum volume and color, and respiratory distress (accessory muscle use)
- Evaluate severity by using appropriate additional investigations such as pulse oximetry, laboratory assessment, C-reactive protein (CRP), and arterial blood gases
- Establish the cause of the event (viral or bacterial infection or environmental of other)

Omnious features that should guide need for hospitalization:
- Severe symptoms such as sudden worsening of breathlessness at rest, high respiratory rate, declining oxygen saturation, confusion, and drowsiness
- Acute respiratory failure
- Onset of new physical signs (e.g., cyanosis peripheral edema)
- Failure of an exacerbation to improve with initial medical management
- Presence of serious comorbidities (e.g., heart failure and newly onset arrhythmias)

Flowchart 1: Grading of the severity of COPD exacerbation.

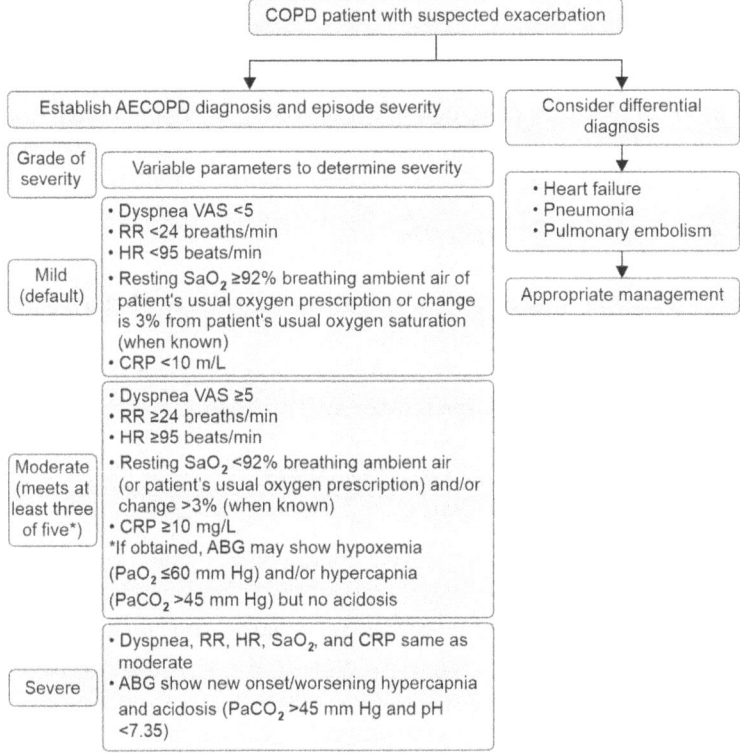

(ABG: arterial blood gases; CRP: C-reactive protein; HR: heart rate; PaO$_2$: arterial pressure of oxygen; RR: respiratory rate; SaO$_2$: oxygen saturation; VAS: visual analog scale)

- Insufficient home support or remote location of the patient's residence

Management of severe but not life-threatening exacerbations:
- Assess severity of symptoms, blood gases, and chest radiograph
- Administer supplemental oxygen therapy, obtain serial arterial blood gas, venous gas, and pulse oximetry measurements

BRONCHODILATORS
- Escalate doses and/or frequency of short-acting bronchodilators
- Combine short-acting beta 2-agonists and anticholinergics

- To consider use of long-acting bronchodilators when patient becomes stable
- Use spacers or air-driven nebulizers as appropriate
- To consider oral corticosteroids
- Consider antibiotics (oral) when signs of bacterial infection are present
- To consider noninvasive mechanical ventilation (NIV)

Following are always applicable:
- Monitoring fluid balance
- Subcutaneous heparin or low-molecular-weight heparin for thromboembolism prophylaxis
- Look for comorbid-associated conditions and treat (e.g., heart failure, arrhythmias, and pulmonary embolism).

INDICATIONS FOR TRANSFER TO INTENSIVE CARE UNIT

- Severe dyspnea that has inadequate response to initial emergency therapy
- Altered to mental status (confusion, lethargy, and come)
- Persistent or worsening hypoxemia (PaO_2 <40 mm Hg) and/or severe/worsening respiratory acidosis (pH <7.25) despite supplemental oxygen and noninvasive ventilation
- Requirement for invasive mechanical ventilation
- Hemodynamic instability leading to necessity of vasopressors.

PHARMACOLOGICAL TREATMENT

The three classes of medications most commonly used for COPD exacerbations are bronchodilators, corticosteroids, and antibiotics.

Bronchodilators

Despite absence of high-quality evidence from RCTs, it is recommended that short-acting inhaled beta-agonists, with or without short-acting anticholinergics, are the initial bronchodilators for acute treatment of a COPD exacerbation. A systemic review of the route of delivery of short-acting bronchodilators failed to show any significant differences in FEV_1 between using metered dose inhalers (MDI) (with or without a spacer device) or nebulizers to deliver the agent. Although the latter may be an easier delivery method for more sick patients, it is recommended that patients do not receive continuous nebulization, but use the MDI inhaler one or two puffs every 1 hour for two or three doses and then every 2-4 hours based on the patient's response. Although, there are no clinical studies that have evaluated the use of inhaled long-acting bronchodilators (either β_2-agonists or anticholinergic or combinations) with or without inhaled corticosteroids (ICS) during an exacerbation, it is recommended to persist with these treatments during the exacerbation or to start these medications as soon as possible before hospital discharge. Intravenous methylxanthines (theophylline or aminophylline) are not recommended for use in these patients due to risk of adverse side effects. If a nebulizer is chosen to deliver the bronchodilator agent, air-driven bronchodilator nebulization is preferable to oxygen-driven in acute exacerbations of COPD in view of avoid the potential risk of increasing the $PaCO_2$ associated with oxygen-driven bronchodilator administration.

Glucocorticoids

Mostly data from hospital-based studies indicate that systemic glucocorticoids in COPD exacerbations expedite recovery time and improve lung function (FEV_1). They also improve oxygenation, reduce risk of early relapse, treatment failure, and the length of hospitalization. A dose of 40 mg prednisone-equivalent per day for 5 days is recommended. One observational study suggests that longer courses of oral corticosteroids for COPD exacerbations may be associated with an increased risk of pneumonia and consequent. Therapy with oral prednisolone is equally effective to intravenous administration. Nebulized budesonide alone may be a viable alternative for treatment of exacerbations in some patients, and provides similar benefits to intravenous methylprednisolone, although the choice between these options may be individualized. Even short bursts of corticosteroids are not devoid of the subsequent increased risk of pneumonia, sepsis, and death, and use should be restricted to patients with significant exacerbations. Contemporary studies suggest that glucocorticoids may be less useful to treat acute

COPD exacerbations in patients with lower count blood eosinophils and further trials of steroid-sparing treatment regimens are required.

Antibiotics

Antibiotics should be prescribed to patients with exacerbations of COPD who have three cardinal symptoms: Increase in dyspnea, sputum volume, and sputum purulence; have two of the cardinal symptoms, if increased purulence of sputum is one of the two symptoms; or require mechanical ventilation (invasive or noninvasive). A meta-analysis demonstrated that ≤5 days of antibiotic treatment had the same clinical and bacteriological efficacy to longer conventional treatment in outpatients with COPD exacerbations. Furthermore, shorter exposure to antibiotics may decrease the risk developing antimicrobial resistance and complications associated with this therapy. The recommended length of antibiotic therapy is 5–7 days. A duration of ≤5 days of antibiotic treatment is recommended for outpatient treatment of COPD exacerbations.

The choice of the antibiotic should be based on the local bacterial resistance pattern. Usually, initial empirical treatment is an aminopenicillin with clavulanic acid, macrolide, tetracycline, or, in selected patients, quinolone. In patients with recurrent exacerbations, severe airflow obstruction, and/or exacerbations requiring mechanical ventilation, cultures from sputum or other materials from the lung should be undertaken, as gram-negative bacteria (e.g., *Pseudomonas* species) or resistant pathogens that are not sensitive to the above-mentioned antibiotics may be present. The route of administration (oral or intravenous) depends on the patient's ability to eat and the pharmacokinetics of the antibiotic, although oral route is preferred whenever suitable. Improvements in breathlessness and sputum purulence suggest clinical success.

Respiratory Support

Oxygen Therapy

This is a key component of hospital treatment of an exacerbation. Supplemental oxygen should be titrated to improve the patient's hypoxemia with a target saturation of 88–92%.

High-flow Nasal Therapy

A meta-analysis, albeit based on poor quality studies, showed no clear benefit. High-flow nasal therapy (HFNT) has been reported to improve oxygenation and ventilation, decrease hypercarbia, prolong the time to next moderate exacerbation, and improve health-related quality of life scores in patients with acute hypercapnia during an exacerbation or in select patients with stable hypercapnic COPD, receiving long-term oxygen therapy. HFNT did not prevent intubation in an RCT conducted in patients hospitalized with an acute exacerbation. It should be noted that European Respiratory Society (ERS) Clinical Practice Guidelines recommend trialing NIV prior to use of HFNT in patients with COPD and hypercapnic ARF. There is a need for well-designed, prospective, randomized and controlled multicenter trials to study the impact of HFNT in people with COPD suffering from episodes of either acute or chronic hypercapnic respiratory failure.

INDICATIONS FOR NONINVASIVE MECHANICAL VENTILATION IN AECOPD

At least one of the following

- Respiratory acidosis ($PaCO_2$ ≥45 mm Hg and arterial pH ≤7.35)
- Severe dyspnea with clinical signs suggestive of respiratory muscle fatigue, increased work of breathing, or both, such as use of respiratory accessory muscles, paradoxical motion of the abdomen, or retraction of the intercostal spaces
- Persistent hypoxemia despite supplemental oxygen therapy

INDICATIONS FOR INVASIVE MECHANICAL VENTILATION

- Unable to tolerate NIV or NIV failure
- Status postrespiratory or cardiac arrest
- Diminished consciousness, psychomotor agitation poorly controlled by sedation
- Massive aspiration or persistent vomiting
- Persistent inability to expectorate respiratory secretions

- Severe hemodynamic compromise without response to fluids and vasoactive drugs
- Severe ventricular or supraventricular arrhythmias
- Life-threatening hypoxemia in patients unable to tolerate NIV

DISCHARGE PLAN

- Full review of clinical and laboratory data
- Assess maintenance therapy and understanding by the patient
- Reconfirm inhaler technique
- Ensure safe withdrawal of acute medications (steroids and/or antibiotics)
- Assess need for continuing any oxygen therapy
- Chalk out management plan for comorbidities and follow-up
- Ensure follow-up arrangements both early and late

TABLE 3: Prevention of COPD exacerbations.

Intervention class	Intervention
Bronchodilators	• LABAs • LAMAs • LABA + LAMA
Corticosteroid-containing regimens	• LABA + IS • LABA + LAMA + ICS
Anti-inflammatory (nonsteroid)	Roflumilast
Anti-infectives	• Vaccines • Long-term macrolides
Mucoregulators	• N-acetylcysteine • Carbocysteine • Erdosteine
Various others	• Smoking cessation • Rehabilitation • Lung volume reduction • Vitamin D resuscitation • Shielding measures (e.g., mask wearing, minimizing social contact, and frequent hand washing)

(ICS: inhaled corticosteroids; LABA: lung-acting beta-agonists; LAMA: lung-acting muscarinie agonists)

MANAGEMENT OF COMORBIDITIES IN CHRONIC OBSTRUCTIVE PULMONARY DISEASE

KEY POINTS

- COPD often coexists with other diseases (comorbidities) that may have a significant impact on disease course and survival
- In general, the presence of comorbidities should not alter COPD treatment and conversely comorbidities should be treated as per usual standards regardless of the presence of COPD
- Cardiovascular diseases are common and important comorbidities in COPD
- Lung cancer is frequently seen in people with COPD and is a major cause of death
  - Annual low-dose CT (LDCT) scan is recommended for lung cancer screening in people with COPD due to smoking according to recommendations for the general population
  - Annual LDCT is not recommended for lung cancer screening in people with COPD not due to smoking, but due to inadequate data to demonstrate benefit over harm
- Osteoporosis and depression/anxiety are frequent; important comorbidities in OPD are often underdiagnosed, and are associated with poor health status and prognosis
- Gastroesophageal reflux (GERD) is associated with an increased risk of exacerbations and poorer health status
- When COPD is a part of a multimorbidity care plan, attention should be directed to ensure simplicity and affordability treatment and to minimize polypharmacy

SUGGESTED READING

1. Celli BR, Fabbri LM, Aaron SD, Agusti A, Brook R, Criner GJ, et al. An Updated Definition and Severity Classification of Chronic Obstructive Pulmonary Disease Exacerbations: The Rome Proposal. Am J Respir Crit Care Med. 2021;204(11):1251-8.
2. Halpin DMG, Celli BR, Criner GJ, Frith P, López Varela MV, Salvi S, et al. The GOLD Summit on chronic obstructive pulmonary disease in low- and middle-income countries. Int J Tuberc Lung Dis. 2019;23(11):1131-41.
3. Lindenauer PK, Stefan MS, Shieh MS, Pekow PS, Rothberg MB, Hill NS. Outcomes associated with invasive and noninvasive ventilation among patients hospitalized with exacerbations of chronic obstructive pulmonary disease. JAMA Intern Med. 2014;174(12):1982-93.
4. The Global Strategy for Diagnosis, Management and Prevention of COPD (updated 2024), the Pocket Guide (updated 2024) and the complete list of references examined by the Committee. [online] Available from https://goldcopd.org/2024-gold-report/ [Last accessed March, 2025].

CHAPTER 17
Mechanical Ventilation

Soumitra Kumar, Sumit Sen Gupta

The primary goal of ventilator support is the maintenance of adequate but not necessarily normal gas exchange, which must be achieved with minimal injurious effects. There have been two paradigm shifts in the management of ventilation in a patient over the last few years:

1. Noninvasive ventilation, which has been shown to decrease infective complications in a number of specific diseases, is increasingly being used in a variety of conditions.
2. Shift away from trying to maintain "normal" physiology to an approach, which minimizes injurious effects while maintaining "adequate" gas exchange.

As a corollary "standard" ventilatory settings are of less use than a disease or condition specific ventilatory protocol. Here, we will try to focus on the basic set-up of ventilation and assist control mode of volume-cycled ventilation along with some disease specific protocols. Weaning protocols will also be addressed.

NONINVASIVE POSITIVE PRESSURE VENTILATION

Modes of Noninvasive Positive-pressure Ventilation (NIPPV)

Continuous Positive Airway Pressure (CPAP)

- The ventilator delivers *one constant airway pressure* throughout the respiratory cycle (e.g., 5 cmH$_2$O). This is equivalent providing positive end-expiratory pressure (PEEP) with the help of air supply source.
- This is useful in respiratory failure (e.g., related to cardiogenic pulmonary edema and OSA).

Bilevel Positive Airway Pressure (BIPAP)

- The ventilator delivers *two pressure levels* and cycles between them.
- *Expiratory positive airway pressure (EPAP):* It is the baseline pressure for which safe range is <10-15 cmH$_2$O
- *Inspiratory positive airway pressure (IPAP):* EPAP *plus* added inspiratory pressure support (PS)
- The safe range for this is <20-25 cmH$_2$O.
- This is useful in hypercapnic respiratory failure and also in hypoxemic respiratory failure.

Indications for NIPPV

- *Treatment of respiratory distress in patients with:*
  - Acute chronic obstructive pulmonary disease (COPD) exacerbation resulting in respiratory acidosis (e.g., pH ≤7.35, PaCO$_2$ >45 mm Hg, RR >20-24 breaths/min)
  - Cardiogenic pulmonary edema (without shock or ACS)
  - Asthma exacerbations are a controversial indication.
- *Treatment of acute respiratory failure in patients with:*
  - Immunocompromise (e.g., solid organ and bone marrow transplant)
  - Thoracic trauma
  - Postoperative deterioration
- As a bridge to intubation in patients with challenging preoxygenation (e.g., ARDS)
- *As a bridge to unassisted breathing:*
  - Weaning from invasive mechanical ventilation in patients with acute hypercapnic respiratory failure
  - As a preventive measure after planned extubation in patients deemed to be at high risk for recurrent respiratory failure
- Patients with a prevailing problem that precludes invasive mechanical ventilation

Contraindications for NIPPV

- *Impaired/absent spontaneous breathing and/or patient not likely to co-operative with NIPPV:*
  - Cardiac or respiratory arrest
  - Severe encephalopathy (GCS <10)
  - Uncontrolled agitation
- *Compromised airway protection:*
  - Upper airway obstruction
  - Impedance to clearing of respiratory secretions
  - Severe upper GI bleeding
  - Increased risk of aspiration
- *Impaired sealing of the mask caused by one or more of the following:*
  - Facial trauma
  - Facial surgery
  - Deformity
- *High possibility of adverse impact from positive pressure:*
  - Recent upper airway or upper gastrointestinal surgery
  - Hemodynamic instability or cardiac arrhythmia
- *Varieties of interface to be chosen:*
  - Oronasal mask
  - Total face masks
  - Nasal mask or nasal pillows
  - Helmet
- *Modes of NIPPV settings:*
  - *BIPAP mode:*
    - *Low-to-high approach:* Begin with low-pressures and adjust upward as needed and tolerated
    - Start EPAP at 3–5 cmH_2O
    - Start IPAP at 10 cmH_2O
    - *High-to-low approach:* Begin with high pressures and adjust downward as needed and tolerated
      - Start EPAP at 5–8 cmH_2O
      - Start IPAP at 20–25 cmH_2O
  - *CPAP mode:* Set PEEP to 5–12 cmH_2O
    - Titrate FiO_2 (between 30 and 50%) to the desired oxygenation target (e.g., SpO_2 88–92% for COPD)

- *Monitoring and adjustments:*
  - Initially, start with NIPPV for 30-60 minutes
  - Titrate initial pressures (PEEP/EPAP and IPAP) to achieve targets:
    - ↓ Work of breathing and dyspnea
    - ↓ Respiratory rate (RR)
    - ↑ Tidal volume (VT)
    - ↓ Patient-ventilator dyssynchrony
  - Check ABG after 20-30 minutes:
    - If SpO_2 is low, increase FiO_2 and PEEP/EPAP.
    - If $PaCO_2$ is high, increase IPAP.
  - If patient's condition worsens, be prepared to switch to invasive mechanical without any delay.

Complications of NIPPV

- Air leaks
- Aspiration and risk of aspiration pneumonia
- Ventilator-associated lung injury—"barotrauma or pneumothorax"
- Severe gastric distention that may necessitate NG tube insertion
- Abrasions/ulcerations at site of interface
- Mucus plugging
- Mucosal dryness

INVASIVE VENTILATION

Invasive ventilation is positive pressure ventilation administered through an invasive airway device, e.g., endotracheal (ET) or tracheostomy tube.

Targets of invasive ventilation are:
- Reduce work of breathing (WOB)
- Treat life-threatening hypoxemia and hypercarbia
- Ensure aggressive bronchopulmonary hygiene and protect airway
- *Prevent multiorgan dysfunction:*
  - *Hazards of invasive ventilation:* The ET tube and ventilator tubing/circuit increase instrumental dead space, which leads

to higher airway resistance and pressure, thereby raising the risk of ventilator-induced lung injury.

Indication for Invasive Mechanical Ventilation
- Hypercapnic respiratory failure
- Hypoxemic respiratory failure
- Hemodynamic compromise:
  - Early mechanical ventilation offloads the heart by reducing the MVO_2 required to maintain the work of breathing
  - Useful in conditions with increased systemic oxygen demand and/or ↓cardiac output (e.g., polytrauma, burns, septic shock, severe MI, and cardiogenic shock)
  - However, the benefits must be weighed against the hemodynamic risks of positive-pressure ventilation
- *Hyperventilation therapy:* Short-term measure to treat patients with increased ICP
- GCS ≤8

Contraindications

There are no absolute contraindications, but relatively contraindicated in patients with advanced directives against mechanical ventilation.

The classical approach of initiating mechanical ventilation based on some parameters is mentioned in **Table 1**. This is only a guidance.

TABLE 1: Initiation of mechanical ventilation.

	Mode	FiO$_2$	PEEP	VT (mL/kg)	RR/min	Flow rate
Normal lung	ACV/PSV	0.5	5	8–12	10	60
Asthma	ACV	0.5	0	5–7	8–14	60
AECOPD	ACV/PSV	1.0	5	5–7	24	60
ARDS	ACV	1.0	10–15	4–6	24	60
Restriction	ACV	0.5	5	5–7	20	60

(ACV: assist control ventilation; AECOPD: acute exacerbation of chronic obstructive pulmonary disease; ARDS: acute respiratory distress syndrome; FiO$_2$: fraction of inspired oxygen; PEEP: positive end-expiratory pressure; RR: respiratory rate; VT: tidal volume)

Precautions during Intubation
- Prevent aspiration from full stomach
- Care to protect spinal cord during difficult airway access
- Anticipate adverse drug reactions

Prerequisites for Ventilation
- Assess risk of intubation by MACOCHA scoring **(Table 2)**
- *Ensure equipment required is ready:* ABCD
- For airway, use MABLES (mask, airway tube, bougie, laryngoscope handle with blade, ET size, suction in functioning condition)
- Bag mask ventilation
- Circulation to be ensured with patent IV access
- Drugs including anesthetic agents, muscle relaxants, and vasopressors must be present at the bedside.

Adjunctive care of ventilated patients include sedation, analgesia, and muscle relaxants.
- *This is targeted toward following benefits:*
    - To decrease patient discomfort
    - To suppress respiratory drive
    - To decrease muscular resistance to mechanical ventilation
    - To decrease patient-ventilator dyssynchrony
- *Sedation:*
    - *To be started immediately after intubation for patient comfort:* It should be titrated to provide patient comfort.
    - *Agents that are commonly used are:*
        - Propofol
        - Midazolam

TABLE 2: MACOCHA score.

Criteria	Score
Mallampati score III/IV	5
Obstructive sleep apnea	2
Reduced mobility of cervical spine	1
Limited mouth opening <3 cm	1
Coma	1
Severe hypoxemia <80%	1

- Dexmedetomidine
- Ketamine
- *Analgesia:*
  - Spontaneously breathing patients should be monitored for respiratory depression.
  - *Agents:*
    - Fentanyl (off-label)
    - Morphine (off-label)
- *Muscle relaxants:*
  - Allow a higher level of ventilatory control when desired (e.g., in refractory ARDS)
  - Should only be used in sedated patients
  - *Agents used include:*
    - Atracurium
    - Rocuronium
    - Vecuronium
    - Pancuronium
    - Cisatracurium
- *Maintenance of bronchopulmonary hygiene:*
  - Oral and airway hygiene
  - Tracheal suctioning
  - Mucolytics
  - Bronchoscopy
  - Chest physiotherapy

Supportive Care
- Orogastric or nasogastric tube infection
- Pressure score prophylaxis
- VTE prophylaxis
- Consider stress ulcer prophylaxis though routine use is controversial.

VENTILATOR SETTINGS
Basic Ventilation Settings
- *Tidal volume (VT):* The volume of air delivered to by the ventilator or taken by the patient per breath
  - Set by the clinician in volume-controlled modes (e.g., 8–12 mL/kg ideal body weight)

- Measured by the ventilator in pressure-controlled or pressure-supported modes (e.g., PRVC and PSV)
- *Respiratory rate (RR):* Breaths taken or delivered per minute by the ventilator
  - Set by the clinician in the absence of patient-initiated breaths (e.g., 10-15 breaths/min)
  - Determined by the patient in spontaneous breathing modes
  - Common setting is a combination of patient-triggered assisted breaths and a clinician-set back-up RR.
- *Fraction of inspired oxygen (FiO_2): The fraction of oxygen (by volume) in the inspired air*
  - FiO_2 of room air = 21%
  - FiO_2 up to 100% can be delivered in perfectly sealed ventilator circuits.
- *Positive end-expiratory pressure:* It is the positive pressure in the lungs maintained over the entire inhalation and expiration phased. It is measured in centimeters of water (cmH_2O). It reopens collapsed or unstable alveoli and improves ventilation perfusion matching:
  - Institution of PEEP is typically justified when an arterial oxygen pressure (PaO_2) of 60 mm Hg cannot be achieved with an FiO_2 of 60%.
  - Almost all patients need a minimum amount of PEEP (3-5 cmH_2O)
  - Higher PEEP is indicated in conditions involving a right-to-left pulmonary shunt pathology.

Adverse effects of PEEP include:
- Ventilator-induced lung injury
- Patient-ventilator dyssynchrony
- Hemodynamic compromise with higher PEEP

MODES OF VENTILATION (TABLE 3)
Volume Controlled

Volume controlled (VC) respiration involves a preset VT inspiratory rate and inspiratory/expiratory time. It is ideal for post-anesthesia phase immediately postintubation, for respiratory failure and neuromuscular dysfunction.

TABLE 3: Ventilatory parameters at a glance.

Parameter	Expanded form	Details
FiO_2	Fraction of inspired oxygen	Ranges from 21 to 100%, depending upon ABG values
VT	Tidal volume	To be set at 8 mL/kg body weight, except 6 mL/kg for ALI/ARDS
f	Frequency respiration	Set at 12–14 breaths/min
MV	Minute volume = tidal volume × respiratory rate	Helps in setting upper and lower limit alarms
PEEP	Positive end-expiratory pressure	Set at 5–10 cmH_2O initially; higher PEEP may be used ARDS
T_{insp}	Inspiratory time	On average for a rate of 12 breaths/min, it is set at 1.7s
I:E ratio	*Inspiratory:* Expiratory time	Usually set at 1:2, but reversal may improve oxygenation. However, it allows gas trapping, creating auto PEEP. In ALI, a 1:1 I:E ratio may be used to improve VT delivery

(ABG: arterial blood gas; ALI: acute lung injury; ARDS: acute respiratory distress syndrome; MV: mechanical ventilation; PEEP: positive end-expiratory pressure; VT: tidal volume)

Pressure Control

Pressure control (PC) is the preferred mode of ventilation in lungs with low compliance that have high airway pressures. PC ventilation ensures a positive pressure during inspiration followed by exhalation at the end of inspiratory time. It helps in gas exchange while connecting V/Q mismatch.

Synchronized Intermittent Mandatory Ventilation

Synchronized intermittent mandatory ventilation (SIMV) is the mode with a preset inspiratory rate and VT, but the patient may take spontaneous breaths if capable, during the assisted breath time interval provided by the machine. If not, mandatory breaths are taken according to the preset rate. It emphasizes upon a patient–ventilator synchrony.

Pressure Support

Pressure support is used as a weaning modality, where patient can breathe spontaneously and thus may control parameters such as VT, and inspiratory rate and time. The presence of a positive inspiratory pressure supports spontaneous respiration and thereby facilitates weaving.

INVASIVE VENTILATION IN ASTHMA

Intubate: Not too early, not too late:
- Drowsy/comatose
- Respiratory arrest
- Respiratory fatigue and decreased respiratory effort
- Decision is clinical
- No objective criteria
- Never based elderly on arbitrary levels of measured parameters (e.g., pCO_2)
- Do not wait until patient moribund, i.e., avoid crash intubation

Ventilation Strategy

Minimize Dynamic Hyperinflation

- VE 115 mL/kg
- VT <8 mL/kg
- Frequency 8–14 breaths/min
- I:E ratio 1:3
- Flow rate 80–100 L/min
- PPLAT >25 cmH_2O, end inspiratory pressure <35 cmH_2O
- Ignore peak pressure
- No/minimal extrinsic PEEP
- Permissive hypercapnia as long as pH >7.15

Pressure support has been used to ventilate patients with asthma in some centers with reasonable outcome.

Problems with Ventilation in Asthma

- Pneumothorax
- Severe dynamic hyperinflation

If patient develops severe hypoxia and hypotension on the ventilator:
- Apnea test—disconnect from ventilator for 1 minute to relieve DHI

- Always X-ray before putting a needle in for pneumothorax unless SBP <70 mm Hg since the consequences of an iatrogenic pneumothorax may be disastrous

Practical problems during ventilation:
- 125 mg/day of methylprednisolone or equivalent plus neuromuscular blockade may cause severe respiratory myopathy
- Large volume nebulization required

Acute Cardiogenic Pulmonary Edema Protocol

Intubate and ventilate if there is refractory shock or cardiorespiratory arrest. If not, be guided by BP and ABGs.
- If systolic BP is >180 mm Hg, start conventional treatment—if oxygenation worsens or there is significant acidosis, institute noninvasive ventilation
- *If systolic BP is <180 mm Hg and:*
  - If there is hyercapnia or acidosis, immediately start noninvasive ventilation
  - If there is normocapnia or hypocapnia and no acidosis, start conventional treatment—ventilate noninvasively if patient worsens

If no improvement, intubate and invasively ventilate.

ACUTE EXACERBATION OF CHRONIC OBSTRUCTIVE PULMONARY DISEASE

Preferably ventilated noninvasively; when intubated, the goals are:
- To rest the patient (and respiratory muscles) completely for 36–48 hours
- To avoid excessive ventilation (which may cause significant posthypercapnic alkalosis)
- To avoid excessive ventilator support (which may contribute to weakness of the diaphragm switch to PS within 48 hours).
- In less severity ill patients, PS ventilation may be used from the outset.

  In patients with COPD, peak airway pressures tend to be only modestly elevated [as they have relatively smaller increases in inspiratory resistance (compared with asthma), with their expiratory flow limitation arising largely from loss of elastic recoil]. Auto-PEEP and its consequences are common. Be careful of the odd patient with COPD who behaves like acute asthma with markedly raised peak airway pressures—in these patients a protocol similar to the asthma protocol may be used.

WEANING

- You do not wean the patient—the patient weans himself if you allow him to do it.
- Weaning should be considered as early as possible in patients receiving mechanical ventilation; a majority of patients can be successfully weaned on the first attempt. SBT (spontaneous breathing trial) is the major diagnostic test to determine if patients can be successfully extubated. The initial SBT should last 30 minutes and consist of either T-tube breathing or low levels of PS (5-8 cmH$_2$O) with or without 5 cmH$_2$O PEEP. SIMV should be avoided as a weaning modality.
- The initial assessment involves calculation of the rapid shallow breathing index (RSBI). In general, patients should be considered for an RSBI calculation and subsequent SBT earlier rather than later, since physicians frequently underestimate the ability of patients to be successfully weaned. Discontinuation of sedation is a critical step that can be achieved by either daily interruption of sedation or continuous titration of sedation to a level that allows the patient to be adequately responsive. Avoid paralyzing the patient at any stage unless absolutely necessary.

Criteria for Attempting Spontaneous Breathing Trials

Clinical Assessment

- Adequate cough
- Absence of excessive tracheobronchial secretion
- Resolution of acute phase for which the patient was intubated
- Stable metabolic status

Objective Measurements

- Adequate oxygenation SaO$_2$ >90% on FiO$_2$ 0.4 (or PaO$_2$/FiO$_2$ <150 mm Hg)

- PEEP <8 cmH$_2$O
- Stable cardiovascular status
- Heart rate <120 beats/min
- Systolic BP 90–160 mm Hg
- No or minimal vasopressors
- Frequency 35 breaths/min
- RSBI = <105 breaths/min (fR = Respiratory frequency)
- No significant respiratory acidosis
- No sedation or adequate mentation on sedation (or stable neurologic patient)

These criteria should be viewed as considerations for probable weaning rather than strict criteria that must all be met simultaneously.

If these criteria are met, a SBTs is attempted. If the patient succeeds, the patient is extubated.

Criteria for Failure of Spontaneous Breathing Trial

- Agitation and anxiety
- Depressed mental status
- Diaphoresis
- Cyanosis
- Evidence of increasing effort
- Increased accessory muscle activity
- Facial signs of distress
- Dyspnea

Objective Measurements

- PaO$_2$ <50–60 mm Hg on FiO$_2$ 0.5 or SaO$_2$ <90% or significant desaturation
- PaCO$_2$ >50 mm Hg or an increase in PaCO$_2$ >8 mm Hg
- pH <7.32 or a decrease in pH >0.07 pH units
- fR/VT >105 breaths/min
- fR >35 breaths/min or increased by >50%
- Heart rate >140 beats/min or increased by >20%
- Systolic BP >180 mm Hg or increased by >20%
- Systolic BP <90 mm Hg
- Cardiac arrhythmias

In patients failing attempts at SBT, PSV or assist-control ventilation should be favored. NIV techniques to shorten the duration of intubation should be considered in selected patients, especially those with hypercapnic respiratory failure due to COPD. NIV should not be routinely used as in the event of extubation failure and should be used with caution in patients with hypoxic respiratory. Consider early tracheostomy.

COMPLICATIONS OF VENTILATION

Ventilator-associated Pneumonia

Ventilator-associated pneumonia (VAP) occurs in approximately 1% of intubated patients per day. Assessment for VAP starts with calculation of the Clinical Pulmonary Infection Score (CPIS) as given here.

Clinical Pulmonary Infection Score Calculation

- *Temperature (°C):*
  - More than or equal to 36.5 and less than or equal to 38.4 = 0 point
  - More than or equal to 38.5 and less than or equal to 38.9 = 1 point
  - More than or equal to 39 and less than or equal to 36 = 2 points
- *Blood leukocytes, mm^3:*
  - More than or equal to 4,000 and less than or equal to 11,000 = 0 point
  - Less than 4,000 or more than 11,000 = 1 point + band forms more than or equal to 50% = add 1 point
- *Tracheal secretions:*
  - Absence of tracheal secretions = 0 point
  - Presence of nonpurulent trachea secretions = 1 point
  - Presence of purulent tracheal secretions = 2 points
- *Oxygenation:* PaO_2/FiO_2, mm Hg
  - Less than 240 or acute respiratory distress syndrome (ARDS defined as Pa/FiO_2 ≥200, pulmonary arterial wedge pressure ≤18 mm Hg and acute bilateral infiltrates) = 0 point
  - More than or equal to 240 and no ARDS = 2 points.

- Pulmonary radiography:
  - No infiltrate = 0 point
  - Diffuse (or patchy) infiltrate = 1 point
  - Localized infiltrate = 2 points
- Progression of pulmonary infiltrate:
  - No radiographic progression = 0 point
  - Radiographic progression [after congestive heart failure (CHF) and ARDS excluded] = 2 points
- *Culture of tracheal aspirate:*
  - Pathogenic bacteria cultured in rare or light quantity or no growth = 0 point
  - Pathogenic bacteria cultured in moderate or heavy quantity = 1 point
  - Same pathogenic bacteria seen on Gram stain, add 1 point.

Clinical Pulmonary Infection Score at baseline was assessed on the basis of the first five variables, i.e., temperature, blood leukocyte count, tracheal secretions, oxygenation, and character of pulmonary infiltrate. CPIS at 72 hours was calculated based on all seven variables and took into consideration the progression of the infiltrate and culture results of the tracheal aspirate. A score >6 at baseline or at 72 hours was considered suggestive of pneumonia.

If CPIS ≥6, start empirical antibiotics according to presence or absence of risk factors for multidrug-resistant (MDR) bacteria after sending of quantitative lower respiratory tract secretions for culture and sensitivity (quantitative or semiquantitative ET aspirate is perfectly acceptable).

Risk Factors for Multidrug-resistant Pathogens Causing Ventilator-associated Pneumonia

- Antimicrobial therapy in preceding 90 days
- Current hospitalization of 5 days or more; high frequency of antibiotic resistance in the community or in the specific hospital unit
- *Presence of risk factors for HCAP:*
  - Hospitalization for 2 days or more in the preceding 90 days
  - Residence in a nursing home or extended care facility
  - Home infusion therapy (including antibiotics)

Flowchart 1: Empiric treatment of ventilator-associated pneumonia (VAP) in adults with normal kidney function.

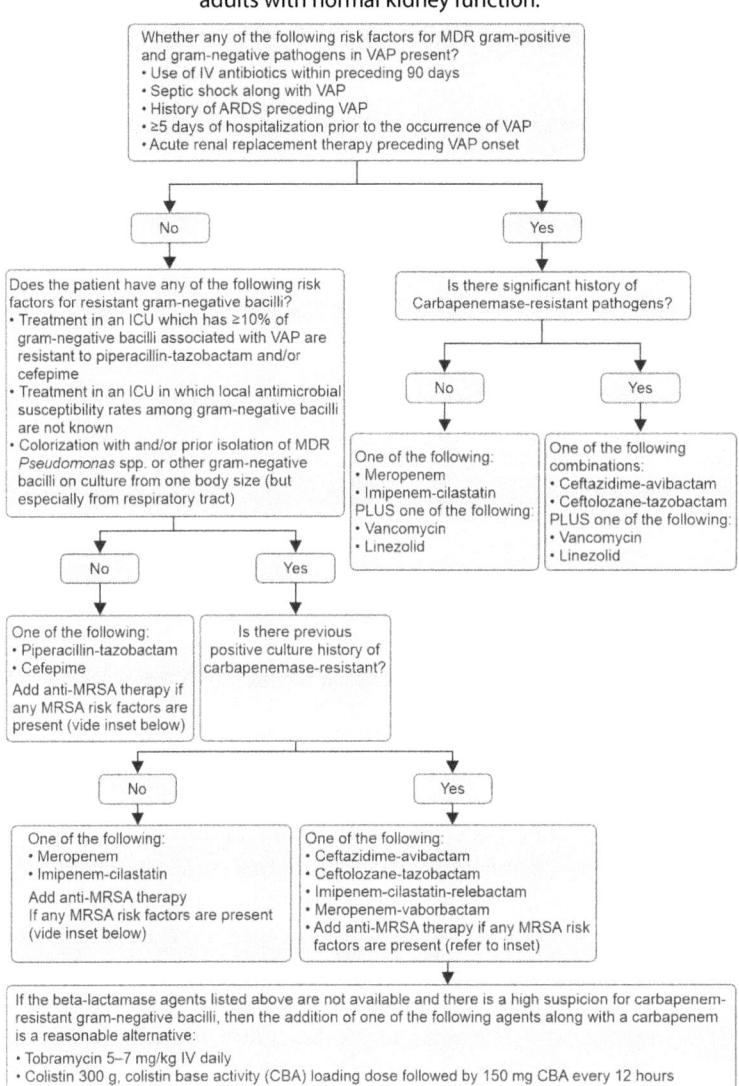

Contd...

Contd...

> **Inset:**
> **Dosing of preferred antibiotics:**
> | | |
> |---|---|
> | • Piperacillin–tazobactam | 4.5 g IV every 6 hours |
> | • Cefepime | 2 g IV every 6 hours |
> | • Meropenem | 1 g IV every 8 hours |
> | • Imipenem–cilastatin | 500 mg IV every 6 hours |
> | • Ceftazidime–avibactam | 2.5 g IV every 8 hours |
> | • Ceftolozane–tazobactam | 3 g IV every 8 hours |
> | • Imipenem–cilastatin–relebactam | 1.5 g IV every 6 hours |
> | • Meropenem-vaborbactam | 4 g IV every 8 hours |
>
> Add anti-MRSA therapy if patient has one of the following risk factors for MRSA:
> - Treatment in a unit in which >10–20% of *Staphylococcus aureus* isolates associated with VAP are methicillin-resistant
> - Treatment in a unit in which the prevalence of MRSA is not known
> - Colonization with and/or prior isolation of MRSA on culture from anybody site (but especially the respiratory tract)

> **Anti-MRSA therapy consists of one of the following:**
> | | |
> |---|---|
> | Vancomycin | • Generally 15–20 mg/kg every 8–12 hours |
> | | • For most patients with normal kidney function |
> | | • Adjustments of intervals should be based on AUC-guided (preferred) or trough-guided |
> | | • Serum concentration monitoring the vancomycin loading dose is based on actual body weight: The dose is rounded to the nearest 250 mg increment and not exceeding 2,000 mg. Within this range, we use a higher dose for cortically ill patients. |
> | Linezolid | 600 mg IV every 12 hours |

(ARDS: acute respiratory distress syndrome; AUC: area under the curve; MDR: multidrug-resistant; MRSA: methicillin-resistant *Staphylococcus aureus*)

- Chronic dialysis within 30 days
- Home wound care
- Family member with MDR pathogen
- Immunosuppressive disease and/or therapy

■ Piperacillin–tazobactam or cefepime are generally preferred, because they are more likely to have activity against gram-negative bacilli than levofloxacin. However, levofloxacin 750 mg IV daily may be preferred, if there is a high suspicion for *Legionella* spp. infection and local resistance rates of *Staphylococcus aureus*, *Pseudomonas aeruginosa*, and other gram-negative bacilli to fluoroquinolones are low. The Infectious Diseases Society of America (IDSA)/American Thoracic Society (ATS) guidelines also include imipenem and meropenem as options, but we generally reserve these agents for patients with a high likelihood of infection with extended spectrum beta-lactamase (ESBL)-producing gram-negative bacilli.

- Prolonged infusions of broad-spectrum beta-lactams for empiric and targeted therapy of gram-negative bacilli is preferred in critically ill patients as well as in patients with infections caused by gram-negative bacilli that have elevated but susceptible minimum inhibitory concentrations to the chosen agent.
- Vancomycin and antipseudomonal beta-lactams, particularly piperacillin–tazobactam, have been associated with acute kidney injury, although the risk is uncertain. Patients receiving vancomycin with piperacillin–tazobactam should be closely monitored for renal injury. In such case, alternative antibiotic combinations should be used.
- If none of the mentioned beta-lactam beta-lactamase agents are available, combination therapy of a carbapenem (e.g., meropenem, and imipenem–cilastatin) with another anti-gram-negative agent (e.g., aminoglycosides, antipseudomonal fluoroquinolone, polymyxin/colistin, or aztreonam) is an appropriate alternative. The IDSA/ATS guidelines recommend either an antipseudomonal fluoroquinolone or an aminoglycoside for the second agent for gram-negative bacilli. However, an aminoglycoside over a fluoroquinolone to be preferred. If there is no concern for *Legionella*, aminoglycosides are more likely to have in vitro activity against gram-negative bacilli in those with risk factor for resistance. Monitoring drug concentrations and adjustment of doses and/or intervals are required.
- Ceftaroline is an alternative agent when neither linezolid nor vancomycin can be used. However, it does not have activity

Flowchart 2: Confirmed VAP by MCR gram-negative pathogen.

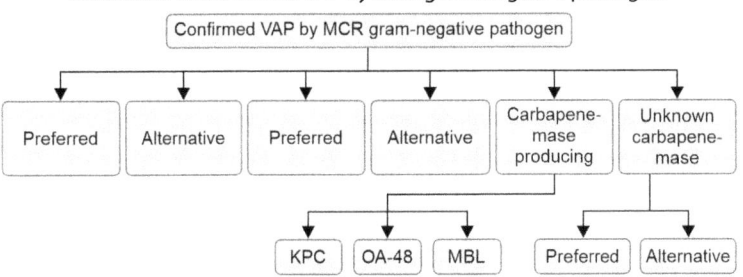

(KPC: *Klebsiella pneumoniae* carbapenemase; MBL: metallo-β-lactamase; VAP: ventilator-associated bacterial pneumonia)

against *P. aeruginosa*. If using in combination with another beta-lactam agent for empiric therapy of VAP, we close monitoring for allergic reactions, antibiotic-associated diarrhea, and renal function is advisable.

Recommendations for Management of Ventilator-associated Pneumonia Caused by Multidrug-resistant Gram-negative Pathogens

Spectrum of activity of empiric therapy: All empiric therapy regimens for VAP and nonventilation-associated hospital-acquired pneumonia (rVHAP) should include agents with activity against *S. aureus*, *P. aeruginosa*, and other gram-negative bacilli. Regimens are stratified based on the patient's presence of MDR pathogen risk factors. Occasionally, consideration for other pathogens is warranted, as is mentioned below.

- *Legionella* spp.: Patients who have compromised immune systems, diabetes mellitus, renal disease, structural lung disease, or have been recently treated with glucocorticoids are at increased susceptibility for *Legionella* spp. pneumonia. However, since nosocomial *Legionella* pneumonia is quite rare, generally empiric anti-*Legionella* therapy (e.g., with azithromycin or a fluoroquinolone) is added for patients in whom the clinical syndrome is consistent with *Legionella* pneumonia (e.g., severe illness and bilateral patchy infiltrates), when there is a known *Legionella* spp. outbreak, or if the patient is not improving on initial empiric therapy. Nosocomial cases of nvHAP and VAP due to *Legionella* spp. attributable to contamination of the hospital water supply have been reported.
- *Anaerobes:* Anaerobes are rarely implicated in VAP, and antianaerobic therapy is generally not required empiric treatment against anaerobes (beta-lactamase inhibitor). We consider empiric treatment against anaerobes (beta-lactam-beta-lactamase inhibitor, a carbapenem, metronidazole, moxifloxacin, or clindamycin) in patients with frank and/or gross aspiration (inhalation of vomitus), poor dentition, recent abdominal surgery, presence of possible lung abscess, or if not improving on initial empiric therapy (see "no clinical improvement after 48–72 hours" below). Antianaerobic empiric

therapy may also be considered if a good quality (e.g., from BAL) Gram stain demonstrates polymicrobial organisms or polymicrobial oral flora as those findings increase the likelihood of anaerobic bacterial presence.
- *Stenotrophomonas maltophilia:* We do not generally administer empiric therapy for *Stenotrophomonas* species unless it has been detected on the patient's previous respiratory cultures, there is an outbreak of *Stenotrophomonas* spp. present at the institution, or the patient is not improving on initial empiric therapy.
- *Viruses and fungi:* It is important to keep in mind that not all hospital-acquired pneumonia (HAP)/VAP are caused by bacteria. Viruses [e.g., coronavirus disease-2019 (COVID-19), influenza] and fungi can present with similar clinical features, especially if patients are severely immunocompromised. Routinely test for circulating respiratory viruses in patients with suspected HAP is indicated, particularly during respiratory viral surges and seasons.
- *Role of prior culture data:* Prior respiratory isolates should also guide antibiotic selection. A patient with a history of a pathogen in their sputum (e.g., *Acinetobacter* spp.) should receive empiric therapy with activity against the previous isolate if they have go on to develop severe pneumonia.

At 72 hours, recheck clinically and recalculate CPIS:
- Clinical improvement but cultures are negative—consider stopping antibiotics.
- Clinical improvement and cultures positive—deescalate treatment if possible.
- No clinical improvement—search for other diagnoses, complications, and sites of infection and other pathogens
- Duration of treatment is for 8 days, except for MRSA or *Pseudomonas*.

Prevention of Ventilator-associated Pneumonia

General prophylaxis:
- Compliance with alcohol-based hand disinfection and universal precautions
- Surveillance of ICU infections

Intubation and mechanical ventilation:
- Intubation and reintubation should be avoided.
- Noninvasive ventilation should be used whenever possible.
- Orotracheal intubation and orogastric tubes are preferred over nasotracheal intubation and nasogastric tubes to prevent nosocomial sinusitis and to reduce the risk of VAP.
- Continuous aspiration of subglottic secretions can reduce the risk of early-onset VAP, and should be used, if available.
- The ET tube cuff pressure should be maintained at >20 cmH_2O to prevent leakage of bacterial pathogens around the cuff into the lower respiratory tract.
- Contaminated condensate should be carefully emptied from ventilator circuits and condensate should be prevented from entering either the ET tube or in-line medication nebulizers.
- Decrease the use of sedation and utilize weaning protocols to accelerate extubation.
- Maintaining adequate staffing levels in the ICU can reduce length of stay, improve infection control practices, and reduce duration of mechanical ventilation.

Aspiration, Body Position, and Enteral Feeding
- Patients should be kept in the semirecumbent position (30–45°).
- Enteral nutrition is preferred over parenteral nutrition.

Modulation of Colonization: Oral Antiseptics and Antibiotics
- Routine prophylaxis of HAP with oral antibiotics [selective decontamination of the digestive tract (SDD)], with or without systemic antibiotics, reduces the incidence of ICU-acquired VAP, has helped contain outbreaks of MDR bacteria, but is not recommended for routine use, especially in patients who may be colonized with MDR pathogens.
- Modulation of oropharyngeal colonization by the use of oral chlorhexidine has prevented ICU-acquired HAP in selected patient populations, such as those undergoing coronary bypass grafting, but its routine use is not recommended until more data become available.

- Use daily interruption or lightening of sedation to avoid constant heavy sedation and try to avoid paralytic agents, both of which can depress cough and thereby increase the risk of HAP.

Stress Bleeding Prophylaxis, Transfusion, and Hyperglycemia

- Comparative data from randomized trials suggest a trend toward reduced VAP with sucralfate, but there is a slightly higher rate of clinically significant gastric bleeding, compared with H2 antagonists. If needed, stress bleeding prophylaxis with either H2 antagonists or sucralfate is acceptable.
- Transfusion of red blood cell and other allogeneic blood products should follow a restricted transfusion trigger policy; leukocyte-depleted red blood cell transfusions can help to reduce HAP in selected patient populations.
- Intensive insulin therapy is recommended to maintain serum glucose levels between 80 and 110 mg/dL in ICU patients to reduce nosocomial blood stream infections, duration of mechanical ventilation, ICU stay, morbidity, and mortality.

Barotrauma (Pneumothorax and Pneumomediastinum)

The incidence of macrobarotraumas is currently approximately 5–10% in ARDS patients, a substantial decline over the years.

High plateau pressure is the most likely culprit—a ventilatory strategy that allows unlimited plateau pressure associated with a very high rate of barotraumas. The occurrence of barotrauma is significantly reduced when plateau pressures are <35 cmH_2O, but plateau pressure is a risk factor for barotrauma only when it is too high. At the levels of plateau pressure used in the ARDS network protocol, the only risk factor for barotraumas is PEEP.

Hypotension during Initiation of Positive-Pressure Ventilation

Positive-pressure ventilation raises intrathoracic pressure during inspiration, decreasing venous return. PEEP, especially when applied to compliant lungs, further impedes venous return.

Hypotension immediately following intubation and initiation of mechanical ventilation is a common clinical consequence caused by the mechanisms just listed, particularly in the presence caused by hypovolemia. The abrupt blunting of sympathetic tone by induction of anesthesia is another mechanism, and hypotension caused by decreased venous tone, such as that seen with sepsis, spinal cord injury, or hypoglycemia, also may occur. Hypotension in these settings usually responds to crystalloid infusion, with the addition of pressors if necessary.

Hypotension (in a Previously Stable, Intubated Patient)

The list of causes of hypotension in mechanically ventilated patients is extensive. The major categories are:

- Hypovolemia may be due to inadequacies in fluid resuscitation, inadequate maintenance hydration, or increased fluid losses. Following the administration of fluids and stabilization of blood pressure, potential sites of fluid or blood loss must be investigated.
- Impediments to venous return include PEEP, dynamic hyperinflation, tension pneumothorax, or massive PE.
- Cardiac dysfunction due to myocardial ischemia/infarct or arrhythmias. An electrocardiogram, ideally compared with an old tracing, aids in determining appropriate concern for ischemia.
- The systemic inflammatory response syndrome (SIRS) should be treated initially with crystalloid infusion and appropriate antibiotic therapy. If there is no response, pressors should be added.
- The effects of medications: The use of benzodiazepines, narcotics, or anesthetic agents such as propofol or etomidate can cause blood pressure lability because of their vasodilatory properties. Acute allergic reactions to medications also can cause hypotension, along with bronchospasm, laryngeal edema, and urticaria.

Initial evaluation of the hypotensive patient should include a review of the other vital signs; a direct physical examination with special attention to volume status; use of the Trendelenburg position to maintain mean arterial blood pressure >70 mm Hg; administration of fluids, if necessary; and the use of pressors if the patient is not responsive to fluid administration. The clinical course before the episode then should be reviewed and other data gathered if warranted.

Acute Respiratory Distress (Fighting the Ventilator)
Assess for Ventilator Malfunction
Right mainstem bronchus intubation at the time of initial placement or secondary to tube migration. Contralateral atelectasis, worsening gas exchange, and increased risk for barotrauma from overinflation of the ipsilateral lung all can arise from right mainstem intubation. Auscultation, followed by tube repositioning, is the best initial management. A chest radiograph must confirm tube placement.

The tube also may migrate above the vocal cords, presenting as low VTs, the sudden ability to phonate, and escape of air from the nose and mouth. Tube migration results from inadequate external fixation coupled with excessive neck movement. Neck flexion or extension may move the tube up to 5 cm. (Confirming adequate tube placement by a chest radiograph reduces the incidence of unrecognized ET tube migration).

Cuffs can rupture/leak (presenting as low delivered VT, inability to maintain PEEP, and a decreased volume of cuff air).

Lower airway obstruction also results in acute respiratory distress. Copious or thick secretions can plug the ET tube or small airways, resulting in atelectasis and inadequate oxygenation. Observation of the amount and consistency of secretions during suctioning assists in the diagnosis. Treatment involves the removal of secretions to maintain lung inflation by aggressive suctioning, chest physiotherapy, or even bronchoscopy.

Bronchospasm, pneumonia (discussed earlier), and pulmonary edema can also lead to dyspnea and other patient discomfort. Physical examination and serial chest radiographs help guide therapy.

Dynamic hyperinflation, or auto-PEEP, occurs in patients with airway collapse. Air-trapping arises from the inability to exhale a delivered VT before the next breath is delivered (so-called stacking breaths). During assist-control ventilation, the patient must generate a preset negative inspiratory pressure to trigger the ventilator. If

auto-PEEP is present, the patient must generate a force equal to the level of auto-PEEP plus the necessary circuit pressure drop to trigger the ventilator. Measures to prevent or reverse auto-PEEP include:
- *Prolong expiratory time:*
  - Increase peak inspiratory flow rates
  - Use nondistensible ventilator tubing that decreases the total VT delivered, so it can be delivered during a shorter period.
- *Minimize expiratory airflow obstruction:*
  - Use larger diameter ET tubes
  - Treat bronchospasm aggressively (bronchodilators and steroids), suction frequently to remove secretions
- *Employ appropriate ventilatory strategies:*
  - Lower VTs
  - Remedy respiratory alkalosis with lower rates or VTs
  - Use PEEP to reduce the inspiratory force necessary to trigger the ventilator, thereby decreasing work of breathing.

Pneumothorax

Inadequate pain relief or sedation: This is a diagnosis of exclusion, and administration of sedatives, and especially muscle relaxants, to a patient with new onset of acute respiratory distress during mechanical ventilation without first excluding specific life-threatening causes is contraindicated.
- Narrowing of the inspiratory passages due to fluid or kinking in the ventilatory inspiratory tubing, smaller gauge ET and

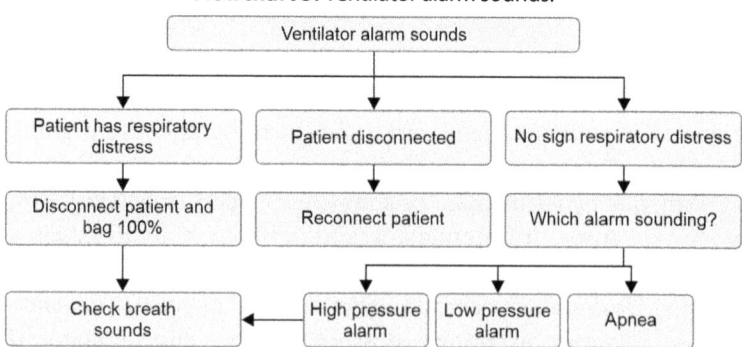

Flowchart 3: Ventilator alarm sounds.

Flowchart 4: Check breath sounds.

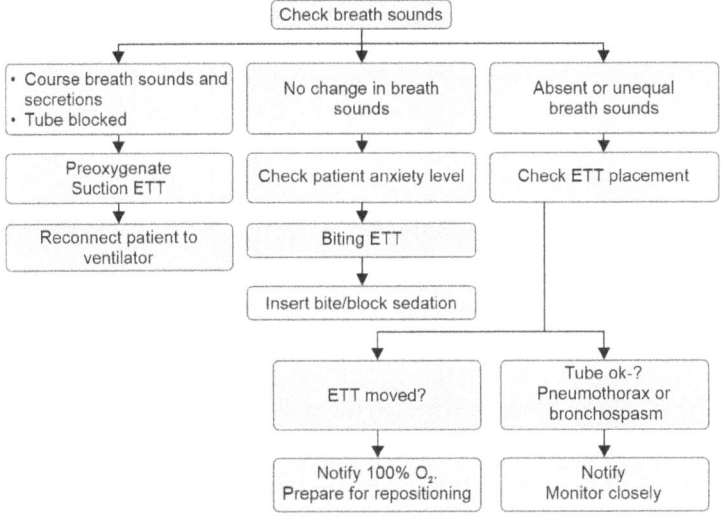

(ETT: endotracheal tube)

Flowchart 5: High pressure alarm.

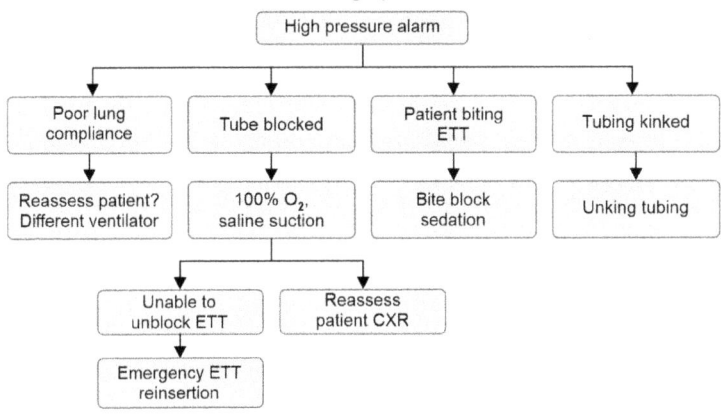

(CXR: chest X-ray; ETT: endotracheal tube)

tracheostomy tubes, neoplasms, stenosis, or foreign bodies in the trachea
- Bronchospasm secondary to underlying intrinsic airway hyperreactivity, worsened by concurrent infection, aspiration, repetitive trauma from suction catheters, or heart failure

- Decreased respiratory system compliance also acts to elevate inspiratory pressures. Recall that compliance corresponds to the change in volume for a given change in pressure. During volume-cycled ventilation, lowering the compliance means a higher pressure will be required to deliver the VT; with pressure-targeted ventilation, the peak inspiratory pressure is fixed and a drop in compliance results in decreased delivered VT. Common causes of decreased compliance include cardiogenic pulmonary edema, early onset of the ARDS, dynamic hyperinflation (from auto-PEEP or an inappropriately high VT), and progression of pneumonia. Splinting of intercostal muscles, often because of pain, can also alter chest wall mechanics by inhibiting lung expansion. Atelectasis during mechanical ventilation may reduce compliance by overdistending the remaining lung.

Extrinsic lung compression: Although there are multiple causes, the most potentially serious is barotrauma (i.e., pneumothorax). Barotrauma, defined for this purpose as ventilator-associated extra-alveolar air, results from alveolar over distention and rupture or other sources of lung parenchymal injury. Such injuries can occur from penetrating trauma, surgical procedures, bronchoscopy with transbronchial biopsy, thoracentesis, and as a complication of central line placement. Pneumothorax can present in a variety of ways, ranging from changes noticed only on a chest radiograph, to alterations in bedside monitoring, and finally to the cardiovascular collapse associated with tension pneumothorax. Chest radiographs may provide early clues, and there are several subtle radiographic signs, including an increased overall lucency in one hemithorax (suggesting an anterior pleural air collection), visualization of the epicardial fat pad, and a "deep sulcus sign." Alterations in bedside monitoring include unexplained hypoxemia, a rise in peak inspiratory pressure, or a decrease in respiratory system compliance.

The clinical syndrome of tension pneumothorax is the most dramatic presentation of barotrauma.

Physical signs include unilaterally diminished breath sounds, contralateral tracheal shift, tachycardia, hyper-resonance to percussion, jugular venous distention, and hypotension. Treatment of tension pneumothorax involves rapid placement of a needle into the pleural space to allow air to escape, followed by a thoracostomy tube.

Many practical measures can be employed to reduce the incidence of barotrauma, including the use of small VTs, the cautious use of PEEP in high-risk patients, monitoring closely for dynamic hyperinflation, and following changes in compliance. Pneumothoraces may result in continued air leak (bronchopleural fistula).

Acute large pleural fluid collections can raise inspiratory pressure by inhibiting lung expansion as can abdominal processes such as gastric distention, ileus, or ascites.

HYPOXIA

The ET or tracheostomy tube may be malpositioned, occluded with secretions, or kinked. Excessive PEEP can overdistend normal alveoli, worsening V/Q mismatching by diverting blood flow to poorly ventilated lung. The ventilator itself may malfunction, resulting in varied oxygen delivery and VTs. An oxygen meter should be used to confirm the delivered FiO_2.

Progression of underlying pulmonary disease can also worsen oxygenation. ARDS, pneumonia, sepsis, and COPD exacerbations can lead to poor oxygenation. Cardiogenic pulmonary edema, from fluid overload, myocardial ischemia, or decreased cardiac output, worsens V/Q mismatch and shunt. Clinical assessment of fluid balance aids the diagnosis and diuresis may correct the problem.

Pulmonary thromboembolism may occur in up to 10% of critically ill patients.

Aspiration of oropharyngeal or gastric contents can lead to bronchospasm and nosocomial pneumonia. VAP is another cause of hypoxia.

Tracheal suctioning, body position changes can help, especially in those with unilateral lung disease, Thoracocentesis has been associated with a drop in PaO_2 in some studies, possibly because of re-expansion pulmonary edema. Chest physiotherapy, which includes postural drainage, percussion, and coughing, may induce bronchospasm or move secretions into larger, more proximal airways causing hypoxia. Bronchoscopy occasionally induces hypoxemia because of bronchospasm or hypoventilation, but also acts to improve oxygenation in some through the removal of secretions.

BLOOD FROM THE ENDOTRACHEAL TUBE

The most common cause is iatrogenic, in the form of suction catheter-related trauma. Necrotizing pneumonia and tracheobronchitis,

TABLE 4: Interpretation of ventilator alarms.

Alarm		Possible causes
High PIP	P_{plat} elevated	Decreased lung compliance due to one of the following: • Pulmonary edema or ARDS • Air trapping • Pleural effusion or pneumothorax • Accidental right mainstem bronchus intubation • DHI

	P_{plat} low or normal	Increased airway resistance due to one of the following:
		• Ventilator malfunction or obstruction
		• Filter obstruction
		• Endotracheal tube obstruction; possible causes include:
		  – ETT too small
		  – Kinked ETT
		  – Patient biting the ETT
		  – Mucus plug or secretions
		  – Foreign body aspiration
		  – Bronchospasm

Low pressure		• Measurement issue or equipment failure (e.g., with the ventilator itself or the power source)
		• Air leak:
		  – Accidental ETT displacement or extubation
		  – Tubing disconnection
		  – ETT cuff leak

High RR respiratory rates		• Hypoxemia • Hypercapnia • Metabolic acidosis • Hypermetabolic state • Anxiety • Fever • Pain • Medications

(ARDS: acute respiratory distress syndrome; DHI: dynamic hyperinflation; ETT: endotracheal tube; PIP: peak inspiratory pressure; RR: respiratory rate)

especially combined with aggressive suctioning, can cause hemorrhage. Another common cause of hemorrhagic secretions is pulmonary edema. Classically, patients who develop cardiogenic pulmonary edema produce pink, frothy sputum. The condition can be severely exacerbated into impressive hemorrhage if a concomitant coagulopathy exists or excessive suction trauma occurs. Pulmonary thromboembolism presents with hemoptysis in a small percentage of patients. Pulmonary artery catheters are also associated with pulmonary artery dissection and rupture. These arise from distal placement and inflation of the balloon. Patients with this condition typically develop hemoptysis and a radiographically well-defined mass near the catheter tip. Prolonged use of pulmonary artery catheters may induce erosion through the arterial wall, with resulting hemorrhage. Erosions secondary to the ET tube cuff also occur rarely. Cuff-associated trauma occurs when cuff pressure exceeds the capillary perfusion pressure of 20–30 mm Hg, causing tissue ischemia and necrosis. Erosions in the trachea or, more proximally, in the larynx also induce hemorrhage. The most dramatic example is tracheoinnominate artery fistula, which presents as an acute eruption of bright red blood from the ET tube. Close monitoring of the cuff volume and pressure is the best prophylaxis.

The last major cause of hemorrhagic secretions is the underlying disease. A variety of illnesses may result in pulmonary hemorrhage, a few examples being vasculitic syndromes and Goodpasture syndrome. Primary or metastatic neoplasms may erode into vessels, inducing pulmonary hemorrhage. Disseminated intravascular coagulation, often associated with the sepsis syndrome, or other forms of acquired coagulopathy rarely result in significant spontaneous hemorrhage, but, in combination, can cause impressive bleeding. Tuberculosis or bronchiectasis may also present with hemoptysis. Rarely leptospirosis may present with hemoptysis.

SUGGESTED READING

1. Goligher EC, Ferguson ND, Brochard LJ. Clinical challenges in mechanical ventilation. Lancet. 2016;387(10030):1856-66.
2. Kapil S, Wilson JG. Mechanical Ventilation in Hypoxemic Respiratory Failure. Emerg Med Clin North Am. 2019;37(3):431-44.

3. Kelly CR, Higgins AR, Chandra S. Noninvasive Positive-Pressure Ventilation. N Engl J Med. 2015;372(23):e30.
4. Page D, Ablordeppey E, Wessman BT, Mohr NM, Trzeciak S, Kollef MH, et al. Emergency department hyperoxia is associated with increased mortality in mechanically ventilated patients: a cohort study. Critical Care. 2018;22(1):9.
5. Papazian L, Aubron C, Brochard L, Chiche JD, Combes A, Dreyfuss D, et al. Formal guidelines: management of acute respiratory distress syndrome. Ann Intens Care. 2019;9(1):69.
6. Scott JB, De Vaux L, Dills C, Strickland SL. Mechanical Ventilation Alarms and Alarm Fatigue. Respir Care. 2019;64(10):1308-13.
7. Silva PL, Rocco PRM. The basics of respiratory mechanics: ventilator-derived parameters. Ann Transl Med. 2018;6(19):376-6.

Chapter 18

Acute Respiratory Distress Syndrome

Sumit Sen Gupta

Acute respiratory distress syndrome (ARDS) is a clinical syndrome of acute hypoxemic respiratory failure (AHRF) due to lung inflammation, not caused by cardiogenic pulmonary edema. It was first described in 1967, and within 1988, a more explicit clinical definition quantified the severity of physiologic respiratory impairment (the lung injury score). Since then, the clinical definition of ARDS has been revised, first by an American-European Consensus Conference convened in 1992 by the American Thoracic Society (ATS) and the European Society of Intensive Care Medicine and subsequently by the ARDS Definition Task Force convened in Berlin in 2012 by the European Society of Intensive Care Medicine.

Summary of key differences between the new global definition of ARDS and the Berlin definition together with the rationale for updating specific diagnostic criteria.

BERLIN DEFINITION

- Acute onset within 1 week of known insult or new or worsening respiratory symptoms
- Bilateral operation on chest radiography or computed tomography not fully explained by effusions, lobar/lung collapse, or nodules
- Three severity categories defined by $PaO_2:FiO_2$
- Requirement for invasive or noninvasive mechanical ventilation such that PEEP ≥5 cmH_2O) is required for all categories of oxygenation severity except mild, which can also be met with CPAP ≥5 cmH_2O

RATIONALE FOR UPDATING CRITERIA

- Onset may be more indolent for some insults, such as COVID-19.
- Chest radiography and computed tomography not available in some clinical settings

- Pulse oximetric measurement of SpO_2, FiO_2 is widely used and validated as a surrogate for PaO_2, FiO_2, HFNO increasingly being used in patients with severe hypoxemia who otherwise meet ARDS criteria.
- Invasive and noninvasive mechanical ventilation not available in resource-limited settings

HOW THIS IS ADDRESSED IN THE GLOBAL DEFINITION?

- The inclusion of patients with HFNO will capture patients with indolent courses, and therefore the timing criterion has not been changed.
- Ultrasound can be used to identify bilateral loss of lung aeration (multiple B lines and/or consolidations) as long as operator is well tolerated in the use of ultrasound.
- SpO_2 and FiO_2 can be used for diagnosis and assessment of severity if SpO_2 is ≤97%.
- New category nonintubated ARDS created for patients on HFNO at ≥30 L/min who otherwise meet ARDS criteria.
- Modified definition of ARDS for resource-limited settings does not require PaO_2, FiO_2, or HFNO.

CAUSES OF ACUTE RESPIRATORY DISTRESS SYNDROME

- *More common:*
  - Sepsis and sepsis syndrome
  - Acid aspiration
  - Multiple transfusions for hypovolemic shock
- *Less common:*
  - Near-drowning
  - Pancreatitis
  - Air or fat emboli
  - Cardiopulmonary bypass
  - Pneumonia
  - Drug reaction or overdose
  - Leukoagglutination

TABLE 1: Diagnostic criteria for the new global definition of ARDS.

Criteria that apply as ARDS categories

Risk factors and origin of edema	Precipitated by an acute predisposing risk factor, such as pneumonia, nonpulmonary infection, trauma, transfusion, aspiration, or shock. Pulmonary edema is not *exclusively or primarily* attributable to cardiogenic pulmonary edema/fluid overload, and hypoxemia/gas exchange abnormalities are not primarily attributable to atelectasis. However, ARDS can be diagnosed in the presence of these conditions if a predisposing risk factor for ARDS is also present
Timing	Acute onset or worsening of hypoxemic respiratory failure within 1 week of the estimated onset of the predisposing risk factor or new or worsening respiratory symptoms
Chest imaging	Bilateral opacities on chest radiography and computed tomography or bilateral B lines and/or consolidations on ultrasound not fully explained by effusions, atelectasis, or nodules/masses

Criteria that apply to specific ARDS categories

	Nonintubated ARDS	Intubated ARDS	*Modified definition for resource–limited settings*
Oxygenation	$PaO_2, FiO_2 \leq 300$ mm Hg or $SpO_2, FiO_2 \leq 315$ (if $SpO_2 \leq 97\%$)	• Mild: $200 < PaO_2, FiO_2 \leq 300$ mm Hg or $235 < SpO_2, FiO_2 \leq 315$ (if $SpO_2 \leq 97\%$) on HFNO with flow of ≥ 30 L/min or • Moderate: $100 < PaO_2, FiO_2 \leq 200$ mm Hg NIV CPAP with at least 5 cmH$_2$O or $148 < SpO_2, FiO_2 \leq 200$ mm Hg (if end-expiratory pressure $SpO_2 \leq 97\%$) • Severe: $PaO_2, FiO_2 \leq 100$ mm Hg or $SpO_2, FiO_2 \leq 148$ mm Hg (if $SpO_2 \leq 97\%$)	$SpO_2, FiO_2 \leq 315$ (if $SpO_2 \leq 97\%$). Neither positive end-expiratory pressure nor a minimum flow rate of oxygen is required for diagnosis in resource-limited settings

- Inhalation injury
- Infusion of biologics (e.g., interleukin 2)
- Ischemia-reperfusion (e.g., post-thrombectomy and post-transplantation)

ARDS (WITH BRONCHOALVEOLAR LAVAGE FINDINGS)

Cardiogenic Pulmonary Edema

- *Acute interstitial pneumonia:*
  - Organizing diffuse alveolar damage
  - Idiopathic (Hamman-Rich syndrome), CVD, cytotoxic drugs, and infections [neutrophilia (>10%)]
- *Acute eosinophilic pneumonia:*
  - Eosinophilic infiltration and diffuse alveolar damage
  - Idiopathic, drugs [eosinophilia (>25%)]
- *Acute cryptogenic organizing pneumonia:*
  - Organizing pneumonia
  - Idiopathic, CVD, drugs, radiation, and infections [neutrophilia, and sometimes lymphocytosis (>25%), eosinophilia (>25%)]
- *Diffuse alveolar hemorrhage:*
  - Pulmonary capillaritis, bland hemorrhage, diffuse alveolar damage
  - Vasculitides, CVD, coagulopathies, diffuse infections (RBCs, hemosiderin-laden macrophages)
- *Acute hypersensitivity pneumonitis:*
  - Granulomatous and cellular pneumonitis with diffuse alveolar damage
  - Environmental and workplace antigens [lymphocytosis (>25%) and sometimes neutrophilia (>10%)]
  - Tuberculosis is rarely a cause of ARDS
  - Neurogenic pulmonary edema

Chest X-rays in ARDS

The initial film may be normal. Within 12–24 hours, bilateral, scattered, and parenchymal homogeneous opacities are present.

Although they represent extravascular lung water, these abnormalities generally are unaccompanied by the findings typically associated with cardiogenic pulmonary edema; that is, cardiomegaly, vascular redistribution or engorgement, or pleural effusion. Rapid progression to dense homogeneous opacification may occur within the next 24-48 hours.

If patients survive this period, there is progression into a chronic phase. Following several days of persistent homogeneous opacification, some areas of lucency are seen scattered throughout the lungs. The "white-out" and ground-glass opacities give way to a more heterogeneous, linear, or reticular pattern. The heterogeneous pattern remains stable for days or weeks. In approximately 10% of cases, persistent chronic fibrosis, and low lung volumes remain as a constant chest film abnormality. In other patients, various degrees of resolution may occur, with a strong tendency toward reversion to normal.

MANAGEMENT OF ARDS
High-flow Nasal Oxygen

- In nonmechanically ventilated patients with AHRF not due to cardiogenic pulmonary edema or acute exacerbation of chronic obstructive pulmonary disease (COPD), what is the role of does HFNO compared to conventional oxygen therapy reduce mortality or intubation?
  - It is recommended that nonmechanically ventilated patients with AHRF not due to cardiogenic pulmonary edema or acute exacerbation of COPD receive HFNO as compared to conventional oxygen therapy to reduce the risk of intubation.
  - *It is not possible at this point to make a recommendation* for or against the use of HFNO over conventional oxygen therapy to reduce mortality.
  - This recommendation applies also to AHRF from COVID-19.
- In nonmechanically ventilated patients with AHRF not due to cardiogenic pulmonary edema or acute exacerbation of COPD, does HFNO compared to noninvasive ventilation reduce mortality or intubation?

It is not possible to make a recommendation for or against the use of HFNO compared to continuous positive airway pressure (CPAP)/ noninvasive ventilation (NIV) to reduce intubation or mortality in the treatment of unselected patients with AHRF not due to cardiogenic pulmonary edema or acute exacerbation of COPD.

It is suggested that CPAP/NIV may be considered instead of HFNO for the treatment of AHRF due to COVID-19 to reduce the risk of intubation (*weak recommendation, high level of evidence*), but *no recommendation* can be made for whether CPAP/NIV can decrease mortality compared to HFNO in COVID-19.

No recommendation; high level of evidence of no effect.

CPAP/Noninvasive Ventilation

- In nonmechanically ventilated patients with AHRF not due to cardiogenic pulmonary edema, obesity hypoventilation or acute exacerbation of COPD does CPAP/NIV, as compared to conventional oxygen therapy reduce mortality or intubation?
  - *It is not possible to make a recommendation* for or against the use of CPAP/NIV compared to conventional oxygen therapy for the treatment of AHRF (not related to cardiogenic pulmonary edema or acute exacerbation of COPD) to reduce mortality or to prevent intubation.
  - *It is suggested* that the use of CPAP over conventional oxygen therapy may reduce the risk of intubation in patients with AHRF due to COVID-19.
  - In this population, *it is not possible* for or against the use of CPAP over conventional oxygen therapy to reduce mortality.
  - *It is not possible to make a recommendation* for or against the use of helmet interface for CPAP/NIV as compared to face mask to prevent intubation or reduce mortality in patients with AHRF.
  - *It is not possible to make a recommendation* for or against the use of NIV compared to CPAP for the treatment of AHRF.

Invasive Ventilation

In adult patients ARDS and COVID-19-related ARDS, does low tidal volume ventilation alone compared with more traditional approaches to ventilation decrease mortality?

Acute Respiratory Distress Syndrome

Protective Ventilation

The recognition of ventilator-induced lung injury (VILI) leads to the concept of "protective ventilation" as many of the pathophysiological consequences of VILI mimic those of ARDS. This development heralded current use of low Vt ventilation strategies with appropriate levels of PEEP to limit lung distention and atelectrauma.

It is strongly recommend to use of low tidal volume ventilation strategies (i.e., 4–8 mL/kg PBW), compared to larger tidal volumes (traditionally used to normalize blood gases), to reduce mortality in patients with ARDS not due to COVID-19.

This recommendation applies also to ARDS from COVID-19.

The key research questions to be addressed in future trials include investigation of (1) the optimal manner to assess whether a given ventilator strategy is likely to worsen VILI, (2) the manner in which we determine optimal Vt (e.g., based on PBW, on driving pressure, or an alternative approach), (3) personalized lung-protective ventilatory strategies based on the physiology of individual patients, and (4) other approaches to remove $PaCO_2$ if the current ventilator strategy is highly likely to worsen VILI.

In patients with ARDS undergoing invasive mechanical ventilation, does *routine* PEEP titration using a higher $PEEP/FiO_2$ strategy compared to a lower $PEEP/FiO_2$ strategy reduce mortality?

Summary of the Evidence on this Issue

Three multicenter randomized clinical trials were identified that compared a higher versus lower $PEEP/FiO_2$ strategy: ALVEOLI, LOVS, and EXPRESS.

ALVEOLI (n = 549) and LOVS (n = 983) each evaluated higher versus lower $PEEP/FiO_2$ titration tables, which specified allowable combinations of PEEP and FiO_2 with instructions to target the lowest allowed combination.

The primary outcome for all three trials was some modulation of mortality, which was not significantly different in any of the three trials nor in the meta-analysis (pooled risk ratio for hospital mortality 0.93; 95% CI 0.83–1.04).

Thus it is not possible to make a recommendation for or against routine PEEP titration with a higher $PEEP/FiO_2$ strategy versus a lower $PEEP/FiO_2$ strategy to reduce mortality in patients with ARDS.

This statement applies also to ARDS from COVID-19.
- In patients with ARDS undergoing invasive mechanical ventilation, does *routine* PEEP titration based principally on respiratory mechanics compared to PEEP titration-based principally on a standardized PEEP/FiO$_2$ table reduce mortality?
  - *It is not possible to make a recommendation* for or against PEEP titration guided principally by respiratory mechanics, compared to PEEP titration-based principally on PEEP/FiO$_2$ strategy, to reduce mortality in patients with ARDS. This statement applies also to ARDS from COVID-19.
- In patients with ARDS undergoing invasive mechanical ventilation, does use of prolonged high-pressure recruitment maneuvers (RM), compared to not using prolonged high-pressure RMs, reduce mortality?
  - *It is recommend not to* use of prolonged high-pressure recruitment maneuvers (defined as airway pressure maintained ≥35 cmH$_2$O for at least 1 minute) to reduce mortality of patients with ARDS.
  - This recommendation applies also to ARDS from COVID-19.
- In patients with ARDS undergoing invasive mechanical ventilation, does *routine* use of brief high-pressure recruitment maneuvers, compared to no use of brief high-pressure recruitment maneuvers, reduce mortality?
  - *It is being suggested not to go* for *routine* use of brief high-pressure recruitment maneuvers (defined as airway pressure maintained ≥35 cmH$_2$O for <1 minute) to reduce mortality in patients with ARDS.
  - This suggestion applies also to ARDS from COVID-19.
- In intubated patients with ARDS, does prone position compared to supine position reduce mortality?
  - In 2013, the PROSEVA trial demonstrated a clear protective effect of prone ventilation in patients with moderate-to-severe ARDS. In 2017, the ESICM and the ATS provided recommendations for the use of prone ventilation in ARDS based on both aggregated and individual patient data meta-analysis that included the largest four trials. In the aggregated data meta-analysis, the overall result was nonsignificant; however, in studies that used duration of proning longer than

12 hours or included patients with PaO_2/FiO_2 ≤200 mm Hg, a statistically significant mortality reduction was found.
- *It is being recommended to use* prone position as compared to supine position for patients with moderate-to-severe ARDS (defined as PaO_2/FiO_2 <150 mm Hg and PEEP ≥5 cmH_2O, despite optimization of ventilation settings) to reduce mortality.
- This recommendation applies also to ARDS from COVID-19.

- In patients with moderate-to-severe ARDS, when should prone positioning be started to reduce mortality?
  - *It is recommended that* starting prone position in patients with ARDS receiving invasive mechanical ventilation early after intubation, after a period of stabilization during which low tidal volume is applied and PEEP adjusted and at the end of which the PaO_2/FiO_2 remains <150 mm Hg; and proning should be applied for prolonged sessions (16 consecutive hours or more) to reduce mortality.
  - This recommendation applies also to ARDS from COVID-19.

- In nonintubated patients with AHRF, does awake prone positioning (APP) as compared to supine positioning reduce intubation or mortality?
  - *It is suggested that* awake prone positioning as compared to supine positioning for nonintubated patients with COVID-19-related AHRF to reduce intubation.
  - *It is not possible to* for or against APP for nonintubated patients with COVID-19-related AHRF to reduce mortality.
  - *It is not possible to* for or against APP for patients with AHRF not due to COVID-19.

- Does the *routine* use of a continuous infusion of neuromuscular blocking agents (NMBA) in patients with moderate-to-severe ARDS not due to COVID-19 or moderate-to-severe ARDS due to COVID-19 reduce mortality?
  - *It is recommended not to go for* the *routine* use of continuous infusions of NMBA to reduce mortality in patients with moderate-to-severe ARDS not due to COVID-19.
  - *It is not possible to* for or against the *routine* use of continuous infusions of NMBA to reduce mortality in patients with moderate-to-severe ARDS due to COVID-19.

ROLE OF ECMO IN ARDS

In adult patients with severe ARDS or COVID-19 does venovenous extracorporeal membrane oxygenation (VV-ECMO) compared with conventional ventilation improve outcomes?

It is recommended that patients with severe ARDS not due to COVID-19 as defined by the EOLIA trial eligibility criteria, should be treated with ECMO in an ECMO center which meets defined organizational standards, adhering to a management strategy similar to that used in the EOLIA trial.

Summary of the Evidence

Two randomized controlled trials comprise the basis of these recommendations. The CESAR trial included 180 patients, and the EOLIA trial included 249 patients with ARDS. The EOLIA inclusion criteria were as follows: A PaO_2/FiO_2 <50 mm Hg for >3 hours, or a PaO_2/FiO_2 of <80 mm Hg for >6 hours, or a pH of <7.25 with a $PaCO_2$ of ≥60 mm Hg for >6 hours, with the respiratory rate increased to 35 breaths/min and mechanical ventilation settings adjusted to keep a plateau pressure of ≤32 cmH_2O.

The EOLIA and CESAR trials were found to be clinically homogenous enough to be meta-analytically combined. However, as per the RoB2 tool, there was a high risk of bias with the CESAR trial, as about one-quarter of patient in the intervention arm did not receive ECMO.

Meta-analysis identified a significant decrease in 60-day mortality in patients receiving VV-ECMO compared to conventional mechanical ventilation (RR 0.72; 95% CI 0.57–0.91; moderate confidence). The protective effect was consistent across the 90-day mortality outcomes as well as a composite outcome of mortality and therapeutic failure at 60 days.

This recommendation applies also to patients with severe ARDS due to COVID-19.

In adult patients with ARDS, does extracorporeal carbon dioxide removal ($ECCO_2R$) compared with conventional ventilation improve outcomes?

In meta-analysis of these two trials, $ECCO_2R$ did not reduce mortality (RR 1.03; 95% CI, 0.82–1.3; high confidence). Patients

TABLE 2: Comparison between 2017 and 2023 ARDS guidelines.

	Observations
Definition	No comparison possible as the 2017 guidelines did not include a definition domain
Phenotypes	No comparison possible as the 2017 guidelines did not features an ARDS phenotype domain
High-flow nasal oxygen	No comparison possible as the 2017 guidelines did not make any recommendations on high-flow nasal oxygen
Noninvasive ventilation	No comparison possible as the 2017 guidelines did not make any recommendations on noninvasive ventilation
Tidal volume	In agreement with the use of low tidal volume strategies. 2023 guidelines extend this recommendation to patients with COVID-19
Positive end-expiratory pressure	*2017:* Suggest that adult patients with moderate or severe ARDS receive higher rather than lower levels of PEEP *2023:* Analysis of data does not permit to make a recommendation for or against higher PEEP strategy
Recruitment maneuvers (RM)	*2017:* Suggest that adult patients with ARDS receive RMs *2023:* Recommend against RMs due to increased mortality and risks
Oscillatory ventilation	*2017:* Recommend that HFOV not be used routinely in patients with moderate or severe ARDS *2023:* Not addressed this issue given the absence of studies since 2017 and the lack use of HFVO in adults
Prone position	Agreement with the use of prone position in ARDS. Additions in 2023 are the use of awake proning and the use in COVID-19
Neuromuscular blockade	No comparison available as the 2017 guidelines did not make recommendations on neuromuscular blockade
Extracorporeal membrane oxygenation	*2017:* Commented that additional evidence is necessary to make a definitive recommendation *2023:* Recommend ECMO in patients with severe ARDS
Extracorporeal CO_2 removal	No comparison possible as the 2017 guidelines did not include recommendations on extracorporeal CO_2 removal 2023 guidelines recommend against $ECCO_2R$ in ARDS

receiving ECCO$_2$R had fewer ventilator-free days to day 28 (mean difference—1.21; 95% CI – 3.77–1.34; moderate confidence). There were no randomized controlled trials in patients with COVID-19.

It is recommended not to go for the use of ECCO$_2$R for the treatment of ARDS not due to COVID-19 to prevent mortality outside of randomized controlled trials.

This recommendation applies also to patients with severe ARDS due to COVID-19.

Weaning from Invasive Ventilation

- *Conduct a CPAP trial daily when:*
  - FiO$_2$ <0.50 and PEEP <8.
  - PEEP and FiO$_2$ < values of previous day
  - Patient has acceptable spontaneous breathing efforts (may decrease ventilation rate by 50% for 5 minutes to detect effort).
  - Systolic BP >90 mmHg without vasopressor support
    - *Conducting the Trial:* Set CPAP = 5 cmH$_2$O, FiO$_2$ = 0.50
    - *If RR <35 for 5 minutes:* Advance to pressure support weaning as mentioned below:
    - If RR >35 in <5 minutes may repeat trial after appropriate intervention (e.g., suctioning, analgesia, and anxiolysis)
    - If CPAP trial not tolerated: Return to previous A/C settings
- *Pressure support (PS) weaning procedure:*
  - Set PEEP = 5, and FiO$_2$ = 0.50
  - Set initial PS based on RR during CPAP trial:
    a. If CPAP RR <25: Set PS = 5 cmH$_2$O and go to step 3d.
    b. If CPAP RR = 25–35: Set PS = 20 cmH$_2$O then reduce by 5 cmH$_2$O at 5 minutes intervals until RR = 26–35 then go to step 3a.
    c. *If initial PS not tolerated:* Return to previous A/C settings
  - *Reducing PS:*
    a. Reduce PS by 5 cmH$_2$O q1–3 hours.
    b. If PS <10 cmH$_2$O not tolerated, return to previous A/C settings (Reinitiate last tolerated PS level next and go to step 3a)
    c. If PS = 5 cmH$_2$O not tolerated, return to PS = 10 cmH$_2$O. If tolerated, 5 or 10 cmH$_2$O may be used overnight with further attempts at weaning the next morning.

Acute Respiratory Distress Syndrome

  d. If PS = 5 cmH$_2$O tolerated for >2 hours assess for ability to sustain unassisted breathing below.
- *Unassisted breathing trial*:
  - Place on T-piece, tracheal collar, or CPAP <5 cmH$_2$O
  - Assess for tolerance as below for 2 hours.
    - SpO$_2$ >90% and/or PaO$_2$ >60 mm Hg
    - Spontaneous TV >4 mL/kg PBW
    - RR <35/min
    - pH >7.3
    - No respiratory distress (distress = 2 or more)
      - HR >120% of baseline
      - Marked accessory muscle use
      - Abdominal paradox
      - Diaphoresis
      - Marked dyspnea
  - If tolerated consider extubation
  - If not tolerated resume PS 5 cmH$_2$O.

Supportive Treatment

Treat the cause:
- Aggressive treatment of sepsis
- Source control
- Fix all fractures as appropriate.

Early goal directed therapy, e.g., early antibiotics in septic shock. After the initial 48 hours conservative fluid strategy:
- Maintain PCWP 8-12 mm Hg
- *Ensure euvolemic state:*
  - Prophylaxis for DVT, GI bleed, and aspiration
  - Maintain glucose about 200 mg/dL with IV insulin infusions
  - Minimize blood transfusions

Patient should be paralyzed for the first 48 hours if necessary and subsequently be on sedation only with daily holidays from sedation when appropriate.

CURRENT AMERICAN THORACIC SOCIETY GUIDELINES (2024) FOR ARDS

- *Strong recommendation against:*
  - Prolonged recruitment maneuvers (as per 2024 guideline)

- High-frequency oscillatory ventilation (same as in 2017 guideline)
- Conditional recommendation in favor:
  - Neuromuscular blockade (as per 2024 guideline) (in severe ARDS)
  - VV-ECMO (as per new 2024 guideline) (in severe ARDS)
  - Systemic corticosteroids (as per new 2024 guideline) (in all stages of ARDS)
  - High PEEEP (as per new 2024 guideline) (in moderate and severe ARDS)
- Strong recommendation in favor:
  - Prone positioning (as in 2017 guideline) (in moderate or severe ARDS)
  - Lung protective ventilation (same as in 2017 guideline) (in all stages of ARDS) [goal VT 6 mL/kg, predicted body weight (range 4–8) + P_{Plat} ≤30 cmH$_2$O]

Systemic Corticosteroids

- Optimal regimen and type of corticosteroid is ill-defined
- For patients with corticosteroid-responsive etiologies, regimen should be used as applicable to the specific condition.
- For other conditions, regimes used in prior RCTs to be used.
- For patients that improve rapidly, discontinuation is to be considered at time of extubation.
- On the contrary, there is increased risk of harm when initiated >14 days of mechanical ventilation.

NEUROMUSCULAR BLOCKING AGENT

- Cisatracurium has been used most frequently used in clinical trials, but optimal agent is unknown.
- Mortality is reduced with use of NMBAs when compared to deep sedation, there is no mortality benefit when compared to light sedation.
- NMBAs may have greater utility in patients with ventricular dyssynchrony not mitigated by ventilator changes.

SUGGESTED READING

1. Combes A, Bréchot N, Luyt CE, Schmidt M. Indications for extracorporeal support: why do we need the results of the EOLIA trial? Med Klin Intensivmed Notfmed. 2018;113:21-5.
2. Grasselli G, Calfee CS, Camporota L, Poole D, Amato MBP, Antonelli M, et al; European Society of Intensive Care Medicine Taskforce on ARDS. ESICM guidelines on acute respiratory distress syndrome: Definition, phenotyping and respiratory support strategies. Intensive Care Med. 2023;49(7):727-59.
3. Liu X, Jiang Y, Jia X, alma X. Identification of distinct clinical phenotypes of acute respiratory distress syndrome with differential responses to treatment. Crit Care. 2021;25:320.
4. Matthay MA, Thompson BT, Ware LB. The Berlin definition of acute respiratory distress syndrome: should patients receiving high- flow nasal oxygen be included? Lancet Respir Med. 20221;9:933-6.
5. Matthay MA, Zemans RL, Zimmerman GA, Arabi YM, Beitler JR, Mercat A, et al. Acute respiratory distress syndrome. Nat Rev Dis Primers. 2019;5(1):18.
6. McNamee JJ, Gillies MA, Barrett NA, Perkins GD, Tunnicliffe W, Young D, et al. Effect of lower tidal volume ventilation facilitated by extracorporeal carbon dioxide removal vs standard care ventilation on 90-day mortality in patients with acute hypoxemic respiratory failure: the REST randomized clinical trial. JAMA. 2021;326:1013-23.
7. Munshi L, Mancebo J, Brochard LJ. Noninvasive respiratory support for adults with acute respiratory failure. N Engl J Med. 2022;387:1688-98.
8. Ranieri VM, Rubenfeld G, Slutsky AS. Rethinking ARDS after COVID-19. If a "better" definition is the answer, What is the question? Am J Respir Crit Care Med. 2023;207(3):255-60.
9. Weatherald J, Parhar KKS, Duhailib ZA, Chu DK, Granholm A, Solverson K, et al. Efficacy of awake prone positioning in patients with COVID-19 related hypoxemic respiratory failure: systematic review and meta-analysis of randomized trials. BMJ. 2022;379:e071966.

CHAPTER 19

Management of Gastrointestinal Bleeding

Debashis Dutta

INITIAL ASSESSMENT AND RESUSCITATION

Gastrointestinal bleeding (GIB) is a common medical emergency globally with mortality rate of 7% at hospital admission, which escalates to 26% if bleeding occurs during hospitalization for other causes. Management of comorbidities also has a significant impact on clinical outcomes. So, the obvious implication is that in unstable patients, it is of great value to have multidisciplinary coordination between gastroenterology, surgery, anesthesiology, transfusion medicine, interventional radiology, and intensive care medicine.

The initial approach to the patient presenting with GIB includes clinical evaluation and simultaneous hemodynamic and cardiopulmonary stabilization. It is important to look for signs of liver disease (LD) and other comorbidities and patient medications such as oral anticoagulants (OACs), antiplatelet therapy (APT), and nonsteroidal anti-inflammatory drug (NSAID). Prior abdominal or vascular surgeries, such as abdominal aortic repair, are also important in the context of differential diagnosis. Vital signs must be monitored in accordance to clinical severity, rapidly of evolution, and hospitalization level. It is not early to quantify blood loss in GIB. In an initial phase, normal hemoglobin (Hb) and blood pressure (BP) do not exclude significant hemorrhage. In this stage, tachycardia is the best marker of severity, unless the patient is on beta-blocker therapy.

The emphasis should be on complications of the etiology of active hemorrhage (hematemesis, melena, persisting/remaining hematoche zia, or live/bright blood in the nasogastric tube) and LD existence. When hematochezia is associated with significant hemodynamic instability, upper GIB (UGIB) must be considered. In patients with chronic LD (CLD), a portal hypertensive cause of GIB is the assumed hypothesis and specific measures should be initiated early (even before etiologic confirmation), including vasopressor therapy and prophylactic antibiotic therapy.

CLINICAL PRESENTATION

Are there signs of active bleeding? (hematemesis, melena, hematochezia*, fresh blood on nasogastric tube, syncope, hemodynamic instability, and others)

Hematochezia + hemodynamic instability: Consider UGIB.

IMMEDIATE EVALUATION/STABILIZATION

- Shock index (SI = HR/SBP) with consideration of specific situations (e.g., β-blocker therapy)
- Simultaneous evaluation and initiation of resuscitation measures

ABCDE approach, depending on clinical case:
- *A—Airway:* Ensure airway patency and stability.
  - Orotracheal intubation is indicated in cases of massive bleeding and decreased level of consciousness. Prevent aspiration of gastric contents, etc.
- *B—Breathing:* Check respiratory rate, SpO_2 and consider O_2 supplementation.
- *C—Circulation:*
  - Noninvasive monitoring of BP, HR (tachycardia is an early indicator), and urine output are indicated in all patients with GIB.
  - Insert two peripheral venous lines (16–18 g).
  - *Collect blood sample:* CBC, PTT, coagulation panel (PT, aPTT, and Fib), VET, biochemistry, and ABG
  - *Infuse warm fluid crystalloids (polyelectrolytes):* PRBC in cases of severe bleeding or lack of no response to crystalloids
  - Further blood transfusion should be goal-directed by targets.
  - *Evaluate blood loss:* It is important to quantity.
  - Central venous catheterization
  - Consider dynamic ultrasonographic evaluation of the interior vena cava.
  - Consider metabolic + electrolyte imbalances and other perfusion indexes.

D—Disability: Neurological state of consciousness and coordination

E—Exposure: Attention to room and body temperature. Maintain normothermia consider blood and

IV fluids + body warmers, warm blankets, and heating environment.
- Nasogastric/orogastric intubation is not routinely recommended
- Nil by mouth
- *Avoid:* Fluid overload and excessive transfusion

Flowchart 1: Approach to severe bleeding.

```
┌─────────────────────────────────────┐
│          Severe bleeding            │
└─────────────────────────────────────┘
                  ↓
```

Consider (according to clinical presentation and availability):
- CT with angiogram
- Massive bleeding protocol activation
- Insert arterial + venous catheters
- If no hemodynamic response to crystalloids + PRBC → give noradrenaline 0.–0.2 µg/kg/m (maximum 2 µg/kg/m) if MAP not recovered
- Transfer to the ICU if patient is hemodynamically unstable and/or has significant risk factors/comorbidities

Seek and arrange multidisciplinary approach

Clinical team: Gastroenterology, transfusion medicine, anesthesiology, surgery, intervention radiology, and intensive medicine

Evaluate past-medical history

Clinical evaluation—history of:
- Previous GIB, known gastrointestinal (GI) disease or prior GI surgery and recent digestive endoscopy
- Radiotherapy
- Aortic surgical/endovascular therapy and aortic aneurysm (? aortic fistula)
- Previous vomiting before bleeding ? ? (Mallory–Weiss)
- Severe abdominal pain (ischemia and GI perforation)
- Wasting syndrome (neoplasia)
- *Comorbidities:* Chronic liver, renal, and ischemic heart disease—coronary stent/CABG

Past drug history

Drugs that interfere with coagulation:
- Anticoagulants
- Antiplatelet drugs
- NSAID

Contd...

Contd...

> Viscoelastic test (VET)
> Laboratory workup in accordance with clinical presentation

- FBC and CS (PT, aPTT, and fibrinogen) (according to bleeding severity)
- BUN, creatinine—BUN/creatinine ratio (BUN mg/dL)/(creatinine mg/dL) >30 indicates that urea is disproportionately high, meaning low renal perfusion or blood in small bowel
- Glucose, ionogram, Ca^{++}, phosphate, magnesium, CRP, and hs-cTnI
- AST, ALT, bilirubin, and albumin
- Pretransfusional tests and reserve/transfuse PRBC
- *ABG:* If severe clinical status, estimate Hb, acid-basis + lactate evaluation
- *Monitor every 30–60 minutes or according to bleeding severity:* ABG, FBC, CS, ICA

> Further tests in accordance with clinical requirements

- ECG and chest X-ray (individualized)
- Urgent fluoroscopic/CT angiography in patients with history suggestive of aortoenteric fistula, severe bleeding refractory to hemodynamic stabilization, persistent bleeding with negative upper endoscopy and not responding to hemodynamic stabilization measures, suspicion of visceral perforation, other individualized conditions

GOALS OF RESUSCITATION

- Hemodynamic
  - *MAP:* 65–90 mm Hg
  - *Heart index:* 2–4 L/m/m^2
  - SaO_2 >92%
  - SvO_2 >70%
  - Temperature >36°C
- Therapeutic
  - Stop bleeding
  - Correct anemia
  - *Avoid:*
    - Coagulopathy, hemodilution, hypothermia, acidosis, and hypocalcemia
  - *Correct:*
    - Coagulopathy guided by viscoelastic test
- Laboratory values
  - Hb ≥ 9 g/dL

- Htc > 24–28%
- Platelets >50 × 10^9/L
- Fibrinogen >2.0 g/L
- INR/PT/aPTT <1.5 × NV
- *In severe bleeding*:
  - Ca^{++} >1.2 mmol/L
  - pH >7.2

TABLE 1: Comorbidities that aggregate GI bleeding episodes.

Liver cirrhosis/ portal hypertension (PHT)	If liver cirrhosis suspected or confirmed, consider specific therapy before endoscopic confirmation	• Start immediately vasopressors (terlipressin/ octreotide/somatostatin), if not contraindicated • Start prolactic antibiotic • *Monitoring:* MELD, Child–Pugh, in pretransplant evolution status on list? • Collect blood + Urine + ascites for bacteriological tests • Consider prophylaxis for hepatic encephalopathy • Consider Sengstaken-Blakemore balloon if clinical situation is not controlled
Chronic renal disease	• Anemia • Platelet dysfunction • Thrombocytopenia	• Dialysis without heparin • *Correct anemia:* Ideally HTC 30% (Grade 1C) • *Fibrinogen concentrate:* 25–50 mg/kg (2–4 g) IV • *Desmopressin:* 0.3 mg/kg IV
Ischemic coronary disease	• Maintain Hg ≥8–≥9 g/dL • Proceed according to ongoing therapy, mostly with APT • Mostly submitted to β-blockers, interferes with shock index • Consider further case of drugs (oral anticoagulants, heparin APT) and stents	

- Lactate <4 mmol/L
- Base deficit <-3

Endoscopic approach is not dependent on complete correction until target values are reached
- Transfusional therapy
  - Hb <7 g/dL → PRBC
  - Platelets <50,000/μ → Platelet concentrate (PC)
  - Fib: <1.5-2.0 g/L → Human fibrinogen concentrate (FC)
  - INR >1.5/PT/aPTT >1.5 → PC/fresh frozen plasma (FFP)
- Markers of poor prognosis
  - Temperature <35°C
  - Base deficit >-6 mmol/L
  - pH <7.2
  - Lactate >4 mmol/L
  - Ca^{++} <1.1 mmol/L
  - PaO_2 <60 mm Hg
  - O_2 saturation< 90 mm Hg
  - Platelets <50 × 10^9/L
  - Fibrinogen <1.5 g/L
  - PT INR >1.5/aPTT >1.5 × NV

APPROACH TO VARICEAL UPPER GASTROINTESTINAL BLEEDING

Mortality rate: 10-20% at 6 weeks

Immediately start: Vasoactive drugs and prepare for endoscopy
- Culture examination and diagnostic paracentesis in case of ascites

Vasoactive drugs: Drugs doses—
- *Terlipressin* 1-2 mg IV 6/6 hours up to 4/4 hours until bleeding controls, then 1 mg in 4/4 hours to avoid rebleeding during 2-5 days
- *Somatostatin* bolus 250 μg/h (3 mg/50 α, 4 cc/h) during 2-5 days
- *Octreotide* bolus 50 μg IV, perfusion 50 μg h (600 μg/50, 4 cc/h) during 2-5 days
- *PPI:* Pantoprazole 40 mg IV q12 h
- *Ceftriaxone* prophylaxis doses 1 g IV per day for up to 7 days

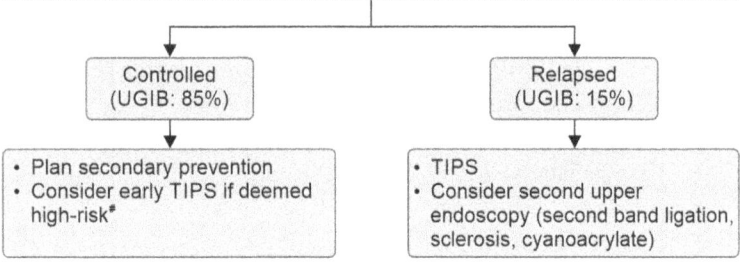

Flowchart 2: Upper GI endoscopy.

(GOV: gastroesophageal varices; TIPS: transjugular intrahepatic portosystemic shunt)

- Preferred in advanced cirrhosis and cases of high guideline resistance
- *Erythromycin* 250 mg IV 30–120 minutes before in absence of contraindications as QT prolongation
- *Lactulose* 25 mL q12 h titrate to 2–3 bowel movements or enema if no oral or enteric route

NONVARICEAL UPPER GASTROINTESTINAL BLEEDING

Initial Risk Assessment and Triage

The severity of blood loss can be assessed by the hemodynamic status and signs that include blood pressure, orthostatic hypotension, tachycardia, respiratory rate, urine output, and sensorium. Several systems (like Baylor, Cedars-Sinai, Rockall, Blatchford, and AIMS65) are in use based on clinical and laboratory parameters for assessment

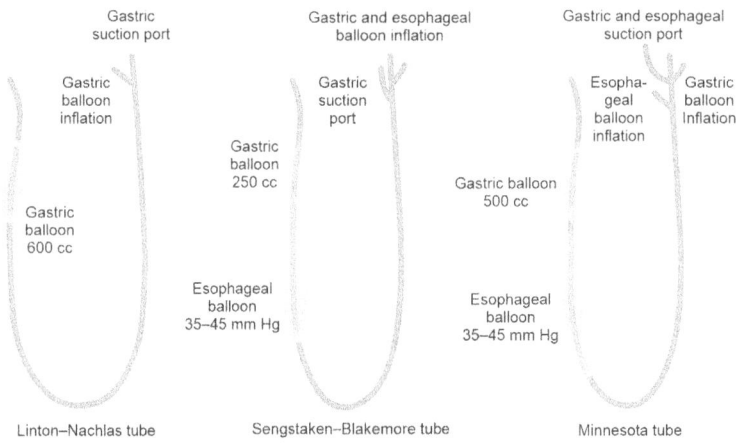

Fig. 1: Different balloon tamponade devices.

TABLE 2: Blatchford score.	
The patients with Blatchford score of 0 can be considered for early discharge. The score can help identify patients who need early intervention.	
Admission risk marker	*Score component*
Blood urea (mg/dL)	
• <18.2	0
• >18.2–<22.4	2
• >22.4–<28	3
• >28–<70	4
• >70	6
Hemoglobin (men—g/dL)	
• 12–<13	1
• 10–<12	3
• 10–<12	6
Hemoglobin (women—g/dL)	
• 10–<12	1
• <10	6
SBP (mm Hg)	
• ≥110	0
• 100–109	1
• 90–99	2
• <90	

Contd...

Contd...

Admission risk marker	Score component
Other markers:	
• Pulse >100/min	1
• Presentation with melena	1
• Presentation with syncope	2
• Hepatic disease	2
• Cardiac failure	3

TABLE 3: Approach to nonvariceal upper GI bleeding.

Blatchford score ≤1	• No need for endoscopy or • Refer to outpatient clinic and the endoscopy (≥24 hours) if not practical in due time, consider inpatient stay
Blatchford score >1 (≥7 predicts the need for endoscopic therapy)	*Prepare UGI endoscopy and start empiric pharmacological management:* • Nil by mouth • Erythromycin 250 mg IV and consider gastric lavage • PPI bolus + infusion – pantoprazole or esomeprazole 80 mg bolus, then 8 mg/h IV • Mortality rate – 10%

BOX 1: Prepare for UGI endoscopy and start empiric treatment (PPI).

Timing:
- Scientifically within 24 hours after hospital admission
- Blatchford score helps to stratify risk
- *Very early (≤12 hours) if:*
  - Persistent hemodynamic instability
  - Intrahospital active bleeding signs
  - Contraindication to anticoagulant suspension
- Early (up to 24 hours) in the remaining conditions

Preparation:
- Nil by mouth
- Erythromycin 250 g IV and consider gastric lavage
- PPI bolus + infusion – pantoprazole or esomeprazole 80 g bolus, 8 mg/h
  - UGI Endoscopy
  - Type of endoscopic lesion and endoscopic stigma of bleeding
  - Rockall score helps to stratify risk
  - Endoscopic treatment—hemostasis
  - Forrest classification, mortality, and rebleeding risk

TABLE 4: Rockall score.

Rockall score	Relapse risk (%)	Death risk (%)
0	4.9	0
1	3.4	0
2	5.3	0.2
3	11.2	2.9
4	14.1	5.3
5	24.1	10.8
6	32.9	17.3
7	43.8	27
≥8	41.8	41.1

TABLE 5: Forest classification.

Type of endoscopic lesion and endoscopic stigma of bleeding	Forest classification:
	• Acute hemorrhage
	  – *Forrest Ia:* Spurting hemorrhage
	  – *Forrest IIb:* Oozing hemorrhage
	• Signs of recurrent hemorrhage
	  – *Forrest IIc:* Flat pigmented hematin coffee ground base on ulcer base
	• Lesions without active bleeding
	  – *Forrest III:* Lesions without signs of recent hemorrhage or fibrin-covered clean ulcer base

If high-risk rebleeding lesions: • *Forest Ia, Ib, IIa:* High-risk stigma endoscopic hemostasis • *Forest IIb:* Careful clot removal and hemostasis versus PPI	• Indication for endoscopic hemostatic treatment • Dilute adrenalin injection, bipolar coagulation, TTS Clips, and argon plasma coagulation
Mortality and rebleeding risk	See Rockall score
If after endoscopic treatment first	• Refer to previous points • Second endoscopy and endoscopic treatment
Rebleeding	• Refer to previous points • Consider angiography, surgery or endoscopic rescue treatment, as hemospray or OTSC

TABLE 6: Forrest classification of nonvariceal upper gastrointestinal bleeding lesions and approximate prevalence.

Forrest class	Definition	Lesional risk of continued bleeding	Prevalence	Risk of rebleeding without endoscopic treatment	Medical treatment	Endoscopic treatment
Ia	Active spurting bleed	High-risk	7%	90–100% [including oozing bleed (Forrest 1b)]	High-dose PPI IV for 72 hours	Yes
Ib	Oozing bleed	High-risk	27%	80–85%	High-dose PPI IV for 72 hours	Yes
IIa	Nonbleeding visible vessel	High-risk	26%	40–50%	High-dose PPI IV for 72 hours	Yes
IIb	Adherent clot	High-risk	11%	20–30%	High-dose PPI IV for 72 hours	After clot removal
IIc	Flat-pigmented spot	Low-risk	4%	5%	Low-dose PPI PO	No
III	Clean-base ulcer	Low-risk	25%	3%	Low-dose PPI PO	No

Management of Gastrointestinal Bleeding

and triage of patients presenting with upper GI bleeding. Of these, following are most established and recommended.

- Blatchford Score at first-assessment (clinical score)
- The full Rockall score after endoscopy (clinical and endoscopy)

Choice of endoscopic hemostatic therapy for bleeding ulcers:
- Endoscopic hemostatic therapy is recommended with bipolar electrocoagulation, heater probe, or injection of absolute ethanol for patients with UGIB due to ulcers (strong recommendation, moderate-quality evidence).
- Endoscopic hemostatic therapy is recommended with clips, argon plasma coagulation, or soft monopolar electrocoagulation for patients with UGIB due to ulcers (conditional recommendation, very-low to low-quality evidence).
- It is recommended that epinephrine injection should not be used alone for patients with UGIB due to ulcers but rather in combination with another hemostatic modality (strong recommendation very-low-to-moderate-quality evidence).
- Endoscopic hemostatic therapy is recommended with hemostatic powder spray TC-325 for patients with actively bleeding ulcers (conditional recommendation, very-low-quality evidence).
- Over-the-scope clips as hemostatic therapy are suggested for patients who develop recurrent bleeding secondary to ulcers after previously successful endoscopic hemostasis (conditional recommendation, low-quality evidence).

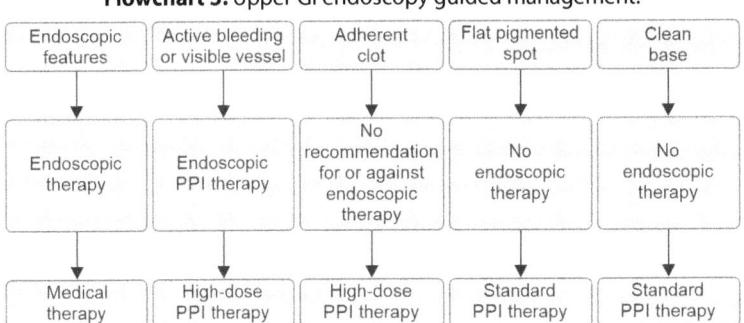

Flowchart 3: Upper GI endoscopy guided management.

Flowchart 4: Approach to lower GI bleeding.

Resuscitation and risk assessment

Oakland score

Age (Years)	Points
<40	0
40–69	1
≥70	2

Gender	Points
Female	0
Male	1

Previous LGB admission	
No	0
Yes	1

Digital rectal examination (DRE)	
No blood	0
Blood	1

Oakland score <8
- With no other indications for hospital admission
- Suitable for immediate discharge and outpatient investigation

Oakland score >8
- Prepare lower endoscopy

Systolic BP	Points
<90	5
90–119	4
120–129	3
130–159	2
≥160	0

Hemoglobin (bpm) points	Points
<7	22
7–8.9	17
9–10.9	13
11–12.9	8
13–15.9	4
≥16	0

Heart rate (bpm)	Points
<70	0
70–89	1
90–109	2
≥110	3

↓

Clinical history and physical examination

- Digital rectal examination is mandatory
- Assess severity
  - Heart rate
  - Blood pressure (BP)
  - Blood tests
    ◊ Hemoglobin
    ◊ Prothrombin time
    ◊ BUN and creatinine
      BUN/creatinine >30—consider UGIB
- Calculate Oakland score
- Risk factor for poor outcome

↓

Contd…

Contd...

```
Risk factors for poor outcome—consider
ICU admission
```

- Hemodynamic instability at admission
  - Heart rate >100
  - Systolic BP <100 mm Hg
  - Syncope
- Persistent bleeding
- Rebleeding
- Nontender abdomen
- History of diverticulosis or angiectasia
- High Charlson Comorbidity Index
- Age >60 years
- Laboratory alterations
  - Creatinine >1.7 mg/dL
  - Hematocrit <35%
  - PT >1.2 control
  - Hypoalbuminemia
- Current aspirin use

BOX 2: Approach to middle GI bleeding.

Overt gastrointestinal bleeding: Negative upper and lower endoscopy
- *Clinical assessment:* Clinical history and physical examination
- *Assess severity:*
  - Heart rate
  - Blood pressure
  - *Blood tests:*
    - Hemoglobin
    - Prothrombin time
    - Blood urea nitrogen (BUN) and creatinine
- Clinical history can suggest the etiology:
  - *Aortic stenosis:* Heyde syndrome
  - *Family history of cancer at an early age:* Lynch syndrome
  - *Telangiectasias of lips and/or oropharynx:* Rendu–Osler–Weber syndrome
  - *Herpetiform dermatitis:* Celiac disease
  - *History of abdominal and aortic aneurysm repair:* Aortoenteric fistula

Flowchart 5: To calculate shock index (SI).

> 1—unstable GI bleeding or suspected active bleeding:
- Consider UGIB—UGI endoscopy, if feasible (if patient is stable after initial resuscitation)
  - If possible, manage as appropriate (4)
- Perform CT angiogram (CTA) (If UGI endoscopy is not feasible or deemed unnecessary)
  - If positive:
    - Treatment with intervention radiology or endoscopic method:
      ◊ *Success:* Consider elective upper-to-lower GI (LGI) endoscopy
      ◊ *Failure:* Consider intervention radiology (after endoscopy attempt) or surgery
  - If negative, admit for LGI endoscopy.

SI >1, unstable GI bleeding or suspected active bleeding:
- Consider IGIB – UGI endoscopy

↓

SI >1 — Unstable GI bleeding or suspected active bleeding

- Consider IGIB — UGI endoscopy, if feasible (if patient is stable after initial resuscitation)
  - If positive – manage as appropriate
- Perform CT angiogram (CTA) (if UGI endoscopy not feasible or deemed unnecessary)
  - If positive:
    Treatment with intervention radiology or endoscopic method
    ◊ Success — consider elective upper or lower GI (LGI) endoscopy
    ◊ Failure — consider intervention radiology (after endoscopic attempt) or surgery
  - If negative — admit for LGI endoscopy

↓

SI = 1, stable GI bleeding

Calculate Oakland risk score:
- *Minor bleeding (Oakland ≤8):* Discharge, further investigation in outpatient department
- *Major bleeding (Oakland >8)*
  - Consider UGI endoscopy (15% of cases of suspected LGIB turn out to be UGIB)
  - If bright rectal bleeding, consider anorectal inspection
  - Admit for colonoscopy after antegrade preparation
    ◊ Ongoing bleeding and/or risk factors <24 hours
    ◊ Not ongoing bleeding and/or no risk factors, next available list
      ☐ If a lesion is found, treat endoscopically
      ☐ If no lesion is found:
        Further bleeding: CTA, capsule endoscopy RBC scintigraphy
        No further bleeding: Discharge and follow-up

↓

Individual variables

Contd...

Contd...

- Ongoing bleeding
- SBP <100 mm Hg
- Prothrombin time >1.2 control
- Altered mental status
- Unstable comorbid illness (any organ system abnormality that ordinarily would require ICU admission)

↓

UGI endoscopy

- Type of endoscopic lesion and endoscopic stigmata of bleeding
- Endoscopic treatment—hemostasis
- BLEED—rebleeding and mortality risk

↓

Type of endoscopic lesion and endoscopic stigma of bleeding	• Diverticula with active bleeding • Bleeding hemorrhoids • Anal fissure • Polyps/postpolypectomy • Carcinoma • Angiodysplasia • Dieulatory lesion • Rectal or colonic ulcers • Active colitis (ischemic, infectious, inflammatory, and radiation-induced)
If high-risk bleeding lesions	• Indication for endoscopic hemostatic treatment • Pharmacological—dilute adrenalin injection and sclerosing agents (conditional use) • Thermal—bipolar coagulation and argon plasma coagulation • Mechanical—endoscopic hemoclips and ligation
Second rebleeding	• Consider angiography, surgery or endoscopic rescue treatment as hemospray or over-the-scope clips (OTSC)
Red flag signs	• For endoscopic treatment, mechanical methods are preferable (higher risk of perforation with thermal method) • Surgery without previous identification of the bleeding or, at least, of the exact location of bleeding to be reviewed as the last recourse—high mortality

Flowchart 6: Suspected variceal lower GI bleeding.

> *Immediately start:*
> Vasoactive drugs and prepare for endoscopy

↓

> Exclude variceal upper GI bleeding

> Start vasoactive and other relevant drugs
> *Vasoactive drugs:*
> Drugs doses:
> - *Terlipressin:* 1–2 mg IV 6/6 hours up to 4/4 hours until bleeding controls, then 1 mg in 4/4 hours to avoid rebleeding during 2–5 days
> - *Somatostatin* bolus 250 µg/h (3 mg/50, α, 4 cc/h) during 2–5 days
> - *Octreotide* bolus 50 µg IV, perfusion 50 µg/h (600 µg/50, 4 cc/h) during 2–5 days
> - *PPI:* Pantoprazole 40 mg IV q12 hours
> - *Ceftriaxone* prophylaxis doses 1 g IV per day up to 7 days
> - Preferred in advanced cirrhosis and cases of high guideline resistance
> - *Erythromycin* 250 mg IV 30–120 minutes before in absence of contraindications as QT prolongation
> - *Lactulose* 25 mL q12h titrate to 2–3 bowel movement or enema if no oral or enteric route

↓

> Variceal lower gastrointestinal bleeding

↓

> Lower GI endoscopy

- *If confirmation of variceal hemorrhage:*
  - Endoscopic therapy (sclerotherapy, variceal band ligation, or cyanoacrylate injection)
  - Maintain vasoactive drugs (3–5 days) and antibiotic prophylaxis
- *If massive bleeding:* Abdominal angiography with intravascular embolization or surgery

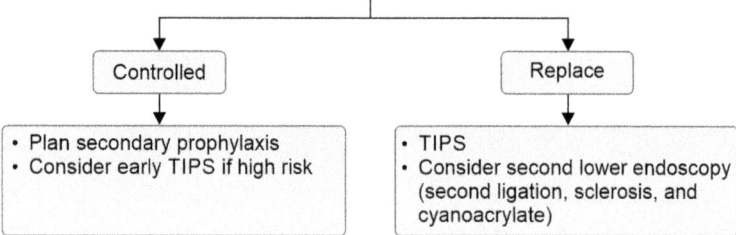

Controlled	Replace
• Plan secondary prophylaxis • Consider early TIPS if high risk	• TIPS • Consider second lower endoscopy (second ligation, sclerosis, and cyanoacrylate)

If feasible, perform heart echocardiography before cyanoacrylate injection

Management of Gastrointestinal Bleeding

Flowchart 7: Hemodynamic status.

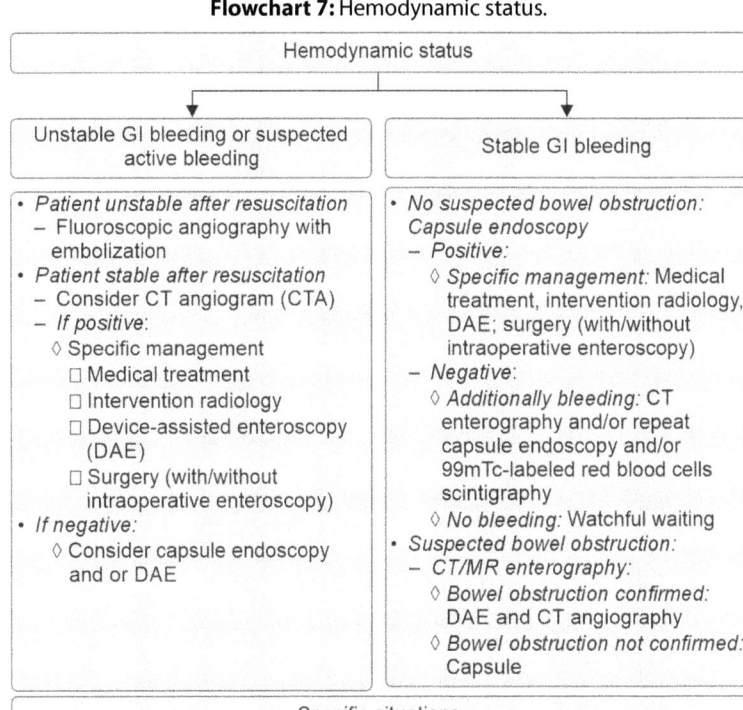

Patients with GI tract bypass: DAE could be necessary to evaluate the excluded luminal segment.
Suspected Meckel's diverticulum:
Consider ^{99m}Tc-pertechnetate scan, particularly if:
- Negative endoscopic examination (capsule endoscopy and/or DAE)
- Negative CT angiography/CT enterography

Heyde's syndrome: Aortic valve replacement or repair
Multiple small bowel angiodysplasias:
- Endoscopic treatment
- If failure/rebleeding: Consider medical treatment including octreotide or thalidomide

TABLE 7: Anticoagulation management in GIB.

VKA (po)
- Evaluate INR: INR >2
- Do not delay endoscopy if (INR ≤1.5)

- Discontinue VKA
- Vitamin K 5–10 IV
- PCC 15–30 IU/kg IV

DOAC (po)
- Evaluate type, dose, time from last intake
- Evaluate coagulation and renal clearance

- Discontinue DOAC
- Last intake <2–4 hours: Oral
- Dialysis: Dabigatran

- Dabigatran
- Idarucizumab 2 × 2.5 g IV

LMWH
- Discontinue perfusion
- Protamine sulphate 1 mg/1 mg enoxaparin

- FXa inhibitors
- PCC: 25–30 IU/kg IV

Heparin (IV)
- Consider UFH or LMWH

UFH
- Discontinue perfusion
- Protamine sulphate 1 mg/100 IU heparin

TABLE 8: Antiplatelet management in GIB.

Antiplatelet therapy (APT)	Acetylsalicylic acid (Aspirin)	Thienopyridines
• Aspirin • Thienopyridines • Double therapy (DAPT)	Do not discontinue (In consultation with cardiologists)	Discontinue + Platelet concentrate (PC) (1 pool of PC or 1 platelet apheresis unit/ 60–70 kg) in cases of severe GIB (individualized approach)

TABLE 9: Resumption of antiplatelets (APT) after bleeding in patients with coronary stent/ACS.

High or very high thrombotic risk (ACS or stenting <30 days)	Minor or major bleeding	• Suggest maintaining aspirin at small dose without interruption • Consider restarting second API drug as soon as possible, after stabilization
Moderate thrombotic risk (ACS or PCI with 2nd generation DES application at 1–12 months before)	Minor or major bleeding	• Suggest restarting aspirin at small dose, as controlled, preferable within 3 days • Consider restarting the second APT, if thrombotic risk is higher than bleeding risk
If patient has bleeding both with DAPT and after new-generation DES application	Within 3 months	Consider restarting DPT until 3 months
	After 3 months and if maintains recurrent bleeding risk	Consider restarting only one APT (aspirin or clopidogrel)
Biovascular scaffolds (BVS) Bioabsorbable DES plus bleeding	—	• *Patients with ACS under DAPT developing major bleeding:* Only one APT should be considered, according to absence of risk of stent thrombosis • DAPT can be necessary until 12 months after BVS application

Flowchart 8: Coagulopathies related to GI bleeding.

Massive bleeding transfusion

↓

- *Blood loss:* TBV/24 hours or >50% of the TBV/3 hours
- *Transfusion:* 3 PRBC/1 hour; 4 PRBC in <4 hours and hemodynamic instability, ±anticipated ongoing bleeding; ≥10 PRBC/24 hours
- *Ongoing bleeding:* 150 mL/min; 1.5 mL/kg/min in 20 min
- Plus circulatory insufficiency besides all resuscitation/fluid therapy

↓

Packed red blood cell (PRBC):
- *Trigger:* Hb <7 g/dL; <8 g/dL, if heart disease
- In nonmassive GIB, a restrictive strategy of RBC transfusion is recommended

↓

Bleeding persists, despite control of previous conditions?
PRBC
1–2 PRBC units according to clinical situation
Continuous Hb monitoring can be used as a trend monitor (Evidence C)
Maintain target:
Hb: 7–9 g/dL and 8–10 g//dL
In patients without and with heart disease (Grade 1A), even during active bleeding (Grade 2C)

↓

- Clinical suspicion of hyperfibrinolysis (HF), e.g., GI-bleeding ulcer, acute bleeding, and LD
- Confirmation of HF may be done by ROTEM analysis
  - EXTEM ML ≥15% of FIBTEM ML ≥10% (L160 ≤85%)
  - EXTEM LI30 and APTEM T
  - APTEM LI30 and ML better than in EXTEM LI30 and ML (>25% improvement)

↓

YES

↓

Tranexamic acid (TXA):
- *Loading dose:* 1 g IV/10 min
- Maintenance 1 g IV/8 hours severe bleeding in GIB, TXA reduces mortality but not rebleeding

↓

Consider fibrinogen deficiency:
- Fibrinogen <1.5–2.0 g/L and/or
- Blood loss ≥1.0–1.5 L and ongoing bleeding
- Confirm by ROTEM analysis if possible

↓

YES

↓

Fibrinogen concentrate (FC)
Initial dose: 25–50 mg/kg (Grade 2C)

Contd...

Contd...

Thrombocytopenia/platelet dysfunction (PDF)
- Platelet <50 × 10/L
- *PD:* Liver cirrhosis, Child–Pugh B/C, renal disease, APT, and vWD

↓
| YES |
↓

Platelet concentrate (PC)
1 PC pool or 1 platelet apheresis unit per 60–70 kg

↓

Acute uremic bleeding or acquired bleeding disorders with induced PDF:
- Associated with renal disease (Grade 2C) and APT (Grade 2C)
- PD usually not evaluated only by clinical decision according to renal function (CrC) and bleeding severity assessment
- *Caution:* Pediatric/geriatric patients because of its antidiuretic effects, to avoid fluid overload and electrolyte abnormalities ($\downarrow Na^+$)

↓
| YES |
↓

Desmopressin (DDAVP):
- 0.3 µg/kg/50–100 mL saline 0.9% IV, over 30 minutes as a single dose; maximum dose—24 µg
  Note: DDAVP—pick effect after 30–60 minutes (IV) testing only 6 g; loose efficacy if repeated within 12–24 hours

↓

- If severe bleeding and multiple blood components were transfused, especially in an ongoing bleeding and liver cirrhosis
- If ionized calcium (Ca^+) <1.2, if magnesium is low

↓
| YES |
↓

Calcium chloride:
- 0.5–1.0 g IV per 500 mL of transfused blood
  Magnesium sulfate

↓

Consider deficit of other coagulation factors (thrombin formation deficit):
- TP/INR or aPTT >1.5 × normal and acute/active bleeding + acute liver failure (ALF) (Grade 2C), LD
- Volume blood loss: ≥150–200% (≥1.5 TBV)
                    <100% (<10 TBV) in liver disease

↓
| YES |
↓

Contd...

Contd...

↓

Prothrombin complex concentrate (PCC)
20–30 IU/kg
Vitamin K (10–20 mg)
If deficiency, especially if decompensated liver cirrhosis or/and
Fresh frozen plasma (FFP)
Initially, 10–15 mL/kg; if severe bleeding up to 20 mL/kg
Note: Must be volume restrictive, because fluid overload increases portal hypertension/worsens bleeding

↓

If variceal bleeding

↓

Consider (Factor V) and natural anticoagulant deficit:
- Suspicion by underlying clinical disease and bleeding severity
- Levels are usually low in LD, mainly in cirrhosis, Child–Pugh C, and ALF
- FV <25% and severe acute/bleeding

↓

YES

↓

FFP
Up to 12 mL/kg
In these situations, FEP (↓FV) and FC (↓Fib.) can be associated to PCC to improve clinical efficacy
Note: Must be volume-restrictive, because fluid overload increases portal hypertension/worsens bleeding
Bleeding persists, despite control of the above conditions

↓

For all types of gastrointestinal bleeding

↓

Consider FXIII deficit (clot instability not related to HF)
- Consider that FXIII activity is likely to be critically reduced (<30–<60%) in cases of ongoing or diffuse bleeding and low clot strength (clot instability) not related with hyperfibrinolysis and despite adequate fib. concentration

↓

FFP
12–20 mL/kg
or
FXIII concentrate
30 IU/kg or 1.250 IU

↓

Bleeding persists, despite control of the above conditions?
Persistent bleeding (uncontrollable)? → rVIIa *"Life-threatening bleeding"*
- *Previously correct:* HF, pH, Ca^{2+}, temperature, fibrinogen, and platelets
- *Without heparin effect (ROTEM and VET)*

↓

YES

↓

Contd...

Management of Gastrointestinal Bleeding

Contd...

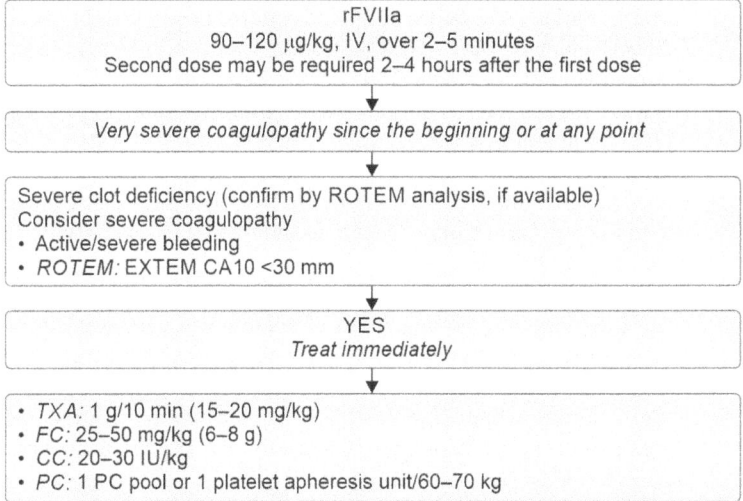

Flowchart 9: Overview of GI bleeding management approach.

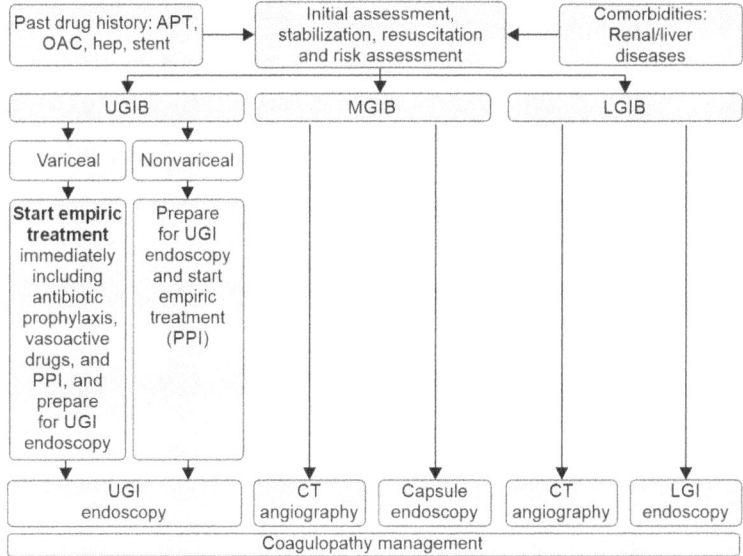

(APT: antiaggregant platelet therapy; CT: computed tomography; Hep: heparin; LGI: lower gastrointestinal; LGIB: lower gastrointestinal bleeding; MGIB: middle gastrointestinal bleeding; OAC: oral anticoagulant; PPI: proton pump inhibitor; UGI: upper gastrointestinal; UGIB: upper gastrointestinal bleeding)

SUGGESTED READING

1. Laine L, Barkun AN, Saltzman JR. Martel M, Leontiadis GI. ACG Clinical Guideline: Upper Gastrointestinal and ulcer bleeding. Am J Gastroenterol. 2021;116(5):899-917.
2. Lau JY. The value of risk scores to predict clinical outcomes in patients with variceal and nonvariceal upper gastrointestinal bleeding. Clin Endosc. 2021;54(2):145-6.
3. Lau JYW, Yu Y, Tang RSY, Chan HCH, Yip HC, Chan SM, et al. Timing of endoscopy for acute upper gastrointestinal bleeding. N Engl J Med. 2020;382(14):1299-308.
4. Oakland K, Chadwick G, East JE, Guy R, Humphries A, Jairath V, et al. Diagnosis and management of acute lower gastrointestinal bleeding: Guidelines from the British Society of Gastroenterology. Gut. 2019;68(5):776-89.
5. Padhi S, Kemmis-betty S, Rajesh S, Hill J, Murphy MF; Guideline Development Group. Blood transfusion: Summary of NICE Guidance. BMJ. 2015;351:h5832.
6. Rodrigues A, Carrilho A, Almeida N, Baldaia C, Alves Â, Gomes M, et al. Interventional algorithm in Gastrointestinal Bleeding: An Expert Consensus Multimodal Approach Based on a Multidisciplinary Team. Clin Appl Thromb Hemost. 2020;26:1-19.
7. Wuerth BA, Rockey DC. Changing epidemiology of upper gastrointestinal hemorrhage in the last decade: A nationwide analysis. Dig Dis Sci. 2018;63(5):1286-93.

20 CHAPTER

Stroke

Soumitra Kumar, Jayanta Roy

Stroke is the second leading cause of death worldwide (9.5% cause of all deaths) and the leading cause of adult disability. World Health Organization (WHO) has defined stroke as "rapidly developing clinical signs of focal (or global) disturbance of cerebral function, with symptoms lasting 24 hours or longer or leading to death, with no apparent cause other than of vascular origin". This definition proved useful for decades in clinical as well as epidemiological studies. Stroke can be of two types—ischemic and hemorrhagic. Ischemic stroke can be arterial or venous in origin. Hemorrhagic stroke includes bleed in the brain parenchyma, within the ventricle or into the subarachnoid space.

In this chapter, management of ischemic stroke and intracerebral hemorrhage (ICH) has been discussed. Treatment of subarachnoid bleed will not be discussed here.

Stroke is one of the leading causes of disability and death in India. The estimated adjusted prevalence rates of stroke are between 84 and 262 strokes per 100,000 persons in rural areas and between 334 and 424 strokes per 100,000 persons in urban areas.

Stroke incidence and mortality are higher in Asian countries than in western countries.

ISCHEMIC STROKE

Pre-hospital Evaluation and Triaging

There is a need to generate a mass stroke awareness program to help identify symptoms of stroke. The facial drooping, arm weakness, speech difficulties, and onset time (FAST) test can help detect and improve reaction to stroke patient awareness, thereby reducing the door-to-needle time.

The Cincinnati Pre-hospital Stroke Scale is an attempt at simplifying 15-item National Institutes of Health Stroke Scale (NIHSS) and evaluates the presence or absence of facial palsy, asymmetric arm weakness, and speech abnormalities in potential stroke patients.

The Los Angeles Pre-hospital Stroke Screen (LAPSS) is a longer instrument consisting of four history items, blood glucose measurement, and three examination items designed to detect unilateral motor weakness (facial droop, hand grip, and arm strength). Based on the results of a few studies, LAPSS demonstrated identification of acute cerebral ischemia and ICH with a high degree of sensitivity or specificity.

The most widely used causative system is the Trial of Org 101.72 in acute stroke treatment (TOAST) classification. With the advances in modification system (CCS) and Chinese ischemic stroke sub-classifications (CISS) system, have been developed to enhance he accuracy of TOAST. The A-S-C-O (Atherosclerosis, Small-vessel disease, Cardiac source, other cause) phenotypic classification system makes efforts to identify the most likely etiology but not neglecting the possibility of other potential multiple causes.

The recommendations regarding the ideal time for each step have been presented in **Table 1**.

Door-to-Needle Time (Door-to-Groin Puncture Time)

Definitive management with thrombolysis is the only effective treatment for eligible acute ischemic stroke patients coming within 4.5 hours of symptoms onset with improved functional outcomes at 3 and 6 months.

For every 15-minute reduction of the door-to-needle time (arrival to emergency room to thrombolysis), there is 5% lower odds of in-hospital mortality. In patients with a door-to-needle time of ≤60 minutes, the unadjusted mortality rate was 8.6% versus 10.4% in patients with a door-to-needle time of >60 minutes ($p < 0.0001$).

The Recognition of Stroke in the Emergency Room (ROSIER) tool incorporates all FAST items and additionally examines visual field deficit, leg weakness, loss of consciousness or syncope, and seizure activity. A ROSIER score, the total of all seven items, of ≥1 suggests a stroke or TIA, whereas a ROSIER score of ≤0 indicates no stroke.

TABLE 1: Major etiologic classification systems for ischemic stroke.

Publication year	TOAST (1993)	CCS (2007)	A-S-C-O (2009)	CISS (2011)
Type of system	Causative	Causative and phenotypic	Phenotypic	Causative
Major subtypes	1. Large artery	1. Supra-aortic large artery atherosclerosis	1. Atherosclerosis	1. Large artery atherosclerosis
	2. Cardioembolism	2. Cardio-aortic embolism	2. Cardioembolism	2. Cardiogenic stroke
	3. Small vessel occlusion	3. Small artery occlusion	3. Small vessel disease	3. Penetrating artery disease
	4. Other determined etiology	4. Other causes	4. Other causes	4. Other etiologies
	5. Undetermined etiology	5. Undetermined cause		5. Undetermined etiology

Complications of Late Diagnosis and Treatment

In an acute ischemic stroke, very large numbers of neurons, synapses, and nerve fibers are beyond the scope of retrieved every moment when untreated. Quantitative estimates of the speed of neural circuitry loss in human ischemic stroke underscores the time urgency of acute stroke care. A typical patient with untreated stroke loses 1.9 million neurons each minute. Compared with the normal rate of neuron loss in brain aging, the ischemic brain ages at the rate of 3.6 years each hour in absence of definitive treatment. For every 15-minute reduction of the door-to-needle time (arrival to emergency room to thrombolysis), there is a 5% lower odds of in-hospital mortality. Each 15-minute reduction in treatment delay can provide an average equivalent of 1 month of additional disability-free life.

Of the five stent retriever studies, two studies demonstrated a 6-hour window after stroke onset while the third study specified 6 hours to start treatment. Time-dependent data available from the Multicenter Randomized Clinical Trial of Endovascular Treatment for Acute Ischemic Stroke (MR CLEAN) study demonstrated absence of benefit of treatment beginning after 6 hours.

Transient Ischemic Attack

The arbitrary nature of the 24-hour time limit and lack of specific pathophysiologic contraindication lead to reduction to the 1-hour time limit and later on further led to a tissue-based definition driven by advances in neuroimaging. As per the AHA-endorsed revised definition, transient ischemic attack (TIA) is defined as "a transient episode of neurologic dysfunction" caused by focal cerebral, spinal cord, or retinal ischemia, without acute infarction.

ACUTE TRANSIENT EVENT (TRANSIENT ISCHEMIC ATTACK) MANAGEMENT

This topic covers the management of a TIA from the initiation of first symptoms suggesting a possible onset of an acute cerebrovascular event. In people who have a history of TIA, the incidence of subsequent stroke is as high as 11% over the next 7 days and 24–29%

over the following 5 years. Several studies have demonstrated the relation between TIA and an accentuated long-term stroke risk. The short-term risk of stroke has also been demonstrated to be particularly high, exceeding 10% in a span of 90 days.

- Patients with a suspected TIA should be assessed as soon as possible in view of the risk of subsequent stroke by using a validated scoring system such as *ABCD*. This score can be assessed even by a nurse or a primary physician.

  ABCD2 score:
  - Age ≥60 years (+1)   Duration of symptoms <10 minutes
  - BP ≥140/90 (+1)   Duration of symptoms 10–15 minutes + 1 >60 minutes + 2
  - *Clinical features of TIA:*

    For example, unilateral (+2) Weakness (+2)/speech turbulence (+1)/others (0) – history of diabetes +1

- *Patients with suspected TIA who are at a high risk of stroke (an ABCD2 score of 4 or above) should receive:*
  - Aspirin or clopidogrel (each as a 300 mg loading dose and 75 mg thereafter) and statin immediately.
  - Admission to a hospital for observation and investigations.
  - Specialist assessment and investigation (carotid Doppler, echocardiogram) within 24 hours of onset of symptoms.
  - Adequate measures for secondary prevention introduced as soon as a specific risk factor is identified.
- *Patients with crescendo TIA (two or more TIAs in a week), atrial fibrillation or those on anticoagulants should be treated as being at high risk of stroke* even though they may have an ABCD2 score of 3 or less.
- *Patients with suspected TIA who are at low risk of stroke (e.g., ABCD2 score of 3 or below) should receive:*
  - Aspirin or clopidogrel (each as a 300 mg loading dose and 75 mg thereafter) and a statin, e.g., simvastatin/atorvastatin/rosuvastatin 40 mg started immediately
  - Specialist assessment and investigations as soon as possible, but not >1 week of onset of symptoms.

- Measures of secondary prevention to be instituted as soon as the diagnosis is confirmed, including discussion of the individual risk factors.
- *In patients who have a suspected TIA who require brain imaging (that is, those in whom vascular territory or pathology is uncertain) should be subjected to undergo diffusion-weighted MRI and CT scan.*

GENERAL MANAGEMENT AND SUPPORTIVE CARE OF ISCHEMIC STROKE

Definitive Treatment

Intravenous Thrombolysis

Recombinant tissue-type plasminogen activator: Intravenous recombinant tissue-type plasminogen activator remains the only approved treatment globally for patients within the first 4.5 hours of the onset of acute stroke. Recombinant t-PA was first approved in 1996 based on the results of a two-part National Institute of Neurological Disorder and Stroke (NINDS) rtPA Study for use within the first 3 hours after the onset of stroke. Four subsequent trials, the European Cooperative Acute Stroke Study (ECASS I and ECASS II) and the Alteplase Thrombolysis for Acute Non-interventional Therapy in Ischemic Stroke (ATLANTIS A and B) showed results similar to the NINDS study. In a pooled individual patient level analysis of these four trials, a benefit of therapy in the 3- to 4.5-hour window was observed. The results of ECASS III trials showed improved outcomes for carefully selected patients treated 3-4.5 hours after a stroke. The Third International Stroke Trial (IST-3) demonstrated some benefit of IV rtPA administered within 6 hours of symptom onset. A meta- analysis of 12 IV rtPA trials with 7,012 enrolled patients confirmed the benefits of IV rtPA administered within 6 hours from symptom onset [odds ratio (OR), 1.17; 95% confidence interval (CI), 1.06–1.29; $p = 0.001$] compared with placebo, and reinforced the importance of timely treatment by showing highest benefit in patients treated within 3 hours from symptom onset (OR, 1.53; 95% CI, 1.26–1.86; $p < 0.0001$).

Treatment with IV rtPA initiated within 1.5 hours of symptom onset was associated with an OR of 2.81 (95% CI, 1.75-4.50) for beneficial outcome at 3 months compared with placebo. The OR for favorable outcome at 3 months for treatment with IV rtPA initiated within 1.5-3 hours was 1.55 (95% CI, 1.12-2.15) compared with 1.40 (95% CI, 1.05-1.85) within 3-4.5 hours and 1.15 (95% CI, 0.90-1.47) within 4.5-6 hours. The clinical trial evidence indicates the vital importance of minimizing the total ischemic time and restoring blood flow to jeopardized but not yet infarcted tissue as soon as possible.

The ECASS I predicted an increased risk of cerebral hemorrhage and poor clinical outcomes in patients with early signs or infarction in more than one-thirds of the MCA territory and undergoing IV thrombolysis within 6 hours of stroke onset. Ischemia involving more than one-thirds of the MCA territory on images obtained within the 0- to 6-hour window implies a relative contraindication to IV thrombolytic therapy.

All three randomized stroke trials [NINDS, Echoplanar imaging thrombolytic evaluation trial (EPITHET), and Third International Stroke Trial (IST-3)] that included patients ≥80 years of age provided evidence of the benefits of alteplase for elderly patients with acute ischemic strokes. Evidence from these clinical trials suggested that there should be no upper limit of the NIHSS score for patients otherwise eligible for alteplase presenting to medical attention within 3 hours of onset of symptoms. The ECASS III trial included thrombolytic therapy in the extended window period from 3 to 4.5 hours with the addition of four exclusion criteria: (1) Age >80 years, (2) NIHSS score >25, (3) history of diabetes and prior stroke, and (4) taking oral anticoagulants. Prevalence of symptomatic intracranial hemorrhage (sICH) is variable (0-36%) but is overall higher in patients taking anticoagulants despite sub-therapeutic INR at the time of thrombolysis.

RECOMMENDATIONS FOR THROMBOLYTIC THERAPY

- Intravenous alteplase should not be administered to patients whose CT reveals any type of acute intracranial hemorrhage.

- IV alteplase (0.9 mg/kg; maximum dose 90 mg) is recommended for selected patients who may be treated within 3 hours of onset of ischemic stroke.
- IV alteplase is recommended for administration to patients in the time window of 3-4.5 hours after stroke onset taking into account additional exclusion criteria: age >80 years, NIHSS score >25, history of diabetes and prior stroke, and those taking oral anticoagulants.
- For patients with severe stroke and those with mild but disabling stroke symptoms, IV alteplase is indicated within 3 hours of symptom onset of ischemic stroke.
- In patients eligible for IV alteplase, benefit of therapy is time dependent, and treatment should be initiated soonest. The door-to-needle time should be <60 minutes from arrival at hospital (emergency department).
- IV alteplase may be used in patients who have a history of warfarin use and an INR of ≤1.7 but not in those with an INR of >1.7.
- In patients who have received a dose of low molecular weight heparin (LMWH) within the previous 24 hours, IV alteplase is contraindicated.
- The use of IV alteplase in patients taking direct thrombin inhibitors and direct factor Xa inhibitors has not been firmly established and relevant laboratory investigation must be consulted to assess the residual anticoagulant effect.
- IV rtPA may be considered reasonable in some cases if patients have a normal thrombin time (TT), activated partial thromboplastin time (aPTT), and prothrombin time (PT), but this should be assessed by further research.

TENECTEPLASE

The study of tenecteplase versus alteplase for thrombolysis (clot dissolving) in acute ischemic stroke
"NOR-TEST" has been of the recent trials to be presented.
Three phase II trials have evaluated the efficacy and safety of tenecteplase in doses of 0.1, 0.25, and 0.4 mg/kg against alteplase in acute ischemic stroke. A meta-analysis of these trials ($n = 291$)

showed no significant difference between any dose of tenecteplase and alteplase for either efficacy or safety endpoints. 1,107 ischemic stroke patients were randomly assigned to tenecteplase, 0.4 mg/kg bolus, or alteplase, 0.9 mg/kg infusion within 4.5 hours of symptom onset. The drugs were comparable on outcomes using modified Rankin score 0-1 suggesting no major difference between two drugs. The rates of intracerebral hemorrhage were similar in two groups. TRACE 2 and ACT trials (both phase three trials) recently provided robust results that 0.25 mg/kg tenecteplase was not inferior to alteplase with a similar safety profile within 4.5 hours of symptom onset. Latest 2023 European Stroke Organization guideline has strongly recommended that 0.25 mg/kg tenecteplase can be used as an alternative to 0.3 mg/kg alteplase for patients with acute ischemic stroke or stroke due to large vessel obstruction (LVO) within 4.5 hours of onset. One of the major advantages of tenecteplase is its ease of its administration. Recent trials have provided evidence for extension of time window for tenecteplase up to 12 hours, using advanced imaging techniques for patient selection. Further studies are needed for its use in an extended treatment window (4.5-24 hours), in minor strokes and in combination with endovascular therapy.

ENDOVASCULAR REVASCULARIZATION RECOMMENDATIONS

Early reperfusion is vital for the good outcome of reperfusion therapy. The recanalization efficacy of IV rtPA is not as high as that of endovascular treatment especially when there is occlusion of larger intracranial arteries such as the internal carotid artery (ICA) or proximal MCA. A recanalization rate of only 6% and 30% was observed with IV rtPA in the terminal ICA and M1, respectively.

In addition, a large proportion of patients still present >4.5 hours after the onset of stroke symptoms and are thereby excluded from rtPA therapy. These limitations of rtPA therapy have necessitated widespread use of endovascular therapy to treat patients having contraindications for rtPA therapy to improve recanalization rates. Especially in the Indian context, endovascular therapy is one of the viable options because of poor availability of resources and delayed presentation (outside door-to-needle window period) after stroke onset. However, dearth of available facilities and scarcity of competent operators remain an obstacle.

Endovascular revascularization includes intra-arterial fibrinolysis, mechanical clot retrieval with the Mechanical Embolus Removal in Cerebral Ischemia (MERCI) Retrieval System (Concentric Medical, Inc, Mountain View, CA, USA), mechanical clot aspiration with the Penumbra System (Penumbra, Inc, Alameda, CA, USA), and acute angioplasty and stenting. Different intra-arterial agents have been used for thrombolytic treatment of acute ischemic stroke. These include tissue plasminogen activator (tPA), urokinase (UK), and pro-urokinase (pro-UK). Mechanical thrombectomy devices are classified into two major groups based on their mechanism of action—those that use an approach distal (retrievers) or proximal to thrombi (aspiration devices). The MERCI was the first stroke mechanical thrombectomy device approved by the FDA in 2004. The aspiration devices include the Penumbra System (Penumbra Inc.), the QuickCat (DSM Inc., PA, USA), and PRONTO (Vascular Solutions Inc., MN, USA) extraction devices.

Recent times have seen completion of major trials of endovascular therapy leading to its acceptance as a treatment for proximal large vessel occlusive stroke. A meta-analysis of eight trials included 1,313 patients who underwent endovascular thrombectomy and 1,110 patients who received standard medical care with tPA. Endovascular therapy was associated with a significant proportional treatment benefit across modified Rankin scale (mRS) scores. Functional independence at 90 days (mRS score, 0-2) occurred among 557 of 1,293 patients (44.6%; 95% CI, 36.6-52.8%) in the endovascular therapy group versus 351 of 1094 patients (31.8%; 95% CI, 24.6-40.0%) in the standard medical care group. Compared with standard medical care, endovascular thrombectomy was associated with significantly higher rates of angiographic revascularization at 24 hours $p < 0.001$) but no significant difference in rates of symptomatic intracranial hemorrhage within 90 days [70 events (5.7%) vs. 53 events (5.1%); OR, 1.12; 95% CI, 0.77-1.63; $p = 0.56$] or all-cause mortality at 90 days.

Recommendations

- All patients eligible for IV thrombolysis should receive IV rtPA even if endovascular treatments have a scope.
- Reduction in time from symptom onset to reperfusion with endovascular therapies is associated with better clinical outcomes. Achievement of reperfusion to thrombolysis in cerebral infarction (TICI) grade 2b/3 as early as possible and within 6 hours of stroke onset may ensure benefit.
- Patients should receive endovascular therapy with a stent retriever if they meet all the following criteria:
  - Pre-stroke mRS score 0–1,
  - Acute ischemic stroke receiving IV rtPA within 4.5 hours of onset according to guidelines from professional medical societies,
  - Causative occlusion of the ICA or proximal MCA (M1),
  - Age ≥18 years,
  - NIHSS score ≥6,
  - ASPECTS score ≥6, and
  - Treatment can be initiated (groin puncture) within 6 hours of symptom onset.
- When treatment is initiated beyond 6 hours from symptom onset, the effectiveness of endovascular therapy becomes uncertain for patients with acute ischemic stroke who have established occlusion of the ICA or proximal MCA (M1).
- In properly selected patients with anterior circulation occlusion who have contraindications to IV rtPA, endovascular therapy with stent retrievers completed within 6 hours of stroke onset is deemed reasonable.
- The technical target of the thrombectomy procedure should be a TICI 2b/3 angiographic result, so as to maximize the probability of a good functional clinical outcome.
- If endovascular therapy is contemplated, a noninvasive intracranial vascular study is strongly recommended during the initial imaging evaluation but IV rtPA should not be delayed (if indicated in eligible patients).
- When mechanical thrombectomy is pursued, stent retrievers such as Solitaire and Trevo are generally preferred to coil

retrievers such as MERCI. The relative effectiveness of the Penumbra system versus stent retrievers has not been clarified.

ROLE OF ANTICOAGULANTS

Anticoagulants are prescribed in an effort to prevent first or recurrent stroke, especially in patients with cardio-embolism due to valvular atrial fibrillation, Rheumatic mitral stenosis (moderate to severe) and mechanical prosthetic valve. Several clinical trials have demonstrated increased risk of bleeding complication with early administration of unfractionated heparin or LMWH. Early administration of anticoagulants does not show reduction in risk of early neurological worsening or early recurrent stroke. Early anticoagulation reduction in risk of early neurological worsening or early recurrent stroke. Early anticoagulation should be avoided when potential contraindications to anticoagulation are present, such as a large infarction (based on clinical syndrome or brain imaging findings), uncontrolled hypertension, or other bleeding conditions. Nonvitamin K antagonists (dabigatran, rivaroxaban, apixaban, and edoxaban) have been shown to prevent stroke or systemic embolization in patients with atrial fibrillation and have been approved by the US FDA for preventing stroke and systemic embolism in patients with atrial fibrillation.

Recommendations

- Urgent anticoagulation, with the goal of preventing early recurrent stroke, halting neurological worsening, or improving outcomes after acute ischemic stroke, is not recommended for the treatment of patients with acute ischemic stroke.
- Initiation of anticoagulant therapy within 24 hours of treatment with IV rtPA is not recommended.

ANTIPLATELETS

Various oral antiplatelet agents including aspirin, clopidogrel, and dipyridamole are in routine use for treatment of acute ischemic stroke. CAST and IST trial showed reduced early recurrence and improved outcome in acute ischemic stroke if aspirin 325 mg per day has been initiated with 48 hours of onset. Early treatment with aspirin plus extended release dipyridamole for TIA or ischemic stroke within 24 hours of symptom onset (EARLY) trial and Fast Assessment of Stroke and Transient Ischemic Attack to Prevent Early Recurrence (FASTER) trial suggested that in patients who received fibrinolytic therapy, both early and late initiation of antithrombotic therapy for the secondary prevention of recurrent stroke appeared to be safe.

However, data regarding usefulness of other antiplatelet agents, including clopidogrel alone or in combination with aspirin, for treatment of acute ischemic stroke are limited and those assessing safety of antiplatelet agents when given within 24 hours of IV fibrinolysis are lacking. The relative indications for the long-term administration of antiplatelet agents to prevent recurrent stroke are included in various guidelines and advisory statements. Inhibitors of the platelet glycoprotein IIb/IIIa receptor such as abciximab and other parenterally administered glycoprotein IIb/IIIa receptor blockers are being evaluated in patients with acute ischemic stroke. However, more research is needed to determine the role of these agents in acute ischemic stroke management.

Recommendations
- Oral administration of aspirin (initial dose of 325 mg) within 24-48 hours after acute ischemic stroke onset is recommended as part of overall management.
- Administration of aspirin (or other antiplatelet agents) as an adjunctive therapy is recommended after 24 hours of IV tPA.

SURGICAL INTERVENTIONS
Carotid Endarterectomy

Carotid endarterectomy (CEA) involves removal of the source of thromboembolic debris resulting in reduction in stroke recurrence and restoration of normal perfusion pressure to the ischemic penumbra in the brain. Delay in intervention may reduce the potential benefit of revascularization. However, early intervention may also lead to transformation of ischemic infarction to hemorrhagic infarction and increased edema or hyperfusion syndrome from sudden restoration of normal perfusion pressure to the brain.

Recommendations

Usefulness of emergent or urgent CEA when clinical indicators or brain imaging suggests a small infarct core with large territory at risk (e.g., penumbra), compromised by inadequate flow from a critical carotid stenosis or occlusion, or in the case of acute neurological deficit after CEA, in which acute thrombosis of the surgical site is suspected, is not well-established and needs further evidence.

TREATMENT OF ACUTE NEUROLOGICAL COMPLICATIONS

Ischemic Brain Edema

Delayed deterioration caused by edema of the infarcted tissue often takes place after acute cerebral infarction. Cerebral edema occurs in all infarcts especially in large volume infarcts. edema may produce a range of clinical findings from being clinically undetectable and not associated with new neurological symptoms to precipitous fatal worsening, depending on stroke location, infarct volume, patient age, and degree of pre-existing atrophy. Cytotoxic edema normally peaks 3–4 days after injury, but early reperfusion of a large volume of necrotic tissue can accelerate and precipitate malignant worsening of the edema resulting in with decreased cerebral perfusion pressure within the first 24 hours. Careful observation is required in patients with severe stroke or posterior fossa infarctions to enable early intervention to tackle potentially life-threatening edema.

Medical Management

Treatment of cerebral edema aims to reduce or minimize edema formation before clinically significant increases in intracranial pressure (ICP) occurs and the interventions may include the following:
- Restriction of free water to avoid hypo-osmolar fluid
- Osmotherapy includes IV mannitol (0.25–0.5 g/kg) and/or glycerol or 3% normal saline

- Acute IV bolus of 40 mg of furosemide
- Avoidance of excess glucose administration
- Minimization of hypoxemia and hypercarbia
- Correction of hyperthermia
- Avoidance of antihypertensives, particularly those that induce cerebral vasodilatation
- Elevation of the head end of the bed to 20°-30° to assist in venous drainage
- Lowering of ICP management when edema produces increased ICP including hyperventilation, hypertonic saline, osmotic diuretics, intraventricular drainage of cerebrospinal fluid, and decompressive surgery.

The mortality rate in patients with increased ICP remains as high as 50-70% despite intensive medical management. Hence, the above interventions should at best need to be considered as temporizing, extending the window for definitive treatment as mentioned below.

Decompressive Surgery

The secondary involvement of the frontal and occipital lobes during a primary brain stem compression, presumably attributable to anterior cerebral and posterior cerebral artery compression against dural structures, can significantly limit the chances for a meaningful clinical recovery or even survival. Surgical decompression with decompressive hemicraniectomy performed within 48 hours of stroke onset in patients of 18-60 years of age with malignant infarctions significantly reduced mortality from 78 to 29% and significantly increased favorable outcomes. Similar benefit was observed in patients with dominant and non-dominant hemisphere infarctions, but the outcome was influenced by older patients who had worse outcomes. Surgical decompression can reduce mortality from 80% to ≈20% but the decision to perform decompressive surgery should be individualized due to the risk of survival with moderate-to-severe disability.

Recommendations

- Patients with major infarctions are at high risk for brain edema and increased ICP. Measures to lessen the risk of edema and close

- monitoring of the patient for signs of neurological worsening during the first few days after stroke are recommended.
- Decompressive surgical evacuation of a space-occupying cerebellar infarction is effective in preventing and treating herniation and brain stem compression.

HEMORRHAGIC TRANSFORMATION

Ischemic infarction may be accompanied by petechial hemorrhage occurring in patients not treated with recanalization strategies or symptomatic hemorrhage in patients after IV rtPA and IA recanalization strategies and anticoagulant use. It can also occur in patients not undergoing reperfusion therapies and hence they too require similar vigilance, especially in patients with larger strokes, older age, or with a cardioembolic origin. Most hemorrhages occur within the first 24 hours after IV rtPA; majority of hemorrhages that occur within the first 12 hours are fatal. The symptoms include worsening neurological symptoms, decreasing mental status, headache, increased blood pressure and pulse, and vomiting.

If a patient demonstrates signs of symptomatic hemorrhage, any remaining IV rtPA should be withheld immediately. An emergent non-contrast CT scan and a complete blood count, coagulation parameters (PT, aPTT, and INR), and fibrinogen levels should be tested. Antithrombotics may be used safely after hemorrhagic infarction as suggested by a study by Kin et al. (PLos ONE, 2014).

As mentioned in a case report, no further hematoma expansion was reported after use of tranexamic acid in the treatment of an IV rtPA-associated hemorrhage in a Jehovah's Witness stroke patient. Evacuation may be considered for large hemorrhages but smaller hematomas may be tolerated without clinical relevance since cerebellar hemorrhagic conversion is more likely to become symptomatic.

Seizures

Some of the studies reported the following incidences of seizures after ischemic infarction:
- Varied incidences with most reports indicating an incidence of <10%

- Increased incidence in patients with hemorrhagic transformation
- Varied incidences of recurrent and late-onset seizures.

There is little information that is available regarding the effects of prophylactic anticonvulsants after acute ischemic stroke or is long-term use after a stroke-related seizure.

STROKE REHABILITATION

The rehabilitation depends on the patient's status and requirements and accordingly may work on improving one or more of the following skills:
- Self-care skills such as feeding, grooming, bathing and dressing, etc.
- Skills related to morbidity such as transferring, walking, or self-propelling a wheelchair
- Communication skills in terms of speech and language
- Cognitive skills such as memory or solving of problems
- Social interactions with other people

The rehabilitation techniques or services may thereby include one or more of the following:
- Nursing care and support
- Physical therapy
- Occupational therapy
- Speech-language therapy
- Audiology care
- Recreational support
- Nutritional care
- Overall rehabilitation counseling
- Psycho-social support
- Educating the family with regard to patient rehabilitation

MANAGEMENT OF SPONTANEOUS INTRACEREBRAL HEMORRHAGE

Initial Clinical Assessment of ICH

- A severity score assessed by neurological examination findings should be conducted as part of the initial assessment. The National Institute of Health Stroke Score is recommended for

awake or drowsy patients or a Glasgow Come Scale (GCS) in patients who are obtunded, semi or fully comatose.
- Patients with declining GCS and/or equal to <8 should be quickly evaluated for airway protection by endotracheal intubation.
- Patients with reduced level of consciousness (LOC), pupillary changes, and/or other signs suggestive of herniation should have temporizing measures to manage presumed rise in ICP, such as temporary hyperventilation, and hyperosmotics (e.g., mannitol or 3% saline).

■ Patients with suspected ICH should undergo CT as soon as possible after initial stabilization to confirm diagnosis, location, and extent of hemorrhage.

■ In patients with confirmed acute ICH, intracranial vascular imaging is recommended *for majority of patients* to exclude an underlying lesion such as an aneurysm or arteriovenous malformation or cerebral sinus venous thrombosis (Evidence Level B).
- Factors that increase the information from angiography include age <50 years, female sex, lobar, or infratentorial location of ICH, accompanying intraventricular hemorrhage, negative neuroimaging markers of cerebral small vessel disease, negative history of hypertension, or impaired coagulation.
- Whenever index of suspicion is high for an underlying vascular lesion, the vascular imaging should be performed simultaneously with as brain imaging.

■ Evaluation of patients with acute ICH should include questions about medication history (Evidence Level C) and antithrombotic therapy, measurement of platelet count, partial thromboplastin time, and international normalized ratio.
- The resolution of CT angiography is preferred over MR angiography when screening for underlying vascular anomalies.
- Clinical signs of increased ICP include reduced LOC, dilated unresponsive pupils, new cranial nerve VI palsies, or other false localizing neurological signs, worsening headache and/or nausea/vomiting, and elevated blood pressure with

reduced heart rate and irregular/decreased respirations (Cushing's reflex).
- Potential unstable patients requiring greater monitoring frequency (i.e., neurovital signs hourly for first 24 hours) include patients with large (>30 cc) ICH volume, depressed or declining GCS (<12), worsening neurological disability, infratentorial location, associated intraventricular hemorrhage or hydrocephalus, refractory hypertension, and/or neuroimaging markers of ICH expansion.
- The use of tranexamic acid has been shown to be safe in a large phase 3 trial (TICH-2) but there was no effect on the primary outcome of functional status at 90 days. Post-hoc prespecified subgroup analyses showed better functional status in patients with baseline SBP less than 170 mm Hg. However, this post-hoc finding has yet to be confirmed. Overall, the clinical role of tranexamic acid for spontaneous ICH remains unclear, and there is no evidence for its use in the setting of anticoagulant-related ICH.

Symptoms of Intracerebral Hemorrhage

It should be emphasized that clinical evaluation cannot reliably differentiate intracerebral hemorrhage from ischemic stroke; brain imaging is required. More frequent symptoms of ICH may include:
- Alteration in LOC (present in approximately 50% of patients)
- Nausea and vomiting (approximately 40–50%)
- Sudden, severe headache (approximately 40%)
- Seizures (approximately 6–7%)
- Sudden weakness or paralysis of the face, arm or leg, or numbness, particularly on one side of the body
- Sudden visual impairment
- Impairment of balance or coordination
- Difficulty in comprehension, speaking (slurring, confusion), reading, or writing

Presentation
- The typical presentation of ICH is abrupt onset of a focal neurological deficit that progresses over minutes to hours

with accompanying headache, nausea, vomiting, decreased consciousness, and elevated blood pressure.
- Patients may also present with aforementioned symptoms upon awakening from sleep. Neurologic deficits are related to the site of parenchymal hemorrhage, e.g., ataxia is the initial deficit noted in cerebellar hemorrhage, whereas weakness of a body part may be the initial symptom with a basal ganglia hemorrhage.
- Rapid progression of neurologic deficits and sensorium can be expected in 50% of patients with ICH.

Neuroimaging

- Hemorrhage volume (cc) can be quickly estimated using the formula ABC/2 where A is the greatest hemorrhage diameter in centimeters on an axial slice, B is the largest diameter perpendicular to A, and C is the approximate number of CT slices with hemorrhage multiplied by the slice thickness in cm (i.e., 5 mm slice thickness = 0.5 cm).
- Urgent repeat CT should be performed in patients when there is clinical deterioration or worsening sensorium. A repeat CT at 24 hours shall be considered despite the absence of clinical deterioration to document hematoma expansion (occurring in ~30% of acute ICH) and to evaluate extent of mass effect, new intraventricular hemorrhage, or evolution of hydrocephalus.
- Presenting clinical and imaging factors that are predictive of hematoma expansion and consequent worse outcomes include short time from symptom onset to baseline imaging (i.e., 6 hours), larger hematoma volume, and antithrombotic therapy. Additional imaging predictors of hematoma expansion including heterogeneous hematoma density or regions of intrahematomal hypodensity, ill-defined hematoma shape and satellite hematomas, amongst others, on non-contrast CT as well as intrahematomal contrast extravasation (Spot Sign) on CTA. However, these markers are yet to be established as useful for clinical interventions.
- Early pronounced vasogenic edema that is disproportionate to presumed there of onset of ICH may be suggestive of underlying hemorrhagic infarction, hemorrhagic tumor, or cerebral venous

sinus thrombosis. CT hyperattenuation within a major dural venous sinus or cortical vein draining region of ICH should arouse suspicion of cerebral venous sinus thrombosis.

Recommended Additional Urgent Neuroimaging to Confirm Intracranial Hemorrhage Diagnosis

- In cases where CTA is not obtained as part of the initial acute stroke protocol, noninvasive angiography (CTA or gadolinium-enhanced MRA) of the intracranial circulation should be considered and, carried out promptly on most patients presenting with ICH to identify potential underlying vascular lesions or spot sign/extravasation.
- If suspected, CT venography can be performed to evaluate for cerebral venous sinus thrombosis.

Recommended Additional Etiological Neuroimaging

Magnetic resonance imaging should be the imaging of choice to evaluate potential underlying mass lesions, hemorrhagic transformation of an ischemic infarct, and cavernous malformations.

Magnetic resonance imaging can in addition provide information on microangiopathic changes to suggest the diagnosis of spontaneous ICH from underlying cerebral small vessel disease due to chronic hypertension and/or cerebral amyloid angiopathy (CAA).

- Magnetic resonance imaging with MR venogram and GRE/SWI may be considered to exclude cerebral venous thrombosis (CVT).
- DSA should be considered in specific cases where there exists continued high suspicion of underlying vascular anomaly despite normal CTA and MRI, or noninvasive studies are suggestive of an underlying lesion.
- In cases where significant suspicion persists for an underlying lesion responsible for the index ICH, delayed repeat imaging with MRI and DSA following hematoma resolution (usually three months post-ICH) can be used to detect an underlying lesion that may have initially been unidentified, such as tumors, cavernous malformations, or small vascular anomalies initially overlapped or hidden by the hematoma.

Blood Pressure Management

- Blood pressure should be measured on initial arrival to the Emergency Department and every 15 minutes thereafter until desired blood pressure target is achieved and maintained for the first 24 hours.
- SBP lowering to a target of <140 mm Hg systolic does not worsen neurological outcomes (relative to a target of 180 mm Hg systolic) (Evidence Level A); however, clinical benefit is yet to be established.
- Subsequent blood pressure monitoring should be adjusted to the individual patients according to stability of the vital signs and ICP.
- There is a lack of strong evidence to guide choice of initial blood pressure lowering agents.
- Factors that may favor a lower target within this range (i.e. <140 mm Hg) may include—presentation within 6 hours of symptom onset; presenting SBP no >220 mm Hg; anticoagulation therapy; presence of neuroimaging markers of expansion and/or normal renal function.
- Parenteral labetalol, hydralazine, nicardipine, and/or enalapril (oral or intravenous) may be considered for acute blood pressure reduction.

Management of Anticoagulation

- Patients presenting with anticoagulant-related ICH should first have their anticoagulation stopped immediately and should be subjected to immediate reversal, without any consideration of the underlying indication for anticoagulation.
- Beyond initial investigations, further management should be based on the specific antithrombotic agent used.
- Warfarin should be reversed immediately with appropriate PCC dosage PCC dosed and in conjunction with intravenous vitamin K 10 mg.
- For patients on direct oral anticoagulants (DOACs), level of about anticoagulation activity can be assessed from identifying time of last dose, creatinine clearance, and anti-factor Xa level, if available.

- Andexanet alfa is not yet commercially available but has been shown to reverse the anticoagulant effect of Factor Xa inhibitors in a non-randomized single-arm clinical trial. It could be considered once commercially available.
- Factor Xa inhibitors (apixaban, edoxaban, and rivaroxaban) should be stopped immediately and PCC administered at a dose of 50 U/kg with a *maximum* dose of 3,000 U.
- Dabigatran should be withheld immediately and reversed with idarucizumab; patients should be given a total dose of 5 g, in two intravenous bolus doses of 2.5 g each, given no >15 minutes apart.

The doses should be given successively. There is no requirement for time delay between doses.

  - If idarucizumab is not available, use of FEIBA (anti-inhibitor coagulant complex; activated PCC) is recommended at 50 U/kg to a maximum of 2,000 U.
  - If both agents are not available, four-factor PCC at a dose of 50 U/kg to a *maximum* dose of 3,000 U is to considered with priority.
    - If the patient has received therapeutic LMWH within the past 12 hours, administering protamine is to be considered.
    - If the patient is receiving intravenous heparin infusion at the time of ICH, infusion should be immediately terminated and protamine dosage as appropriate is to be considered.
    - Antiplatelet agents [e.g., acetylsalicylic acid (ASA), clopidogrel, dipyridamole/ASA, and ticagrelor] should be stopped immediately too.
      - Platelet transfusions are not recommended (in the absence of significant thrombocytopenia) and may in fact be harmful.

Surgical Management of Intracranial Hemorrhage

- External ventricular drainage (EVD) is to be considered in patients with an altered consciousness LOC and hydrocephalus due to either intraventricular hemorrhage or mass effect.

- Surgical evacuation is not recommended if symptoms are stable and there are no signs of herniation.
  - Intraventricular thrombolysis to treat spontaneous intraventricular hemorrhage with or without associated ICH is not recommended overall. Treatment may improve survival but does not ensure chances of survival without major disability.
- Acute surgical intervention is to be considered in patients with supratentorial hemorrhages and which appear to be surgically accessible clinical signs of herniation (e.g., decreasing LOC, pupillary changes), particularly in the following subgroups:
  - Young patients (<65 years of age)
  - Superficial ICH location (≤1 cm from the cortical surface)
  - Associated vascular or neoplastic lesion
- Patients with cerebellar hemorrhage may be considered for neurosurgical consultation, particularly in the setting of altered LOC, new brainstem symptoms, or diameter of 3 or more centimeter.
  - EVD placement should occur in conjunction with hematoma evacuation in the setting of concurrent hydrocephalus.
- The clinical benefit of minimally invasive clot evacuation is yet to be established.
- Routine use of stereotactic thrombolysis and drainage (MISTIE) technique (tPA) is not recommended based on current evidence.
- Patients with significant hydrocephalus and normal LOC should be monitored closely and could be considered for EVD at earliest signs of decreasing LOC.
- Based on the findings of one RCT (MISTIE III), stereotactic thrombolysis appears to be safe and reduce mortality compared to medical management alone but does not improve functional outcomes. Successful hematoma volume reduction to <15 mL may be associated with functional outcome benefit.
- Endoscopic evacuation of deep and superficial ICH also reduces hematoma volume. Small randomized and non-randomized series have suggested benefit. The impact on functional outcomes is currently under evaluation in larger randomized clinical trials.

Flowchart 1: Algorithm for management of cerebral hemorrhage.

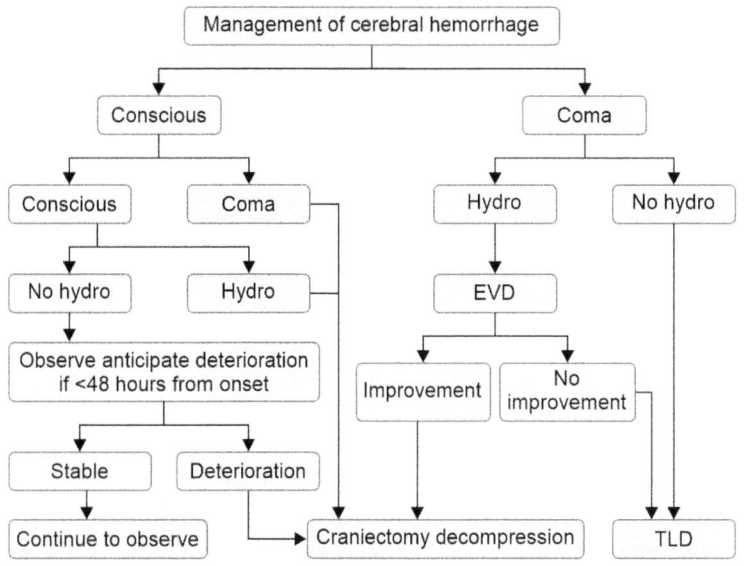

(EVD: external ventricular drainage; TLD: treatment limiting decisions)

- Endoscopic evacuation without the use of thrombolysis is being investigated. Its routine use is not recommended outside the framework of a clinical trial.

VENOUS THROMBOEMBOLISM PROPHYLAXIS

- In the acute phase of ICH, patients should be started on intermittent pneumatic compression devices, beginning the day of admission.
- Graduated compression stockings are not recommended for DVT prevention.
- Chemoprophylaxis (LMWH) can be initiated after 48 hours provided there is documentation of hematoma stabilization on neuroimaging.
  - Documentation hematoma stabilization implies an additional scan that is separated by at least 24 hours from the baseline scan.

Seizure Management
- People with ICH are at a greater risk of seizures at presentation and should be monitored clinically.
- Continuous EEG is to be considered for the diagnosis of non-convulsive status epilepticus in patients with depressed sensorium that is out of proportion to the size and location of ICH.
- New-onset seizures in patients admitted to hospital with ICH should be treated with antiepileptic medications if they are not self-limiting.
- A single, self-limiting seizure occurring at the onset or within 24 hours after an ICH (considered an "immediate" post-stroke seizure) should not be considered for long-term anticonvulsant medications. Short-term anticonvulsant therapy can be considered in such cases on an individual basis.
- Patients who have an immediate post-ICH seizure should be observed for recurrent seizure activity during routine monitoring of neurological status. Recurrent seizures in patients with ICH should be approached as per treatment guidelines for seizures in other neurological conditions.
- Prophylactic use of anticonvulsants in patients with ICH is not recommended.

Increased Intracranial Pressure
- In cases of suspected elevated ICP, conservative methods to lower ICP [such as elevation of head of bed 30°, methods of neuroprotection (e.g., euthermia and euglycemia), analgesia, and mild sedation] are advisable.
- There is inadequate evidence to recommend the routine prophylactic use of hyperosmotic agents in ICH.
  - Hyperosmotic agents (mannitol and/or 3% normal saline) can be considered as a temporizing measure to decrease ICP in ICH patients with clinical signs of herniation prior to surgical intervention.
- Use of corticosteroids to treat ICP in ICH may not provide any benefits and may be actually harmful, therefore it not recommended.

SECONDARY STROKE PREVENTION IN AN INDIVIDUAL AFTER AN EPISODE OF INTRACEREBRAL HEMORRHAGE

Risk Evaluation

- Persons at risk of stroke and patients who have had an ICH should be assessed for vascular disease risk factors (such as diet, sodium intake, waist-to-hip ratio, sedentary lifestyle, alcohol intake, blood pressure, and smoking).
- Patients who have suffered from an ICH should be assessed for underlying etiology and risk of recurrence.
  - The assessment of recurrent risk for an ICH should be based on clinical factors (including age, hypertension, ongoing anticoagulation, and prior lacunar stroke) and neuroimaging (lobar location of index ICH suggestive of cerebral artery aneurysm, presence of associated subarachnoid hemorrhage in convexal position, and presence and number of cerebral microbleeds and/or cortical superficial siderosis as in aged on susceptibility weighted or gradient echo MRI sequences).

Lifestyle Management

For individuals with intracerebral hemorrhage, healthcare professionals should recommend increased physical activity, healthy diet, reductions of alcohol consumption, cessation of smoking, and cessation of cocaine/amphetamine use where relevant.

Blood Pressure Management Following ICH

Long-term blood pressure should be aggressively monitored, treated, and controlled to sustain a target blood pressure consistently <130/80 mm Hg.

Use of Antithrombic Therapy Following ICH

- In ICH patients with an indication for anticoagulant treatment, the decision to initiate or resume anticoagulation should be individualized keeping in mind both patient's risk of recurrent hemorrhage and thromboembolism.

- If anticoagulation is deemed essential and where DOAC treatment is indicated (i.e., atrial fibrillation), DOAC therapy is favored over warfarin. This is based, however, primarily on their reduced rates of ICH in atrial fibrillation randomized trials where ICH patients were excluded.
- DOACs should not be used in patients with mechanical heart valves and intracerebral hemorrhage.
- Where indicated, antiplatelet monotherapy can be considered in patients deemed too high risk for anticoagulation.
- In patients with an indication for continued antiplatelet treatment, resuming antiplatelet therapy is reason able.
- The optimal timing and strategy regarding antithrombotic therapy (antiplatelet or anticoagulant) following an intracerebral hemorrhage is not well-defined and should be individualized to the patient.

Statin Therapy in Intracerebral Hemorrhage

- There is no role for statin therapy in the secondary prevention of ICH. Statin therapy should not be initiated for secondary prevention of intracerebral hemorrhage.
- For intracerebral hemorrhage patients who have a clear concomitant indication for cholesterol lowering treatment, statin therapy should be individualized and should take into account the patient's overall thrombotic risk as well as the probable risk of increased ICH with statin therapy.

CEREBRAL VENOUS THROMBOSIS

Cerebral venous thrombosis, which includes thrombosis of the cerebral veins and the dural sinuses, is a rare disorder that is associated with significant morbidity and mortality. Cerebral venous thrombosis can present with variable signs and symptoms that include a headache, benign intracranial hypertension, subarachnoid hemorrhage, focal neurological deficit, seizures, unexplained altered sensorium, and meningoencephalitis.

Etiology

Many risk factors lead to the development of cerebral venous thrombosis. At least one risk factor was identified in more than 85% of patients with cerebral venous thrombosis, and multiple risk factors are found in >50% of patients with cerebral venous thrombosis. In general, cerebral venous thrombosis is common in any condition that leads to a prothrombotic state, including pregnancy, the post-partum state, or oral contraceptive therapy. In the International Study on Cerebral Vein and Dural Sinus Thrombosis (ICSVT), genetic and acquired thrombophilia were present in 34% of patients with cerebral venous thrombosis. Inherited thrombophilia includes protein C and protein S deficiencies, antithrombin deficiency, factor V Leiden mutation, prothrombin gene mutation *20210*, as well as hyperhomocysteinemia.

Acquired thrombophilia should be kept in mind in patients with a history of nephrotic syndrome (due to loss of antithrombin) or antiphospholipid antibodies. Additional causes and risk factors associated with cerebral venous thrombosis include chronic inflammatory disease states such as systemic lupus erythematosus, inflammatory bowel disease, malignancy, and vasculitides such as Wegener's granulomatosis. Local infections such as otitis and mastoiditis, which can lead to thrombosis of the adjacent sigmoid and transverse sinuses, have also been implicated in developing cerebral venous thrombosis. Cerebral venous thrombosis has also been seen in a patient with a head injury, after certain neurosurgical procedures, direct injury to the sinuses or jugular veins, such as jugular vein catheterization, and even after a lumbar puncture.

Neuroimaging

Non-contrast computed tomography (CT): The easy availability with which this test can be obtained make it the first test that should be acquired in any patient presenting with an atypical headache, focal neurologic deficit, seizures, altered mental status, or coma. A classic sign of cerebral venous thrombosis is the *cord sign*, a curvilinear hyperdensity within a cortical vein in the presence of thrombosis that can be seen for up to 2 weeks following thrombus formation.

Other direct signs include hyperdensity with a triangular shape in the superior sagittal sinus, also known as the *dense triangle sign*.

Computed tomography venography (CTV): While MRI does have a better sensitivity and specificity when compared to computed tomography, diagnostic and confirmatory venography is required to exclude cerebral venous thrombosis.

Magnetic resonance imaging and magnetic resonance venography (MRV) are considered the gold standard in diagnosing cerebral venous thrombosis as they have a higher sensitivity than computed tomography. MRI is superior to CT when evaluating for parenchymal edema as a result of cerebral venous thrombosis. MRI findings are variable depending on age of the thrombus, as signal intensities change based on thrombus age.

Cerebral angiography: If the diagnosis is still in question after using MRI and MRV, then intra-arterial angiography is indicated.

Management

Management initially focuses on identifying and safe-guarding against life-threatening complications of cerebral venous thrombosis, including increased ICP, seizures, and coma. If a patient has seizures and has a lesion such as a hemorrhage or infarction on neuroimaging, then specific anticonvulsant therapy, as well as seizure prophylaxis, should be initiated. If a seizure does not occur, then seizure prophylaxis is not recommended. In the case of raised ICP, the head of the bed should be elevated, and administration of dexamethasone and mannitol should be done promptly to reduce increased ICP.

This is followed by admission to the intensive care unit or stroke unit for close ICP monitoring, with a neurosurgical consultation if the patient deteriorates and requires surgical decompression. Finally focus should be shifted to specific therapy, which includes anticoagulation and, in certain cases, catheter-directed fibrinolysis, and surgical thrombectomy.

Anticoagulation

Anticoagulation has been a topic for debate due to the potential for hemorrhagic transformation of cerebral infarcts before administering anticoagulation. The goal of anticoagulation is to prevent thrombus propagation, help recanalize the lumen of occluded cerebral veins, and to prevent the complications of deep venous thrombosis and pulmonary embolism in patients who already have thrombus burden and are susceptible to develop additional thrombi. The results of two randomized controlled trials, which compared anticoagulation with placebo, although statistically insignificant, showed that anticoagulation had a favorable outcome more often than controls. They also showed that anticoagulation was safe and not contraindicated, even in patients with cerebral hemorrhage.

Based on these randomized controlled trials and other observational studies, anticoagulation is considered as a safe and effective treatment of cerebral venous thrombosis. It should be started immediately upon diagnosis of cerebral venous thrombosis. Anticoagulation with intravenous unfractionated heparin or subcutaneously administered low-molecular-weight heparin is recommended as a bridge to oral anticoagulation with a vitamin K antagonist. There are no outcome differences while comparing unfractionated heparin (UFH) or LMWH. The European Stroke Organization (ESO) guidelines recommend unfractionated heparin in patients with compromise keeping in mind the probability of requiring emergent reversal.

The target goal of treatment is an international normalized ratio of 2.0-3.0 cerebral venous thrombosis 3-6 months in patients with provoked cerebral venous thrombosis and 6-12 months in patients with unprovoked cerebral venous thrombosis. Indefinite anticoagulation is recommended in patients with recurrent cerebral venous thrombosis, those who develop deep vein thrombosis and pulmonary embolism in addition to cerebral venous thrombosis, or those with first-time cerebral venous thrombosis of even in the setting of severe thrombophilia.

A recent meta-analysis shows that direct oral anticoagulations, mainly dabigatran are also similarly effective in cerebral venous thrombosis and may use used in place of vitamin K antagonists.

Thrombolysis

Although most patients see clinical improvement with anticoagulation therapy, a small subset of patients do not, and these individuals actually deteriorate clinically despite anticoagulation. In these cases, where the prognosis is poor, systemic and catheter-directed thrombolysis is indicated in patients with large and extensive cerebral venous thrombi who clinically deteriorate despite treatment with anticoagulation.

Surgical Intervention

Surgical thrombectomy is reserved for cases of severe neurological deterioration despite maximal medical therapy. In the case of large venous infarcts and hemorrhages causing a mass effect with risk of herniation, decompressive surgery has been to improve clinical outcomes, especially if done early, although this is questionable. Decompressive surgery is life-saving, with favorable outcomes observed in >50% of patients, with a high mortality rate of approximately 20%.

SUGGESTED READING

1. Badhiwala JH, Nassiri F, Alhazzani W, Selim MH, Farrokhyar F, Spears J, et al. Endovascular Thrombectomy for Acute Ischemic Stroke: A Meta-analysis. JAMA. 2015;34(17):1832-43.
2. Chen PH, Gao S, Wang YJ, Xu AD, Li YS, Wang D. Classifying Ischaemic Stroke from TOAST to CISS. CNS Neurosci Ther. 2012;18(6):452-6.
3. Cheng NT, Kim AS. Intravenous Thrombolysis for Acute Ischemic Stroke within 3 hours versus between 3 and 4.5 hours of Symptom Onset. Neurohospitalist. 2015;5(3):101-9.
4. Hoh BL, Ko NU, Amin-Hanjani S, Chou SH-Y, Cruz-Flores S, Dangayach NS, et al. Management of Patient with Aneurysmal Subarachnoid Hemorrhage: A Guideline from the American Heart Association/American Stroke Association. Stroke. 2023;54(7):e314-70.
5. Logallo N, Novotny V, Thomassen L. The Norwegian Tenecteplase Stroke Trial (NOR-tEST): randomized controlled trial of Tenecteplase vs. Alteplase in acute ischaemic stroke (abstract). Eur Stroke J. 2017: 2(IS):3-97.
6. Powers WJ, Rabinstein AA, Ackerson T, Adeoye OM, Bambakidis NC, Becker K, et al. Focused Update of the 2019. Guidelines for the Early Management of Patients with Acute Ischemic Stroke regarding Endovascular Treatment: A Guideline for Healthcare Professionals from the American Heart Association/American Stroke Association. Stroke. 2019:50:e344-e418.

7. Saposnik G, Barinagarrementeria F, Brown RD, Bushneli B, Cushman M, deVeber G, et al. Diagnosis and Management of Cerebral Venousthrombus: a statement for healthcare professionals from the American Heart Association/American Stroke Association. Stroke. 2011;42(4):1158-92.
8. Shoamanesh A, Patrice Lindsay M, Castellucci LA, on behalf of the Canadian Stroke Best Practices Advisory Committee in collaboration with the Canadian Stroke Consortium and the Canadian Hemorrhagic Stroke Trials Initiative Network (CoHESIVE). Canadian stroke best practice recommendations: Management of Spontaneous Intracerebral Hemorrhage, 7th edition. Update 2020. Intern J Stroke. 2020;16(3):321-41.
9. Specogna AV, Turin TC, Pattern SB, Hill MD. Hospital treatment costs and length of stay association with hypertension and multimorbidity after hemorrhagic stroke. BMC Neurol. 2017;17:158.

Acute Kidney Injury

Soumitra Kumar, Arghya Majumder

DEFINITION

Acute renal failure (ARF) is defined as sudden rapid decline in renal function over a period of hours to days causing retention of nitrogenous waste products and failure to maintain fluid and electrolyte homeostasis. However, this definition failed to describe the dynamic process extending across the phases of initiation, maintenance, and recovery.

Due to significant heterogeneity in definitions in prior studies, during the past 20 years efforts have been made by the acute disease quality initiative (ADQI) group to develop consensus definitions of ARF which has been re-christened as acute kidney injury in particular for use in epidemiologic studies and clinical trials.

PARAMETERS FOR EARLY DETECTION OF IMPAIRMENT OF RENAL FUNCTION

- Careful review of flow sheet-vital signs, records of intake and urine output, medication, contrast imaging if any
- Daily weight of the patient to check for cumulative balance
- Supine and standing BP to check for postural hypotension dehydration
- Regular estimation of plasma urea, creatinine and electrolyte, s-sodium, potassium

RISK FACTORS

- CKD (eGFR <60 mL/min/1.73 m^2)
- Age >75 years
- Sepsis causing shock; infections causing rhabdomyolysis—influenza, leptospirosis
- Cardiac failure
- Liver disease

Flowchart 1: Severity of AKI staging.

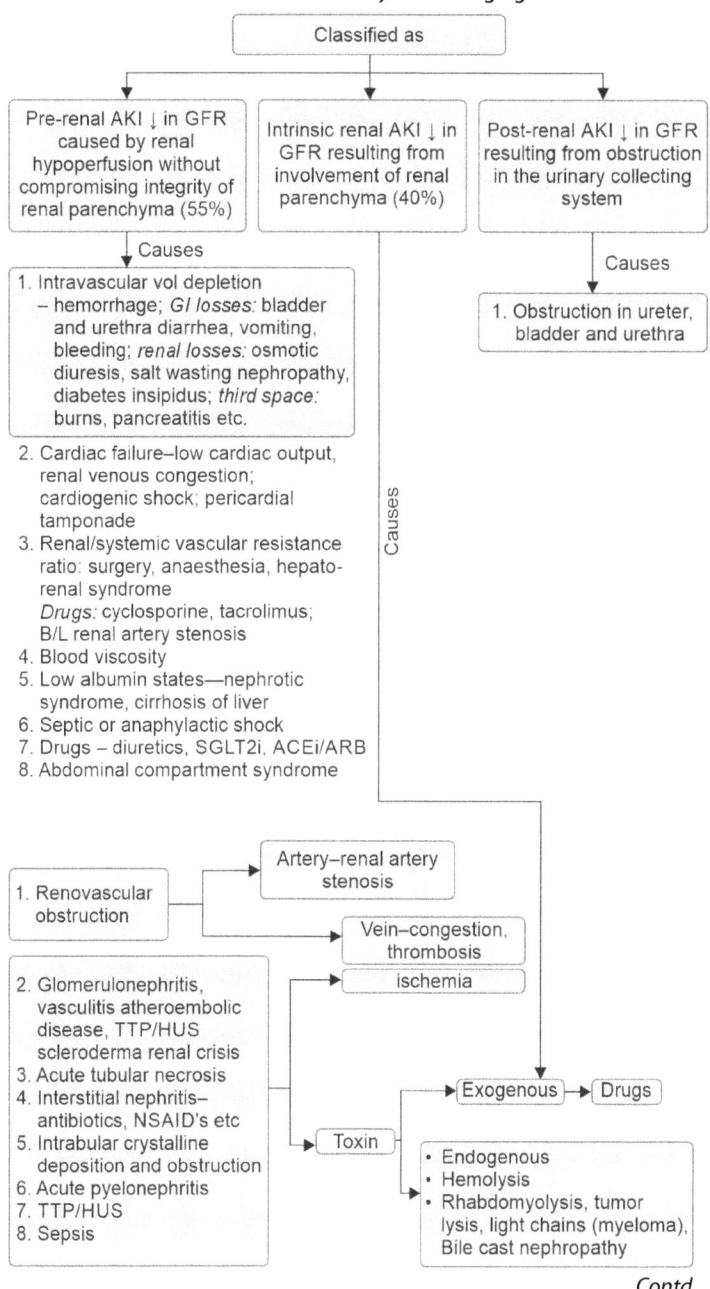

Contd...

Acute Kidney Injury

Contd...

AKI stage	Serum creatinine criteria	Urine output criteria
AKI stage I	Increase of serum creatinine by ≥0.3 mg/dL (B/L ≥26.4 mmol/L) or Increase to 15–1.9 times from baseline	Urine output <0.5 mL/kg/h for 6–12 hours
AKI stage II	Increase of serum creatinine to 2.0–2.9 times	Urine output <0.3 mL/kg/h for from baseline ≥24 hours
AKI stage III	Increase of serum creatinine ≥3.0 times from baseline or serum creatinine ≥4.0 mg/dL (≥354 mmol/L) treatment with RRT *or* in patients <18 years, decrease in estimated GFR to <35 m/min per 1.73 m^2	or anuria for ≥12 hours

(AKI: acute kidney injury; GFR: glomerular filtration rate; KDIGO: Kidney Disease Improving Global Outcomes; RRT: renal replacement therapy)

- Diabetes mellitus
- Drugs affecting renal function
- Hypovolemia
- Atherosclerotic peripheral vascular disease

Possibility of chronic kidney disease is suggested by:
- A history of preexisting chronic kidney disease
- Previous biochemical examination is suggestive of impaired renal function.
  USG—bilateral echogenic, shrunken kidneys.
  However, CKD with normal sized-kidney may be found in rapidly progressively glomerulonephropathy (RPGN); leukemic infiltration, scleroderma, renal crisis, diabetic nephropathy, Polyarteritis Nodosa (PAN), amyloidosis, ADPKD, and HIVAN.
- *Anemia:* Hypocalcemia/hyperphosphatemia—suggestive of secondary hyperparathyroidism.
  History of vague ill health of some month duration, history of nocturia, pruritus, skin pigmentation, anemia, hypocalcemia, hyperphosphatemia, renal osteodystrophy, and band keratopathy are signs of chronicity.

Flowchart 2: Urine analysis and renal indices charts based on urinary sediment.

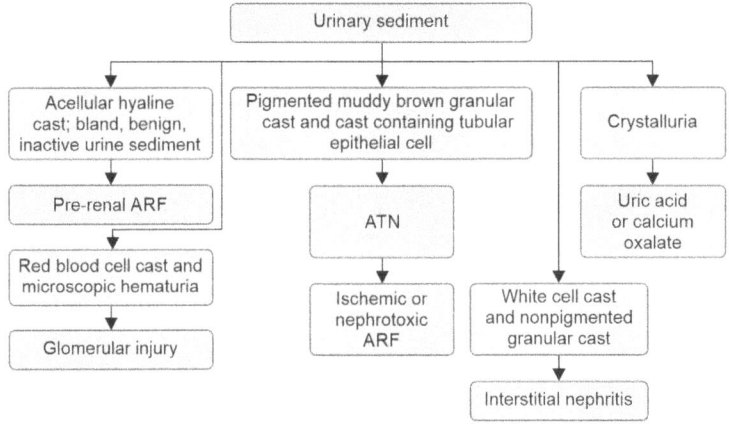

Flowchart 3: Classification and possible etiology of AKI based on urinary output.

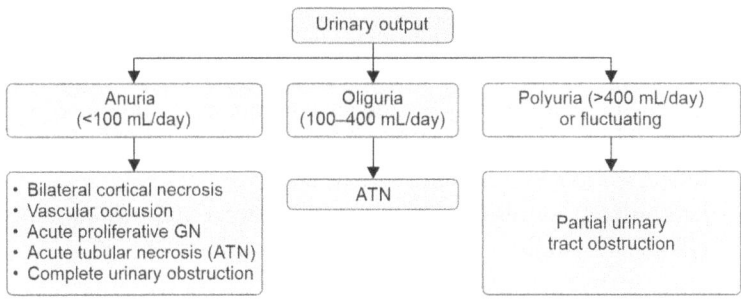

(AKI: acute kidney injury; ARF: acute renal failure; ATN: acute tubular necrosis; GN: glomerulonephritis)

CHECKLIST FOR ASSESSMENT OF A PATIENT WITH SUSPECTED TO HAVE DEVELOPED ACUTE KIDNEY INJURY

- Clear evidence of genuine and recent decline in GFR.
- Sequence of deterioration in renal function with its relation to possible causative factor in history.
- Documentation of potential nephrotoxins—contrast, NSAID's, aminoglycosides, vancomycin, cisplatin, etc.

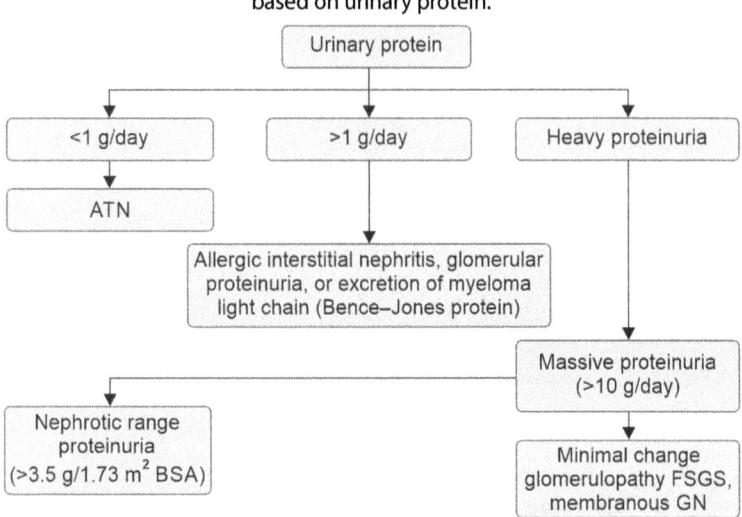

Flowchart 4: Urine analysis and renal indices charts based on urinary protein.

(ATN: acute tubular necrosis; BSA: body surface area; FSGS: focal segmental glomerulosclerosis; GN: glomerulonephritis)

- Estimation of adequacy of renal perfusion prior to or during decline in renal function by clinical assessment of volume status.
- Probe for extrarenal manifestation—purpura in vasculitis, livedo reticularis in atherothrombotic disease, etc.
- Examination of urine → volume, sediment, composition, and chemical analysis.
- Renal imaging—USG.
- Consideration of the necessity for kidney biopsy.
- Detection of biochemical abnormalities common in AKI.

DIAGNOSIS

History
- History of fluid loss—GI, renal, skin/heat stroke, history of trauma, and bleeding
- History of thirst, dryness of mucosa, and oliguria
- History of use of diuretics or other potential nephrotoxic drugs, history of contrast imaging
- History of Syncope or dizziness—suggestive of dehydration

Flowchart 5: Imaging modalities in diagnosis of AKI.

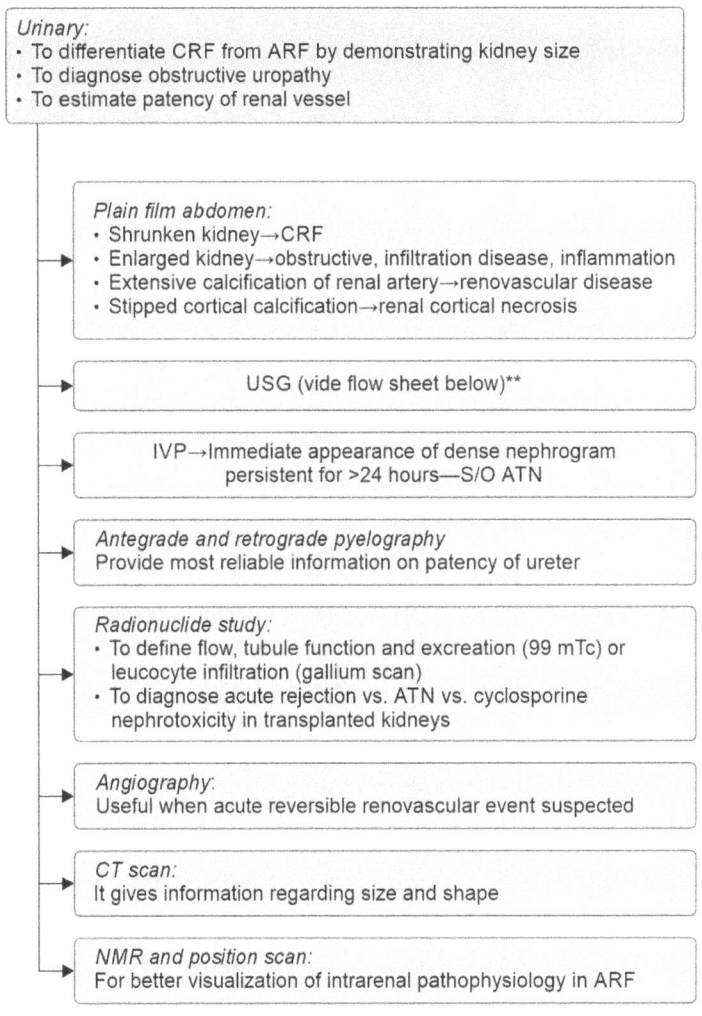

- Breathlessness, peripheral oedema—suggestive of heart failure, nephrotic syndrome, and cirrhosis
- Color, volume, and frequency dysuria
- History of fever, rash, joint pain suggestive of SLE, history of abdominal pain suggestive of acute pancreatitis, abdominal compartment syndrome, history of pain in the limbs suggestive of rhabdomyolysis, and abdominal pain or pain in the limbs

Flowchart 6: Ultrasound for AKI.

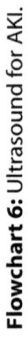

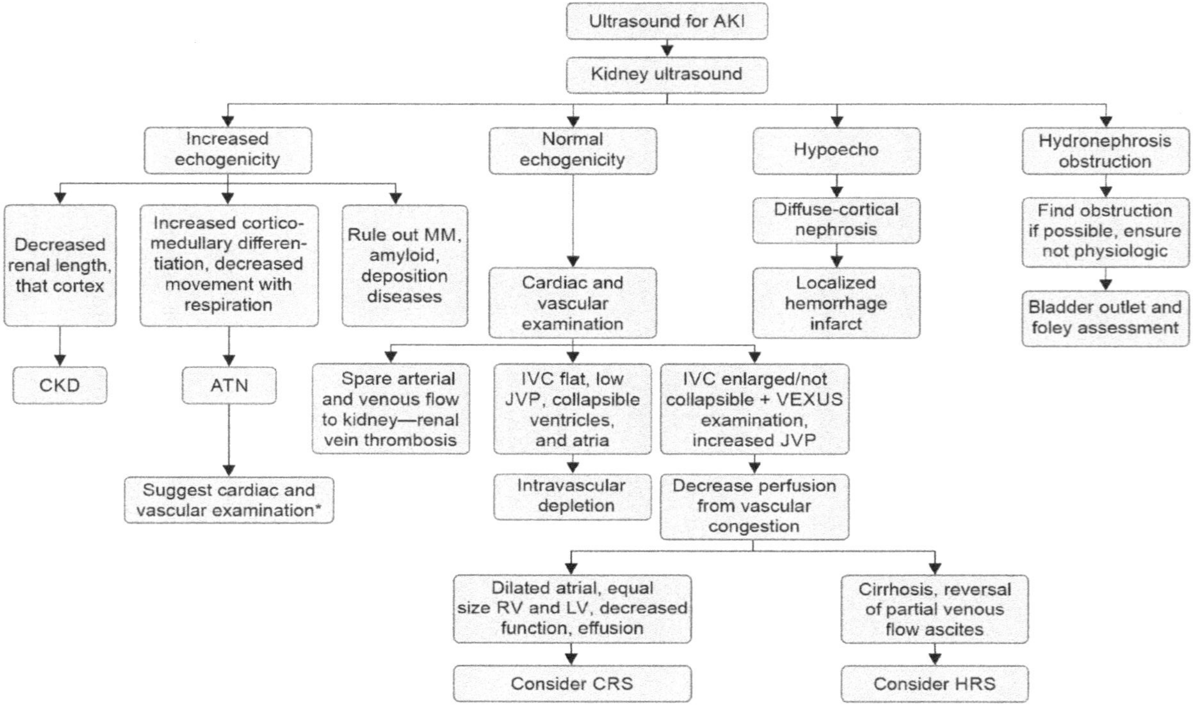

Following this flow sheet and starting with a kidney ultrasound, one can determine most causes of AKI.

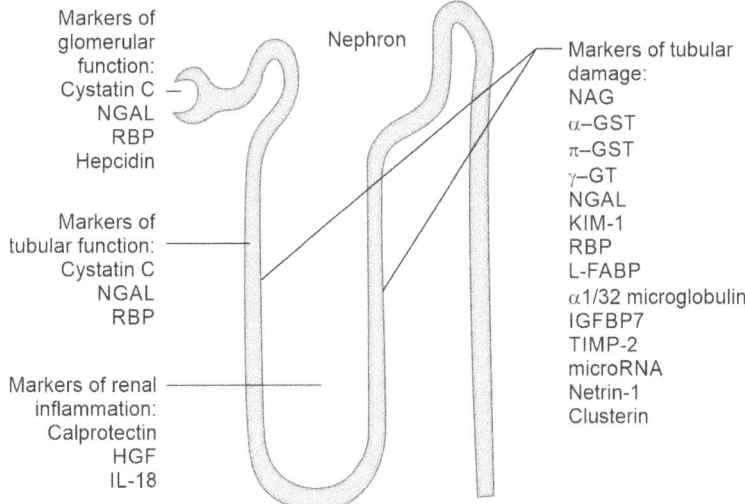

Fig. 1: Markers of glomerular function and tubular damage.

- *Lookout for extrarenal manifestations*
  - History of prostatic disease
  - History of intermittent claudication—suggesting renal artery stenosis
  - History of chronic liver disease
  - History of pregnancy related—pre eclampsia, HELLP, PPH, and septic abortion
  - History suggestive of some infective etiology—falciparum malaria, leptospirosis, etc.
  - History of HIV infection—HIVAN, TTP/HUS, plasmacytic interstitial nephritis, drug-induced rhabdomyolysis, ATN, and crystalluria

Clinical Examination

- *Symptoms*
  - Features of volume depletion—thirst, orthostatic dizziness, progressive fall of urine output, diminished axillary sweating
  - Volume excess—swelling of both legs and periorbital puffiness

Acute Kidney Injury

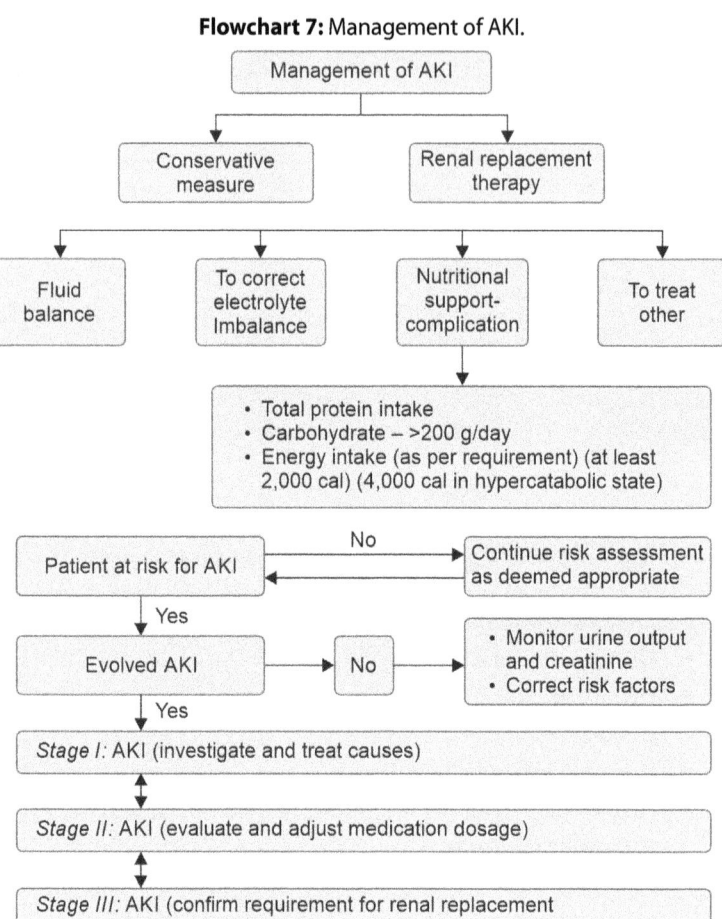

Flowchart 7: Management of AKI.

- Signs A: Volume depletion manifested by:
  - Poor skin turgor
  - Tachycardia
  - JVP
  - Dry mucous membrane
  - Decreased temperature of extremity
  - Postural sign—Decrease of BP >10 mm Hg } on standing
    Increase of Pulse rate >10/min

Acute Kidney Injury

Flowchart 8: Initial conservative approach to management of AKI.

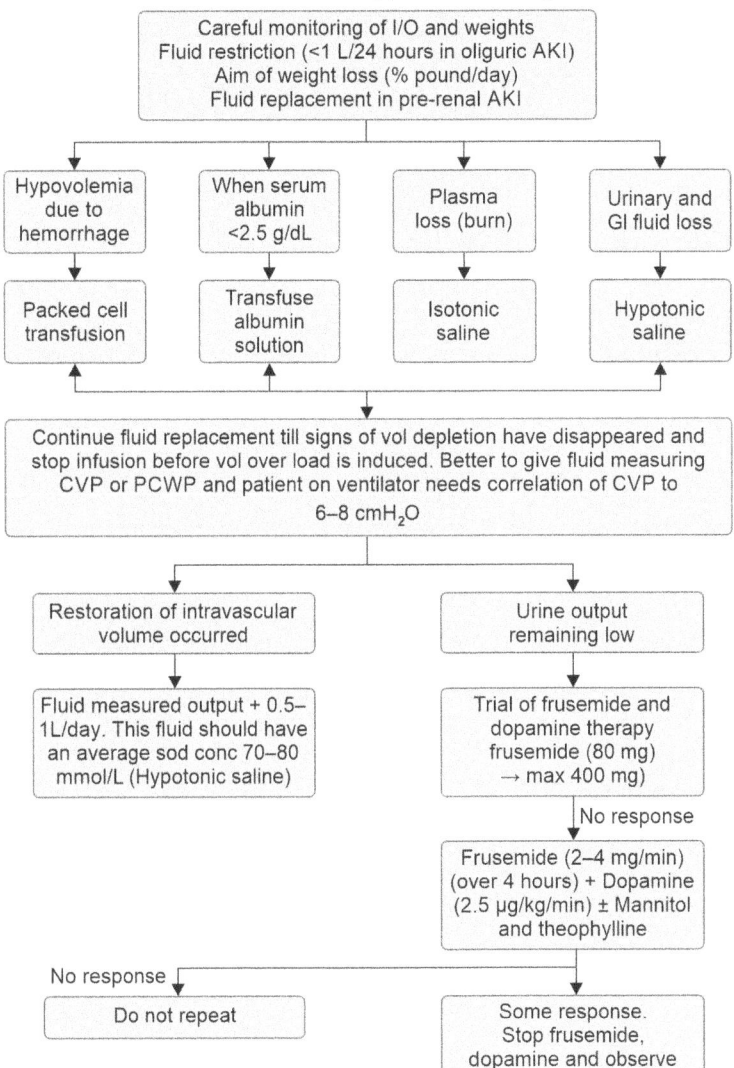

Flowchart 9: Prevent and treat hyperkalemia.

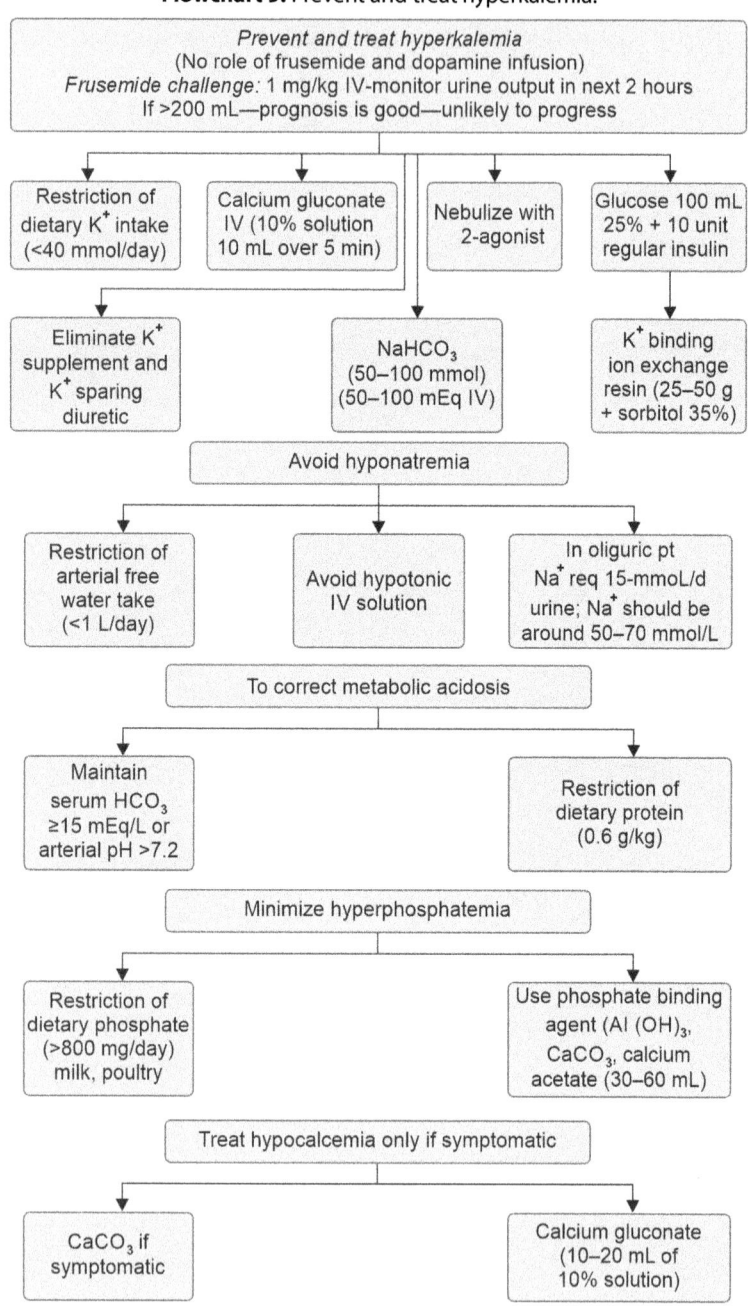

Flowchart 10: To treat other complications.

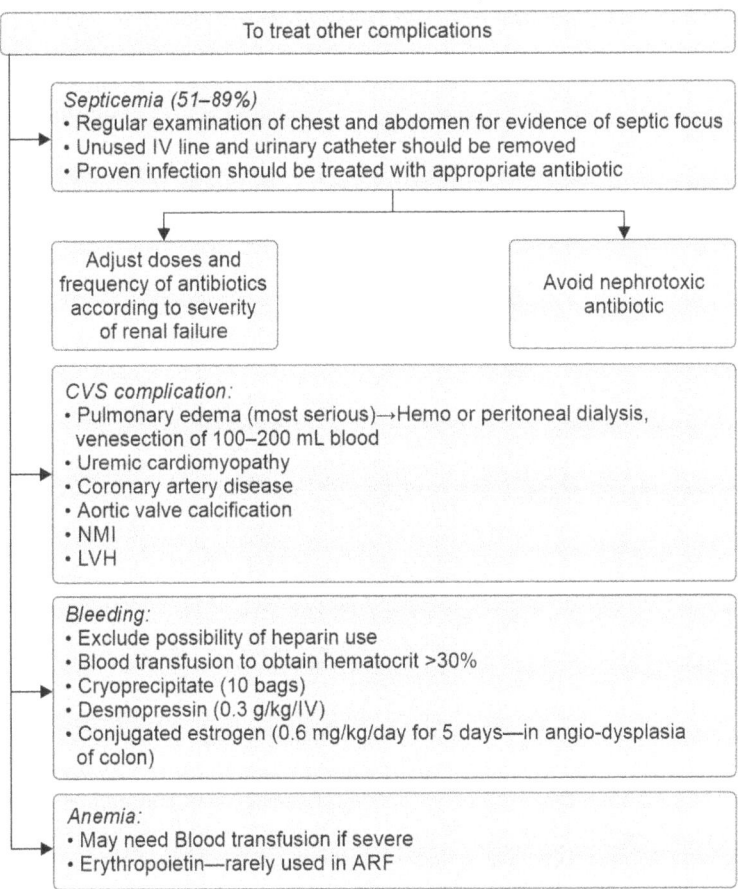

- *Volume excess manifested by:*
  - S3 gallop
  - Cardiomegaly
  - Jugular venous distension
  - Pulmonary congestion
  - Liver congestion
  - Peripheral edema, ascites, and pleural effusion

Flowchart 11: Pathophysiology, medical management, and use of renal replacement therapy in severe acute kidney injury and refractory cardiorenal syndrome.

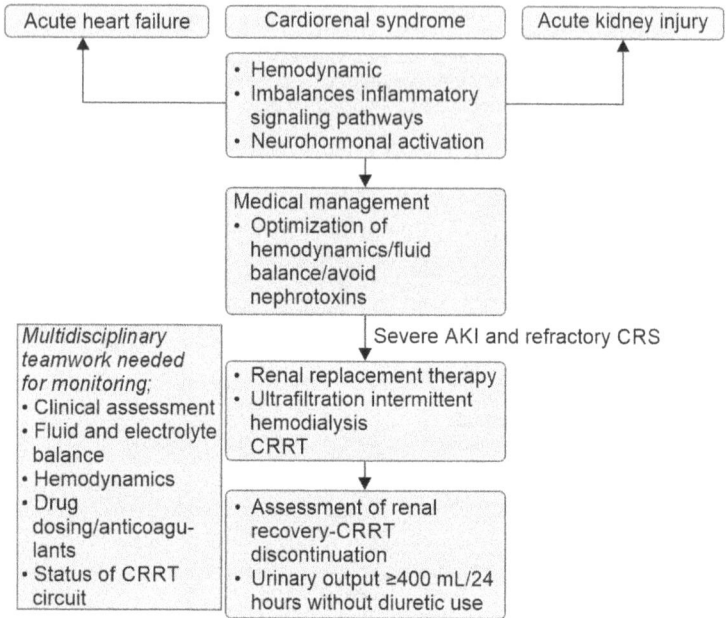

Cardiorenal syndrome (CRS) involves the interplay between hemodynamic, inflammatory, and neurohumoral abnormalities to produce worsening heart and kidney function. Management of patients with CRS involves multidisciplinary care, starting with medical management and avoidance of further acute kidney injury (AKI). For medically refractory CRS and severe AKI, renal replacement therapy, including continuous renal replacement therapy (CRRT), may be necessary.

INVESTIGATIONS

Blood

- CBC–anemia–bleeding, hemolysis, multiple myeloma etc., acute on chronic renal failure
  - Thrombocytopenia—TTP, HUS
  - Peripheral eosinophilia—Churg-Strauss syndrome, PAN, and allergic interstitial nephritis
  - Leukocytosis—sepsis

Acute Kidney Injury

Flowchart 12: Volume management in patients with acute heart failure and CRS.

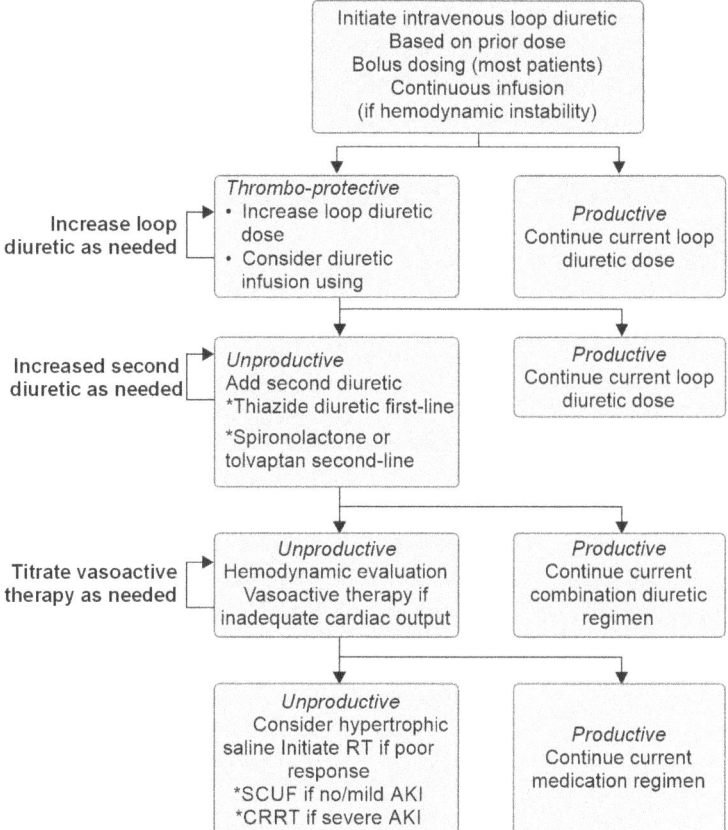

Escalating doses of loop diuretics are the first line of therapy for volume removal, with combination diuretic therapy used for patients who do not respond adequately to loop diuretics. A target urine output of 3–5 L/day has been used in studies of stepped-diuretic therapy. Hemodynamic assessment and vasoactive therapy can be helpful in selected patients with poor response to diuretics, with extracorporeal volume removal for patients in whom medical therapy fails.

(CRRT: continuous renal replacement therapy; RRT: real replacement therapy; SCUF: slow continuous ultrafiltration)

- *Peripheral smear*—schistocytes indicating TMA, sickle cells—in sickle cell crisis
- Reticulocyte count high—indicates hemolysis
- Blood urea, creatinine—baseline value and daily rate of rise—rise in urea > creatinine—dehydration, GI bleed, and steroid therapy
  - Rise in creatinine >urea—indicates CKD

TABLE 1: Comparison of recent consensus AKI definitions.

AKI stage	Urine output	KDIGO	AKIN	RIFLE
1	<0.5 mL/kg/h for 6–12 h	Scr. to 1.5–1.9 × baseline over 7 days or ≥0.3 mg/dL absolute increase over 48 h	Scr. to 1.5–2 × baseline or ≥0.3 mg/dL absolute Scr. increase within 48 h	*Risk:* Scr. to ≥1.5 × increase within 7 days, sustained for ≥24 h
2	<0.5 mL/kg/h for ≥12 h	Scr. to 2.0–2.9 × baseline	Scr. to >2–3 × baseline	*Injury:* Scr. to ≥2 × increase
3	<0.3 mL/kg/h for ≥24 h or anuria for ≥12 h	Scr. to ≥3.0 × baseline, or Scr. increase to ≥4.0 mg/dL or initiation of RRT	Scr. to >3.0 × baseline, or Scr. increase to ≥4.0 mg/dL (with increase of 0.5 mg/dL) or initiation of RRT	*Failure:* Scr. to ≥3.0 × increase or Scr. increase to ≥4.0 mg/dL (with increase of 0.5 mg/dL) or initiation of RRT *Loss:* Complete loss of kidney function for >4 weeks *ESKD:* Complete loss of kidney function >3 months

If a patient does not have a baseline serum creatinine report within 1 week of their admission or presentation it has been considered acceptable to use a reference serum creatinine value within 3 months (acceptable up to 1 year). If reference serum creatinine is not available within 3 months and AKI is suspected, has to be repeated within 24 hours.

TABLE 2: Differentiating points between AKI and CKD.

	Chronic	Acute
History of kidney disease, hypertension, and abnormal urinalysis	√	o
Small kidney size	√	o
Urinalysis with broad cast	√	o
Return of renal function to normal with time	o	√
Signs of chronicity	√	o
Hyperkalemia, anemia acidemia, and hyperphosphatemia	+++	+ (more common)
Low carbamylated Hb%	o	√

(Non-enzymatic carbamylation of hemoglobin occurs in direct relationship to magnitude and duration in BUN. A carbamylated hemoglobin level >80–100 µg carbamyl naline per gram Hb suggests more acute cause than chronic).

- *Electrolytes*
    - Hypercalcemia (multiple myeloma), hypocalcemia, and hyperphosphatemia (may indicate acute on CKD)
    - Marked phosphate with low calcium—rhabdomyolysis (CPK rise), hyperuricemia tumor lysis syndrome (CPK normal, uric acid high K)—high Na- may indicate dehydration,- low Na and K- may indicate use of diuretics -low Na, high K- may be due to use of ARNI, ARB with diuretics
    - Anion gap and osmolal gap—may indicate methanol, ethylene glycol poisoning
    - *Serology:* Serum C3, C4, complement, cANCA, pANCA, anti-GBM, and cryoglobulin
    - *Liver function tests*—high bilirubin may indicate bile cast nephropathy
    - Serum protein electrophoresis—may indicate a M band suggestive of myeloma
    - *Very high glucose*—may indicate hyperosmolar non-ketotic coma and presence of ketone in urine-diabetic ketoacidosis
    - Very high uric acid may indicate uric acid-induced interstitial nephritis
    - Raised PT or APTT may indicate DIC

TABLE 3: Compromised kidney perfusion.

Type	Instances of specific causes
(i) Prerenal causes	
Hypovolemia	Increased losses (hemorrhage, burns, massive vomiting or diarrhea), and poor oral intake
Diminished cardiac output	Heart failure, cardiac tamponade, and massive pulmonary embolism
Systemic vasodilation	Sepsis, SIRS, and hepatorenal syndrome
Renal vasomodulation/shunting	Medications (NSAID, ACEi/ARB, cyclosporine, and iodinated contrast), hypercalcemia, hepatorenal syndrome, and abdominal compartment syndrome
(ii) Intrarenal causes	
Microvascular pathologies	Thrombotic microangiopathies (TTP, HUS, aHUS, DIC, APS, malignant hypertension, scleroderma renal crisis, preeclampsia/HELLP syndrome, and drug-induced), cholesterol emboli
Glomerular	Rapidly progressive (crescentic) GN—anti–glomerular basement membrane; immune complex diseases—IgA nephropathy, postinfectious, lupus, mixed cryoglobulinemia with MPGN; pauci-immune glomerulonephritis—ANCA-associated vasculitides—GPA, MPA, EGPA (Churg–Strauss); ANCA-negative; nephrotic-range proteinuria with associated AKI—HIV-associated nephropathy (secondary FSGS); other causes of nephrotic-range proteinuria that commonly associate with AKI—minimal change disease with ATN/AIN; membranous nephropathy + crescentic GN or renal vein thrombosis; myeloma + multiple different pathologies, but in particular light chain cast nephropathy

Contd...

Contd...

Tubulointerstitial causes	AIN—medications, infection, lymphoproliferative disease; pigment nephropathy—rhabdomyolysis (myoglobin), massive hemolysis (hemoglobin); crystal nephropathy—uric acid (tumor lysis), acyclovir, sulfonamides, protease inhibitors (indinavir, atazanavir), methotrexate, ethylene glycol, acute phosphate nephropathy, oxalate nephropathy; myeloma-associated AKI (cast nephropathy); ATN—ischemia (shock, sepsis), inflammatory (sepsis, burns), medications
(iii) Postrenal causes	
Bladder outlet	Benign prostatic hypertrophy, cancer strictures, and blood clots
Ureteral	Bilateral obstruction (or unilateral with one kidney) —stones, malignancy, retroperitoneal fibrosis
Renal pelvis	Papillary necrosis (NSAIDs), stones

(ACEI: angiotensin-converting enzyme inhibitor; AKI: acute kidney injury; ANCA: antineutrophil cycloplasmic antibody; APS: antiphospholipid; AR: angiotensin receptor blocker; ATN/AIN: acute tubular necrosis/acute interstitial nephritis; DIC: disseminated intravascular coagulation; EGPA: eosinophilic granulomatosis with polyangiitis; FSGS: focal segmental glomerulosclerosis; GN: glomerulonephritis; GPA: granulomatosis with polyangiitis; HELLP: hemolysis, elevated liver enzymes, low platelet count syndrome; HIV: human immunodeficiency virus; HUS: (atypical) hemolytic uremic syndrome; MPA: microscopic polyangiitis; MPGN: membranoproliferative glomerulonephritis; NSAID: nonsteroidal anti-inflammatory drug; SIRS: systemic inflammatory response syndrome; TTP: thrombotic thrombocytopenic purpura)

Urine Examination

- *Urine sediment*—eosinophil cast in allergic interstitial nephritis, muddy brown cast in ATN, bile casts in cholemic nephritis, and light chain casts in myeloma
- *Crystals*—ca oxalate crystals in ethylene glycol intoxication, uric acid crystals in urate nephropathy
- *Pigments*—hemoglobin—in hemolysis, myoglobin in rhabdomyolysis
- *RBCs*—in infection, post infective GN, granulomatosis with polyangiitis

TABLE 4: Key medications requiring dose adjustment (or discontinuation) in AKI.

- Analgesics (morphine, meperidine, gabapentin, and pregabalin)
- Antiepileptics (lamotrigine)
- Antivirus (acyclovir, ganciclovir, and valganciclovir)
- Antifungals (fluconazole)
- Antimicrobials (almost all antimicrobials need close adjustment in AKI with important exceptions of azithromycin, ceftriaxone, doxycycline, linezolid, moxifloxacin, nafcillin, and rifampin)
- Diabetic agents (sulfonylureas and metformin)
- Allopurinol
- Baclofen
- Colchicine
- Digoxin
- Lithium
- Low-molecular-weight heparin
- NOACs

TABLE 5: Biochemical examination of urine (clues from chemical analysis of urine with regard to etiopathogenesis of AKI).

Diagnostic index	Prerenal	Intrinsic
• Concentration		
– Specific gravity	>1.020	<1.010
– Uosm (mOsm/kg H_2O)	>500	<350
– U_{osm}/P_{osm}	>13	<1.1
– Free water clearance (mL/min)	< (-20)	> (–l)
• GFR and tubule reabsorptions		
– U/P urea	>8	<3
– U/P creatinine	>40	<20
– Creatinine clearance (mL/min)	>20	<20
– BUN/Plasma creatinine	>20	~10
• Tubule handling of solute		
– U_{Na} (mEq/L)	<20	>40
– Fe_{Na} (%)	<1	>1
– Renal failure index	<1	>1
• Urinary markers of tubule damage		
– β_2 microglobulin (mg/24 h)	<1.0	>50

(BUN: blood urea nitrogen; GFR: glomerular filtration rate)

TABLE 6: Biomarkers.

	Sample	Cardiac surgery	Contrast nephropathy	Kidney transplant
NAGL	Plasma	Early	Early	Early
Cystatin C	Plasma	Intermediate	Intermediate	Intermediate
NAGL	Urine	Early	Early	Early
IL-18	Urine	Intermediate	Absent	Intermediate
KIM-1	Urine			Intermediate

(KIM-1: kidney injury molecule-1; NAGL: neutrophil gelatin-associated lipocalin)

- WBCs in infection, interstitial nephritis
- *Protein*—urine protein by creatinine ratio high in nephrotic syndrome
- Urine leukocyte esterase or nitrite positive—in infection
- *Urine biochemistry*—urine sodium, FeNA, specific gravity, osmolality etc.

USG: Can differentiate—pre, post, or renal AKI; stones; presence of CKD, ADPKD

CT/MRI: May reveal retroperitoneal fibrosis occluding both ureters, renal vein thrombosis, etc.

Radionuclide scanning: DMSA may highlight pyelonephritis scars, DTPA may delineate renovascular disease or post renal obstruction

MCUG: To detect reflux

Cystoscopy: Retrograde or antegrade pyelography—to identify obstruction due to papillary necrosis, cancer etc.

Renal angiography: To exclude renal artery thrombosis and dissection

Renal biopsy:
- ATN not resolving in 4 weeks
- Suspicion of acute GN, vasculitis, myeloma, and anti GBM disease
- All kidney transplants with AKI

Biomarkers:

TABLE 7: Comparison of renal replacement therapy modalities.

	IHD	SLED	SCUF	CVVH	CVVHD	CVVHDF	PD
Blood flow (mL/min)	250–400	100–200	<100	200–300	100–200	100–200	—
Dialysate flow (mL/min)	500–800	100–200	0	0	16.7–33.4	16.7–33.4	0.4
Filtrate (L/day)	0–4	0–4	0–4	24–96	0	24–48	2.4
Replacement fluid (L/day)	0	0	0	21.6–90	4.8	23–44	0
Dialysate buffer	Bicarbonate	Bicarbonate	—	—	Lactate bicarbonate none (Titrate)	Lactate bicarbonate none (titrate)	Lactate bicarbonate
Replacement fluid buffer	—	—	—	Lactate bicarbonate	—	Lactate bicarbonate	—
Mechanism of clearance	Diffusion	Diffusion	Convection	Convection	Diffusion	Both	Both
Urea clearance (mL/min)	180–340	75–90	1.7	16.7–67	21.7	30–60	8.5
Duration (hours)	3–4	8–12	Variable	>24	>24	>24	

TABLE 8: Comparison of various modalities of renal replacement therapy.

Types

Hemodialysis	Peritoneal dialysis	Hemofiltration (CAVH and CVVH)
Indication: • Catabolic patient • Hemodynamically stable • Nonhypotensive • Diagnosed intraabdominal ds • Recent abdominal surgery	*Indication:* • Noncatabolic patient • Hemodynamically unstable patient • Poor vascular access • Active hemorrhage	Continuous process so that 1 L of plasma ultrafiltrate is removed per hour (12–18 L/24 h); rate of ultrafiltration maintained 7–15 mL/min
Disadvantage: • Can impose substantial hemodynamic stress not tolerated by patient • CVS abnormality	*Disadvantage:* • Not useful in patient of ARF following abdomen surgery since it needs intact peritoneum • Pain (56%), hemorrhage (30%) leakage (14%), restricted ability to clear fluid and uremic waste (39%) peritoneal infection. Difficulty making dialysate flow, protein loss limit its use	*Disadvantage:* • Anticoagulation required for very extended interval of time with risk of bleeding • Needs to accurately control quite large input and output volume ↓ Not recommended for routine management of ARF; used only for patient with refractory fluid overload, complicated ARF, acid base, and electrolyte derangement

In hepatic failure, acetate dialysis is contraindicated.
(CAVH: continues arteiro-venous hemofiltration; CVVH: continues veno-venous himodialysis; CVH: chronic villus sampling; ds: diagnostic score)

TABLE 9: Detection of biochemical abnormalities common in AKI.

	Non-hypercatabolic	Hypercataboli
1. Daily rise in BUN	10–20 mg/dL	20–100 mg/dL
2. Daily rise in serum creatinine	0.5–1.0 mg/dL	>2 mg/dL
3. Daily rise in serum potassium	<0.5 mEq/L	≥2 mEq/L
4. Daily rise in serum HCO_3^-	<1 mEq/L	>2 mEq/L

(AKI: acute kidney injury; BUN: blood urea nitrogen)

TABLE 10: Cardiorenal syndrome—pathophysiology and its management.

"Cardiorenal syndrome" (CRS) refers specifically to a spectrum of disorders involving both the heart and kidneys, wherein acute or chronic dysfunction in one organ may induce acute or chronic dysfunction in the other organ.

Type CRS	Nomenclature	Description	Examples
1	Acute cardiorenal syndrome	Acute heart failure resulting in AKI	*Situations:* Cardiogenic shock and AKI, ADHF, and AKI
2	Chronic cardio-renal syndrome	Chronic heart failure resulting in CKD	*Situations:* Chronic heart failure
3	Acute reno-cardiac syndrome	AKI resulting in acute heart failure	*Situations:* Heart failure in the setting of AKI from volume overload, inflammatory surge and accompanying metabolic disturbances
4	Chronic reno-cardiac syndrome	CKD resulting in chronic heart failure	*Situations:* Myocardial remodeling and heart failure from CKD-associated cardiomyopathy
5	Secondary cardio-renal syndrome	Systemic process resulting in heart	*Situations:* Diabetes, amyloidosis, sepsis, and cirrhosis

TABLE 8: Comparison of various modalities of renal replacement therapy.

Types

Hemodialysis	Peritoneal dialysis	Hemofiltration (CAVH and CVVH)
Indication: • Catabolic patient • Hemodynamically stable • Nonhypotensive • Diagnosed intraabdominal ds • Recent abdominal surgery	*Indication:* • Noncatabolic patient • Hemodynamically unstable patient • Poor vascular access • Active hemorrhage	Continuous process so that 1 L of plasma ultrafiltrate is removed per hour (12–18 L/24 h); rate of ultrafiltration maintained 7–15 mL/min
Disadvantage: • Can impose substantial hemodynamic stress not tolerated by patient • CVS abnormality	*Disadvantage:* • Not useful in patient of ARF following abdomen surgery since it needs intact peritoneum • Pain (56%), hemorrhage (30%) leakage (14%), restricted ability to clear fluid and uremic waste (39%) peritoneal infection. Difficulty making dialysate flow, protein loss limit its use	*Disadvantage:* • Anticoagulation required for very extended interval of time with risk of bleeding • Needs to accurately control quite large input and output volume ↓ Not recommended for routine management of ARF; used only for patient with refractory fluid overload, complicated ARF, acid base, and electrolyte derangement

In hepatic failure, acetate dialysis is contraindicated.
(CAVH: continues arteiro-venous hemofiltration; CVVH: continues veno-venous himodialysis; CVH: chronic villus sampling; ds: diagnostic score)

TABLE 9: Detection of biochemical abnormalities common in AKI.

	Non-hypercatabolic	Hypercataboli
1. Daily rise in BUN	10–20 mg/dL	20–100 mg/dL
2. Daily rise in serum creatinine	0.5–1.0 mg/dL	>2 mg/dL
3. Daily rise in serum potassium	<0.5 mEq/L	≥2 mEq/L
4. Daily rise in serum HCO_3^-	<1 mEq/L	>2 mEq/L

(AKI: acute kidney injury; BUN: blood urea nitrogen)

TABLE 10: Cardiorenal syndrome—pathophysiology and its management.

"Cardiorenal syndrome" (CRS) refers specifically to a spectrum of disorders involving both the heart and kidneys, wherein acute or chronic dysfunction in one organ may induce acute or chronic dysfunction in the other organ.

Type CRS	Nomenclature	Description	Examples
1	Acute cardiorenal syndrome	Acute heart failure resulting in AKI	*Situations:* Cardiogenic shock and AKI, ADHF, and AKI
2	Chronic cardio-renal syndrome	Chronic heart failure resulting in CKD	*Situations:* Chronic heart failure
3	Acute reno-cardiac syndrome	AKI resulting in acute heart failure	*Situations:* Heart failure in the setting of AKI from volume overload, inflammatory surge and accompanying metabolic disturbances
4	Chronic reno-cardiac syndrome	CKD resulting in chronic heart failure	*Situations:* Myocardial remodeling and heart failure from CKD-associated cardiomyopathy
5	Secondary cardio-renal syndrome	Systemic process resulting in heart	*Situations:* Diabetes, amyloidosis, sepsis, and cirrhosis

TABLE 11: Diuretic regimen.

	Current diuretic regimen		Suggested diuretic regimen	
Step	Furosemide dose	Thiazide	Furosemide dose (IV)	Metolazone
1	≤80 mg/day	+/–	40 mg + 5 mg/h	0
2	81–160 mg/day	+/–	80 mg + 10 mg/h	5 mg QD
3	161–240 mg/day	+/–	80 mg + 20 mg/h	5 mg BD
4	>240 mg/day	+/–	80 mg + 30 mg/h	5 mg BID

TABLE 12: Indications of real replacement therapy (RRT).

Acute RRT indications in common medical emergencies	Proposed cardiac intensive care unit (CICU)
A: Severe metabolic acidosis (i.e., severe lactic acidosis with refractory shock and multiorgan failure)	Patients with severe cardiac and/or valvular dysfunction and borderline blood pressure with AKI and volume overload
E: Severe electrolyte disturbances, most commonly hyperkalemia	Cardiogenic shock or heart failure with pulmonary edema on mechanical ventilation and high FiO_2 (>80% to 90%) despite diuretic therapy
I: Intoxication with dialyzable drugs or toxins	Precardiac surgical volume removal to improve likelihood of chest closure and prevent postoperative right ventricular failure
O: Medically refractory volume overload	Refractory cardiorenal syndrome with progressive AKI (e.g., stage 2–3 AKI plus volume overload with inadequate diuretic response)
U: Severe azotemia or symptoms of uremia	

CRITERIA FOR KIDNEY BIOPSY

Indication: (Required in only 20% Patients)

- Equivocal case history
- Renal sign suggestive of glomerular, vascular or interstitial lesion
- Patient with extra-renal manifestation
- Prolonged renal failure (beyond 6 weeks)

> **BOX 1:** Drugs—medications currently associated with acute tubular necrosis (ATN).
> - Aminoglycosides (tobramycin and gentamycin)
> - NSAIDs (ibuprofen, naproxen, ketorotac, and celecoxib)
> - ACEi (captopril, lisinopril, benazepril, and ramipril)
> - ARB (losartan, valsartan, candesartan, and irbesartan)
> - Amphotericin
> - Cisplatin
> - Foscarnet
> - Iodinated contrast
> - Pentamidine
> - Tenofovir
> - Zoledronic acid
>
> *Note:* Diuretics are not a classic cause of ATN, but they can aggravate the effects of some of the aforementioned medications.

- To confirm diagnosis of drug-induced interstitial nephritis by diffuse inflammatory infiltrate with prominent component of eosinophil and plasma cell
- When urine sediment contains red cell cases

Novel Biomarkers

Biomarkers are Needed

- Differentiate type of AKI
- To identify etiology
- Early diagnosis
- Predict severity
- Monitoring course and response to therapy

The various AKI biomarkers are:
Cystatin C–13 kD cysteine protein that is a potential alternative to serum creatinine in measurement of GFR. It is filtered solely by glomerulus, well-secreted in tubules; completely reabsorbed by the tubules and generated at a constant rate by all cells in body which serve a reasonable basis for GFR calculation. It is increased about 1–2 days earlier than serum creatinine in AKI patients. It also has a prognostic value with regard to the need for kidney transplant and in-hospital mortality.

TABLE 13: Comparison between CRRT modalities (i.e., CVVH) and Intermittent RRT Modalities (i.e., IHD) can be included.

	Continuous RRT modalities	**Intermittent RRT modalities**
Indication	• Hemodynamic instability • Volume control • Intracranial hypertension	• Severe acid-base and electrolyte imbalances • Intoxication • Refractory filter clotting
Advantage	• Hemodynamic stability • Stable, effective, and predictable volume control • Stable and predictable control of chemistry • Stable intracranial pressure • Disease modification by cytokine removal • Potentially imported chances of renal recovery	• (Relatively) inexpensive • Flexible timing allows for mobility/transport • Rapid correction of fluid overload • Rapid removal of dialyzable drugs • Minimizes anticoagulant exposure • Rapid correction of acidosis and electrolyte abnormality
Disadvantage	• Anticoagulation requirements • Reduced patient mobility • Higher cost	• Intradialytic hypotension • Potential nephrotoxicity • Risk of bowel and coronary ischemia

(CVVH: continuous veno-venous hemodialysis; IHD: intermittent hemodialysis)

Fluid Balance to Correct Electrolyte Imbalance
Salient Features

- Prevent and treat hyperkalemia
- Avoid hyponatremia
- Correct metabolic acidosis
- Minimize hyperphosphatemia and
- Treat hypocalcemia, only if symptomatic

Nutrition
Goals
- To prevent protein energy wasting
- To preserve lean body mass and nutritional status
- To avoid complications
- Improve immune status and wound healing
- Improve antioxidant and endothelial function
- Reduce mortality

Nutritional Requirement
- Total energy intake should be 20–30 kcal/kg/day in stage of AKI
- Energy:
  - Non-protein calories–25 kcal/kg/day
  - Carbohydrate–5 g/kg/day
  - *Fat:* 0.8–1.2 g/kg/day
- Protein:
  Conservative therapy (mild catabolism)–0.8 g/kg/day
  Extra-corporeal therapy, moderate catabolism: 1–1.5 g/kg/day
  CRRT or SLED, *severe catabolism:* 1.5–2 g/kg/day

RENAL REPLACEMENT THERAPY
Indications of Renal Replacement Therapy
Biochemical Indications
- Refractory hyperkalemia
- Serum urea
- Refractory metabolic acidosis pH <7.15
- *Refractory electrolyte abnormalities:* Hyponatremia, and hypernatremia of hypercalcemia. Tumor lysis syndrome with hyperuricemia and hyperphosphatemia. Urea cycle defects and organic acidosis resulting in hyperammonemia

Clinical Indications
- Urine output <0.3 mL/kg for 24 hours or complete anuria for 12 hours
- AKI with multiple organ failure

- Refractory volume overload
- End organ involvement pericarditis, encephalopathy, neuropathy, myopathy, and uremic bleeding
- Severe poisoning or drug overdose

Classification

- *Intermittent therapy*
  - Intermittent hemodialysis (IHD)
  - Sustained low efficacy dialysis (SLED)/extended daily dialysis (EDD)
- *Continuous therapy*
  - Slow continuous ultrafiltration (SCUF)
  - Continuous arterio-venous hemofiltration (CAVH)
  - Continuous arterio-venous hemodialysis (CAVH)
  - Continuous veno-venous hemodialysis (CVVHD)
  - Continuous veno-venous hemofiltration (CVVH)
  - Continuous arterio-venous hemodiafiltration (CAVHDF)
  - Continuous veno-venous hemofiltration (CVVHDF)

There is no consensus as to which modality is superior, each having its own strengths and weaknesses; by and large continuous therapies are used in hemodynamically unstable patients. The use of peritoneal dialysis in acute kidney injury is decreasing primarily because of the widespread availability of dialysis machines. However, PD has its unique advantages which includes the capacity to be performed anywhere.

CONTRAST-INDUCED ACUTE KIDNEY INJURY

Contrast-induced AKI (CI-AKI, also referred to as contrast-associated AKI) is a specific form of AKI that usually manifests as a transient small increase in serum creatinine (Scr) concentration within a few days of exposure to intravascular iodinated contrast. Despite its usually self-limited course, CI-AKI is associated with increased short- and long-term mortality, as well as progressive CKD. Recently, the degree to which radiocontrast affects the kidney has been debated because several studies (both meta-analyses and cohort studies) have suggested that in the aggregate population, the risk for AKI after contrast administration is perhaps overemphasized.

Management of CI-AKI aims primarily at prevention. Consideration should be given to alternative non-contrast studies if possible. Those who undergo iodinated contrast studies should have treatment with nonsteroidal anti-inflammatory drugs and other nephrotoxins discontinued, ideally at least 24 hours before the procedure. Low- or iso-osmolar radiocontrast should be used, at the lowest possible volume required. Isotonic intravenous fluid administration reduces the risk for CI-AKI and should be used in those at elevated risk. Typical regimens consist of a 1-mL/kg/h infusion 12 hours before and 12 hours after contrast exposure, or 3 mL/kg/h 1 hour before and 1.5 mL/kg/h for 4 to 6 hours post-procedure. With regard to fluid selection, although small studies suggested a benefit to the use of isotonic sodium bicarbonate solution, a large randomized clinical trial of isotonic bicarbonate versus normal saline solution (factorialized with N-acetylcysteine vs. placebo) in high-risk patients undergoing angiography showed no benefit with bicarbonate or N-acetylcysteine with regard to a composite end point of death, RRT, and 50% reduction in GFR at 90 days. There have been a variety of other pharmacotherapies evaluated for CI-AKI prevention, none of which is clearly beneficial. Hemodialysis after administration of contrast is ineffective for preventing CI-AKI and may cause harm.

Prevention of Acute Kidney Injury Includes

- Early recognition of "at risk" patients
- Maintaining adequate hydration to achieve effective circulatory volume
- Avoid nephrotoxic agent
- Recognize and treat sepsis promptly
- Follow contrast nephropathy guidelines in CKD

A pooled analysis of studies of long-term risk for CKD and dialysis dependence found a pooled hazard ratio of 8.8 for CKD and 3.1 for end-stage kidney disease in patients with AKI compared with those without AKI.

It is currently recommended that all patients who experience AKI have their kidney function re-evaluated 3 months after AKI to identify those with new/worsening CKD, which should be managed accordingly. Even those who return to their baseline kidney function should be considered at elevated risk for the development of CKD. At this time, it is unclear whether any intervention or increase in monitoring would reduce the risk for poor outcomes in these patients.

SUGGESTED READING

1. Bucaloiu ID, Kirchner, HL, Norfolk ER, Hartie JE, Perkins RM. Increased risk of death and de novo CKD following reversible AKI. Kidney Int. 2012;81:477-85.
2. Darmon M, Ostermann M, Cerda, J, Dimopoulos MA, Forni L, Hoste E, et al. Diagnostic work-up and specific causes of AKI. Intensive Care Med. 2017;43:829-40.
3. Lewington AJP, Kanayasundarum NS. (2010). Clinical Practice Guidelines for Acute Kidney Injury. Available from http://www.renal.org/clinical/guidelines section/acute kidney injury aspx; [Last accessed March, 2025].
4. Moore PK, Hsu RK, Liu KD. Management of Acute Kidney Injury: Core Curriculum 2018. Am J Kidney Dis. 72(1):136-48.
5. Rangaswami J, Bhalla V, Blair JEA, Chang TI, Costa S, Lentine KL, et al. Cardiorenal syndrome: classification, pathophysiology, diagnosis, and treatment strategies: a scientific statement from the American Heart Association. Circulation 2019;139:e840-78.
6. Wang C, Pei YY, Ma YH, Ma XL, Liu ZW, Zhu JH, et al. Risk factors for acute kidney injury in patients with acute myocardial infarction. Chin Med J (Engl). 2019;132(14):1660-5.

CHAPTER 22

Endocrine Emergencies

Ajitesh Roy

Endocrine emergencies are dealt by internists more than by endocrinologists, so a thorough knowledge of handling these patients is mandatory for all emergency physicians and internists.

Commonly encountered endocrine emergencies may be enlisted as follows:
- *Diabetes related endocrine emergencies:*
  - Diabetic ketoacidosis (DKA)
  - Hyperglycemic hyperosmolar state (HHS)-HONK
  - Hypoglycemic states
- *Nondiabetes-related endocrine emergencies:*
  - Adrenal crisis
  - Pheochromocytoma with acute presentation
  - Pituitary apoplexy
  - Thyroid storm
  - Myxedema coma
  - Hypercalcemia
  - Hypocalcemia
- *Others:* Hyponatremia and hypernatremia

ADRENAL CRISIS

It is a state of acute adrenal insufficiency (primary or secondary). It usually occurs when It usually manifested with shock but there are some other nonspecific features:
- Nausea or vomiting with or without pain abdomen
- Hyperpigmentation in case of primary
- Severe fatigue
- Fever
- Hyponatremia
- hyperkalemia (in case of primary)
- Hypoglycemia

In a known case of primary adrenal insufficiency, risk of a crisis is 6–8 per 100-patient years. In a recent prospective study on adrenal insufficiency patients, it was shown that overall mortality due to crisis is 0.5/100-patient years. Some adrenal insufficiency patients are yet unexplainably prone to have repeated episodes of adrenal crisis whereas the rest remain without such even for decades.

Primary Adrenal Crisis
- Adrenal infection—histoplasmosis and tuberculosis
- Autoimmune
- Adrenal infiltration—metastasis, lymphoma, and sarcoidosis
- Adrenal hemorrhage—*Meningococcus sepsis* (Waterhouse-Friderickson Syndrome), antiphospholipid syndrome, anticoagulant therapy, and disseminated intravascular coagulation (DIC)
- Drug induced—ketoconazole and etomidate

Secondary Adrenal Insufficiency
Pituitary tumor and mass lesion affecting hypothalamopituitary region, pituitary irradiation, autoimmune hypophysitis, pituitary apoplexy, and combined pituitary hormone deficiency.

Sign and Symptoms
- *Glucocorticoid deficiency:* Fatigue, lack of energy, myalgia, joint pain, fever, anemia, hypoglycemia, postural hypotension, and hyponatremia
- *Mineralocorticoid deficiency:* Abdominal pain, nausea, vomiting, dizziness, and postural hypotension
- *Adrenal androgen deficiency:* Lack of energy, dry and itchy skin, loss of libido, loss of axillary, and pubic hair.

PITUITARY APOPLEXY
Definition
Classical pituitary apoplexy refers to a clinical syndrome, characterized by sudden onset of headache, vomiting, visual impairment, and decrease consciousness caused by hemorrhage and/or infarction of the pituitary gland (UK guideline 2010).

Flowchart 1: Diagnostic approach to adrenocortical insufficiency.

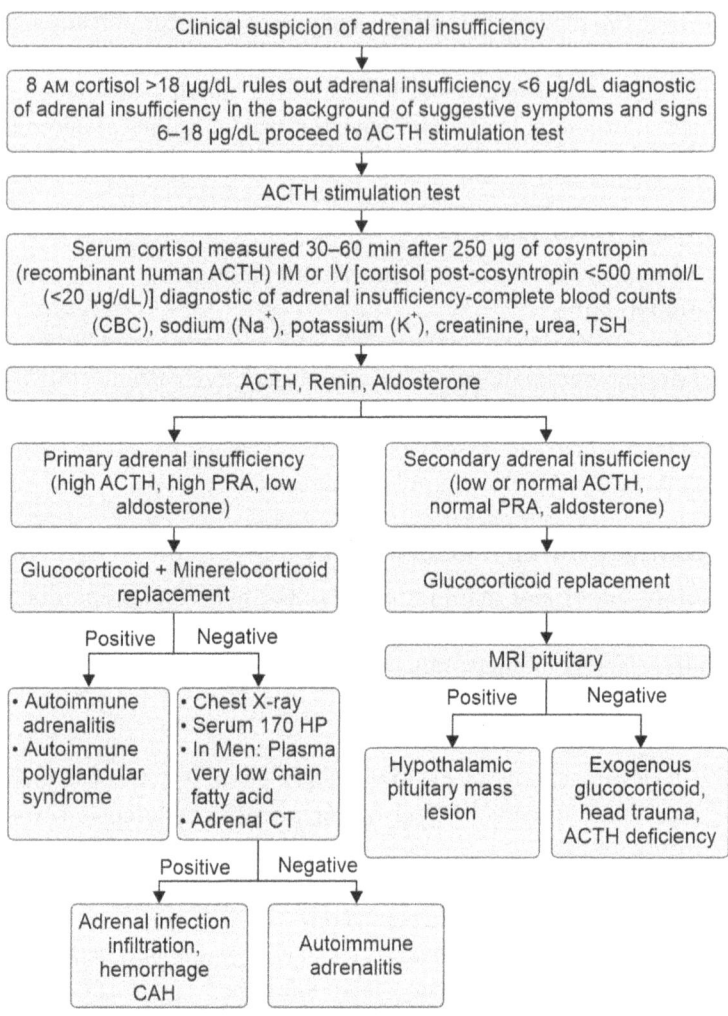

It is due to acute hemorrhage or infarction of pituitary gland. Vascular supply of anterior pituitary gland is derived from the branches of the internal carotid arteries (superior and inferior hypophyseal arteries) which form the hypophyseal portal passing through the pituitary stalk. Apoplexy is believed to be due to compression of this portal system by enlarging pituitary resulting in compromised blood supply.

> **BOX 1:** Treatment: Acute adrenal insufficiency.
> - Infuse 1 liter of isotonic saline or 5% dextrose in isotonic saline as quickly as possible. Repeat fluid bolus resuscitation, followed by maintenance fluids
> - Give hydrocortisone (100 mg intravenous bolus) followed by 50 mg intravenously every 6 hours
> - Continue intravenous isotonic saline at a slower rate for next 24–48 hours
> - Search for and treat possible infectious precipitating causes of the adrenal crisis
> - Taper parenteral glucocorticoid over 1–3 days, if precipitating or complicating illness permits, to oral glucose saline infusion is stopped or hydrocortisone dose is tapered to <40 mg daily
>
> *Prevention of adrenal crisis is done by patient education and appropriate dose adjustment of glucocorticoids under stressful situations such as minor and major surgical procedures, infection, and fever.*

History and Clinical Features

Patient usually presents with headache, nausea, vomiting, diminished visual acuity, or visual field defects, (diplopia and ptosis) due to cavernous sinus involvement (third, fourth, ophthalmic, and maxillary division of fifth and sixth cranial nerves).

Headache occurs in >90% of patients (often retro-orbital). Vomiting occurs in about 70% of patients simultaneously with headache.

Visual acuity and field defects occur in 50-60% of patients and according to level of compression on optic nerve, chiasma, or tract.

- If the optic chiasma is compressed, the defect is bitemporal superior quadrantanopia (earliest field defect).
- Optic tract involvement may occur if the chiasma is *prefixed* and result in bitemporal homonymous hemianopia (common).
- When the optic chiasma is *postfixed*, the pituitary may compress optic nerve with ipsilateral visual acuity loss and a central scotoma on visual field testing.
- Extraocular muscle paresis is common (80%) and usually result from compression of cranial nerves in the cavernous sinus, which gives symptoms and signs of ptosis, diplopia, and strabismus.
  - Involvement of third cranial nerve—most common

- Involvement of IV cranial nerve—less common
- Involvement of VI cranial nerve (isolated)—least common
- Involvement of cranial nerve V. This may produce facial pain and sensory loss over the face.
- *Carotid artery:* It may be compressed leading to stroke. Blood in subarachnoid space may cause spasm of cerebral arteries, meningismus, stupor, and coma.
- *Hypothalamus:* Involvement of hypothalamus may alter thermal regulation.

Precipitating Cause

- Pregnancy—due to temporary enlargement of pituitary which compromises blood supply followed by postpartum pituitary necrosis of a nontumorous gland due to arterial spasm due to postpartum hemorrhage. This is also defined as Sheehan's syndrome. An inability to lactate after delivery due to prolactin deficiency and amenorrhea secondary to gonadotrophin deficiency are seen. Also central Hypothyroidism and hypoadrenalism are observed.
- Coagulopathy, anticoagulant therapy
- *Head trauma*: Pituitary stalk injury
- Hypertension
- Major surgery especially CABG
- Endocrine stimulation test such as insulin tolerance test
- Rapid Initiation of DA-agonist

Management

Strong clinical suspicion is essential to diagnose pituitary apoplexy as in only 40% of cases there are definite precipitating factors present.

Liasion with endocrinologist and neurosurgery is essential component for successful management of these patients.

Medical

- Secondary adrenal insufficiency occurs in about two-thirds of these patients. Glucocorticoids are therefore the mainstay therapy to prevent mortality and morbidity.

- IV hydrocortisone 100 mg bolus followed by 2–4 mg/h IV infusion (alternatively 50 mg 6 hourly IM) to continue until the patient is stable. IV infusion is preferred to intermittent IV doses due to saturation kinetics followed by cortisol binding globulin which results in reduced drug availability.
- Blood samples for hormonal profile (cortisol, TSH, fT4, estradiol in women, testosterone in men, prolactin, IGF-1, FSH, and LH) electrolytes, renal function, liver function, counts, and coagulation profile should be drawn before starting steroid.
- Quick tapering to oral steroid in the form of oral hydrocortisone 20–30 mg/day in three divided doses should be started and continued once acute episode is over.
- After collection of blood samples and administration of bolus steroid diagnosis should be confirmed by an urgent MRI pituitary (if contraindicated, a dedicated CT scan of pituitary gland).
- Fluid balance and electrolyte status should be assessed closely and blood counts, urea, creatinine, sodium, potassium, plasma, and urine osmolality should be checked at least once daily.
- Every patient should undergo an endocrine review after 4–8 weeks following the event.
- Thyroid hormone replacement for secondary hypothyroidism.
- Sex hormone replacement in gonadotropin deficiency.

Surgical

Cases with severe neuro-ophthalmic signs or deteriorating neurological status or visual impairment should be considered for surgery. Visual outcome is usually good after surgery.

PHEOCHROMOCYTOMA AND HYPERTENSIVE CRISIS

Pheochromocytoma is an endocrinologist's curiosity but it is often a nightmare for anesthetist. An undiagnosed or improperly treated pheochromocytoma can cause severe morbidity or even mortality.

Hypertensive crisis in pheochromocytoma is an hypertensive emergency.

Treatment

- Phenoxybenzamine/oral prazosin, an α-adrenoceptor blocker is mostly used for preoperative control of blood pressure.
- Liberal salt intake and hydration are allowed to avoid severe orthostasis.
- Beta(β)-blockers are often used to control arrhythmias. But, a β-blocker should never be used before first blocking α-adrenoceptor-mediated vasoconstriction by an α-blocker, because loss of $β_2$-adrenoceptor-mediated vasodilatation and unopposed α-adrenoceptor-mediated vasoconstriction may precipitate hypertensive crisis.
- CCBs and ARBs/ACE-i have also been used with success.
- Phentolamine may be used to treat hypertensive crisis. It can be given by:
  - IV boluses of 2.5–5 mg at the rate of 1 mg/min; it can be repeated every 5 minutes until desired effect is reached.
  - IV continuous infusion by dissolving 100 mg of phentolamine in 500 mg of 5% dextrose and infusion rate is adjusted according to blood pressure response.
  - Sodium nitroprusside—IV sodium nitroprusside could be infused alternatively at the rate of 0.5–5 μg/kg/min.
  - Cardiac arrhythmias should be managed with lidocaine (50–100 mg intravenously) or esmolol (50–200 μg/kg/min intravenously).
- Postoperative hypotension can be avoided by adequate crystalloids and hypoglycemia (which can occur in 10–15% of patients) by glucose containing infusion.

THYROID STORM/THYROTOXIC CRISIS

Thyrotoxic crisis is an acute, life-threatening, hypermetabolic state induced by iatrogenic or spontaneous release of thyroid hormones in a patient with uncontrolled thyrotoxicosis. Rarely, thyroid hormones storm may be the initial presentation of thyrotoxicosis. The morbidity rate in undiagnosed and untreated case is 90% which could be reduced to <20% by early diagnosis and treatment.

Thyroid storm can be triggered by many different events usually in patients with underlying Grave's disease and toxic multinodular goiter.
- Infection
- Surgery
- Cardiac events
- DKA
- Radioactive iodine
- Sudden stoppage of antithyroid drugs
- Vigorous palpation of thyroid gland

Though these patients are not able to give history but following history from a family member may help in the diagnosis.
- Weight loss (15%)
- Palpitation
- Tremor
- Nervousness, anxiety, and emotional lability
- Heat intolerance
- Psychosis
- Menstrual irregularities
- Disorientation
- Dyspnea
- Bowel movements hyperactivity

Clinical Examination
- Fever
- Relative tachycardia
- Profuse sweating
- Dehydration
- Goiter
- Fine tremor
- Warm, moist skin
- Widened pulse pressure
- Congestive cardiac failure
- Atrial fibrillation
- Exophthalmos
- Thyroid bruit

Management

In a known case of thyrotoxicosis high suspicion should be kept for thyroid storm. Thyroid storm is a clinical diagnosis, thus the diagnosis has been augmented by few diagnostic systems. Two standard systems are BWPS (Burch–Wartofsky point scale) and JTA (Japanese Thyroid Association) category (TS1 and TS2), the former being a more sensitive one.

In BWPS, seven clinical parameters are taken (temperature, heart rate, presence of atrial fibrillation, severity of congestive cardiac failure, GI dysfunction, CNS disturbances, and precipitating history status) and scored according to severity.

Total score >45 is consistent with thyroid storm, 25–44 is impending thyroid storm, and <25 makes the diagnosis unlikely.

Laboratory Confirmation

- Treatment should be started immediately without waiting for the reports. Several laboratory features (except elevated T_4 and T_3 and low TSH) may be associated with thyroid storm such as:
- Leukocytosis
- Hypokalemia
- Hyperglycemia
- Hypercalcemia
- Liver function abnormalities
- ECG-sinus tachycardia, atrial fibrillation
- Chest X-ray shows CCF or infection.

Treatment

Treatment is aimed at the following broad areas of interest:
- Blockade of thyroid hormone synthesis and secretion
- Blockade of peripheral action at tissue level
- Reversal of decompensation
- Correction of precipitating event or intercurrent illness
- Definitive therapy
    - Once thyroid storm is suspected, treatment should not be delayed.

TABLE 1: Treatment of thyroid storm.

Drugs	Dosage	Effect
PTU	250 mg every 4 hours	• Inhibit hormonogenesis • Blocks T_4 to T_3 conversion
MMZ	20 mg every 6 h/d	Inhibit hormonogenesis
Propranolol (alternative drug: Esmolol infusion)	60 mg every 4–6 hours	Blocks T_4 to T_3 conversion in high doses; monitor invasively in cardiac failure patients
SSKI[a] (alternative drug: Lugol's solution)	5 drops (0.25 mL or 250 mg) orally every 6 hours	• Inhibit hormonogenesis • Inhibit release of thyroid hormone
Hydrocortisone[b] (alternative drug:	300 mg intravenous load, then 100 mg every 8 hours	May block T_4 to T_3 conversion

Note:
[a]Not to start until 1 hour after antithyroid drug
[b]Prophylactically used against relative adrenal insufficiency
Patients not responding (or intolerant to antithyroid drugs) to therapeutic measures may be treated with surgery (with or without plasmapheresis/plasma exchange)
(MMZ: methimazole; PTU: propylthiouracil; SSKI: saturated solution of potassium iodide)

- Patient should be intubated, if level of consciousness is profoundly altered.
- Supplemental oxygen to maintain oxygen saturation.
- Aggressive fluid replacement according to electrolyte levels.
- Appropriate electrolyte replacement according to electrolytes levels.
- Fever is controlled with cooling with cooling measures and paracetamol. Aspirin should be avoided as it interferes with thyroid hormone binding with the circulating proteins resulting in increased free T_3 and T_4.

Aggressively treat infections or any other precipitant: Iodide should not be used in pregnancy with thyroid storm as it can lead to goiter in fetus. PTU should be preferred in pregnancy on in the first trimester. Carbimazole/methimazole is preferred in the second/third trimester.

Prevention of thyroid storm can be done by recognizing and avoiding the precipitating cause or event, patient education, improving compliance to antithyroid drugs, proper precautions prior to surgery, labor, or other stressors.

MYXEDEMA COMA

It occurs almost exclusively in older patients, especially in winter months, has a high mortality rate, and delay in clinical diagnosis worsens the prognosis. High index of suspicion is the key to diagnosis and better outcome.

Cause

Precipitating factors are:
- Hypothermia
- Infections especially pneumonia
- Myocardial infarction or congestive heart failure
- Cerebrovascular accident (CVA)
- Respiratory depression due to drugs (e.g., anesthetics, sedatives, and tranquilizers)
- Trauma

Clinical Features

Main features are:
- Altered mental state ranging from poor cognitive function through psychosis to coma; sometimes seizures
- Delayed relaxation of deep tendon reflexes or areflexia at times
- Hypothermia (as low as 23°C)
- Absence of fever in spite of severe infection.

Other Features

- Respiratory depression and CO_2 narcosis
- Bradycardia
- Hypotension
- Low voltage on ECG
- Dilutional hyponatremia
- Hypoglycemia
- Anemia
- Raised CPK and LDH

> **BOX 2:** Other aspects of management.
>
> *Supportive measures*
> - Mechanical ventilation—If GCS <8
> - Fluids and vasopressor drugs
> - *Passive rewarming*: Gastric warm saline, perfusion may be used for internal warming
> - Intravenous dextrose
> - Consider empirical antibiotic
> - Monitor for arrhythmias

Thyroid Function Test

Thyroid function test (TSH) values may only be modestly raised (and will be normal or low in secondary hypothyroidism) but free T_4 levels are usually very low.

Treatment

Rapid replacement of thyroid hormones is needed but there is no agreement on whether it should be "high dose" or "low dose". In view of a severe hypometabolic state and unpredictable enteral absorptive function, medications are preferably to be administered IV to get rapid response.

If intravenous levothyroxine is available, administer levothyroxine 200-400 µg intravenously, followed by daily doses of 50-100 µg, and triiodothyronine 5-20 µg intravenously, followed by 2.5-10 µg every 8 hours. Oral thyroxine (LT4 + LT3) in similar doses are given (usually by nasogastric tube) in these part of country because of nonavailability of IV Thyroxine. IV Hydrocortisone 5-10 mg/h should be administered to prevent relative adrenal insufficiency.

DIABETIC EMERGENCIES

Hyperglycemia

Diabetic Ketoacidosis and the Hyperglycemia Hyperosmolar State

Diabetic ketoacidosis and the hyperglycemia hyperosmolar state (HHS) appear as two extremes in the spectrum of diabetic decompensation. They remain the most serious acute metabolic complications of diabetes mellitus and are still associated with excess mortality. Because the approach to the diagnosis and treatment of these hyperglycemic crises are similar, we have opted to address them together.

Diagnosis and Clinical Presentation

A definitive diagnosis of DKA or HHS must be confirmed through laboratory investigation. The clinical presentation can provide helpful information for the preliminary bedside diagnosis. DKA usually occurs in younger, lean patients with type 1 diabetes and develops within a day or so, whereas HHS is more likely to occur in older, obese patients with type 2 diabetes, and an take days or weeks to fully develop. In addition, HHS usually occurs in elderly diabetic patients, often those with decreased renal function who do not have access to water. In both conditions, abdominal pain with nausea and vomiting can develop owing to acidosis per se or to decreased mesenteric perfusion and can be mistaken for an acute surgical abdomen. Kussmaul-Kien respiration (rapid and deep respiration) with breath acetone is typical of DKA but is absent in HHS. DKA and HHS are usually accompanied by hypothermia, a normal or elevated temperature may indicate underlying infection.

Diabetic Ketoacidosis

Introduction

It is characterized by the biochemical triad of:
- Hyperglycemia

TABLE 2: Typical water and serum electrolyte deficits at presentation in DKA and HHS.

Parameter	DKA	HHS
Water, mL/kg	100 (7 L)	100–200 (10.5 L)
Sodium, mmol/kg	7–10 (490–70)	5–13 (350–910)
Potassium, mmol/kg	3–5 (210–300)	5–15 (350–1050)
Chloride, mmol/kg	3–5 (210–350)	3–7 (210–490)
Phosphate, mmol/kg	1–1.5 (70–105)	1–2 (70–140)
Magnesium, mmol/kg	1–2 (70–140)	1–2 (70–40)
Calcium, mmol/kg	1–2 (70–140)	1–2 (70–140)

(DKA: diabetic ketoacidosis; HHS: hyperglycemic hyperosmolar state)

TABLE 3: Laboratory diagnostic criteria for DKA and HHS.

Parameter	Normal range	DKA	HHS
Plasma glucose level, mmol/L	4.2–6.4	≤14	≤34
Arterial pH	7.35–7.45	≤7.30	≤34
Serum bicarbonate level mmol/L	22–28	≤15	>15
Effective serum osmolality mmol/kg	275–295	≤320	>320
Anion gap, †mmol/L	<12	<12	Variable
Serum ketones	Negative	Moderate to high	None of trace

Note:
*If venous pH is used, a correction of 0.03 must be made
†Calculation: [Na^+ – (Cl + HCO_3)]
(DKA: diabetic ketoacidosis; HHS: hyperglycemic hyperosmolar state)

- Ketosis
- Metabolic acidosis.

With appropriate treatment mortality rate is <1% and mostly attributed to the precipitating events like infection etc.

Cause

Relative or absolute insulin deficiency and excess counter regulatory hormones (including glucagon, catecholamines, growth hormones and cortisol, etc.) resulting in decreased insulin glucagon ratio in the background of a number of various precipitating events (see below) modulate a number of enzymatic activities involved in carbohydrate metabolism shifting it toward greater glucose synthesis (by glycogenolysis and gluconeogenesis) and lesser glucose degradation (glycolysis).

Role of Counter Regulatory Hormones

Hypersecretion of epinephrine, glucagon, cortisol, growth hormone promote glycogenolysis, neoglucogenesis (decrease activity of pyruvate kinase), and activating lipolysis.

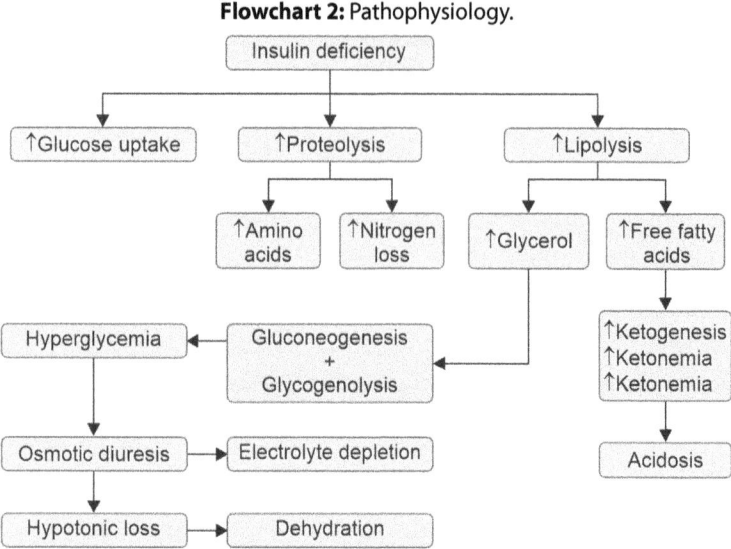

Flowchart 2: Pathophysiology.

History and Clinical Features

History—onset of symptoms < 24 hours

Patients generally give an history of diabetes with poor compliance to treatment (20% of DKA may present without any history of diabetes).

A history of the common event that may precipitate DKA are:
- Stoppage of insulin or inadequate and irregular insulin therapy is the most common cause (33%)
- The history of infection (pneumonia and UTI—30-50 percent of the illnesses that lead to DKA)
- Alcohol abuse
- Trauma
- Tissue ischemia such as AMI and stroke
- Pulmonary embolism
- Drug abuse—corticosteriods, sympathomimetic agents; pentamidine, excessive use of diuretics in elderly
- Pancreatitis
- Eating disorder and mental health disorder

Symptoms of DKA
- Nausea and vomiting
- Thirst, polyuria, polydipsia, and weight loss
- Abdominal pain
- Shortness of breath
- Altered mental status
- Fatigue

Signs
A thorough physical examination with emphasis on the following must be done:
- Presence of any infection
- Patency of airway
- Cardiovascular + respiratory status

Important Signs
- Fruity odor of breath
- Signs of dehydration
  - Loss of skin turgor and dry mucous membrane
  - Tachycardia
  - Hypotension
- *Tachypnea:* Rapid and deep respiration (Kussmaul respiration)
- Abdominal tenderness
- *Sensorium:* Alert to drowsy to comatose (10-15%) (when serum osmolality exceeds 340 mOsmol/kg)
- *Temperature:* Normal to hypothermic

Bedside Assessment
- Determination of capillary blood glucose and ketone
- Qualitative assessment of urine + blood glucose, ketones using reagent stick

Where to Manage?
- If patient is alert to mildly drowsy with moderate dehydration—manage in ward.

- Patient comatose with or without features of hypovolemic shock → manage in intensive care unit.

Initial Investigations (After Transfer to ITU)
- Blood gas analysis—immediate
- Blood glucose
- Urea, creatinine
- Electrolytes
- Urine and/or serum ketones
- Blood count DC
- Cultures of blood, urine, and other body fluids
- Chest X-ray
- ECG
- Serum osmolality
- Other investigations to establish source of infection and eliminate associated conditions such as:
    - Pancreatitis
    - Myocardial infarction
    - Pulmonary embolism, etc.

TABLE 4: Classification of diabetic ketoacidosis.

	Mild	*Moderate*	*Severe*
Plasma glucose	>250 mg/dL	>250 mg/dL	>250 mg/dL
Urine and serum ketosis	Positive	Positive	Positive
Serum osmolality	Variable	Variable	Variable
[Na$^+$] in mEq/L + glucose 18 + BUN/2.8 (normal) 290 ± 5			
Anion Gap Na$^+$ − (Cl$^-$ + HCO) (normal) 7–9 mEq	10–12	>12	>12
Arterial pH	7.25–7.3	7.0–<7.24	<7.0
Sensorium	Alert	Alert—drowsy	Drowsy—comatose

Flowchart 3: Treatment of diabetic ketoacidosis in adults.

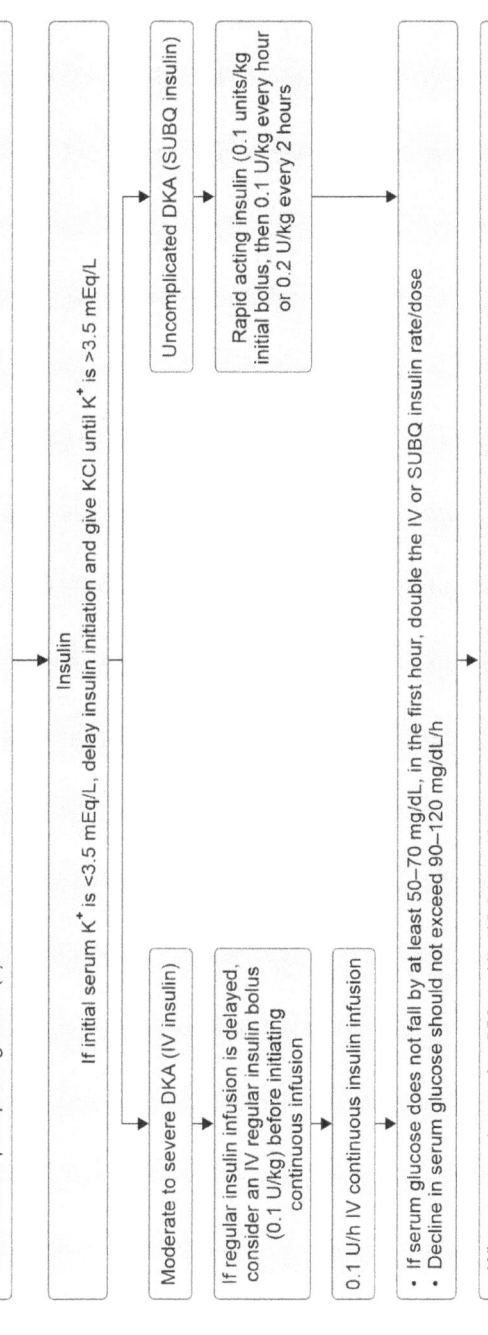

Contd...

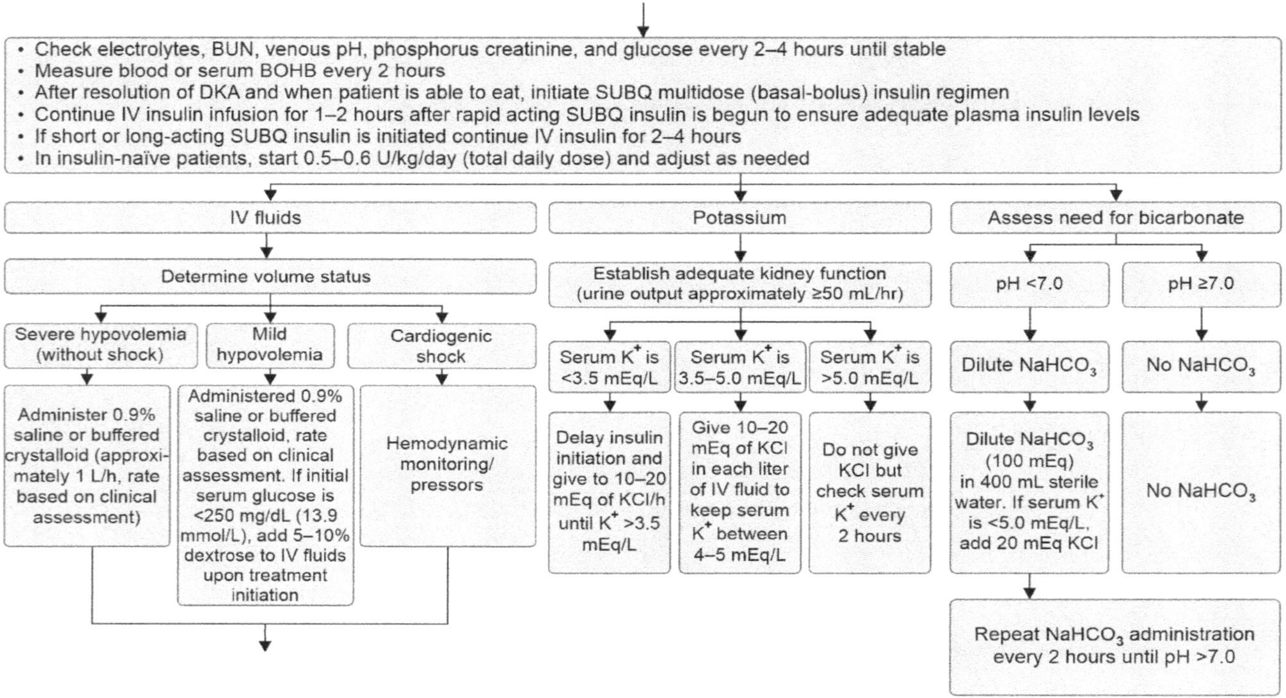

- Check electrolytes, BUN, venous pH, phosphorus creatinine, and glucose every 2–4 hours until stable
- Measure blood or serum BOHB every 2 hours
- After resolution of DKA and when patient is able to eat, initiate SUBQ multidose (basal-bolus) insulin regimen
- Continue IV insulin infusion for 1–2 hours after rapid acting SUBQ insulin is begun to ensure adequate plasma insulin levels
- If short or long-acting SUBQ insulin is initiated continue IV insulin for 2–4 hours
- In insulin-naive patients, start 0.5–0.6 U/kg/day (total daily dose) and adjust as needed

IV fluids

Determine volume status

- **Severe hypovolemia (without shock)**: Administer 0.9% saline or buffered crystalloid (approximately 1 L/h, rate based on clinical assessment)
- **Mild hypovolemia**: Administered 0.9% saline or buffered crystalloid, rate based on clinical assessment. If initial serum glucose is <250 mg/dL (13.9 mmol/L), add 5–10% dextrose to IV fluids upon treatment initiation
- **Cardiogenic shock**: Hemodynamic monitoring/pressors

Potassium

Establish adequate kidney function (urine output approximately ≥50 mL/hr)

- **Serum K⁺ is <3.5 mEq/L**: Delay insulin initiation and give to 10–20 mEq of KCl/h until K⁺ >3.5 mEq/L
- **Serum K⁺ is 3.5–5.0 mEq/L**: Give 10–20 mEq of KCl in each liter of IV fluid to keep serum K⁺ between 4–5 mEq/L
- **Serum K⁺ is >5.0 mEq/L**: Do not give KCl but check serum K⁺ every 2 hours

Assess need for bicarbonate

- **pH <7.0**: Dilute NaHCO₃. Dilute NaHCO₃ (100 mEq) in 400 mL sterile water. If serum K⁺ is <5.0 mEq/L, add 20 mEq KCl. Repeat NaHCO₃ administration every 2 hours until pH >7.0
- **pH ≥7.0**: No NaHCO₃. No NaHCO₃

Contd...

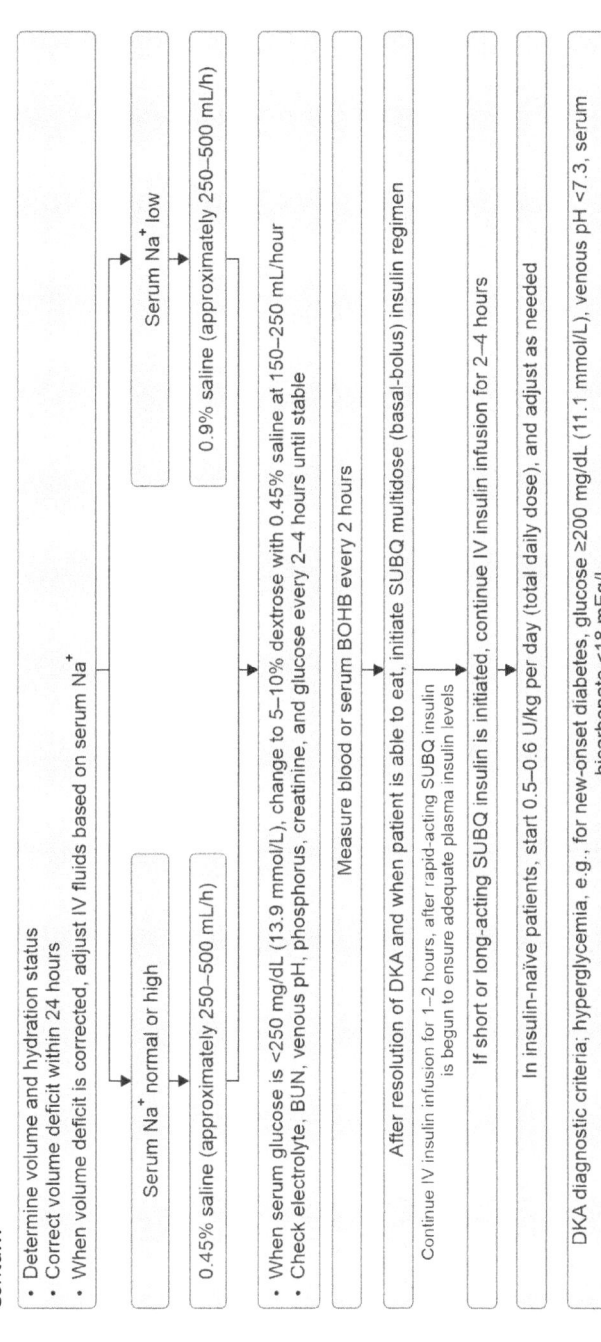

Contd…

- Determine volume and hydration status
- Correct volume deficit within 24 hours
- When volume deficit is corrected, adjust IV fluids based on serum Na⁺

Serum Na⁺ normal or high → 0.45% saline (approximately 250–500 mL/h)

Serum Na⁺ low → 0.9% saline (approximately 250–500 mL/h)

- When serum glucose is <250 mg/dL (13.9 mmol/L), change to 5–10% dextrose with 0.45% saline at 150–250 mL/hour
- Check electrolyte, BUN, venous pH, phosphorus, creatinine, and glucose every 2–4 hours until stable

Measure blood or serum BOHB every 2 hours

After resolution of DKA and when patient is able to eat, initiate SUBQ multidose (basal-bolus) insulin regimen

Continue IV insulin infusion for 1–2 hours, after rapid-acting SUBQ insulin is begun to ensure adequate plasma insulin levels

If short or long-acting SUBQ insulin is initiated, continue IV insulin infusion for 2–4 hours

In insulin-naive patients, start 0.5–0.6 U/kg per day (total daily dose), and adjust as needed

DKA diagnostic criteria; hyperglycemia, e.g., for new-onset diabetes, glucose ≥200 mg/dL (11.1 mmol/L), venous pH <7.3, serum bicarbonate <18 mEq/L

(BOHB: beta-hydroxybutyrate; BUN: bleed urea nitrogen; DKA: diabetic ketoacidosis; HCO₃: bicarbonate; IV: intravenous; K⁺: potassium; KCl: potassium chloride; NA⁺: sodium; NaCl: sodium chloride; NaHCO₃: sodium bicarbonate; STAT: intervention should be performed emergently; SUBQ: subcutaneous)

Endocrine Emergencies

Flowchart 4: Treatment of hyperosmolar hyperglycemic state in adults.

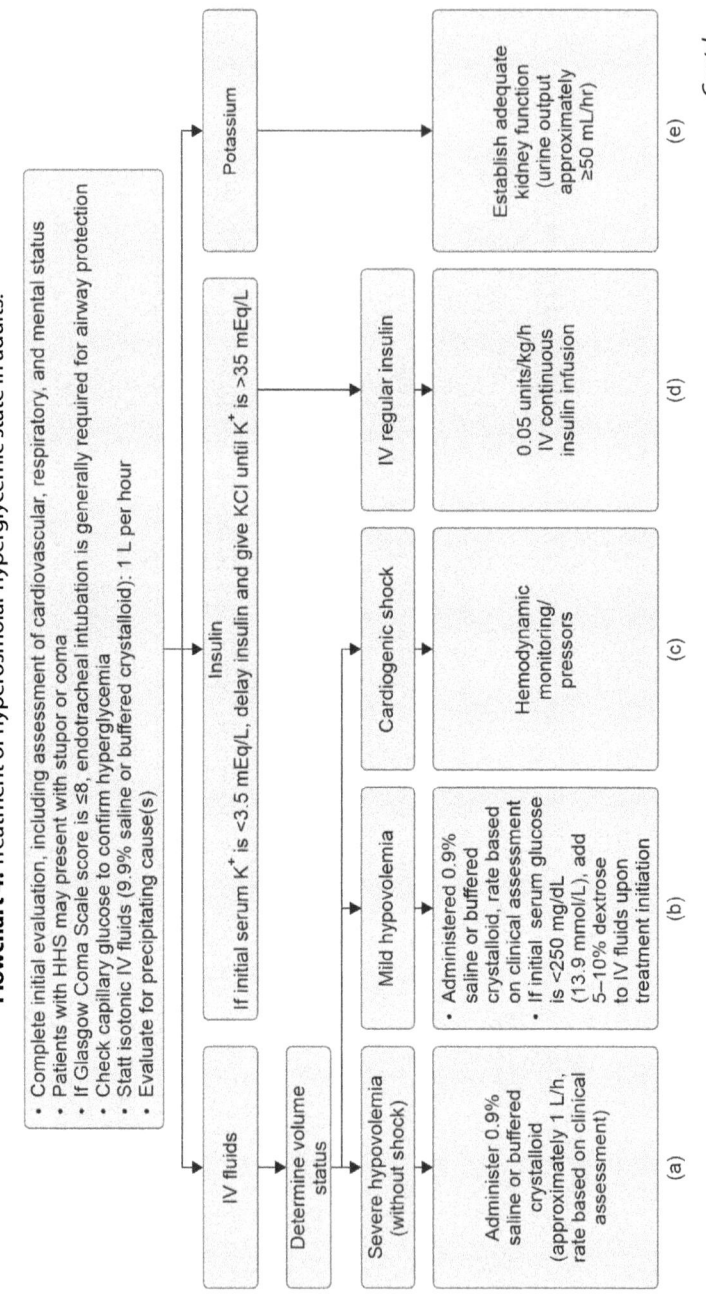

Contd...

Endocrine Emergencies

Contd...

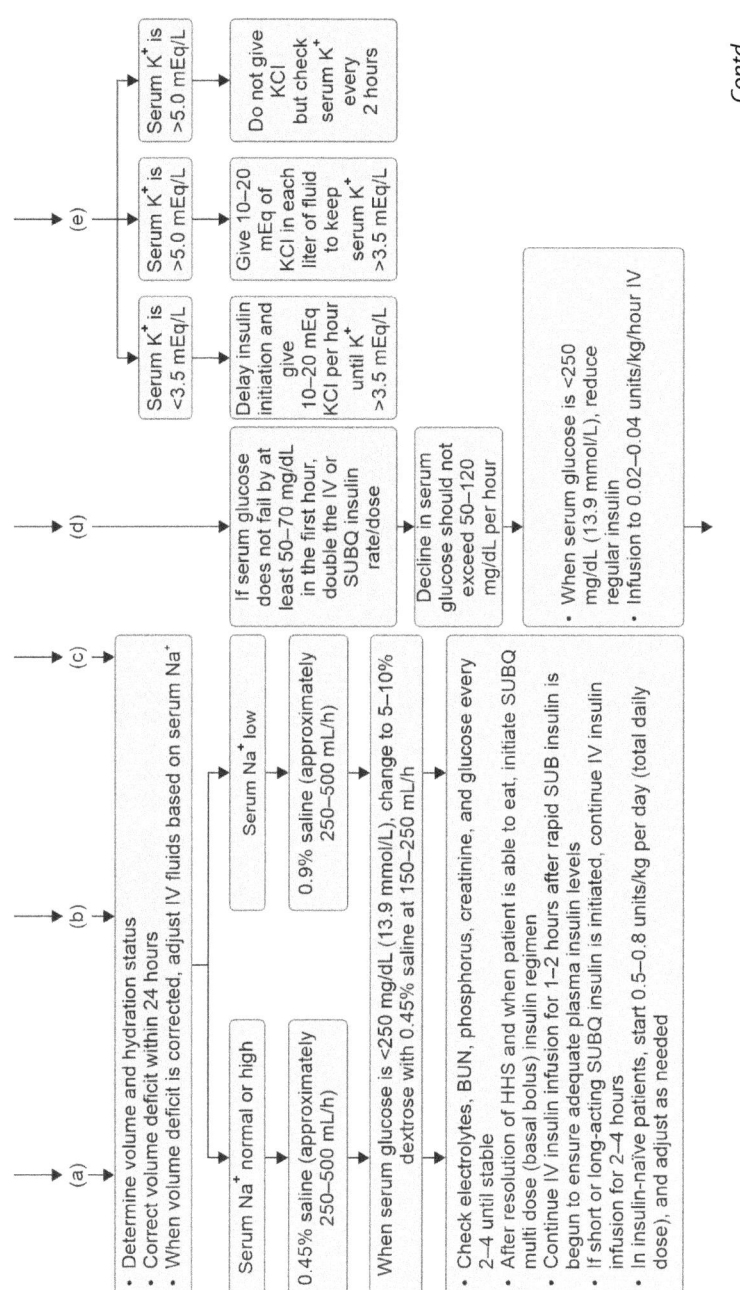

Contd...

Contd...

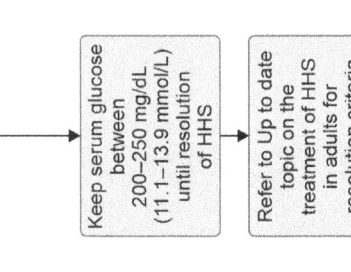

HHS diagnostic criteria: Hyperglycemia (glucose ≥60.0 mg/mmol/L), serum osmolality >300 mOsm/kg, arterial pH >7.3 serum bicarbonate >18 mEq/L, and minimal ketonuria (<2+) or ketonemia (BOHB <3 mmol/L). Normal laboratory values vary; check local laboratory reference ranges for all electrolytes.

(BOHB: beta-hydroxybutyrate; BUN: blood urea nitrogen; DKA: diabetic ketoacidosis; HHS: hyperosmolar hyperglycemic state; IV: intravenous; K^+: potassium; KCl: potassium chloride; Na^+: sodium; NaCl: sodium chloride; STAT: intervention should be performed emergently; SUBQ: subcutaneous)

Contd...

Endocrine Emergencies

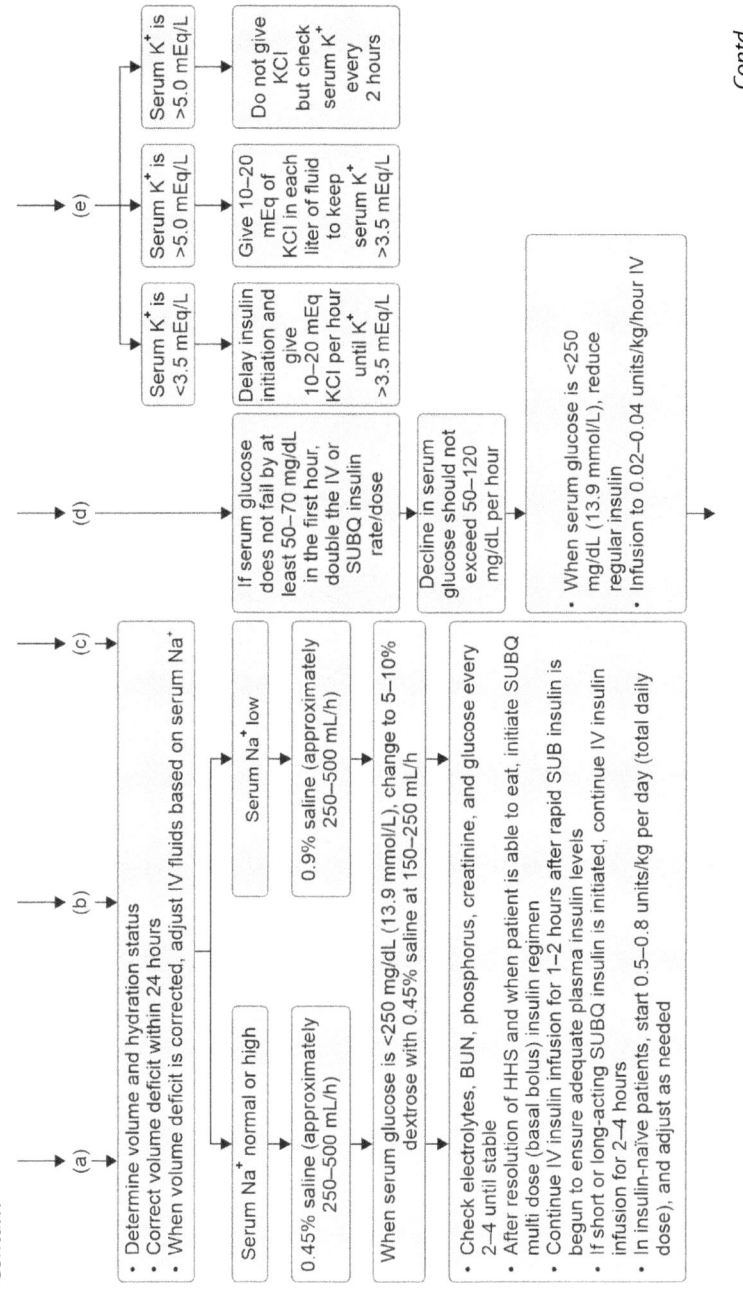

Contd...

Contd...

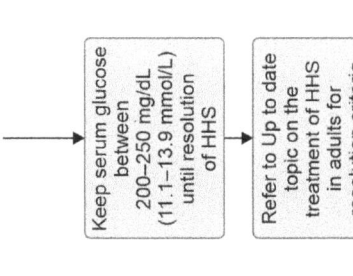

HHS diagnostic criteria: Hyperglycemia (glucose ≥60.0 mg/mmol/L), serum osmolality >300 mOsm/kg, arterial pH >7.3 serum bicarbonate >18 mEq/L, and minimal ketonuria (<2+) or ketonemia (BOHB <3 mmol/L). Normal laboratory values vary; check local laboratory reference ranges for all electrolytes.

(BOHB: beta-hydroxybutyrate; BUN: blood urea nitrogen; DKA: diabetic ketoacidosis; HHS: hyperosmolar hyperglycemic state; IV: intravenous; K⁺: potassium; KCl: potassium chloride; Na⁺: sodium; NaCl: sodium chloride; STAT: intervention should be performed emergently; SUBQ: subcutaneous)

Hyperglycemic Hyperosmolar Non-ketonic State Pathophysiology

- *Precipitating factor:* Too little insulin, infection, severe stress, hypokalemia, renal failure, old age, infancy, drug-cortisone, thiazide, beta-blocker, and calcium channel blockers
- *Sign and symptom*: Hyperosmolar coma, dehydration, increased temperature, convulsion, Kussmaul's breathing, abdominal pain-30%, vomiting-50 to 60%.

Laboratory abnormalities:
- Blood glucose >700 mg/dL
- Serum osmolality >320 mOsm/L
- Serum bicarbonate >15 mEq/L
- pH > 7.3
- Urine ketone—absent
- Sodium—low normal high
- *Leukocytes counts:* 15,000–40,000.

Complications: Infection, DIC, deep-venous thrombosis (DVT), acute myocardial infarction (AMI), CVA, hypoglycemia, and hypokalemia.

Whipple's Triad: Symptoms of hypoglycemia, low plasma glucose concentration, and relief of symptoms with glucose.

TABLE 5: *Treatment*: Fluid replacement, estimated water loss-10% of body weight. Replace 50% of deficit in first 5 hours. Infuse normal saline if hypotension and sodium <140 mEq/L. Infuse ½ NS if Na^+ >145 mEq/L and patient normotensive.

Hours	Vol
0.5–1	1 L
2	1 L
3	500 mL–1 L
4	500 mL–1 L
5	500 mL–1 L
First 5 hours	3.5–5L
6–12 hours	250–500 mL/h
Insulin—same as DKA	

Underproduction:
- *Hormone deficiency*—hypopituitarism, adrenal insufficiency, and catecholamine deficiency
- *Enzyme deficiency*—G-6 phosphatase, liver phosphorylase, and pyruvate carboxylase
- *Substrate deficiency*—ketotic hypoglycemia of infancy, severe malnutrition, and late pregnancy
- *Acquired liver disease*—hepatic congestion, cirrhosis, and hepatitis
- *Drugs*—alcohol, propranolol, and salicylate.

Overutilization:
- *Hyperinsulinism*—insulinoma, beta-cell disorder, exogenous insulin overdose, and sulfonylurea over dose
- *Inappropriate insulin level*—extrapancreatic tumor

Fed state hypoglycemia (reactive hypoglycemia):
- *Early (2-3 hours after meal)*—alimentary hyperinsulinism, postgastrectomy, functional fructose intolerance, and galactosemia
- *Late (3-5 hours after meal)*—counter-regulatory deficiency of growth hormone, glucagon, cortisone, and epinephrine.

Pseudohypoglycemia-chronic leukemia—when leukocyte count is markedly elevated, and there is utilization of glucose by leukocyte. Such hypoglycemia is not associated with symptoms.

Physiologic response to hypoglycemia—decreased insulin, increase glucagon, increase epinephrine, increased cortisol, and growth hormone.

Symptoms: Autonomic failure (adrenergic)—palpitation, sweating, anxiety—tremor, tachycardia, (parasympathetic)—hyperactivity, nausea, hunger (Neuroglycopenia)—headache, fatigue, mental dullness, dizziness, blurring of vision, confusion, amnesia, seizure, and unconsciousness.

Oral Treatment

The 10-20 g of rapidly digested CHO; monitor after 10 minutes; repeat dose if required.

TABLE 6: Comparison of hypoglycemic and hyperglycemic come.

	Hypoglycemic coma	Hyperglycemia coma
Pulse rate	Increased	Increased
Pulse volume	Full	Weak
Temperature	Decreased	Decreased
Respiration	Shallow	Rapid and deep
Blood pressure	Normal	Raised
Skin	Sweating	Dry
Tongue	Moist	Dry
Tissue Turgor	Normal	Decreased
Eye ball tension	Normal	Low
Breath	Normal	Fully odor
Reflux	Brisk	Normal
Urine glucose	Negative	Positive
Plasma glucose	Low	Increased
Bicarbonate	Normal	Low
pH	Normal	<7.3

Parenteral Rx:
- *IV glucose:*
  - If 50% dextrose given then 0.5 mL/kg required to raise blood. Glucose by 5–8 mmol/dL
  - 25% dextrose—1 mL/kg of fluid needed
  - 10% dextrose—2.5 mL/kg required
  - Monitor capillary glucose till hypoglycemia corrected then 5–10% dextrose to be given IV continuously for approximately 48 hours.
- *Parenteral glucagon* for age >5 years 1.0 mg—SC or IM (repeat after 10 minutes if required). Glucagon is contraindicated in sulfonylurea induced hypoglycemia and hypoglycemia secondary to chronic alcoholism.

Complications of Hyperglycemia in the ICU Patient
- Osmotic diuresis
- Fluid and electrolyte imbalances

TABLE 7: Effect of hypoglycemia on internal milieu and clinical features.

<4.2 mmol/L (75.6 mg)	Endogenous insulin production by pancreas suggested
<3.8 mmol/L (68.4 mg)	Secretion of counter regulatory hormones- glucagon, epinephrine, cortisol, and growth hormones
<3.2 mmol/L (57.6 mg)	Secretion of hormones cases autonomic symptoms: • Sweating • Tremor • Tachycardia • Anxiety • Hunger • Nausea • Tingling
<2.5 mmo/L (45 mg)	Signs and symptoms of neuroglycopenia appear: • Dizziness • Headache • Clouding of vision • Blunted mental acuity • Confusion • Abnormal behavior • Convulsions • Loss of consciousness

TABLE 8: Grades of hypoglycemia; detection + therapy.

Grade	Detection	Therapy
1. Asymptomatic	Lab or glucose meter	Adjust daily regimen
2. Mild	Autonomic symptoms	Oral CHO - Self therapy
3. Moderate	Neuroglycopenic + autonomic symptoms	Oral CHO = Self therapy
4. Severe	Neuroglycopenic + autonomic symptoms	Oral/parenteral assistance needed
5. Unawareness	Coma, seizures, neuroglycopenic + autonomic signs detected by someone Use carbohydrate (CHO)	Parenteral CHO

Flowchart 5: Hyperglycemia: Its impact on Infections in the ICU patient.

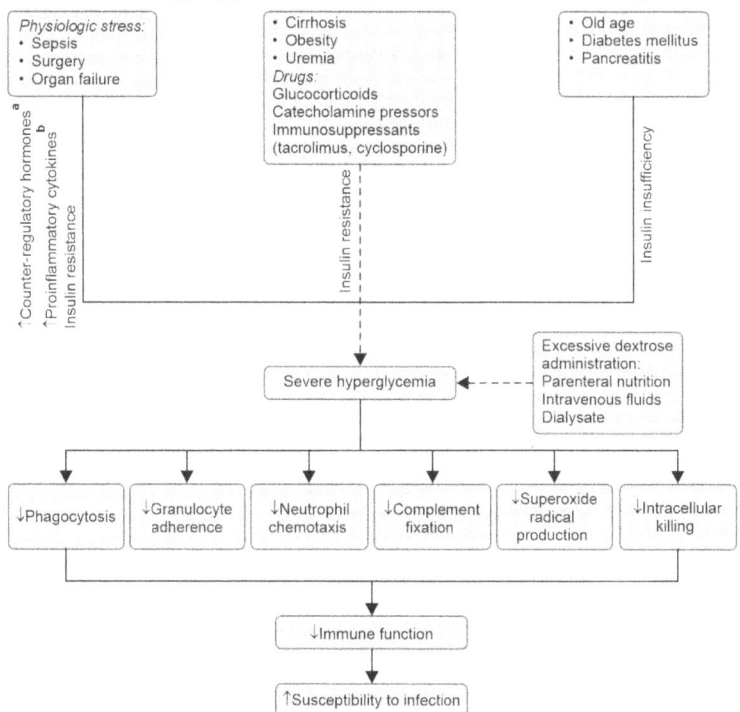

[a] Counter-regulatory hormones are glucagon, catecholamines, cortisol and growth hormone
[b] Proinflammatory cytokines are tumor necrosis factor-α, interleukin (IL)-I, and IL-6

- Hyperosmolar nonketotic coma
- Worsening skeletal muscle catabolism
- Impaired wound healing
- Changes in coagulability and increased CV risk
- Impaired immune function
- Increased susceptibility to infections and increased risk of sepsis.
- Death in certain surgical patients (Butler SO, et al.)

Glycemic Control in ICU

- Initiate resuscitation and check blood glucose.
- *Assess glycemic risk:* Coronary artery disease, renal disease, liver disease, pancreatitis, and obesity

- Frequency of blood glucose (CBG) check—hemodynamically unstable patient—hourly CBG check. After stabilization—prolong the interval. Any change in condition or nutrition delivery regimen—more frequent check.
- *Target blood glucose:* 140–180 mg/dL
- *Insulin delivery route*: OHA or long acting insulin should be stopped. Intravenous regular insulin is treatment of choice. Step down from IV to SC route.
- Avoid hypoglycemia (blood glucose <70 mg/dL) → risk group—renal failure, dialysis, liver failure, and adrenal insufficiency. Check CBG every 15 minutes.
- Avoid large variation in glucose concentration.
- Switch over to S/C insulin (short-acting along with long acting before discharge).

ACUTE HYPERCALCEMIA

Cause

The most common cause is hypercalcemia of malignancy via either extensive bony involvement [lytic skeletal metastasis (myeloma and breast)] or by ectopic production of a PTH-related peptide (PTHrP).

- Hyperparathyroidism, either primary or tertiary (associated with renal failure)—second most common cause.
- *Others*:
  - Vitamin D toxicity
  - Sarcoidosis, TB, silicosis Lymphomas
  - Thiazides
  - Lithium therapy

Manifestations

- Lethargy and mental status changes
- Vomiting
- Polyuria, polydipsia (nephrogenic diabetes insipidus)
- Renal insufficiency
- Ectopic calcification
- Short QT interval on ECG

Treatment

Mild asymptomatic hypercalcemia does not require immediate treatment and management should be based on the underlying cause.

Patients with severe [calcium >14 mg/dL (3.5 mmol/L)] or symptomatic (e.g., lethargy and confused) hypercalcemia require aggressive therapy.

- Volume repletion with intravenous normal saline (administration of isotonic saline at an initial rate of 200-300 mL/h to maintain the urine output at 100-150 mL/h) with close hemodynamic monitoring especially in patients with comorbidities.
- *Calcitonin*—Calcitonin should be administered subcutaneously. The initial dose is 4 U/kg. The serum calcium is repeated in 4-6 hours for a total duration of 24-48 hours.
- Loop diuretics (e.g., frusemide) which has calciuretic effects, should be given only after initial volume expansion.
- Intravenous bisphosphonates Zoledronate 4 mg IV over 30 minutes are extremely effective. Also denosumab could be used in the face of renal insufficiency.
- If sarcoidosis or vitamin A or D intoxication are considered, corticosteroids (prednisolone 40-60 mg/day for 3-7 days or IV hydrocortisone 100-300 mg daily) are the drugs of choice.
- Hemodialysis in refractory cases.

HYPOCALCEMIA

Hypocalcemia must be interpreted relative to plasma albumin concentration; a useful approximation is for every 1.0 mg/dL that the albumin is below 4.0, the calcium is lowered by about 0.8 mg/dL (2 mM) (Normal Ca^{2+} range: 8.4-10.2 mg/dL or 2.1-2.55 mmol/L). Alkalosis will cause more calcium to bind to albumin and will drop ionized calcium further. It is the free or ionized calcium that is physiologically relevant (Ca^{2+} range: 2.24-2.60 mEq/L or 1.12-1.30 mmol/L).

Cause

- Vitamin D deficiency (poor sunlight or malnutrition malabsorption, phenytoin or ketoconazole therapy, renal failure, vitamin D resistance including receptor defects, etc.)

- Hypoparathyroidism (postsurgical—most commonly encountered after total thyroidectomy, agenesis of gland, and autoimmune)
- Reduced glandular function (hypomagnesemia)
- PTH resistance syndrome
- Drugs such as calcium chelators and bisphosphonates
- Acute pancreatitis
- Severe sepsis
- Acute rhabdomyolysis
- Hungry bone syndrome after parathyroidectomy
- Large volume of blood transfusion

Manifestations
- Perioral and digital numbness and paresthesia
- Mental status changes
- Tetany including laryngospasm and carpopedal spasm
- Positive Chvostek sign and Trousseau's sign
- Seizures
- QT prolongation → arrhythmias (Torsade de pointes)
- DCM like presentation

[Clinical symptoms start when adjusted serum calcium falls below 1.9 mmol/L (7.6 mg/dL), although the threshold varies and depends upon the rate of fall.]

Treatment

Since calcium administration in the critically ill can cause hypoxic cell damage, so calcium should be corrected in this setting only if patient is symptomatic.

1 ampoule of calcium gluconate 10% w/v (90 mg or 2.2 mmol) diluted in 50 mL of 5% dextrose or 0.9% NaCl, over 5-15 minutes IV with frequent monitoring of serum levels should be done along with correction of underlying cause. The bolus may be repeated after 10-60 minutes, if needed to resolve symptoms. Continuous IV infusion (10 ampoules of calcium gluconate or 900 mg of calcium in 1,000 mL of D5 or DNS over 24 hours) should be considered for persistent hypocalcemia. IV calcium should be continued until the patient is receiving an effective regimen of oral calcium

and vitamin D. For patients with hypoparathyroidism, calcitriol (in a dose of 0.25–0.5 µg twice daily) and oral calcium (1–4 g of elemental calcium carbonate daily in divided doses) should be initiated as soon as possible.

It is also crucial that hypomagnesemia is corrected with magnesium supplements, since this may potentiate tendency to tetany and arrhythmias. Thus, if the serum magnesium concentration is low, 2 g (16 mEq) of magnesium sulfate should be infused as a 10% solution over 10–20 minutes, followed by 1 g (8 mEq) in 100 mL of fluid per hour.

Hazards of IV calcium therapy are cardiotoxicity, nausea, thrombophlebitis, perspiration, flushing, etc. Patients on digoxin therapy need continuous ECG monitoring during IV calcium administration.

Later investigation should be carried out to determine the cause with long term follow-up.

SUGGESTED READING

1. Bensing S, Hulting AL, Husebye ES, Kämpe O, Løvås K. Management of endocrine disease: epidemiology, quality of life and complications of primary adrenal insufficiency: a review. Eur J Endocrinol. 2016;175(3):R107-116.
2. Briet C, Salenave S, Bonnevillo JF, Laws ER, Chanson P. Pituitary apoplexy. Endocr Rev. 2015;36(6):622-45.
3. Carroll R, Matfin G. Endocrine and metabolic emergencies: thyroid storm. Ther Adv Endocrinol Metab. 2010;1(3):139-45.
4. Gosmanov AR, Gosmanova FO, Kitabchi AE. Hyperglycemic crises: Diabetic ketoacidosis (DKA) and hyperglycemic hyperosmolar state (HHS). Endotext [Internet]. South Dartmouth (MA): MDText.com, Inc.;2018.
5. NICE. (2019). Treatment of hypoglycemia. [online] Available from http://bnf.nice.org.uk [Last accessed March, 2025].

CHAPTER 23

Rheumatological Emergencies

Samar Ranjan Pal

Emergencies in rheumatological diseases present to physicians as multisystem problems in various combinations and in a catastrophic manner with significant morbidity and mortality.

They may be divided into two broad categories:
1. Disease-related emergencies:
    - *Rheumatoid arthritis (RA):*
        - Atlantoaxial dislocation
        - Scleromalacia perforans
        - Vasculitis
        - Infections
        - Disease flare
    - *Systemic lupus erythematosus (SLE):*
        - CNS Lupus
        - Cardiac involvement in the form of peri, myo, and endocarditis
        - Lung involvement in the form of pneumonia and ARDS
        - Vasculitis
        - Pancreatitis
        - Infections
        - Pregnancy and neonatal lupus
    - *Antiphospholipid antibody (APLA):*
        - Catastrophic APLA
        - Thromboembolic events in the form of AMI; retinal vessel thrombosis and PE
        - Thrombotic thrombocytopenic purpura (TTP)/microangiopathic presentation of APLA
    - *Spondyloarthropathy:*
        - Iridocyclitis

- *Vasculitis:*
  - Cerebral vasculitis
  - Mesenteric vasculitis
  - Uveitis and optic neuritis
  - Acute nephritis
  - Hypertensive crisis
  - Visual loss in giant cell arteritis
- *Systemic sclerosis:* Scleroderma renal crisis (SRC)
- *Inflammatory myositis:* Respiratory failure
- *Crystal-induced arthopathies:*
  - Acute gout
  - Acute interstitial nephritis
- *Infection-related arthritis:*
  - Septic arthritis
  - Reactive arthritis
- Hemophilic arthritis
- *Osteoporosis:* Fracture
- *Miscellaneous:*
  - Macrophage activation syndrome (MAS)
  - Pulmonary renal syndrome
  - Symmetric peripheral gangrene (SPG)

2. Drug-related emergencies:
   - *NSAIDs:*
     - GI bleeding
     - Interstitial nephritis
     - Celecoxib: Selective cox-2 inhibitor may cause heart failure, HTN, and peripheral edema.
   - *Steroids:*
     - Addisonian crisis due to withdrawal
     - Psychosis
     - Infections
   - *DMARDs:*
     - Bone-marrow suppression
     - Hepatic failure
     - Stevens–Johnson Syndrome (SJC)

- *Biologic-response modifiers:*
  - Infusion reactions
  - Infections.
    - *Anaphylaxis:* Rituximab and infliximab
    - Reactivation of TB/opportunistic infection like listeria
    - Drug induced Lupus/Demyelination.

APPROACH TO A RHEUMATOLOGIC EMERGENCY

Rheumatological disorders are per se insidious in onset and usually follow chronic pathway. However, clinicians may encounter emergencies in connection to rheumatological disorders. It may present either as emergency medical condition in a patient with rheumatic disease as for example:

- Hypoglycemia in a patient with diabetes mellitus and rheumatoid arthritis taking hypoglycemic agents as well as NSAIDS
- Or, directly related to the inflammatory basis of the rheumatological disorder itself or toxicity from the treatment.

Multiorgan involvement such as lungs, kidney, heart, brain, and joints may present at the emergency in a catastrophic manner; hence, increasing the morbidity and mortality (e.g., SLE with cardiac tamponade, catastrophic antiphospholipid syndrome, etc.) whereas necrotizing vasculitis with inflammation may lead to ischemia, target organ damage, and therefore, vital organ failure in a common basis of pathogenesis.

Many of these conditions are autoimmune and thus, immunosuppression is the prime agent of their management making the patient prone to infection. Again, the biological therapy that inhibits the proinflammatory cytokines as well as B-cell and T-cell activity invites many complications including infection. The challenge is making the difference between the two because the treatments are diametrically opposed as, for example, whether to give immunosuppression or antibiotics.

Assessment of patients presenting with rheumatological emergency starts with detailed history taking of present and past illness; search of related physical signs, and laboratory investigations, and disease activity calculation will help to diagnose the specific cause of underlying emergency.

Primary aim is to save life firstly and then to prevent irreversible organ damage by instituting suitable and aggressive therapy.

Lab investigation has to be done to:
- Diagnose the underlying main disease (If not a diagnosed case)
- Find the nature of the disease, for example,
  - Precipitating cause
  - Organ involvement
  - Extent of disease and damage of underlying emergency
- Rule out mimickers in appropriate settings.

LABORATORY WORK-UP

- *Clinical pathology, microbiology and biochemistry:*
  - Hb%, TC, DC, platelet, ESR, CRP, reticulocyte count, PBS,
    - LDH Coombs' test (DCT), and blood culture
  - Na^+, K^+ Urea, creatinine, uric acid, LFT, triglycerides (Tg), ferritin, blood INR, FDP, D-dimer, fibrinogen,
  - Urine R/E, ME, 24-hour urinary protein, 24 hour urinary uric acid
  - Synovial fluid aspiration for crystals and C/S,
  - Stool for R/E, C/S, OBT, and fecal calprotectin
- *Immunology:*
  - ANF by heparin 2 cell
  - RF
  - c-and-p ANCA against PR3 and MPO
  - Anti-GBM antibody
  - Anti-Ro and La
  - Anti-RNA Polymerase III
  - dsDNA
  - $\beta 2$ glycoprotein [Anticardiolipin (IgG and IgM) antibodies]
  - Cryoglobulin screening and lupus anticoagulant
- *Serology:* HBsAg, anti-HCV and HIV (I and II)
- *Radiology:*
  - Chest X-ray
  - USG (whole abdomen)
  - HRCT—thorax
  - CT—PNS and brain

- MRI brain/spine/sacroiliac joints
- Echo—2D, M-mode with Doppler
- *Endoscopic exploration* (to exclude IBD)

TREATMENT

It is designed according to underlying disease process. Aim is to save life and prevent irreversible organ damage. Basic organ support therapy is common to all disease.

Before starting aggressive therapy with glucocorticoid, infection must be ruled out in each and every case. Comorbidities should also be considered during therapy.

Individual Entities

The most common rheumatological emergency seen in our emergency department is acute monoarthritis.

Acute Arthritis

It may start afresh (de novo) or flare of preexisting arthritic illness. The causes of de novo arthritis can be divided into:
- *Acute monoarthritis:*
  - Gout
  - Septic arthritis
  - Trauma
  - Hemophilic arthritis
- *Acute oligo/poly arthritis:*
  - Reactive arthritis/Reiter's syndrome/Spondyloarthropathy
  - Viral arthritis
  - Rheumatic fever
  - HIV
  - Disseminated gonococcal infection

Acute monoarthritis should be managed as a medical emergency warranting immediate joint aspiration. Synovial fluid should be investigated to rule out pus in the joint including crystal studies, preferably using polarized microscopy.

Synovial Fluid Analysis

Points to remember:
- Sample should be anticoagulated with heparin or liquid EDTA.
- Total and differential WBC counts, culture and sensitivity, Gram's stain, Ziehl-Neelsen's (ZN) stain, and crystal identification should be performed on all fluids.
- Polarized light microscopy is ideal for crystal identification.

Treatment of Acute Gout

- NSAID, if not contraindicated
- Colchicin, 0.6 mg PO BD (Renal insufficiency—dose reduce to OD, may cause myopathy if patient is on calcineurin inhibitor)
- *Corticosteroid:* Intraarticular (knee) or oral (small joints).
    - Allopurinol should not be started in acute gout. If patient is on a stable dose of allopurinol, it can be continued through the attack.

Septic Arthritis

Aspiration/drainage + Antibiotics

Lupus Flare

High-dose steroid therapy is indicated for life-threatening SLE such as vasculitis, CNS lupus, diffuse proliferative glomerulonephritis (DPGN), lupus pneumonia, myocarditis, and hemolytic anemia.
There are 3 regimens that are as follows:
- *Regimen 1:* Daily oral short-acting prednisolone 1-2 mg/kg, daily in divided doses—controls disease rapidly in 5-10 days for hematologic or CNS diseases, serositis, or vasculitis and in 2-10 weeks for glomerulonephritis.
- *Regimen 2:* It includes IV methylprednisolone 500-1,000 mg every day for 3-5 days and then 1-1.5 mg/kg/day of oral glucocorticoid. This controls disease rapidly. A few nonresponders to regimen 1 respond to regimen 2.
- *Regimen 3:* It includes a combination of regimen 1 or 2 with cyclophosphamide (CPM). Many experts believe that it should be included in initial therapeutic regimens in most SLE patients with severe nephritis or other rapidly progressive, life-threatening

organ involvement. When CPM is given IV once a month for 6 months and then discontinued, 50-80% patients can be expected to improve. That improvement is lost in more than half during subsequent 6 months. In contrast, if 6 monthly pulses are given at longer intervals for an additional 12-24 months, number of disease flares and preservation of renal function are better than in groups treated with glucocorticoids alone.

Catastrophic Antiphospholipid Syndrome

Criteria for catastrophic antiphospholipid syndrome (cAPS)
- Definite cAPS:
    - Evidence of vessel occlusion
        - [a]Or occlusive impact on >3 organs, systems, and/or tissues
    - Anatomopathological confirmation
        - [b]Or small-diameter vessel occlusion, at least in one organ or tissues
    - Simultaneous or <1 week event occurrence
    - Anatomopathological confirmation of small-diameter vessel occlusion, at least in one organ or tissue
    - Persistent presence of antipathological antibodies (APA/lupus anticoagulant) ≠ 6 weeks
- Probable cAPS:
    - Two or more organs or systems affected
    - Occurrence of two events in <1 week and the third prior to week 4
    - The four criteria, except for absence of separate lab confirmation
        - [c]of at least 6 weeks due to early patient death

---

[a]Usually, clinical evidence of vascular occlusion is confirmed by imaging techniques, if appropriate. Renal involvement is defined as a 50% rise in plasma creatinine, severe systemic hypertension (>180/100 mm Hg), and/or proteinuria (>500 mg/24 hours).

[b]The anatomopathological confirmation in done based on signs of thrombosis, though occasionally vasculitis may be present.

[c]If the patient had not been previously diagnosed with APS, the lab confirmation requires the presence of antiphospholipid antibodies detected on two or more separate occasions, at least 6 weeks apart (not necessarily at the time of the thrombotic accident), in accordance with the criteria for definite APS.

TABLE 1: Organ system involvement in cAPS.

Organ system	Percentage of involvement
Renal	78%
Pulmonary	66%
CNS	56%
Cutaneous	50%
Gastrointestinal	38%
Hepatic	34%
Adrenal	13%
Urogenital	6%

Treatment:
- *Anticoagulation* with heparin/LMWH followed by oral anticoagulant warfarin to keep INR 2.5 for venous thrombosis and 3.5 for arterial thrombosis.
- *Corticosteroid:* Pulse therapy for 3 days followed by oral prednisolone as daily dose of 1-2 mg/kg. The postulated benefit of steroids may relate to inhibition of the systemic inflammatory response. However, steroids may simply be an ancillary agent since the recovery rate, when used in isolation, was not significant.
- *Plasma exchange (PEX):* It has theoretical benefit as it removes antibodies from circulation; however, no control trials have been shown to prove this. PEX can be done with fresh frozen plasma (FFP)/4% human albumin solutions. However, FFP can increase the level of procoagulant factors and theoretically, may reduce the effectiveness of anticoagulation, as supported by Bortolati et al., who reported two patients with cAPS who worsened with FFP but improved once albumin solution was used in the replacement fluid.
- IVIg 400 mg/kg qd for 5 days
- Rituximab 375 mg/m^2/week × 4 weeks
- Heparin/LMWH or factor Xa inhibitor
- Fondaparinux 7.5 mg S/c
- Rivaroxaban 10 mg OD per oral

Scleroderma Renal Crisis (SRC)

Scleroderma renal crisis (SRC) occurs in 5–10% of systemic sclerosis (SSc) patients.

Risk factors include:
- Early diffuse SSc
- Rapidly progressive skin disease
- Anti-RNA polymerase III, topoisomerase I, and U3 RNP positivity
- Corticosteroid use (Steen and Medsger observed recent history of high dose, e.g., prednisolone/equivalent at >15 mg/day precedes SRC diagnosis)
- Anemia
- Hormone replacement therapy
- Pericardial effusion, cardiac insufficiency, and new cardiac event
- High skin score (modified Rodnan skin score)
- Large joint contracture

Clinical features:
- New onset of significant systemic hypertension
- >150/85 mm Hg and decreases renal function (≥30% reduction in eGFR)
- Minority of the patient may be normotensive, 20% of the patients diagnosed of SRC may precede diagnosis of SSc.

Treatment:
- Aggressive treatment of hypertension in SRC patients is essential to prevent the occurrence of irreversible vascular injury.
- ACE inhibitors are the mainstay of treatment. ACEI is also helpful in normotensive SRC.
- Addition of CCB may be beneficial for patients with inadequate blood pressure control on ACE inhibitors.
- I/V iloprost may also help to reverse microvascular changes.
- Additional oral hypotensive agents (e.g., Labetalol) together with nitrate infusion, if there is pulmonary edema, can be used.
- Plasma exchange is considered if there is substantial thrombotic microangiopathy.
- Renal function is supported by intermittent hemodialysis/continuous veno-venous hemofiltration.

- Renal function following SRC may become normal up to 2 years, so final decision regarding transplant should not be made until at least 2 years after SRC.
- Immunosuppressive, plasmapheresis, and corticosteroids have no role in management.

Macrophage Activation Syndrome/ Hemophagocytic Syndrome

Macrophage activation syndrome (MAS) is potentially life-threatening and dreaded complication of several chronic rheumatic diseases of childhood; characterized by activation and uncontrolled proliferation of T lymphocytes and macrophages leading to cytokine overproduction and widespread hemophagocytosis.

Most commonly seen with systemic onset juvenile idiopathic arthritis (SOJIA), it is also seen in association with SLE, Kawasaki disease, Adult onset Still's disease, Behçet's syndrome, Sjögren syndrome, MCTD, sarcoidosis, PAN, and dermatomyositis.

Clinical features: Sudden onset high fever, hepatosplenomegaly, may be associated with CNS dysfunction in the form of lethargy, irritability, disorientation, headache, seizure, and coma.

Diagnosis:
Diagnostic guidelines for hemophagocytic lymphohistiocytosis (HLH): the HLH-2004 criteria.
- Molecular diagnosis of genetic defect-usually present in primary hemophagocytic syndrome.
- Diagnostic criteria for HLH fulfilled (five out of eight criteria).
  1. Fever ≥38.5°
  2. Splenomegaly
  3. *Cytopenia affecting at least 2 of 3 lineages in peripheral blood:* Hb <9 g/dL, Platelet <1 Lac/cmm, Neutrophil <1,000/cmm
  4. Hypertriglyceridemia ≥265 mg/dL and/or hypofibrinogenemia ≤1.5 g/L
  5. Hemophagocytosis in bone marrow, spleen, and lymph nodes. No evidence of malignancy.
  6. Low or absent NK cell activity
  7. Ferritin ≥500 ng/mL
  8. Soluble CD25 ≥2,400 U/mL

In 2014 a retrospective analysis concluded that guidelines of HLH-2004 are not appropriate for identification of MAS in SOJIA. Preliminary diagnostic guidelines for MAS as a complication of SOJIA-proposed by Ravelli et al. showed the strongest ability to diagnose MAS in SOJIA.

Clinical criteria:
- CNS dysfunction (irritability, disorientation lethargy, headache, seizures or coma)
- Hemorrhages (purpura, easy bruising, mucosal bleeding)
- Hepatomegaly (≥3 cm below the costal arch)

Laboratory criteria:
- Decreased platelet count ≤2.62 L
- Elevated levels of aspartate aminotransferase (>59 U/L)
- Decreased white blood cell count (≤4,000/cmm)
- Hypofibrinogenemia (≤2.5 g/L)

Histopathological criteria:
- Evidence of macrophage hemophagocytosis in bone marrow aspirate
- The presence of two or more laboratory criteria or any two or more clinical and/or laboratory criteria is diagnostic of MAS. Demonstration of hemophagocytosis in bone marrow may be required only in doubtful cases.

Treatment:
- Corticosteroid
- Cyclosporin A (CyA)
- Antithymocyte globulin (ATG)
- Etoposide
- Rituximab
- *Anti-TNF therapy:* Etanercept and anakinra

Pulmonary Renal Syndrome

Causes
- *ANCA associated vasculitis:*
  - Granulomatosis with polyangiitis (Wegener's granulomatosis)
  - Microscopic polyangitis
  - Churg-Strauss syndrome

Flowchart 1: Diagnostic–therapeutic algorithm PRS.

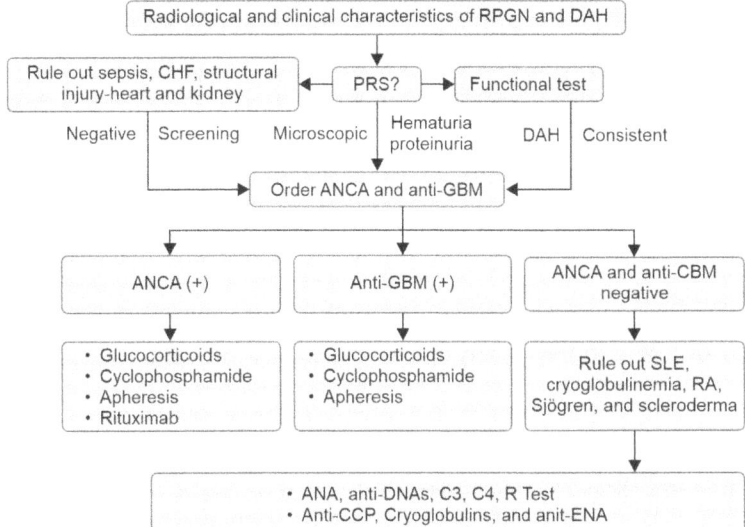

- *ANCA negative vasculitis:*
  - HSP
  - Mixed cryoglobulinemia
  - Behçet's disease
  - SLE
  - Sclerodermal (ANCA +ve)
  - RA
  - MCTD

Treatment:
- Pulse methylprednisolone (1 g) given daily for 3–5 days followed by oral corticosteroids starting at 1–1.5 mg/kg/day.
- Cyclophosphamide can be given either orally (1.5–2.5 mg/kg/day) or as monthly pulses of 0.5–1 g/m^2.
- Plasmapheresis in patients with very severe renal disease defined by a serum creatinine >5 mg/dL or in patients with severe alveolar hemorrhage.
- Other therapies are rituximab (anti-CD20) and MMF

Diffuse Alveolar Hemorrhage

Diffuse alveolar hemorrhage (DAH) is a very serious condition in SLE with mortality ranging from 50 to 90%. It often mimics clinically and radiologically as severe pneumonia or ARDS. The characteristic presentation is abrupt onset of dyspnea, cough, fever, infiltrates, and a dramatic fall in hemoglobin. Hemoptysis is present in only 50% cases.

Treatment:
- High dose steroid with either cyclophosphamide or azathioprine
- Plasmapheresis
- Rituximab (anti-CD20) shown to be effective in different trials

CNS Vasculitis

The term vasculitis refers to the inflammation of the blood vessels, including arteries and veins, regardless of diameter. It results in tissue damage from ischemia and the subsequent activation of the inflammatory cascade that leads to blood vessel occlusion and necrosis. The cause is the direct effect of the antigen–antibody complex that triggers an inflammatory cascade mostly mediated by cytokines.

The rheumatic diseases with manifestations of central and peripheral nervous system vasculitis are classified as follows:
- *Connective tissue diseases:* Systemic lupus erythematous, scleroderma, rheumatoid arthritis, Sjögren syndrome, mixed diseases of the connective tissue, and Behçet's disease.
- *Systemic necrotizing vasculitis:* Polyarteritis nodosa, Churg-Strauss syndrome, microscopic polyangiitis, and Kawasaki disease
- *Systemic granulomatous vasculitis:* Wegener's granulomatosis, lymphomatoid granulomatosis, and lethal mid-line granuloma.

Diagnostic approach for CNS vasculitis: If a cerebral vasculitis of autoimmune origin is suspected, there has to be first a pretest verification—predominantly females, young, no previous history of cardiovascular disease, focal or multiple lesions evidenced in a brain MRI or CT. Always rule out any infectious etiology through a cerebrospinal fluid (CSF) analysis showing pleocytosis with a prevalence of plasmacytoid cells and in lesser numbers, polymorphonuclear (PMN). It is important to know the level of proteins in the CSF since a cytoprotein disassociation (i.e., CSF, pleocytosis with no evidence of elevated proteins or with a very discrete rise) may suggest an autoimmune process. In contrast, an albumin-cytological disassociation suggests a polyradiculoneuritic process such as multiple sclerosis or Guillain–Barré infections, and neoplastic lesions may also be ruled out via the CSF.

Neonatal Lupus

Complete heart block (CHB) can be fatal. Those who survive, develop cardiomyopathy or complete heart block.
- PRIDE study evaluates role in early diagnosis and treatment during pregnancy of anti-Ro antibody-exposed fetuses.
- The conclusion of this study was that first-degree block is no more common than third-degree block but unlike the latter, it may be reversible with dexamethasone in rare cases.
- In a study comprising eight pregnancies in mothers with anti-SSA/Ro antibodies and previous children with CHB treated with 1 g/kg of IVIg at 14th and 18th week of gestation, it prevented CHB in seven cases.

Synovial Rupture

- Aspiration + Intraarticular steroids
- *Atlantoaxial dislocation:* Fusion ± Decompression

CONCLUSION

Proper knowledge of natural history of the disease, its complications, good clinical judgement for early symptom recognition, and solving the dilemma between infection versus inflammation and prompt institution of proper therapy will save multiple lives. Most of the lives are lost due to nonrecognition of the exact underlying causes by the physician. Newer modalities of therapy also hold good promise in controlling these emergencies.

SUGGESTED READING

1. Gutiérrez-González LA. Rheumatological emergencies. Clin Rheumatol. 2015;34(12):2011-92.
2. Handa H, Aggarwal P, Wali JP. Rheumatological emergencies in clinical practice. JIACM. 2000;5(2):135-41.
3. Kumar A, Marwaka V, Grover R. Emergencies in Rheumatology. J Indian Med Assoc. 2003;101(9):520-4.
4. Martin K, Deleveaux S. Cunningham M, Ramaswamy K, Thomas B, Lerma E, et al. The presentation, etiologies, pathophysiology and treatment of pulmonary renal syndrome: a review of the literature. Dis Mon. 2022;68(12):101465.
5. Ramrakkha P, Moore K, Sam A. Rheumatological emergencies. Oxford Handbook of Acute Medicine. UK: Oxford University Press; 2010.
6. Rao URK, Shantaram V. Rheumatological Emergencies. Supplement to JAPI. 2006;54.
7. Walsh M, Merked PA, Peh CA, Szpirt WM, Puéchal X, Fujimoto S, et al. Plasma exchange and glucocorticoids in severe ANCA-associated vasculitis. N Engl J Med. 2020;382(7):622-31.

24 CHAPTER

Antimicrobial Therapy Including Management of Septic Shock

Prabuddha Mukhopadhyay

SEPSIS AND SEPTIC SHOCK

Definitions

The Third International Consensus on Sepsis (Sepsis-3) in 2016 provided the following definitions for sepsis and septic shock.

Sepsis is defined as life-threatening organ dysfunction caused by a dysregulated host response to infection.

For clinical purposes, organ dysfunction is represented by an increase in the Sequential (sepsis-related) Organ Failure Assessment (SOFA) score of two or more.

Septic shock is defined as a subset of sepsis in which profound circulatory, cellular, and metabolic abnormalities are associated with a greater risk of mortality than with sepsis alone.

Clinically, a patient of septic shock can be identified by a serum lactate level >2 mmol/L (>18 mg/dL) and vasopressor requirement to maintain a mean arterial pressure (MAP) of 65 mm Hg or greater in the absence of hypovolemia.

TABLE 1: SIRS criteria and qSOFA score.

SIRS criteria (≥2)	Body temperature >38.0°C or <36.0°C
	Heart rate of >90/min
	Respiratory rate of >20 breaths/min or $PaCO_2$ of <4.3 kPa
	White blood cell count of <4,000 cells/mm³ or >12,000 cells/mm³ or >10% immature bands
qSOFA score (≥2)	Respiratory rate ≥22 breaths/min
	Systolic blood pressure ≤100 mm Hg
	Altered mental state

($PaCO_2$: partial pressure of carbon dioxide in arterial blood; qSOFA: quick sequential organ failure assessment; SIRS: systemic inflammatory response syndrome)

TABLE 2: Sequential Organ Failure Assessment (SOFA) score.

Organ system		0	1	2	Score 3	4
Respiratory	PaO_2/FiO_2 (kPa)	≥53.3	<53.3	<40	<26.7	<13.3
Renal	Creatinine (µmol/L)	<110	110–170	171–299	300–440	>440
Hepatic	Bilirubin (µmol/L)	<20	20–32	33–101	102–204	>204
Hematological	Platelets × 10^3/µL	≥150	<150	<100	<50	<20
Neurological	Glasgow Coma Score	15	13–14	10–12	6–9	<6
Cardiovascular		MAP ≥70 mm Hg	MAP <70 mm Hg	Dopamine <5 or dobutamine	Dopamine 5.1–15, epinephrine ≤0.1 or norepinephrine ≤0.1*	Dopamine >15 or epinephrine >0.1 or norepinephrine >0.1*

*Adrenergic agents (µg/kg/min) given for at least 1 hour.
(FiO_2: fraction of inspired oxygen; MAP: mean arterial pressure; PaO_2: partial pressure of oxygen in the arterial blood)

TABLE 3: Modified Early Warning Score (MEWS).

Score	3	2	1	0	1	2	3
Respiratory rate (breaths/min)		<9		9–14	15–20	21–29	≥30
Heart rate (BPM)		≤40	41–50	51–100	101–110	111–129	≥130
Systolic blood pressure (mm Hg)	≤70	71–80	81–100	101–199		≥200	
Temperature (°C)		<35,0		35–38.4		≥38.5	
AVPU				Alert	Reacting to voice	Reacting to pain	Unresponsive

TABLE 4: Comparison between the criteria of sepsis screening tools on between the criteria of sepsis screening tools.

	SIRS	Single parameter	qSOFA	NEWS aggregate score			
	TWO or more of	ONE or more of	TWO or more of	0	1	2	3
Respiratory rate, breaths per minute (BPM)	>20	≥25	>22	12–20		9–11 or 21–24	≥25
SpO$_2$, scale 1	n/a	n/a	n/a	≥96	94–95	92–93	≤91
SpO$_2$, scale 2	n/a	n/a	n/a	88–92	86–87	84–85	≤83
Oxygen treatment	n/a	Yes	n/a	No	No	Yes	Yes
Blood pressure, mm Hg	n/a	≤90	<100	111–219	101–110	91–100	≤90 or ≥220
Heart rate, beats per minute	>90	≥130	n/a	51–90	91–110 or 41–50	111–130	≥131
ACVPU	n/a	CVPU	CVPU	Alert	Alert	Alert	CVPU
Temperature	>38°C or <36°C	n/a	n/a	36.1°C–38.0°C	38.1–39.0°C or 35.1°C–36.0°C	≥39.1°C	≤35.0°C
White blood count	Yes	N/A	N/A	N/A	N/A	N/A	N/A

(ACVPU: alert, confusion, voice, pain or unresponsive; CVPU: confusion, voice, pain or unresponsive; NEWS: National Early Warning Score; qSOFA: quick Sequential Organ Failure Assessment; SIRS: systemic inflammatory response syndrome; SpO$_2$: peripheral capillary oxygen saturation)

However, the recommendation of the Surviving Sepsis Campaign (SSC): International Guidelines for management of sepsis and septic shock, 2021 is as follows:
- It is recommended not to use background for the recommendation: The qSOFA uses three variables to predict death and prolonged ICU stay in patients with known or suspected sepsis: a Glasgow Coma Score <15, a respiratory rate ≥22 breaths/min, and a systolic blood pressure ≤100 mm Hg. When any two of these variables are present simultaneously, the patient is considered qSOFA positive. Data analysis used to support the recommendations of the Third International Consensus Conference on the Definitions of Sepsis identified qSOFA as a predictor of poor outcome in patients with known or suspected infection, but no analysis was performed to support its use as a screening tool. Since then, numerous studies have investigated the potential use of qSOFA as a screening tool for sepsis. The results have been contradictory as to its usefulness. Studies have shown that qSOFA is more specific but less sensitive than having two of four systemic inflammatory response syndrome (SIRS) criteria for early identification of infection-induced organ dysfunction. Neither SIRS nor qSOFA are ideal screening tools for sepsis, and the bedside clinician needs to understand the limitations of each. In the original derivation study, authors found that only 24% of infected patients had a qSOFA score 2 or 3, but these patients accounted for 70% of poor outcomes. Similar findings have also been found when comparing against the National Early Warning Score (NEWS) and the Modified Early Warning Score (MEWS). Although the presence of a positive qSOFA should alert the clinician to the possibility of sepsis in all resource settings, given the poor sensitivity of the qSOFA, the panel issued a strong recommendation against its use as a single screening tool.

INITIAL RESUSCITATION
Recommendation
Since sepsis and septic shock are medical emergencies, the SSC (2021) recommendations are as follows:
- Treatment and resuscitation must begin immediately.

Best practice statement.
At least 30 mL/kg of intravenous (IV) crystalloid fluid should be given within the first 3 hours of resuscitation.

Weak recommendation, low-quality evidence.
Dynamic measures to guide fluid resuscitation over physical examination or static parameters alone.

Weak recommendation, very low-quality evidence.
Observations: Dynamic parameters include response to a passive leg raising or a fluid bolus, using, stroke volume variation (SVV), and pulse pressure variation (PPV).

Guiding resuscitation to decrease serum lactate in patients with elevated lactate level. However, serum lactate level should be interpreted considering the clinical context and other causes of elevated lactate.

Weak recommendation, low-quality evidence.

Rationale for the Recommendations

The 2016 SSC guideline had issued a recommendation for using a minimum of 30 mL/kg (ideal body weight) of IV crystalloids in initial fluid resuscitation. This fixed volume of initial resuscitation was suggested on the basis of observational evidence. However, there are no prospective intervention studies comparing different volumes for initial resuscitation in sepsis or septic shock. A retrospective analysis of adults presenting to an emergency department with sepsis or septic shock showed that failure to receive 30 mL/kg of crystalloid fluid therapy within 3 hours of sepsis onset was associated with increased odds of in-hospital mortality, delayed resolution of hypotension and increased length of stay in ICU, irrespective of comorbidities, including end-stage kidney disease and heart failure. In the PROCESS, ARISE, and PROMISE trials, the average volume of fluid received pre-randomization was also in the range of 30 mL/kg, justifying that this fluid volume has been recommended in routine clinical practice.

If fluid therapy beyond the initial 30 mL/kg administration is required, clinicians may use repeated small boluses guided by objective measures of SV and/or CO when facilities, e.g., electrocardiography, permit. If facilities for measurement of CO or SV are not available, a >15% increase in pulse pressure could indicate that the patient is fluid responsive, utilizing a passive leg-raise test for 60–90 seconds.

MEAN ATRIAL PRESSURE
Recommendations of SSC 2021
An initial target MAP of 65 mm Hg over higher MAP targets. *Strong recommendation, moderate-quality evidence.*

Rationale for the Recommendation
The recommendation was based principally on a randomized controlled trial (RCT) in septic shock comparing patients who were given vasopressors to target a MAP of 65–70 mm Hg versus a target of 80–85 mm Hg. This study found no difference in mortality, although a subgroup analysis demonstrated a 10.5% absolute reduction in renal replacement therapy (RRT) with higher MAP targets among patients with chronic hypertension. Moreover, higher MAP targets with vasopressors were associated with a higher risk of atrial fibrillation. A meta-analysis of two RCTs on this subject supported that higher MAP targets did not result in better survival in septic shock.

In another recent RCT, the "permissive hypotension" group (mean MAP of 66.7 mm Hg), when compared with the usual care group (mean MAP of 72.6 mm Hg) in patients aged 65 years old or more, had similar 90-day mortality (41% vs. 43.8%).

Given the lack of advantage associated with higher MAP targets and the lack of harm among elderly patients with MAP targets of 60-65 mm Hg. SSC (2021) recommends targeting a MAP of 65 mm Hg in the initial resuscitation of patients with septic shock who require vasopressors.

ADMISSION TO INTENSIVE CARE
Recommendation of Surviving Sepsis Campaign 2021
The patient should be admitted to the intensive care unit (ICU) within 6 hours; if this is not possible in resource-limited countries,

close evaluation of patients and appropriate treatment should not be delayed, irrespective of patient location.

Weak recommendation, low-quality evidence.

◼ INFECTION

Diagnosis of Infection and Recommendation of 2021

For adults with suspected sepsis or septic shock but unconfirmed infection, it is recommended to continuously reevaluate and search for alternative diagnoses and to discontinue empiric antimicrobials if an alternative cause of illness is demonstrated or strongly suspected.

Best practice statement.

Rationale

In previous versions of SSC guidelines, we highlighted the importance of obtaining a full screen was highlighted for infectious agents prior to starting antimicrobials wherever it is possible to do so in a timely fashion. As a best practice statement, it was recommended that appropriate routine microbiologic cultures (including blood) should be obtained before starting antimicrobial therapy in patients with suspected sepsis and septic shock if it results in no substantial delay in the start of antimicrobials (i.e., <45 minutes). This recommendation has not been updated in the SSC 2021 version but remains as valid as before.

The signs and symptoms of sepsis are nonspecific and often mimic multiple other diseases (90-92). There is no "gold standard" test to diagnose sepsis; third or more of patients initially diagnosed with sepsis turn out to have noninfectious conditions. The best practice is to continually assess the patient to determine if other diagnoses are more or less likely, especially because a patient's clinical trajectory can evolve significantly after hospital admission, thereby increasing or decreasing the likelihood of a diagnosis of sepsis. With this uncertainty, there can be significant coclinical questions in determining when it is "scientifically right" to deescalate or discontinue antibiotics.

Clinicians are strongly encouraged to discontinue antimicrobials if a noninfectious syndrome (or an infectious syndrome that does not benefit from antimicrobials) is demonstrated or strongly suspected.

TIME OF ANTIBIOTICS

Recommendations of the Surviving Sepsis Campaign 2021

For adults with possible septic shock or a high likelihood for sepsis, the administration of antimicrobials immediately, ideally within one hour of recognition, is strongly recommended.

Strong recommendation, low quality of evidence (septic shock): *Strong recommendation, very low quality of evidence (sepsis without shock).*

Rationale for the Recommendation

The early administration of appropriate antimicrobials is one of the most effective interventions to reduce mortality in patients with sepsis. Initiating antimicrobials to patients with sepsis or septic shock should, therefore, be treated as an emergency.

The mortality reduction associated with early antimicrobials appears strongest in patients with septic shock, where studies have reported a strong association between time to antibiotics and death in patients with septic shock but weaker associations in patients without septic shock.

Flowchart 1: Recommendations for timing of antibiotics.

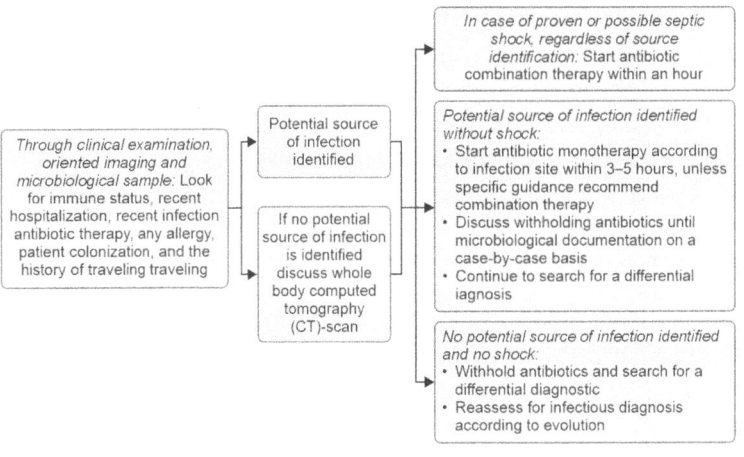

BIOMARKERS TO START ANTIBIOTICS

Recommendations of the Surviving Sepsis Campaign 2021

It recommends against using procalcitonin plus clinical evaluation to decide when to start antimicrobials, as compared to clinical evaluation alone. Weak recommendation, very low quality of evidence.

Rationale for the Recommendation

Procalcitonin is not detectable in healthy states, it escalates sharply in response to proinflammatory stimuli, especially bacterial infections. Theoretically, procalcitonin levels in combination with clinical evaluation may facilitate the diagnosis of serious bacterial infections and prompt early initiation of antimicrobials. In a meta-analysis of 30 studies (3,244 patients), procalcitonin had a pooled sensitivity of 77% and specificity of 79% for sepsis in critically ill patients.

Three RCTs compared procalcitonin-guided protocols for antibiotic initiation vs usual care. A meta-analysis of the three trials ($n = 1,769$ ICU patients) found no difference in short-term mortality, length of ICU stays, or length of hospitalization. Data related to long-term mortality, readmission rates, and hospital-free days were not reported in any of the trials, and no relevant studies on the cost-efficacy of the use of procalcitonin were found very low. Available guidelines for the management of community-acquired pneumonia suggest the initiation of antimicrobials for patients with community-acquired pneumonia regardless of procalcitonin level. With no clear-cut benefit, unassessed costs, and limited availability, the SSC 2021 panel issued a weak recommendation against using procalcitonin to guide antimicrobial initiation in addition to clinical evaluation.

ANTIMICROBIAL CHOICE

Recommendations of the Surviving Sepsis Campaign 2021

For adults with sepsis or septic shock at high risk of methicillin-resistant *Staphylococcus aureus* (MRSA), using empiric

TABLE 5: *Main biomarkers in sepsis:* CRP and procalcitonin.

	C-reactive protein	Procalcitonin
Properties	Acute phase protein (pentraxin)	Hormokine
Normal values	0.08 mg/dL (median)	1 ng/mL
Maximum peak	>50 mg/dL (>1,000 × reference value)	>100 ng/mL (>10,000 × reference value)
Source	Liver	Virtually all cells and macrophages
Time to increase after insult	4–6 hours	3–4 hours
Time to peak concentration	36–50 hours	Around 2 hours
Half-life	19 hours	22–35 hours
Possible confounders	—	—
Steroids	No effect	Frequent false negatives
Immunosuppression	No effect	Frequent false negatives
Neutropenia	No effect	Frequent false negatives
Renal failure	No effect	↑↑
Renal replacement therapy	No effect	↓↓
Chronic liver failure	↓ (70% of the normal)	No effects
Acute liver failure	No CRP increase	No effect
Secondary infection (second hit)	↓ (70% of first episode)	↓↓↓ (10% of first episode)
Bacterial versus viral infections	Poor	Poor

(CRP: C-reactive protein; PCT: procalcitonin)

antimicrobials with MRSA coverage over using antimicrobials without MRSA coverage is recommended as compared with using antimicrobials without MRSA coverage. Weak recommendation, low quality of evidence.

Antimicrobial Therapy Including Management of Septic Shock

Flowchart 2: How to use biomarkers of infection or sepsis at the bedside?

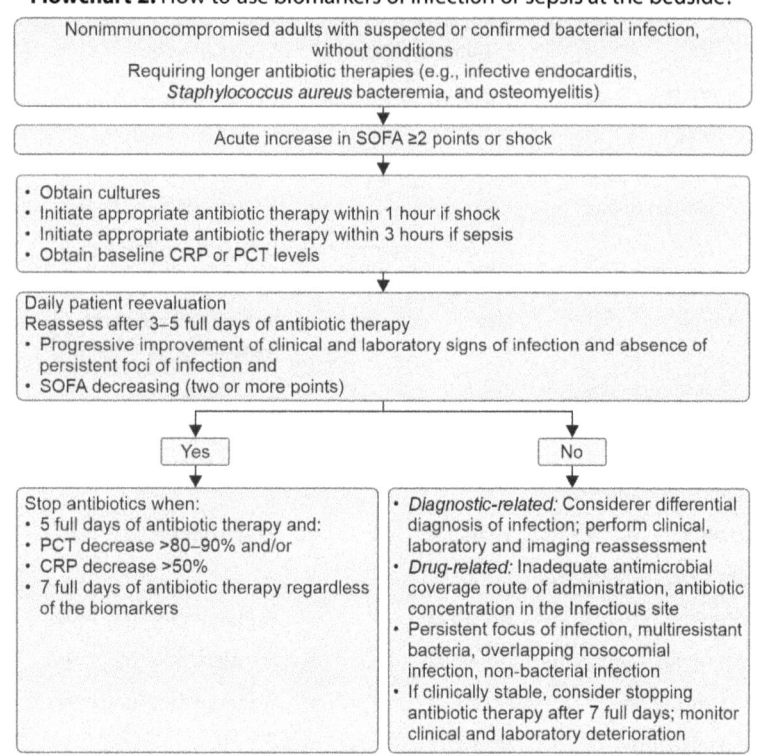

(CRP: C-reactive protein; PCT: procalcitonin; SOFA: Sequential Organ Failure Assessment)

Rationale for the Recommendation

Methicillin-resistant *Staphylococcus aureus* has been found to be accountable for about 5% of culture. The incidence of MRSA varies, however, by region and by patient-related characteristics. Patient-related risk factors for MRSA include prior history of MRSA infection or colonization, recent IV antibiotics, history of recurrent skin infections or chronic wounds, presence of invasive devices, hemodialysis, recent hospital admissions, and severity of illness. As per observational data among patients with documented MRSA infections, delays of >24–48 hours until antibiotic administration resulted in increased mortality in some studies, but uniformly. Among undifferentiated patients with pneumonia or sepsis, broad-spectrum

TABLE 6: Main risk factors for multidrug-resistant pathogens.

MRSA	• Previous infection/colonization by MRSA in the last 12 months • Hemodialysis or peritoneal dialysis • Presence of central venous catheters or intravascular devices • Administration of multiple antibiotics in the last 30 days (in particular with cephalosporins or fluoroquinolones) • Immunodepression • Immunosuppressor treatments • Rheumatoid arthritis • Drug addiction • Patients coming from long-term care facilities or who have undergone a hospital stay in the last 12 months • Close contact with patients colonized by MRSA
ESBL	• Previous infection/colonization with ESBL in the last 12 months • Prolonged hospitalization (>10 days, in particular in ICU/hospice/long-term care facilities) • Presence of permanent urinary catheter • Administration of multiple antibiotics in the last 30 days (particularly with cephalosporins or fluoroquinolones) • Patients with percutaneous endoscopic gastrostomy
Pseudomonas aeruginosa	• Previous infection/colonization with *P. aeruginosa* in the last 12 months • Administration of multiple antibiotics in the last 30 days (particularly with cephalosporins or fluoroquinolones) • Pulmonary anatomic abnormalities with recurrent infections (e.g., bronchiectasis) • Elderly patients (>80 years) • Scarce glycemic control in diabetic subjects • Presence of permanent urinary catheter • Prolonged steroid use (>6 weeks) • Neutropenic fever • Cystic fibrosis
Candida spp.	• Immunosuppression • Presence of central venous catheters or intravascular devices • Patients in total parenteral nutrition • Prolonged hospitalization (>10 days, particularly in an ICU) • Recent surgery (particularly abdominal surgery) • Prolonged wide-range antibiotic administration • Previous necrotizing pancreatitis • Recent fungal infection/colorization

(ESBL: extended-spectrum beta-lactamase; ICU: intensive care unit; MRSA: methicillin-resistant *Staphylococcus aureus*)

TABLE 7: Main empiric antimicrobic therapies according to the site of infection.

	Infection site	I Choice	II Choice	Allergy to penicillin	Risk factors for ESBL+	Risk factors for MRSA
Pulmonary	Community-acquired pneumonia (CAP)	Amoxicillin/clavulanate 2.2 g/TID + Azithromycin 500 mg/die or Clarithromycin 500 mg/BID	Levofloxacin 750 mg/die	Levofloxacin 750 mg/die	Piperacillin/tazobactam 9 g LD followed by 18 g/die + Levofloxacin 750 mg/die or Meropenem 2 g LD followed by 2 g/RID	Levofloxacin 750 mg/die + Linezolid 600 mg/BID or Vancomycin 25–30 mg/kg LD than 20 mg/kg/BID
	Hospital-acquired pneumonia (HAP)	Piperacillin/tazobactam 9 g LD followed by 18 g/die or Cefepime 1 g LD followed by 2 g/TID + Linezolid 600 mg/BID	Levofloxacin 750 mg/die + Linezolid 600 mg/bid	Levofloxacin 750 mg/die + Linezolid 600 mg/bid	Piperacillin/tazobactam 9 g LD followed by 18 g/die + Meropenem 2 g LD followed by 2 g/RID	Piperacillin/tazobactam 9 g LD followed by 18 g/die or Cefepime 1 g LD followed by 2 g/RID + Gentamicin 5–7 mg/kg/die + Linezolid 600 mg/BID or Vancomycin 25–30 mg/kg LD than 20 mg/kg/BID

Contd...

Antimicrobial Therapy Including Management of Septic Shock

Infection site	I Choice	II Choice	Allergy to penicillin	Risk factors for ESBL+	Risk factors for MRSA
Ventilator-associated pneumonia (VAP)	Piperacillin/tazobactam 9 g ID followed by 18 g/die or Cefepime 1 g ID followed by 2 g/TID + Linezolid 600 mg/BID	Levofloxacin 750 mg/die + Linezolid 600 mg/bid	Levofloxacin 750 mg/die + Linezolid 600 mg/bid	Piperacillin/tazobactam 9 g LD followed by 18 g/die + Meropenem 2 g LD followed by 2g/RID	Piperacillin/Tazobactam 9 g LD followed by 18 g/die or Cefepime 1 g LD followed by 2g/tid + Linezolid 600 mg/BID or Vancomycin 25–30 mg/kg LD than 20 mg/kg/bid
Urinary Community	Piperacillin/tazobactam 9 g LD followed by 18 g/die	Ciprofloxacin 500 mg/bid	Ciprofloxacin 500 mg/bid	Piperacillin/tazobactam 9 g LD followed by 18 g/die	Piperacillin/tazobactam 9 g LD followed by 18 g/die or Meropenem 2 g LD followed by 2 g/RID
Urinary Nosocomial	Piperacillin/tazobactam 9 g LD followed by 18 g/die	Meropenem 2 g LD followed by 2 g/RID	Meropenem 2 g LD followed by 2 g/RID	Meropenem 2 g LD followed by 2 g/RID	Meropenem 2 g LD followed by 2 g/RID

Contd...

Infection site		I Choice	II Choice	Allergy to penicillin	Risk factors for ESBL+	Risk factors for MRSA
Abdominal	Community	Amoxicillin/ clavulanate 2.2 g/TID or Ceftriaxone 2 g/die + Metronidazole 500 mg/QID	Piperacillin/ tazobactam 9 g LD followed by 18 g/die	Ciprofloxacin 500 mg/BID + Metronidazole 500 mg/QID	Meropenem 2 g LD followed by 2 g/TID	Meropenem 2 g LD followed by 2 g/TID + Vancomycin 25–30 mg/kg LD than 20 mg/kg/BID
	Nosocomial	Piperacillin/ tazobactam 9 g LD followed by 18 g/die	Meropenem 2 g LD followed by 2 g/TID	Ciprofloxacin 500 mg/bid + Metronidazole 500 mg/QID	Meropenem 2 g LD followed by 1 g/TID	Meropenem 2 g LD followed by 2 g/TID + Tigecycline 100 mg LD followed by 100 mg/bid ± Caspofungin 70 mg LD followed by 50 mg/die

Contd...

Infection site		I Choice	II Choice	Allergy to penicillin	Risk factors for ESBL+	Risk factors for MRSA
CNS	<50 years	Dexamethasone 0.1 mg/kg/QID + Ceftriaxone 2 g/die ± Ampicillin 12 g/die ± Acyclovir 10 mg/kg/TID	Dexamethasone 0.1 mg/kg/QID + Meropenem 2 g LD followed by 2 g/TID ± Acyclovir 10 mg/kg/TID	Dexamethasone 0.1 mg/kg/QID + Meropenem 2 g LD followed by 2 g/TID ± Acyclovir 10 mg/kg/TID	/	/
	>50 years	Dexamethasone 0.1 mg/kg/QID + Ceftriaxone 2 g/die ± Ampicillin 12 g/die ± Acyclovir 10 mg/kg/TID	Dexamethasone 0.1 mg/kg/QID + Meropenem 2 g LD followed by 2g/TID ± Acyclovir 10 mg/kg/TID	Dexamethasone 0.1 mg/kg/QID + Meropenem 2 g LD followed by 2 g/TID ± Acyclovir 10 mg/kg/TID	/	/

Contd...

Infection site		I Choice	II Choice	Allergy to penicillin	Risk factors for ESBL+	Risk factors for MRSA
Skin	Cellulitis	Amoxicillin/ Clavulanate 2.2 g/TID ± Clindamycin 600 mg/QID	Ceftriaxone 2 g/die	Levofloxacin 750 mg/die	Piperacillin/ tazobactam 9 g LD followed by/die + Meropenem 2 g LD followed by 2 g/TID	Daptomycin 8–10 mg/ kg/die or Vancomycin 25–30 mg/kg LD than 20 mg/kg/BID
	Necrotizing fasciitis (NF)	Daptomycin 8–10 mg/kg/die + clindamycin 600 mg/QID + Piperacillin/ tazobactam 9 g LD followed by 18 g/die	/	Daptomycin 8–10 mg/kg/die + Clindamycin 600 mg/QID + Meropenem 2 g LD followed by 2 g/TID	Daptomycin 8–10 mg/kg/die + Clindamycin 600 mg/QID + Meropenem 2 g LD followed by 2 g/TID	Daptomycin 8–10 mg/kg/die + Clindamycin 600 mg/QID + Meropenem 2 g LD followed by 2 g/TID

Contd...

Antimicrobial Therapy Including Management of Septic Shock

Contd...

Infection site	I Choice	II Choice	Allergy to penicillin	Risk factors for ESBL+	Risk factors for MRSA
Gynecological	Clindamycin 600 mg/QID + Gentamicin 5–7 mg/kg/die	/	Clindamycin 600 mg/QID + Gentamicin 5–7 mg/kg/die	Meropenem 2 g LD followed by 2 g/TID	Meropenem 2 g LD followed by 2 g/TID
Undefined	Piperacillin/tazobactam 9 g LD followed by 18 g/die + Daptomycin 8–10 mg/kg/die or Vancomycin 25–30 mg/kg LD then 20 mg/kg/BID ± Caspofungin 70 mg LD followed by 50 mg/die	Daptomycin 8–10 mg/kg/die or Vancomycin 25–30 mg/kg LD than 20 mg/kg/bid + Meropenem 2 g LD followed by 2 g/TID ± Caspofungin 70 mg LD followed by 50 mg/die	Daptomycin 8–10 mg/kg/die or Vancomycin 25–30 mg/kg LD than 20 mg/kg/BID + Meropenem 2 g LD followed by 2 g/TID ± Caspofungin 70 mg LD followed by 50 mg/die	Daptomycin 8–10 mg/kg/die or Vancomycin 25–30 mg/kg LD than 20 mg/kg/BID + Meropenem 2 g LD followed by 2 g/TID ± Caspofungin 70 mg LD followed by 50 mg/die	Daptomycin 8–10 mg/kg/die or Vancomycin 25–30 mg/kg LD than 20 mg/kg/bid + Meropenem 2 g LD followed by 2 g/TID ± Caspofungin 70 mg LD followed by 50 mg/die

regimens, including agents active against MRSA, were associated with higher mortality, particularly among patients without MRSA. The unwanted effects associated with unnecessary MRSA coverage are also substantiated by studies showing a relation between early discontinuation of MRSA coverage and better outcomes in patients with negative nares or bronchoalveolar lavage (BAL) MRSA PCR.

So, to conclude, failure to cover for MRSA in a patient with MRSA may be harmful, but unnecessary MRSA coverage in a patient without MRSA may also be harmful. Data from RCTs, including the evaluation of nasal swab testing to withhold therapy for MRSA, are warranted, and further research on rapid diagnostic tools and clinical prediction rules for MRSA are needed.

The choice of the most appropriate empiric antimicrobial therapy is often challenging; therefore, it might be useful to consider several risk factors for pathogens that most commonly appear as etiological agents of sepsis.

Carbapenem-sparing agents may include cefepime, fluoroquinolones, temocillin and new beta-lactam–beta-lactamase inhibitors:

- Cefepime does not seem to be a reasonable alternative for the treatment of ESBL infection since its efficacy depends on the mechanism of resistance. There is no difference between cefepime and carbapenems when Enterobacteriaceae express AmpC beta lactamase and there is an excess mortality if the resistance is due to an ESBL. A randomized-controlled trial evaluating cefepime versus piperacillin–tazobactam and ertapenem in nosocomial urinary tract infections caused by ESBL-producing *Escherichia coli* was stopped early for a clear failure rate in their cefepime arm:
- There is a scarcity of data on fluoroquinolones. Although there is frequent resistance to their class of antibiotics in ESBL-producing Enterobacteriaceae, it seems possible to use fluoroquinolones when there is no resistance to nalidixic acid, and the minimum inhibitory concentration (MIC) is <0.25 mg/L. Higher MICs were associated with a higher risk of default.
- Temocillin might be an interesting option due to its activity on ESBL and AmpC beta-lactamas; however, there are only a few

data available, and all are retrospective without a control group. A current ongoing randomized-controlled trial will evaluate the efficacy of temocillin in ICU patients with ESBL infection (NCT05565222).
- The new beta-lactam-beta-lactamase inhibitors (ceftazidime-avibactam and ceftolozane-tazobactam) are not used as carbapenem-sparing agents since their etiological impact, as compared to carbapenems impact, is currently not known. Therefore, they are not recommended in this indication.

Recommendation of Surviving Sepsis Campaign 2021

- For adults with sepsis or septic shock and high risk for multidrug-resistant (MDR) organisms, it is suggested to use two antimicrobials with gram-negative coverage for empiric treatment over one gram-negative agent.

  Weak recommendation, very low quality of evidence.
- For adults with sepsis or septic shock and low risk for MDR organisms, it is suggested to use two gram-negative agents for empiric treatment, compared with one gram-negative agent.

  Weak recommendation, very low quality of evidence.
- For adults with sepsis or septic shock, it is suggested to use double gram-negative coverage once the causative pathogen and the susceptibilities are known.

  Weak recommendation, very low quality of evidence.

ANTIFUNGAL THERAPY

Recommendations of the Surviving Sepsis Campaign 2021

- For adults with sepsis or septic shock at high risk of fungal infection, it is suggested to use empiric antifungal therapy over no antifungal therapy.

  Weak recommendation, low quality of evidence.
- For adults with sepsis or septic shock at low risk of fungal infection, we *suggest against* the empiric use of antifungal therapy.

  Weak recommendation, low quality of evidence.

Flowchart 3: Proposed algorithm to decrease antimicrobial consumption in the ICU and potential beneficial effects of reducing antibiotics consumption.

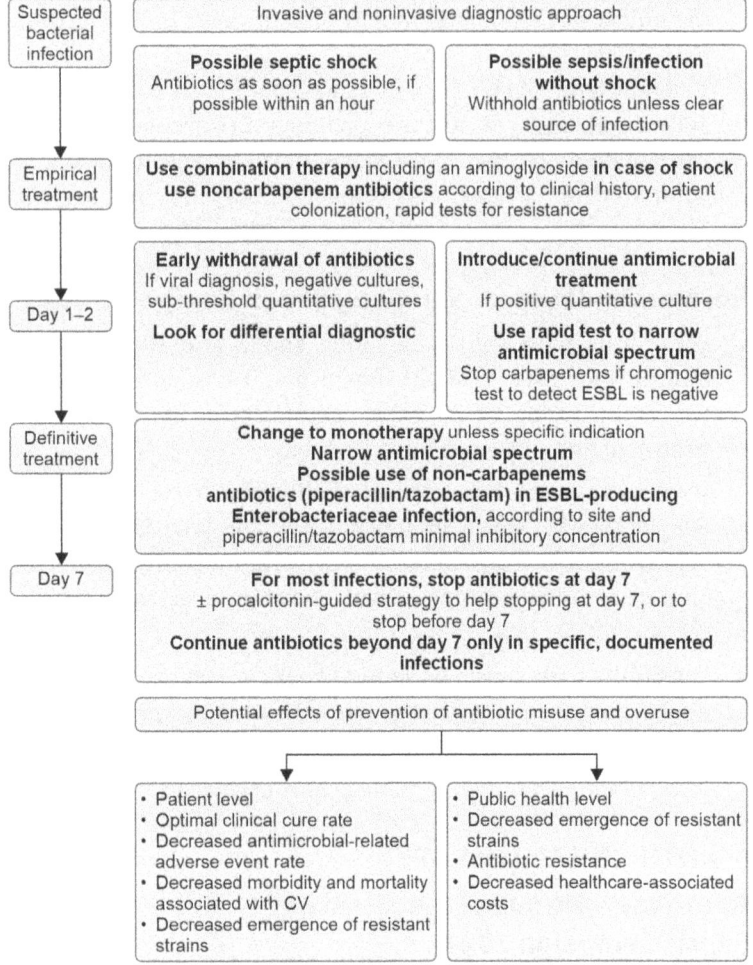

(CV: cardiovascular; ESBL extended-spectrum beta-lactamase)

Rationale for Recommendation

While patients with sepsis or septic shock may not, in general, benefit from empiric antifungals, some patients with particular risk factors for fungal infection may. For example, patients with febrile neutropenia who fail to defervesce after 4–7 days of broad-spectrum antibacterial therapy are at increased risk of having fungal disease.

BOX 1: Bedside principles for optimizing antibiotic prescribing in the ICU.

- Carry out a thorough clinical examination with targeted imaging ± whole body CT scan
- Use invasive diagnostic tools, especially if the patient is severely ill on admission. Microbiological sampling is essential prior to administering antibiotics
- If septic shock is suspected, use broad-spectrum combination therapy within 1 hour
- Without shock, if a potential source of infection is identified, use monotherapy except for specific recommendation (e.g., community-acquired pneumonia)
- Without shock, if sepsis is suspected and no source of infection is identified, withhold antimicrobial treatment. Search for differential diagnosis
- Empiric antibiotic therapy should be selected depending on the identified source and local etiology
- Restrict the use of carbapenems to patients with a high likelihood of ESBL infection. The use of rectal or respiratory ESBL colonization may be useful
- Methodically reassess antibiotic therapy after 48 hours
- De-escalation is to be done as early as possible. For early de-escalation, ESBL-chromogenic tests may be useful
- In the absence of documentation after 48 hours, look for a differential diagnosis
- In most cases, the definite treatment should be a monotherapy. Combination therapy is to be considered for difficult-to-treat pathogens or specific localizations (endocarditis, prosthetic device infection, joint and bone infection, abscess)
- Use prolonged beta-lactam infusion after initial loading dose in severe patients (e.g., shock)
- TDM is recommended for aminoglycosides and vancomycin and, in general, for antibiotics having a narrow therapeutic window or suspected drug toxicity
- Beta-lactams TDM should be used for prolonged therapy and in specific situations (augmented renal clearance, RRT, and ECMO)
- Use short-course (7-day) for most of infections. PCT may be useful to help shorten the duration of antimicrobial treatment

(CT: computed tomography; ECMO: extracorporeal membrane oxygenation; ESBL: extended-spectrum-beta-lactamase; ICU: intensive care unit; PCT: procalcitonin; RRT: renal replacement therapy; TDM: therapeutic drug monitoring)

BOX 2: Risk factors for harboring *Candida* sepsis.

- *Candida* colonization at multiple sites
- Surrogate markers such as serum beta-D-glucan assay
- Neutropenia
- Immunosuppression
- Severity of illness (high APACHE score)
- Longer ICU length of stay
- Central venous catheters and other intravascular devices
- Persons who inject drugs
- Total parenteral nutrition
- Broad-spectrum antibiotics
- Gastrointestinal tract perforations and anastomotic
- Emergency gastrointestinal or hepatobiliary surgery
- Acute renal failure and hemodialysis
- Severe thermal injury
- Prior surgery

(APACHE: Acute Physiology and Chronic Health Evaluation; ICU: intensive care unit)

BOX 3: Risk factors for endemic yeast (*Cryptococcus*, *Histoplasma*, *Blastomyces*, and coccidioidomycosis).

- Antigen markers, such as cryptococcal, *Histoplasma*, and *Blastomyces* assays
- Human immunodeficiency virus (HIV) Infection
- Solid organ transplantation
- High-dose corticosteroid therapy
- Hematopoietic stem cell transplantation
- Certain biologic response modifiers
- Diabetes mellitus

BOX 4: Risk factors for invasive mold infection.

- Neutropenia
- Surrogate markers such as serum and bronchoalveolar lavage galactomannan assay
- Hematopoietic stem cell transplantation
- Solid organ transplantation
- High-dose corticosteroid therapy
- Certain biologic response modifiers
- The decision to start

ANTIVIRAL THERAPY
Recommendation of Surviving Sepsis Campaign 2021
No recommendation on the use of antiviral agents.

Historically, influenza has been one of the more common viral causes of sepsis. However, it is unclear to what extent the primary viral infection, as opposed to bacterial pneumonia coinfection, is the cause of organ dysfunction in these patients. More recently, severe acute respiratory syndrome coronavirus 2 (SARS-CoV-2) (causing COVID-19) is now responsible for many cases of infection and sepsis. The recent pandemic due to SARS-CoV-2 has resulted in the understanding of this condition changing very rapidly.

While there appears to be no overall effect of neuraminidase inhibitors on mortality in patients with influenza-related pneumonia, there may be an effect when they are administered early in the course of the disease.

Immunocompromised patients are particularly vulnerable to viral infections, including patients with neutropenia, human immunodeficiency virus (HIV) infection, hematological malignancies, and hematopoietic stem cell transplantation or solid organ transplants; in these patient's herpes simplex virus, Epstein–Barr, virus, cytomegalovirus, and respiratory viruses such as adenoviruses, can cause severe disease. Tropical and subtropical regions have endemic and epidemic outbreaks of zoonotic viral infections, including those caused by dengue, Ebola, Lassa, Marburg, Sin Nombre, and chikungunya virus. Many of these can manifest with clinical signs of sepsis, particularly in their early stages. Unfortunately, effective therapies are lacking for most of these viruses.

The efficacy of empiric antiviral therapy is unknown, and as for other antimicrobial agents, there is a risk of undesirable effects. Cost-effectiveness is also not established.

DE-ESCALATION OF ANTIBIOTICS
Recommendation of Surviving Sepsis Campaign 2021
For adults with sepsis or septic shock, daily assessment is suggested for de-escalation of antimicrobials over using fixed durations of therapy without daily reassessment for de-escalation.

Weak recommendation, very low quality of evidence.

DURATION OF ANTIBIOTICS
Recommendation of Surviving Sepsis Campaign 2021
For adults with an initial diagnosis of sepsis or septic shock and adequate source control, it is recommended to use shorter over longer duration of antimicrobial therapy.

Weak recommendation, very low quality of evidence.

BIOMARKERS TO DISCONTINUE ANTIBIOTICS
Recommendation of Surviving Sepsis Campaign 2021
For adults with an initial diagnosis of sepsis or septic shock and adequate source control where the optimal duration of therapy is unclear, it is recommended to use procalcitonin AND clinical evaluation to decide when to discontinue antimicrobials over clinical evaluation alone. Weak recom*mendation, low quality of evidence.*

HEMODYNAMIC MANAGEMENT
Fluid Management
Recommendations of Surviving Sepsis Campaign 2021

- For adults with sepsis or septic shock, it is recommended to use crystalloids as first-line fluid for resuscitation.

  Strong recommendation, moderate quality of evidence.
- For adults with sepsis or septic shock, it is recommended to use balanced crystalloids instead of normal saline for resuscitation.

  Weak recommendation, low quality of evidence.
- For adults with sepsis or septic shock, it is recommended to use albumin in patients who received large volumes of crystalloids over using crystalloids alone.

  Weak recommendation, moderate quality of evidence.
- For adults with sepsis or septic shock, it is recommended not to use starches for resuscitation.

  Strong recommendation, high quality of evidence.
- For adults with sepsis and septic shock, it is recommended to use gelatin for resuscitation.

  Weak recommendation, moderate quality.

TABLE 8: Key randomized controlled trials investigating resuscitation with different colloids and crystalloids in critically ill patients, including patients with sepsis and septic shock.

Schortgen et al. 2001

Compared to gelatin, HES 200/0.6 exposure was a independent risk factor for ARF in patients with severe sepsis or septic shock

CHEST 2012

Resuscitation with 6% HES (130/0.4) as compared with saline in the ICU, which did not provide any clinical benefit. No difference in mortality and a higher rate of PRT in the HES groin

SAFE 2004

Use of 4% albumin or 0.9% sodium chloride for fluid resuscitation in critically ill patients results in smaller outcomes, at 28 days. A nonsignificant trend in favor of albumin in sepsis and saline in trauma was observed

CRISTAL 2012

Among ICU patients with hypovolemic and septic shock, there was no mortality benefit at 28 days with colloids over crystalloids for fluid resuscitation

Dubois et al. 2006

A pilot trial suggested that albumin administration may improve organ function in hypoalbuminemic critically ill patients and results in a less positive fluid balance

ALBIOS 2014

Among patients with severe sepsis or septic shock, daily administration of albumin to maintain serum albumin ≥3 g/dL was not associated with a reduction in all-cause mortality at 28 days when compared to no albumin. Potential better hemodynamics with albumin (tertiary outcome)

6S 2012

Patients with severe sepsis who received fluid resuscitation with HES compared with Ringer's acetate had a higher risk of death within 90 days and were more likely to receive renal replacement therapy

ARISS (recruiting)

A multicenter RCT of albumin replacement therapy in septic shock to investigate whether albumin replacement and maintenance of its serum levels at ≥3 g/dL for 28 days to improve survival in patients with septic shock (not sepsis) compared to resuscitation without albumin

(ARF: acute renal failure; HES: hydroxyethyl starch; ICU: interactive care unit; RRT: renal replacement therapy)

VASOACTIVE AGENTS

Recommendations of the Surviving Sepsis Campaign 2021

For adults with septic shock, it is recommended to use norepinephrine as the first-line agent over other vasopressors. *Strong recommendation:* Dopamine. *High-quality evidence for* Vasopressin. *Moderate-quality evidence* Epinephrine. *Low-quality evidence* Selepressin. *Low-quality evidence* Angiotensin II. *Very low-quality evidence.*

In settings where norepinephrine is not available, epinephrine or dopamine can be used as an alternative, but the use and availability of norepinephrine is to be encouraged. Special attention should be given to patients at risk for arrhythmias when using dopamine and epinephrine.

For adults with septic shock on norepinephrine with inadequate MAP levels, it is suggested to add vasopressin instead of escalating the dose of norepinephrine.

Weak recommendation, moderate-quality evidence.
It is recommended to start vasopressin, which is usually started when the dose of norepinephrine is in the range of 0.25–0.5 µg/kg/min.

For adults with septic shock and inadequate MAP levels despite norepinephrine and vasopressin, it is suggested not to add epinephrine.

Weak recommendation, low-quality evidence.
For adults with septic shock, it is suggested not to add terlipressin.

Weak recommendation, low quality of evidence.

Rationale for Recommendation

Norepinephrine is a potent α-1 and β-1 adrenergic receptors agonist, which results in vasoconstriction and increased MAP with minimal effect on heart rate. Dopamine acts in a dose-dependent fashion on dopamine-1, α-1, and β-1 adrenergic receptors. At lower dosages, dopamine causes vasodilation via dopamine-1 receptor activity in the renal, splanchnic, cerebral, and coronary beds. With higher dosages, dopamine's α-adrenergic receptor activity predominates, resulting in vasoconstriction and increased systemic vascular resistance (SVR); its β-1 adrenergic receptor activity can lead to dose-limiting arrhythmias. Norepinephrine is more potent than dopamine as a vasoconstrictor. In a systematic review and meta-analysis of 11 RCTs, norepinephrine resulted in a lower mortality and lower risk of arrhythmias compared with dopamine. Although the β-1 activity of dopamine may be useful in patients with myocardial dysfunction, the higher risk of arrhythmias limits its use.

Epinephrine's action is also dose-dependent with potent β-1 adrenergic receptor activity and moderate β-2 and α-1 adrenergic receptor activity. The activity of epinephrine, at low doses, is primarily driven by its action on β-1 adrenergic receptors, resulting in increased cardiac output (CO), decreased SVR, and variable effects on MAP. At higher doses, however, epinephrine administration results in increased SVR and CO. Potential adverse effects of epinephrine include arrhythmias and impaired splanchnic circulation. The panel issued a strong recommendation for norepinephrine as the first-line agent over other vasopressors.

Vasopressin is an endogenous peptide hormone produced in the hypothalamus and stored and released by the posterior pituitary gland. Its mechanism for vasoconstrictive activity is multifactorial and includes the binding of V1 receptors on vascular smooth muscle, resulting in increased arterial blood pressure.

Studies show that vasopressin concentration is elevated in early septic shock but decreases to the normal range in most patients between 24 and 48 hours as shock continues. This finding has been called "relative vasopressin deficiency" as, in the presence of hypotension, vasopressin would be expected to be elevated. The significance of this finding is unknown.

Unlike most vasopressors, vasopressin is not titrated to response, but it is usually administered at a fixed dose of 0.03 units/min for the treatment of septic shock. In clinical trials, vasopressin was used up to 0.06 units/min. Higher doses of vasopressin have been associated with cardiac, digital, and splanchnic ischemia.

In a systematic review of 10 RCTs, vasopressin with norepinephrine reduced mortality as compared with norepinephrine alone but did not reduce the need for RRT. There was no difference in the risks of digital ischemia or arrhythmias. The threshold for adding vasopressin varied among studies and remains unclear. Starting vasopressin when norepinephrine dose is in the range of 0.25–0.5 µg/kg/min seems sensible. Another meta-analysis of RCTs on distributive shock showed a lower risk of atrial fibrillation with the combination of vasopressin and norepinephrine compared to norepinephrine alone. However, a recent individual patient data meta-analysis of patients with septic shock from four RCTs showed that vasopressin alone or in combination with norepinephrine led to a higher risk of digital ischemia (risk difference but lower risk of arrhythmia compared with norepinephrine alone).

Selepressin is a highly selective V1 agonist, inducing vasoconstriction via stimulation of vascular smooth muscle. It does not share the typical V1b and V2 receptor effects of vasopressin and has, therefore, been postulated as a potentially attractive non-catecholamine vasopressor alternative to norepinephrine.

Selepressin failed to demonstrate clinical superiority over norepinephrine, and it is considered the desirable and undesirable consequences to be in favor of norepinephrine, and a weak recommendation is issued against the use of selepressin as a first-line therapy. Furthermore, it is not currently commercially available.

Angiotensin II is a naturally occurring hormone with marked vasoconstrictor effects, triggered through stimulation of the renin angiotensin system. A synthetic human preparation has recently become available for clinical use and has been studied in two clinical trials.

The SSC panel considered that angiotensin should not be used as a first-line agent, but having demonstrated physiological effectiveness, it may have a role as an adjunctive vasopressor therapy.

Terlipressin is a prodrug and is converted to lysine vasopressin by endothelial peptidases, producing a "slow release" effect and giving an effective half-life of around 6 hours. Terlipressin is more specific for the V1 receptors, and it has been studied in nine clinical trials of patients with sepsis.

The SSC panel, in view of the adverse consequences being higher with the use of terlipressin, has issued a weak recommendation against its use in patients with septic shock.

INOTROPES

Recommendations of SSC 2021

- For adults with septic shock and cardiac dysfunction with persistent hypoperfusion despite adequate volume status and arterial blood pressure, it is suggested to either add dobutamine to norepinephrine or use epinephrine alone.

  Weak recommendation, low quality of evidence.

- For adults with septic shock and cardiac dysfunction with persistent hypoperfusion despite adequate volume status and arterial blood pressure, it is suggested not to use levosimendan.

  Weak recommendation, low quality of evidence.

MONITORING AND INTRAVENOUS ACCESS

Recommendations of the Surviving Sepsis Campaign 2021

- For adults with septic shock, it is suggested to invasive monitoring of arterial blood pressure over noninvasive monitoring, as soon as practical and if resources are available.

  Weak recommendation, very low quality of evidence.

- For adults with septic shock, it is suggested to initiate vasopressors peripherally to restore MAP rather than delaying initiation until a central venous access is secured.

  Weak recommendation, very low quality of evidence.

When using vasopressors peripherally, they should be administered only for a short period of time and in a vein in or proximal to the antecubital fossa.

FLUID BALANCE

Recommendation of Surviving Sepsis Campaign 2021

There is insufficient evidence to make a *recommendation* on the use of restrictive versus liberal fluid strategies in the first 24 hours of resuscitation in patients with sepsis and septic shock who still have signs of hypoperfusion and volume depletion after initial resuscitation.

Fluid resuscitation should be given only if patients present with signs of hypoperfusion.

Rationale for the Recommendation

The existing literature does not provide clear guidance about the best fluid strategy following the initial resuscitation bolus of fluids. The four largest clinical trials in sepsis resuscitation used moderate to large amounts of fluids in the first 72 hours. Although Rivers administered over 13 L of fluids, ProCESS, ARISE, and ProMISe administered approximately 7-8 L in the usual care groups with a reported low mortality rate. However, recent evidence suggests that IV fluids used to restore organ perfusion may actually damage vascular integrity and cause organ dysfunction. Data from observational studies have shown an association between high-volume fluid resuscitation and increased mortality, but these studies are likely affected by incubation variables, i.e., the administration of higher amounts of fluids to sicker patients.

OXYGEN TARGETS

Recommendation of Surviving Sepsis Campaign 2021

There is insufficient evidence to make a recommendation on the use of conservative oxygen targets in adults with sepsis-induced hypoxemic respiratory failure.

Background for the Recommendations

Patients who are undergoing mechanical ventilation in the ICU often receive a high fraction of inspired oxygen and have a high arterial oxygen tension. The conservative use of oxygen may reduce oxygen exposure and diminish lung and systemic oxidative injury. The evidence for the use of conservative oxygen targets [generally defined as partial pressure of oxygen in the arterial blood (PaO_2) 55-70 mm Hg; SpO_2 88-92%] and therapy in patients with sepsis is limited, with three randomized trials in the critically ill population.

HIGH-FLOW NASAL OXYGEN THERAPY
Recommendation of Surviving Sepsis Campaign 2021

For adults with sepsis-induced hypoxemic respiratory failure, it is suggested to use high-flow nasal oxygen over noninvasive ventilation.

Weak recommendation, low quality of evidence.

Rationale for the Recommendation

Acute hypoxemic respiratory failure can result from causes of sepsis, such as pneumonia or nonpulmonary infections resulting in acute respiratory distress syndrome (ARDS). Patients presenting with hypoxia without hypercapnia are treated with high concentrations of inhaled oxygen, which can be delivered via conventional interfaces like nasal prongs, a facemask with a reservoir, or a Venturi mask.

Advanced interventions for patients with severe hypoxia requiring escalation of support include noninvasive ventilation (NIV) or high-flow nasal oxygen (HFNO). Both therapies avoid the complications of intubation and invasive mechanical ventilation. Further to improving gas exchange, NIV may help to reduce the work of breathing in select patients. However, NIV use can be associated with the development of complications, including increased risk of gastric distention and aspiration, facial skin breakdown, excessively high tidal volumes, and patient discomfort related to the inability to eat or effectively phonate during therapy.

High flow nasal oxygen is a noninvasive, high-concentration oxygen delivery interface that confers warming and humidification of secretions, high flow rates to better match patient demand, washout of nasopharyngeal dead space, and modest positive airway pressure effect. The single inspiratory limb of HFNC allows for airflows as high as 60 L/min to achieve inspired oxygen fractions (FiO_2) as high as 95–100%. However, HFNC is less effective at reducing the work of breathing and supplying a moderate or higher level of positive end-expiratory pressure (PEEP). Complications with HFNC are possible; however, they are usually self-limited and do not require discontinuing therapy.

PROTECTIVE VENTILATION IN ACUTE RESPIRATORY DISTRESS SYNDROME

Recommendation of Surviving Sepsis Campaign 2021

For adults with sepsis-induced ARDS, it is suggested to use a low tidal volume ventilation strategy (6 mL/kg) over a high tidal volume strategy (>10 mL/kg).

Strong recommendation, high quality of evidence.

Rationale for the Recommendation

Several meta-analyses suggest decreased mortality in patients with a pressure- and volume-limited strategy for established ARDS. The largest trial of a volume- and pressure-limited strategy showed a 9% absolute decrease in mortality in ARDS patients ventilated with tidal volumes of 6 mL/kg compared with 12 mL/kg predicted body weight (PBW) and aiming for plateau pressure ≤30 cmH_2O.

For adults with sepsis-induced severe ARDS, it is recommended to use an upper limit goal for plateau pressures of 30 cmH_2O, over higher plateau pressures.

Strong recommendation, moderate quality of evidence.

Rationale for the Recommendation

A recent systematic review that included five RCTs also identified a strong relationship between plateau pressure and mortality. The recommendation is also supported by observational data. LUNGSAFE, a large international observational study, which reported that plateau pressure correlated with mortality; however, the relationship between the two was not evident when the plateau pressure was below 20 cmH_2O. A secondary analysis of five observational studies identified a plateau pressure cut-off value of 29 cmH_2O, above which an ordinal increment was accompanied by an increment of risk of death. Hence, it is recommended that the upper limit goal for plateau pressure should be <30 cmH_2O.

Recommendation of Surviving Sepsis Campaign 2021

For adults with moderate-to-severe sepsis-induced ARDS, it is suggested to use higher PEEP over lower PEEP.

Weak recommendation, moderate quality of evidence.

Rationale for the Recommendation

The recommendation is unchanged from 2016.

A patient-level meta-analysis showed no benefit of higher PEEP in *all patients* with ARDS; however, patients with moderate or severe ARDS (PaO_2/FiO_2 ≤200 mm Hg) had decreased mortality with the use of higher PEEP, whereas those with mild ARDS did not. A patient-level analysis of two of the randomized PEEP trials suggested that patients with ARDS who respond to increased PEEP with improved oxygenation have a lower risk of death; this association was stronger in patients with more severe ARDS (PaO_2/FiO_2 <150 mm Hg) compared with patients with less severe ARDS.

LOW TIDAL VOLUME IN NONACUTE RESPIRATORY DISTRESS SYNDROME RESPIRATORY FAILURE

Recommendation of Surviving Sepsis Campaign 2021

For adults with sepsis-induced respiratory failure (without ARDS), it is suggested to use low tidal volume as compared to high tidal volume ventilation.

Weak recommendation, low quality of evidence.
Since, sepsis is an independent risk factor for the development of ARDS, and delays in diagnosing ARDS may result in delayed use of low tidal volumes. It is suggested that low tidal volume ventilation be used in all patients with sepsis who are receiving mechanical ventilation to avoid underuse or delayed use of this intervention. Moreover, the use of low tidal volume ventilation avoids the risk of promoting ventilator-induced lung injury in septic patients in whom the diagnosis of ARDS has been missed.

PRONE VENTILATION

Recommendation of Surviving Sepsis Campaign 2021

For adults with sepsis-induced moderate-severe ARDS, it is recommended to use prone ventilation for >12 hours daily.

Strong recommendation, moderate quality of evidence.

Rationale for the Recommendation

There were no new randomized, controlled trials except one trial, called PROSEVA (Proning Severe ARDS Patients), published in 2013, evaluating the use of prone ventilation in sepsis-induced severe ARDS published since the 2016 guidelines. Therefore, no change in the recommendation was added. This repeated meta-analysis with the inclusion of PROSEVA confirmed the results from the previously published work: In patients with ARDS and a PaO_2/FiO_2 ratio <200, the use of prone compared with the supine position within the first 36 hours of intubation, when performed for >12 hours a day, showed improved survival.

NEUROMUSCULAR BLOCKING AGENTS

Recommendation of the Surviving Sepsis Campaign 2021

For adults with sepsis-induced moderate-severe ARDS, it is recommended to use intermittent neuromuscular blocking agents (NMBA) boluses over NMBA continuous infusion.

Weak recommendation, moderate quality of evidence.

Rationale for the Recommendation

In the 2016 SSC guidelines, we issued a weak recommendation for using NMBA infusion for 48 hours in sepsis-induced moderate to severe ARDS. Since then, several RCTs have been published, the largest of which is the ROSE Trial. A continuous NMBA infusion did not improve mortality when compared with a light sedation strategy with as-needed NMBA boluses but no continuous infusion.

Recommendation of Surviving Sepsis Campaign 2021

For adults with moderate-to-severe sepsis-induced ARDS, it is suggested to use higher PEEP over lower PEEP.

Weak recommendation, moderate quality of evidence.

Rationale for the Recommendation

The recommendation is unchanged from 2016.

A patient-level meta-analysis showed no benefit of higher PEEP in *all patients* with ARDS; however, patients with moderate or severe ARDS (PaO_2/FiO_2 ≤200 mm Hg) had decreased mortality with the use of higher PEEP, whereas those with mild ARDS did not. A patient-level analysis of two of the randomized PEEP trials suggested that patients with ARDS who respond to increased PEEP with improved oxygenation have a lower risk of death; this association was stronger in patients with more severe ARDS (PaO_2/FiO_2 <150 mm Hg) compared with patients with less severe ARDS.

LOW TIDAL VOLUME IN NONACUTE RESPIRATORY DISTRESS SYNDROME RESPIRATORY FAILURE

Recommendation of Surviving Sepsis Campaign 2021

For adults with sepsis-induced respiratory failure (without ARDS), it is suggested to use low tidal volume as compared to high tidal volume ventilation.

Weak recommendation, low quality of evidence.
Since, sepsis is an independent risk factor for the development of ARDS, and delays in diagnosing ARDS may result in delayed use of low tidal volumes. It is suggested that low tidal volume ventilation be used in all patients with sepsis who are receiving mechanical ventilation to avoid underuse or delayed use of this intervention. Moreover, the use of low tidal volume ventilation avoids the risk of promoting ventilator-induced lung injury in septic patients in whom the diagnosis of ARDS has been missed.

PRONE VENTILATION

Recommendation of Surviving Sepsis Campaign 2021

For adults with sepsis-induced moderate-severe ARDS, it is recommended to use prone ventilation for >12 hours daily.

Strong recommendation, moderate quality of evidence.

Rationale for the Recommendation

There were no new randomized, controlled trials except one trial, called PROSEVA (Proning Severe ARDS Patients), published in 2013, evaluating the use of prone ventilation in sepsis-induced severe ARDS published since the 2016 guidelines. Therefore, no change in the recommendation was added. This repeated meta-analysis with the inclusion of PROSEVA confirmed the results from the previously published work: In patients with ARDS and a PaO_2/FiO_2 ratio <200, the use of prone compared with the supine position within the first 36 hours of intubation, when performed for >12 hours a day, showed improved survival.

NEUROMUSCULAR BLOCKING AGENTS

Recommendation of the Surviving Sepsis Campaign 2021

For adults with sepsis-induced moderate-severe ARDS, it is recommended to use intermittent neuromuscular blocking agents (NMBA) boluses over NMBA continuous infusion.

Weak recommendation, moderate quality of evidence.

Rationale for the Recommendation

In the 2016 SSC guidelines, we issued a weak recommendation for using NMBA infusion for 48 hours in sepsis-induced moderate to severe ARDS. Since then, several RCTs have been published, the largest of which is the ROSE Trial. A continuous NMBA infusion did not improve mortality when compared with a light sedation strategy with as-needed NMBA boluses but no continuous infusion.

EXTRACORPOREAL MEMBRANE OXYGENATION

Recommendation of Surviving Sepsis Campaign 2021

For adults with sepsis-induced severe ARDS, it is suggested to use venovenous (VV) extracorporeal membrane oxygenation (ECMO) when conventional mechanical ventilation fails in experienced centers with the infrastructure in place to support its use.

Weak recommendation, low quality of evidence.

Rationale for the Recommendation

Venovenous ECMO is used in patients with severe acute respiratory failure to facilitate gas exchange in the setting of refractory hypoxemia or hypercapnic respiratory acidosis. It may also be used to facilitate a reduction in the intensity of mechanical ventilation. The evidence for the use of VV-ECMO in sepsis-induced ARDS is limited, with two RCTs completed in the last 10 years to assess the potential efficacy of VV-ECMO for severe ARDS.

However, one recent systematic review found that VV-ECMO delivered at expert centers reduced mortality for patients with severe ARDS.

ADDITIONAL THERAPIES

Corticosteroids

Recommendation of the Surviving Sepsis Campaign 2021

For adults with septic shock and an ongoing requirement for vasopressor therapy, it is suggested to use IV corticosteroids.

Weak recommendation; moderate quality of evidence.

The typical corticosteroid used in adults with septic shock is IV hydrocortisone at a dose of 200 mg/day given as 50 mg intravenously every 6 hours or as a continuous infusion. It is suggested that this is commenced at a dose of norepinephrine or epinephrine ≥0.25 µg/kg/min at least 4 hours after initiation.

Rationale for the Recommendations

In the 2016 guidance, the accumulated evidence did not support a recommendation for their use if adequate fluid resuscitation and vasopressor therapy were able to restore hemodynamic stability. Since then, (ADRENAL, APROCCHSS, and VANISH) three large RCTs have been published. An updated meta-analysis found systemic corticosteroid to expedite resolution of shock vasopressor. However, corticosteroid use increased neuromuscular weakness without a definite effect on short- or long-term mortality.

The three trials, however, used different inclusion criteria: in ADRENAL, eligible patients were those on any dose of vasopressor or inotrope for ≥4 hours to maintain a MAP >60 mm Hg and present at the time of randomization. In APROCCHSS, the dose of vasopressor was ≥0.25 µg/kg/min or ≥1 mg/h of norepinephrine or epinephrine, or any other vasopressor for at least 6 hours to maintain a MAP ≥65 mmHg. In the ADRENAL study, hydrocortisone was administered for a maximum of seven days or until ICU discharge or death; in APROCCHSS, hydrocortisone was administered for seven days; in VANISH, 200 mg of hydrocortisone was administered daily for 5 days and then tapered over a further 6 days.

BLOOD PURIFICATION

Recommendations of the Surviving Sepsis Campaign 2021

For adults with sepsis or septic shock, using polymyxin B hemoperfusion is not recommended.

Weak recommendation; low quality of evidence.
There is insufficient evidence to make a recommendation on the use of other blood purification techniques.

RED BLOOD CELL TRANSFUSION TARGETS

Recommendation of the Surviving Sepsis Campaign 2021

For adults with sepsis or septic shock, the use of a restrictive (over liberal) transfusion strategy is recommended.

Strong recommendation; moderate quality of evidence.
A restrictive transfusion strategy typically includes a hemoglobin concentration transfusion trigger of 70 g/L; however, RBC transfusion should not be guided by hemoglobin concentration alone.

Assessment of a patient's overall clinical status and consideration of extenuating circumstances such as acute myocardial ischemia, severe hypoxemia, or acute hemorrhage is required.

IMMUNOGLOBULINS

Recommendation of Surviving Sepsis Campaign 2021

For adults with sepsis or septic shock, the use of IV immunoglobulins is not recommended.

Weak recommendation, low quality of evidence.

STRESS ULCER PROPHYLAXIS

Recommendation of Surviving Sepsis Campaign 2021

For adults with sepsis or septic shock and who have risk factors for gastrointestinal (GI) bleeding, it is suggested to use stress ulcer prophylaxis.

Weak recommendation, moderate quality of evidence.

Rationale for the Recommendation

The current literature search identified one new RCT (494), and the meta-analysis from the previous guideline was updated. This demonstrated no effect on mortality and a reduction in GI hemorrhage in 2016. A sensitivity analysis including only trials at low risk of bias provided similar results. No increase in *Clostridioides difficile* colitis or pneumonia was observed.

A recent meta-analysis published since the finalization of the literature searches has suggested that there is a higher risk of recurrent *Clostridioides difficile* infections with proton pump inhibitors.

VENOUS THROMBOEMBOLISM PROPHYLAXIS

Recommendations of the Surviving Sepsis Campaign 2021

For adults with sepsis or septic shock, using pharmacologic VTE prophylaxis unless a contraindication to such therapy exists is recommended.

Strong recommendation, moderate quality of evidence.

For adults with sepsis or septic shock, using low molecular weight heparin (LMWH) over unfractionated heparin (UFH) for VTE prophylaxis is recommended.

Strong recommendation, moderate quality of evidence.

For adults with sepsis or septic shock, we use mechanical VTE prophylaxis in addition to pharmacological prophylaxis; over pharmacologic prophylaxis alone is not recommended.

Weak recommendation, low quality of evidence.

Rationale

Critically ill patients are at risk for deep vein thrombosis (DVT) as well as pulmonary embolism (PE). The incidence of DVT acquired in the ICU may be as high as 10%, and the incidence of acquired PE may be 2–4%.

No new RCT evidence was identified. Our previous meta-analysis demonstrated a significant reduction in both DVT and PE and no increase in bleeding complications.

On balance, the effect favors the intervention with a moderate quality of evidence. The cost of intervention is not large, and it is likely feasible in countries with low- and middle-income economies. These judgements support a recommendation for the use of pharmacologic venous thromboembolism (VTE) prophylaxis unless a contraindication exists. The recommendation is unchanged from the 2016 guidelines.

RENAL REPLACEMENT THERAPY

Recommendations of the Surviving Sepsis Campaign 2021

In adults with sepsis or septic shock and AKI who require RRT, it is suggested to use either continuous or intermittent RRT.

Weak recommendation, low quality of evidence.

In adults with sepsis or septic shock and AKI, with no definitive indications for RRT, using RRT is not recommended.

Weak recommendation, moderate quality of evidence.

Rationale for the Recommendation

Two systematic reviews and meta-analyses summarized the total body of evidence: they do not show a difference in mortality between patients who receive continuous (CRRT) versus intermittent hemodialysis (IHD). The results remained the same when the analysis was restricted to RCTs.

The recommendation for either intervention is unchanged from the 2016 guidelines.

GLUCOSE CONTROL

Recommendation of Surviving Sepsis Campaign 2021

For adults with sepsis or septic shock, it is recommended to initiate insulin therapy at a glucose level of ≥180 mg/dL (10 mmol/L).

Strong recommendation; moderate quality of evidence.
Following initiation of insulin therapy, a typical target blood glucose range of 144–180 mg/dL (8–10 mmol/L) is set.

Rationale for the Recommendation

Hyperglycemia (>180 mg/dL), hypoglycemia, and increased glycemic variability are associated with increased mortality in critically ill patients. The American Diabetes Association, in its most recent recommendations for glycemic control of critically ill patients, recommended the initiation of insulin therapy for persistent hyperglycemia >180 mg/dL and, thereafter, a target glucose range of 140–180 mg/dL.

NUTRITION

Recommendation of Surviving Sepsis Campaign 2021

For adult patients with sepsis or septic shock who can be fed enterally, we suggest early (within 72 hours) initiation of enteral nutrition.

Weak recommendation; very low quality of evidence.

Rationale for the Recommendation

The early administration of enteral nutrition in patients with sepsis and septic shock has potential physiologic advantages related to the maintenance of gut integrity and prevention of intestinal permeability, dampening of the inflammatory response, and modulation of metabolic responses that may reduce insulin resistance.

LONG-TERM OUTCOMES AND GOALS OF CARE

Patients who survive a protracted period of ICU care for sepsis typically face a long and arduous road to recovery. They require very well-organized and coordinated care to overcome physical and psychosocial rehabilitation challenges. Meta-analysis of randomized studies has assessed rehabilitation programs in survivors of sepsis and other critical illnesses. Whereas such programs can produce small improvements in quality of life and depressive symptoms, they are yet to show any benefit in terms of mortality and physical function. Despite this, referral to rehabilitation programs is suggested for survivors of sepsis.

SUGGESTED READING

1. Evans L, Rhodes A, Alhazzani W, Antonelli M, Coopersmith CM, French C, et al. Surviving Sepsis Campaign: International Guidelines for Management of Sepsis and Septic Shock 2021. Crit Care Med. 2021;49(11):e1063-143.
2. Fleischmann-Struzek C, Mellhammar L, Rose N, Cassini A, Rudd KE, Schlattmann P, et al. Incidence and mortality of hospital- and ICU-treated sepsis: Results from an updated and expanded systematic review and meta-analysis. Intensive Care Med. 2020;46(8):1552-62.
3. Rhodes A, Evans LE, Alhazzani W, Levy MM, Antonelli M, Ferrer R, et al. Surviving Sepsis Campaign: International guidelines for management of sepsis and septic shock: 2016. Crit Care Med. 2017;45(3):486-552.
4. Singer M, Deutschman CS, Seymour CW, Shankar-Hari M, Annane D, Bauer M, et al. The third international consensus definitions for sepsis and septic shock (Sepsis-3). JAMA. 2016;315(8):801-10.

Index

Page numbers followed by *b* refer to box, *f* refer to figure,
fc refer to flowchart, and *t* refer to table.

A

ABCDE bundle 36
Abciximab 286, 294
Abdominal aortic repair 462
Accessory pathway 232
    localization of 228, 228*fc*
Acetate dialysis 541
Acetazolamide 122
Acetylcholine 25
Acetylsalicylic acid 509
Acid-base
    disorder 353-355, 357*f*, 364
        types of 353
    disturbance 353, 357*t*
Acidosis 267, 359*t*
    evidence of 60
    metabolic 353, 356
Activated clotting time 12
Activated partial thromboplastin time 12, 168, 314
Acute aortic
    disease 336, 341
    syndrome 38, 57, 62
Acute asthma
    assessment of 390
    differential diagnosis of 389
    exacerbation 390
    management of 390
Acute cardiogenic pulmonary
    edema 341
    protocol 426
Acute coronary events, global registry of 3, 10
Acute coronary syndrome 1, 1*f*, 2, 3, 3*t*, 4, 4*t*-5*t*, 6*f*, 7, 11*t*, 12, 13*t*, 14, 15*t*, 16, 22, 24, 25, 50, 86, 158, 297, 336, 341
    guidelines 297
    spectrum of 1*f*
Acute heart failure 28, 50, 54, 533*fc*
    classification 51*t*
    diagnostic workup of 50, 55*fc*
    management of 54, 54*fc*
    treatment 62
    triaging of 54*fc*
Acute hyponatremia 369
    treatment of 368
Acute ischemic stroke 197, 488, 490, 498
    management 499
Acute kidney injury 45, 520, 523, 532, 535*t*, 537, 542
    biomarkers 544
    contrast-induced 547
    diagnosis of 525*fc*
    management of 528*fc*, 529*fc*
    prevention of 548
    severe 532*fc*
    staging, severity of 521*fc*
    ultrasound for 526*fc*
Acute mechanical circulatory support 48*fc*
Acute respiratory acidosis 355, 356
    management 364*fc*
Acute respiratory alkalosis 355, 356
Acute respiratory distress syndrome 61, 420, 424, 429, 432, 439, 444, 447, 449*t*, 450, 456, 459, 629, 630
    causes of 448
    diagnosis of 631
    management of 451
    moderate-to-severe 455
Acute stroke 336, 340
    management of 334

Adenosine 276, 293
    injection 215
    receptor blockade 394
    triphosphate test 139
Adrenal androgen deficiency 551
Adrenal crisis 550
    primary 551
Adrenal insufficiency
    acute 553*b*
    secondary 551
Adrenaline 72
Adrenergic agonists 107
Adrenocortical insufficiency 552*fc*
Adult postcardiac arrest care
    algorithm 270*fc*
Advanced cardiac life support 268
    bradycardia 268*fc*
Advanced life support 58, 243
Airflow obstruction
    absence of 406
    severity of 407*b*
Airway 263, 268, 269, 327
    collapse 439
    obstruction 439
    protection 418
Alanine
    aminotransferase 55, 154
    transaminase 190
Albumin concentration 357
Albuterol 392, 403
Alcohol
    drinking, excessive 154
    use, chronic 18
Alkali therapy 377
Alkaline phosphatase 154
Alkalosis
    metabolic 353, 356, 360*t*
    pseudorespiratory 367
    respiratory 354, 363*t*
Allergic interstitial nephritis 532
Alteplase, intravenous 493
Altered mental status 309
Ambulatory blood pressure
    monitoring 135
Ambulatory electrocardiogram
    monitoring 234*fc*
American College of Cardiology 9, 21,
    24, 34

American College of Emergency
    Physicians 9, 21
American Heart Association 9, 21,
    24, 34
American Thoracic Society
    guidelines 459
Amiloride 64
Aminoglycosides 433
Aminophylline 411
    intravenous 394, 395
Amiodarone 177*t*, 178, 188, 220, 232,
    266, 322
    oral 190*t*
Amyloid
    angiopathy, cerebral 507
    cardiomyopathy 102
Anaerobes 434
Analgesia 422
Andexanet alfa 509
Anemia 82, 110, 151, 522
    correction of 335
Anesthetic agents 399
Angina 290
Angiography
    cerebral 516
    invasive 4*fc*
    noninvasive 507
Angiotensin 626
    converting enzyme inhibitor 23,
        24, 26, 67, 104, 117, 377, 537
    receptor
        blocker 23, 24, 26, 104, 117, 537
        neprilysin inhibitor 78, 104
Anion gap approach 354
Ankle swelling 82
Anorexia 84, 338
Antiaggregant platelet therapy 485
Antianaerobic therapy 434
Antiangiogenic therapy 338
Antiarrhythmic drug 176, 182,
    193, 261
    strategy 196
    therapy 143
Antibiotics 412, 436
    de-escalation of 621
    duration of 622
    therapy, prophylactic 462
    time of 605, 605*fc*

Anticholinergics,
        short-acting 404, 410
Anticoagulant 69, 498
    administration of 498
    dose of 161
    drugs 11t
    naïve 284
    oral 5, 18, 19f, 69, 166t, 169fc, 170, 462, 485
    role of 498
    therapy 15t, 164t, 165t, 283, 498, 551
Anticoagulation 175fc, 205t, 208, 302, 312, 513, 516, 589
    co-therapy 19
    management of 480t, 508
    parenteral 312
    post-intracranial bleeding, initiation of 209fc
    strategies 204t
    summary 157
    therapy 16t, 194t
Anticonvulsants 335
Antidromic atrioventricular re-entrant tachycardia 230f
Antifungal therapy 617
Antihypertensive therapy 351
Anti-immunoglobulin E 402
Anti-inflammatory reliever medications 403
Antimicrobial therapy 597, 604, 622
Antineurohormonal drugs 77
Antineutrophil cycloplasmic antibody 537
Antiphospholipid 537
    antibody 582
    syndrome 551
Antiplatelets 498
    agents 499
        oral 498
    drugs 11, 11t
    management 480t
    responsiveness 296
    resumption of 481t
    strategies 14fc, 298t
    therapy 15t, 16, 37, 281, 295, 297, 302, 462
        oral 2

Antipseudomonal beta-lactams 433
Antiseptics, oral 436
Antithrombic therapy, use of 513
Antithrombin
    deficiency 515
    loss of 515
Antithrombotic
    co-therapies 20t
    therapy 2f, 13t, 506
Anti-thymic stromal lymphopoietin 402
Antithyroid drugs 559, 560
Antiviral
    agents, use of 621
    therapy 621
Aorta, severe coarctation of 331
Aortic dissociation 337
Aortic regurgitation 42, 48
Aortic stenosis 42
    severe 67
Aortic valve 175
Apixaban 162, 170, 173, 302, 498, 509
Areflexia 381
Arrhythmias 56, 321, 581
    life-threatening 289
    rapid 50
Arrhythmogenic right ventricular cardiomyopathy 83, 133, 144, 251t
Arterial access 285
Arterial blood 597, 598
    gas 58, 60, 353, 364, 409, 424
    pressure monitoring 35
Arterial oxyhemoglobin saturation 309
Arteriovenous fistula 214
Arteriovenous hemofiltration 541
Artery
    disease, peripheral 172t
    infarct-related 9, 22, 44, 291
Arthopathy, crystal-induced 583
Arthritis
    acute 586
    infection-related 583
    septic 587
Artificial nutrition 33

Aspartate
  aminotransferase 55, 154
  transaminase 190
Aspiration 436
  devices 496
  nasogastric 383
  thrombectomy 286
Aspirin 11, 20, 281, 297, 491, 498
Assist control ventilation 420
Asthma 388, 392*fc*, 395, 407, 425
  acute life-threatening 395
  acute severe 388, 390, 396
  control
    questionnaire 388
    test 389
  drugs for 394
  exacerbations,
    management of 391*fc*
  life-threatening 390
  moderate acute 390
  related death 404
  severe 388, 395
  symptoms 403
  uncontrolled 388
Atenolol 177
Atlantoaxial dislocation 595
Atopic dermatitis,
  moderate-severe 402
Atorvastatin 491
Atracurium 422
Atrial fibrillation 79, 95, 100, 101, 110,
    113, 129, 133, 145, 149, 151,
    155*fc*, 162, 170, 173, 178,
    179, 181, 189, 195, 197, 199,
    232, 233, 302, 304, 494
  catheter ablation 191*t*, 193*t*
  chronic 147
  clinical 145
  initial acute care of 150
  management of 194
  nonvalvular 147
  screening 148
Atrial flutter 150, 153, 158*fc*, 218, 219*t*
  chronic therapy of 221*fc*
  typical 218
Atrial high-rate episode 146, 162, 162*t*
Atrial tachycardia 212, 216, 217, 235

Atriofascicular accessory
    pathway 230*f*
Atrioventricular 43, 129, 133, 181,
    199, 235-237
  block 141*fc*, 142*fc*
  canal defects 332
  junctional arrhythmias 222
  nodal ablation 180*t*
Atrioventricular nodal re-entrant
    tachycardia 212, 213*f*, 214,
    222, 226, 226*fc*
  acute therapy of 226*fc*
  atypical 224*f*
  management of 227*t*
  types, classification of 225*t*
Atrioventricular reciprocating
    tachycardia 212, 214
Atrioventricular re-entrant
    tachycardia 213*f*, 229*f*, 231*t*,
    232, 233, 234*fc*, 238
  acute therapy of 232*fc*
  chronic therapy of 233*fc*
Atropine 43
Attempting spontaneous breathing
    trials, criteria for 427
Automated external defibrillator 264,
    267, 328
Autonomic failure 135*fc*
Autoregulation, cerebral 338
Autoregulatory systems 338
Avibactam 617
Aztreonam 433

B

Bacilli, gram-negative 432, 433
Bacteria, multidrug-resistant 430
Bacterial pneumonia, ventilator-
    associated 433
Balloon tamponade devices 469*f*
Baroreceptor activation therapy 123
Baroreflex activation therapy 123, 125
Barostim neo device 125
Barotrauma 437, 442
  risk for 437, 439
Basic autonomic function tests 134
Basic life support 328
Beclometasone 400, 401

Benzodiazepines 351
Berlin definition 447
Beta 2 adrenoceptor agonists,
    nebulized 392
Beta-blockers 23, 74, 77, 90*t*, 92, 117,
    160, 177, 217, 232
    therapy 463
    treatment 78
Beta-hydroxybutyrate 560, 572
Beta-lactam inhibitor 434
Beta-lactamase inhibitor 434
Bicarbonate 560
Bicuspid aortic valve 43
Bifascicular bundle branch
    block 143*fc*
Bilevel positive airway pressure 417
Bisoprolol 92, 177
Bisphosphonate 384
    zoledronate, intravenous 579
Bivalirudin 12, 284
Blalock-Taussig shunt 331, 333
Blastomyces 620*b*
Blatchford score 469*t*
Bleeding
    events 297
    issues 206*b*
    risk 295
        high 16, 18
    severe 464*fc*
    ulcers 473
Blood 444, 532
    glucose 578
    leukocytes 429
    loss, severity of 468
    pressure 36, 128, 133, 140, 268,
        309, 313, 327, 336, 348, 462,
        468
        management 508, 513
        mean 41*f*
        systolic 5, 29, 51, 54, 68, 104,
            154, 158, 309
    purification 634
    urea nitrogen 55, 538, 542,
        560, 572
Body mass index 114
Bradycardia 43, 139, 301
    pediatric 327*fc*
    severe 50

Brain
    abscess 334
    cells 368
    edema
        ischemic 500
        risk for 501
    natriuretic peptide 55, 158
    parenchyma 487
Brainstem compression, primary 501
Breast 578
Breath sounds 441*fc*
Breathing 263, 268, 269, 327
Breathlessness 82, 525
Bronchiectasis 407
Bronchiolitis 405
Bronchitis 405
Bronchoalveolar lavage 450
Bronchodilators 409, 410, 414
    nebulized 392
Bronchopulmonary hygiene,
    maintenance of 422
Bronchoscopy 442
Bronchospasm 439
Brugada criteria 237*t*
B-type natriuretic peptide 85, 88, 110
Budesonide 400, 401
    nebulized 411
Bumetanide 62, 63

C

Calcitonin 579
Calcium
    channel blockers 117, 160, 250,
        268
    serum 384
    translocation of 394
Cancer 309
Candesartan 92
Candida sepsis 620*b*
Cangrelor 11
Carbamylated hemoglobin level 535
Carbapenem 434
    sparing agents 616
Carbapenemase 433
Carbimazole 559
Carbon dioxide, partial
    pressure of 597

Carbonic anhydrase inhibitor 72
Cardia output 41*f*
Cardiac amyloidosis 102*fc*, 254*t*
Cardiac arrest 9*t*, 47, 260, 264*fc*, 274*fc*, 308, 313, 318, 324
Cardiac care
  acute 321
  unit 158
Cardiac computer tomography 58
Cardiac defects, types of 332
Cardiac dysfunction 82, 627
Cardiac emergencies 332
Cardiac implantable electronic device 124
Cardiac index 33, 43
Cardiac intensive care
  role of 47
  unit 47
Cardiac magnetic resonance 25, 26, 87, 199, 239
Cardiac output 40, 313
Cardiac resynchronization therapy 108, 143
Cardiac surgery 163*t*
Cardiac tamponade 267, 584
Cardiac toxicity 376
Cardinal symptoms 412
Cardiogenic pulmonary edema 336, 447, 450
Cardiogenic shock 29, 31-33, 36, 37, 38*t*, 40, 43, 44, 46*f*, 47, 48, 48*fc*, 50, 286, 288
  classification of 31*b*
  etiology of 34*b*
  specific preparedness plan 33
Cardiomegaly 331
Cardiomyopathy 100, 100*fc*, 199, 250*t*
  aggravated 251*t*
  dilated 87
  hypertrophic 67, 131, 144, 253*t*
Cardiopulmonary arrest 321
Cardiopulmonary exercise test 87, 119
Cardiopulmonary support, mean 310
Cardiorenal syndrome 532, 542*t*
  acute 542
  chronic 542
  secondary 542

Cardiovascular death, risk of 290
Cardiovascular disease 88, 594
Cardiovascular system 381
Cardioversion 177*t*
Carotid
  artery 554
  endarterectomy 499
  sinus
    massage 136
    syndrome 136
  stenosis 500
Carpal tunnel syndrome 109
Carvedilol 92, 177
Catastrophic antiphospholipid syndrome 584, 588
  criteria for 588
Catecholaminergic polymorphic ventricular tachycardia 260, 260*t*
Catecholamines 563
Catheter ablation 182, 220
Cavotricuspid isthmus 153, 221, 222
Cefepime 432, 616
Ceftaroline 433
Ceftazidime 617
Ceftolozane 617
Ceftriaxone 467
Central nervous system 135
  vasculitis 594
Central venous
  pressure 36
  saturation 35
Cerebral edema 368, 369
  risk of 368
  treatment of 500
Cerebral venous thrombosis 514, 515
  development of 515
  treatment of 517
Cerebrospinal fluid 594
Cerebrovascular accident 195, 321, 328, 334
  development of 334
Chemoprophylaxis 511
Chest
  compression 263
  computed tomography angiography 61
  pain 338

radiographs 442
X-ray 60, 158, 441, 450
Chikungunya virus 621
Child-Pugh scoring 205
Chlorthalidone 64
Cholecystectomy 305
Chronic coronary artery disease 172*t*, 247*fc*, 248*fc*
Chronic heart failure 85*t*, 86*t*, 104, 124*fc*, 309
   management of 82
   treatment of 84
Chronic kidney disease 12, 88, 109, 172*t*, 374, 522, 535*t*
   development of 549
Chronic obstructive lung disease
   grades 407*b*
Chronic obstructive pulmonary disease 86, 405, 406*t*, 407, 407*t*, 408, 415, 451
   diagnosis of 406
   exacerbation 405, 408, 420, 426
      prevention of 414*t*
   severity of 409*fc*
   risk of 405
Chronic respiratory acidosis 355, 356, 364
   management 356
Churg-Strauss syndrome 532
Ciclesonide 400
Cilastatin 433
Circulation 268, 327
Cirrhosis 205
Cisatracurium 422
Clevidipine 349
Clindamycin 434
Clinical pulmonary infection score calculation 429
Clonidine 350
Clopidogrel 11, 20, 281, 282, 297, 491, 498
Cocaine 338
   intoxication 351
Coccidioidomycosis 620*b*
Cold intravenous fluids 272
Colistin 433
Colonization, modulation of 436

Coma 591
   hyperglycemic 575*t*
   hypoglycemic 575*t*
   myxedema 560
Combination diuretic therapy 533
Common vasoactive medications 40*t*
Complete blood count 35, 158
Compression 269
   ultrasonography 307
Computed tomography 55, 58, 190, 195, 307, 485, 619
   angiography 4, 58, 87, 307, 309, 310, 312
   non-contrast 515
   venography 516
Confusion 600
Conivaptan 373
Connective tissue diseases 594
Consciousness 338
   apparent loss of 127
   level of 504
   loss of 131, 488
   transient loss of 127, 127*fc*
Continuous positive airway pressure 51, 78, 416
Continuous renal replacement therapy 272, 532, 533
Continuous veno-venous hemodialysis 545
Contraceptive therapy, oral 515
Cord sign 515
Coronary angiography 21*fc*, 62, 138, 292
Coronary artery
   bypass graft 16, 39, 44, 45, 101
      surgery 58, 346
   disease 45, 87, 91, 113, 162, 247
Coronary care unit 351
Coronary disease, ischemic 466
Coronary flow reserve 293
Coronary thrombosis 268
Coronavirus disease-2019 (COVID-19) 447, 453, 455, 621
   infection 59
   vaccination 59
Cortical blindness 338
Corticosteroids 393, 394, 587, 589, 633
   inhaled 400, 401, 411, 414

systemic 393, 403, 460
    use of 512
Cortisol 563
Cough 405, 406
Counter regulatory hormones, role of 563
C-reactive protein 58, 409, 607, 608
Creatinine
    clearance 12, 170, 173, 189, 314
    serum 36
Critical care unit 54
    monitoring 35
Cryoballoon catheter ablation 193
Cryptococcus 620*b*
Crystalloids 623*t*
Crystals 537
Culprit-shock trial 44
Cushing's reflex 505
Cyanosis peripheral edema 408
Cyclic adenosine monophosphate 71, 393
Cyclic guanosine monophosphate 68
Cyclophosphamide 593
Cyclosporine 338
Cystatin 544
Cystoscopy 539
Cytochrome P-450 189
Cytokines, proinflammatory 584
Cytomegalovirus 621

D

Dabigatran 170, 173, 302, 498, 509
Dapagliflozin 92, 114
Decompressive surgery 501
Deep breathing tests 135
Deep sulcus sign 442
Deep vein thrombosis 69, 307, 573
    complications of 517
Defibrillator, types of 324, 326*t*
Dehydration, signs of 565
Delirium 360
    monitoring 37
Dengue virus 621
Desmoteplase 316
Devices 108, 401
Dexamethasone 394, 403

Diabetes
    insipidus
        central 375
        nephrogenic 375
    mellitus 102, 151, 374
        acute metabolic complications of 561
Diabetic decompensation, spectrum of 561
Diabetic ketoacidosis 359, 382, 560-563, 563*t*, 572
    classification of 566*t*
    diagnosis of 562
    symptoms of 565
    treatment of 567*f*
Dialysis, role of 364
Diarrhea, chronic 383
Diastolic filling time 43
Diastolic pulmonary artery pressure 41*f*
Diet 113
Diffuse alveolar hemorrhage 450, 594
Digital ischemia, higher risk of 626
Digitalis glycoside 178
Digoxin 69, 92, 178
Diltiazem 160, 178, 217, 232, 293
Dipyridamole 498, 499
Direct oral anticoagulants 170, 171, 173, 508
    laboratory monitoring 155
Disseminated intravascular coagulation 343, 537
Diuretics 62, 63*t*
    regimen 543*t*
    response 76
Dizziness 338, 524
Dobutamine 40, 70, 72, 107
Dofetilide 188
Dopamine 40, 43, 70, 107, 277, 332, 624, 625
Dronedarone 188
Drug-drug interactions 12
Drugs 154, 544*b*
    intravenous 349*t*
    therapy 187*fc*, 266
Dual antiplatelet therapy 14, 16, 18, 19*f*

Dual chamber pacemaker 140
Dynamic left ventricular tract obstruction 38, 43
Dyspepsia 18
Dyspnea 76, 338, 405, 406
  severe 410, 413

E

Early warning score, modified 599t
Ebola virus 621
Echocardiography 119, 138
  transthoracic 4, 58, 309, 310
Eclampsia 336, 343
  management of 345
  prevention of 344
Edema
  peripheral 82, 525
  pulmonary 50, 79, 339, 341, 439
Edoxaban 170, 173, 302, 498, 509
Effective regurgitant orifice 101
Ejection fraction 103
Electrical cardioversion 79, 185t
Electrocardiogram 3, 4, 6f, 7, 25, 55, 58, 60, 71, 85, 102, 128, 128t, 133, 148, 158, 162, 190, 232, 236, 239, 243, 260, 325, 327
Electrocardiography 141, 268, 269
  monitoring 137
Electrolyte 535
  imbalance 368, 545
  serum 36
Electrophysiology 158
  study 138, 141-143, 234
Elevated jugular venous pressure 82
Embolectomy, surgical 318
Emergency medical services 6f
Empagliflozin 76, 92, 114
Emphysema 405
Empiric antiviral therapy, efficacy of 621
Enalaprilat 350
Encephalopathy 205
  hypertensive 336
  severe hypercapnic 356
Endemic yeast 620b
Endocarditis 57, 62

Endocrine emergencies 550
  nondiabetes-related 550
Endomyocardial biopsy 87
Endoscopic hemostatic therapy 473
Endoscopy 473
Endotracheal intubation 398
  criteria for 79
Endotracheal tube 347, 441, 444
Endovascular revascularization recommendations 495
Endovascular therapy 495
Enoxaparin 12, 21
Enoximone 40, 72
Enteral feeding 436
Enteral nutrition 637
  initiation of 637
Enzyme
  adenylyl cyclase 393
  deficiency 574
Eosinophilia, peripheral 532
Epicardial blood flow, abnormal 292
Epicardial fat pad 442
Epidemiology 337
Epinephrine 40, 71, 107, 266, 271, 275, 293, 313, 624, 633
  action 625
  activity of 625
  administration 625
  hypersecretion of 563
Eplerenone 64, 92
Eptifibatide 11, 294
Ertapenem 616
Erythrocyte sedimentation rate 58
Erythromycin 468
Escherichia coli 616
Esmolol 177, 322, 349
Ethyl glycol poisoning 364
Euglycemia 512
European Heart Rhythm Association 149
  symptom scale 149t
European Society of Cardiology 3, 4, 5, 7-10, 16, 18, 20, 21, 29, 30, 103
  current guidelines of 297
Euthermia 512
Everolimus-eluting stent 285

Exacerbations, life-threatening 409
Excretion 159
Exercise 113
    echocardiography 138
Expiratory positive airway
        pressure 417
Extended spectrum beta-lactamase
    432, 609, 618, 619
Extra-alveolar air, ventilator-
        associated 442
Extracellular fluid 363, 375
Extracorporeal membrane
        oxygenation 31, 39, 313,
        319, 400, 457, 619, 633
    role of 456
Extracorporeal therapy 546
Extraocular muscle paresis 553
Extravascular lung water 451

F

Fanconi's syndrome 386
Fatigue 82
Fatty acid 124
Fenoldopam 349
Fentanyl 23
Ferric carboxymaltose 75
    role of 77
Fever 525
    sudden onset high 591
Fibrinolysis 9t, 19
Fibrinolytic therapy 19, 19t, 21fc, 282,
    287, 499
Field-atrial fibrillation 151
Fighting ventilator 439
Finerenone 116, 122
Flecainide 189, 232
Fluid
    balance 545, 627
    loss 524
    management 622
    replacement 573t
    resuscitation 628
    volume 602
Fluoroquinolone 616
    antipseudomonal 433

Fluticasone
    furoate 400, 401
    propionate 400
        formoterol 401
Focal atrial tachycardia 213
    acute therapy of 216fc
    chronic therapy of 216fc
Fondaparinux 12, 314, 589
Forest classification 471t, 472t
Formoterol 401
Frusemide 63, 384, 579
Fungi 435
Furosemide 62, 65

G

Gastric bleeding 437
Gastroesophageal reflux disease 18
Gastroesophageal varices 468
Gastrointestinal bleeding 462, 482fc
    episodes 466t
    lower 474fc, 485
    management 462
        approach, overview of 485fc
    middle 475b, 485
    upper 467, 485
    variceal lower 478fc
Gastrointestinal endoscopy,
        upper 468fc
Gastrointestinal illness 331
Gastrointestinal manifestations 338
Gastrointestinal system 381
Genetic testing 296
Glasgow come scale 504
Glenn procedure 332, 333
Global anticoagulant registry 151
Glomerular filtration
    markers of 527f
    rate 361, 363, 538
Glomerulonephritis 523, 524, 537
    focal segmental 524, 537
    membranoproliferative 537
Glucagon 563
    like peptide receptor agonist 114
    parenteral 575
Glucocorticoids 411
    deficiency 551

Index 649

Gluconeogenesis 563
Glucose 370
   control 637
   very high 535
Glycemic control 577
Glyceryl trinitrate 136, 137
Glycogenolysis 563
Glycolysis 563
Glycoprotein, trials of 283
Goodpasture syndrome 445
Gore-Tex graft 333
Gout, acute 587
Granulomatosis 537
   eosinophilic 537
Growth hormones 563
Guideline-directed medical therapy 76, 78, 88, 100, 101, 199, 291
Guillain-Barré infections 594

H

Haptoglobin 336
Head
   injury 515
   trauma 554
Headache 338, 360, 591
Heart
   block 100, 595
   catheterization 76, 87
   contractions 124
   rate 43, 142, 158, 409
   type fatty acid-binding protein 309
Heart disease 131, 232
   absence of 261
   congenital 201t, 321
   cyanotic congenital 334
   structural 142, 217, 239
   valvular 101t, 149
Heart failure 28, 30, 33, 51, 82, 83, 83t, 85fc, 86t, 87, 88, 89fc, 100, 101, 103, 104, 108, 120b, 123, 162, 187, 194, 199, 217, 232, 235t, 286, 304, 337, 369, 374, 408
   acute 28, 50, 54, 533fc
      congestive 331
      decompensated 34, 74t, 77
      right 50
      severe 289
   advanced 32, 103b, 104b
   chronic 85t, 86t, 104, 124fc, 309
   congenital 34, 102, 151, 269, 321, 331, 407
   decompensated 50
   diagnosis of 91
   guideline 97t, 103t, 106t
   hypertensive 341
   management of 107t, 120
   recurrence of 50
   stages of 88t
   with mildly reduced ejection fraction 82, 83, 85, 91, 99, 104, 104fc
   with preserved ejection fraction 83, 85, 87, 109, 110, 112t, 199
      diagnosis of 111
      prognosis of 118
      treatment of 113, 116
   with reduced ejection fraction 82, 83, 85, 87, 92t, 100, 102, 178, 187, 189, 199, 217, 232, 236
      comprehensive management of 95fc, 96fc
   worsening 120
Helicobacter pylori infection 18
Hematoma volume, larger 506
Hematopoietic stem cell transplantation 621
Hemodialysis 33
   intermittent 545, 637
Hemodynamic 38
   formulas 38
   instability 311fc, 312fc, 356
   management 622
   monitoring 33
   status 479fc
   support 305
Hemoglobin 594
   concentration 634
   glycated 85, 135
   non-enzymatic carbamylation of 535
   normal 462

Hemolysis 343
  elevated liver enzymes, low
     platelet count syndrome
     336, 348, 537
  intravascular 342
Hemolytic uremic syndrome 342, 537
Hemophagocytic syndrome 591
Hemophilic arthritis 583
Hemoptysis 594
Hemorrhage 462, 513
  cerebellar 510
  cerebral 511*fc*
  intracerebral 169*t*, 513, 514
  intracranial 12, 210*fc*, 315, 318,
     336, 337, 507
  subarachnoid 514
  volume 506
Hemorrhagic secretions, cause of 445
Heparin 284, 485, 589
Hepatic disease 82
Hepatic failure 541
Hepatic function, abnormal 154
Hepatomegaly 331
Hepatosplenomegaly 591
Hepatotoxicity 190
Herniation, clinical signs of 510
High pressure alarm 441*fc*
High-flow nasal cannula 308
High-flow nasal oxygen 395, 396, 451,
     457, 629
  therapy 413, 629
High-resolution chest computed
     tomography 62, 407
High-sensitivity cardiac troponin 1*f*,
     2*f*, 3, 4, 4*fc*, 10, 58
His-Purkinje block 139
Histopathological criteria 592
Histoplasma 620*b*
Hormone deficiency 574
Hudson facemask 392
Human immunodeficiency
     virus 135, 537
  infection 621
Hydralazine 92
Hydrochlorothiazide 63
Hydrocortisone 403
Hydroxyethyl starch 623

Hypercalcemia 383, 535
  acute 578
  causes of 384
  mild asymptomatic 579
Hypercapnia 356, 364, 398
Hypercapnic respiratory failure 396,
     420, 429
Hypercarbia 347
Hypercyanotic spell 328
  management of 329
Hypereosinophilic syndrome 402
Hyperglycemia 394, 437, 561, 562,
     577*fc*, 637
  complications of 575
Hyperglycemic hyperosmolar state
     550, 562, 563, 563*t*
Hyperhomocysteinemia 515
Hyperinflation, dynamic 444
Hyperinsulinism 574
Hyperkalemia 115, 267, 374, 530*fc*
  acute 376
  chronic 376
  diagnosis of 377*fc*
  severe 377
Hyperlactatemia 367
Hypermagnesemia 381
Hypernatremia 373, 394
  etiology of 373*fc*
  hypotonic 370
Hyperosmolar hyperglycemic state
     570, 572
Hyperosmotic agents 512
Hyperphosphatemia 386, 522
Hyperpnea 328
Hypersensitivity pneumonitis,
     acute 450
Hypertension 29, 102, 109, 151, 374,
     466, 504, 513
  chronic 507
  control of 345
  emergency 58
  malignant 336, 338*fc*, 339, 342
  paroxysmal 346
  perioperative management
     of 346*fc*
  poorly controlled 347
  severe 342, 351

asymptomatic
   uncontrolled 337
   treatment of 590
   uncontrolled 154, 337
Hypertensive complications,
   acute 343
Hypertensive crises 336, 337, 346, 555
Hypertensive emergency 50,
   336-339, 348t
   diagnosis of 342
   management of 339
   treatment of 349t
Hypertensive urgencies 337
Hyperthyroidism 190
Hypertonic saline 368
Hyperventilation
   temporary 504
   therapy 420
Hypocalcemia 384, 387, 522, 579
   causes of 385
   mild 385
Hypocapnia, arterial 367
Hypodipsia 373
Hypoglycemia 438, 573, 574, 584
   effect of 576t
   grade of 576t
   reactive 574
   symptoms of 573
Hypokalemia 267, 378, 573
   causes of 380
   diagnosis of 382fc
   life-threatening 378
   mild-to-moderate 380
   severe 380, 381
Hypomagnesemia 383
   mild 383
Hyponatremia 368-370
   acute 369
   chronic 368, 369
   diagnosis of 375fc
   euvolemic 369
   hypervolemic 369, 372
   postoperative 372
Hypophosphatemia 385
Hypoplastic left heart syndrome 331
Hypotension 37, 115, 217, 232, 425,
   437, 438

   orthostatic 141fc, 468
   symptomatic 79
Hypothalamus 554
Hypothermia 267, 272, 347
Hypothyroidism 190
Hypovolemia 267, 438
Hypoxemia 78, 305
   correction of 308
   degree of 393
   effects of 391
   persistent 413
   severe 308
Hypoxia 267, 347, 443
   correction of 318
   severe 425

I

Ibutilide 232, 235
Idiopathic premature ventricular
   complexes 249fc, 250t
Idiopathic ventricular
   fibrillation 255fc
   tachycardia 240
Imipenem 433
Immunofixation electrophoresis 102
Immunoglobulins 635
Immunology 585
Impaired end-organ perfusion,
   markers of 30b
Impella catheter 311
Implantable cardioverter defibrillator
   58, 86, 104, 105, 108, 141,
   143, 171, 257, 260
   discharges 245fc
   implantation 254t
Implantable loop recorder 138, 140,
   141, 143, 247
Infarction, ischemic 502
Infections 573, 604
   diagnosis of 604
Inflammatory disease, chronic 515
Influenza 621
Inhalational anesthetic agents 399
In-hospital therapeutic
   interventions 62
Inodilators 40

Inorganic phosphate concentration 357
Inotropes 40, 70*t*, 72, 627
Inotropic agents, intravenous 107*t*
Inspiratory positive airway pressure 79, 417
Inspired oxygen, fraction of 420, 423, 598
Insulin delivery route 578
Insulin therapy, initiation of 637
Intensive care unit 58, 410, 603, 609, 619, 620
Intensive insulin therapy 437
Interatrial shunt device 118
Intercurrent respiratory illness 331
Intermittent therapy 547
International normalized ratio 154, 170
Interstitial lung disease 190
Interventional therapies 317*fc*
Intestinal permeability, prevention of 638
Intra-aortic balloon pump 32, 39, 43, 46*f*, 80
Intracellular osmoles 368
Intracerebral hemorrhage 169*t*, 513, 514
   management of 487
   spontaneous 503
   symptoms of 505
Intracranial hemorrhage 12, 210*fc*, 315, 318, 336, 337, 507
   surgical management of 509
Intracranial hypertension, benign 514
Intracranial pressure 512
Intubation 396, 436
Invasive coronary angiography 13
Invasive mold infection 620*b*
Invasive monitoring 35
Invasive strategy, selection of 7*fc*
Invasive ventilation 419, 425, 452, 458
   hazards of 419
   targets of 419
Ionotropic support 106*t*
Iron supplementation, intravenous 77
Irritability 591

Ischemia
   asymptomatic 279
   coronary 351
Ischemic attack 151
Ischemic stroke 301, 340, 487, 489*t*, 492
   management of 487
   supportive care of 492
Ischemic ventricular septal rupture 288
Isoproterenol 40, 43
Isosorbide dinitrate 92
Isotonic saline 384
Istaroxime 72
Ivabradine 92, 94

J

Joint pain 525
Jugular vein catheterization 515

K

Kansas city cardiomyopathy questionnaire 123
Ketamine 399
Ketoacidosis 359
Ketoconazole therapy 579
Ketosis 563
Kidney
   biopsy, criteria for 543
   disease, chronic 12, 88, 109, 172*t*, 374, 522, 535*t*
   failure 172*t*
   function 431*fc*, 532
   injury molecule 539
   perfusion 536*t*
Klebsiella pneumoniae 433
Korea Acute Myocardial Infarction National Health Registry Data 45
Kussmaul-Kien respiration 562
Kyoto circling 363

L

Labetalol 339, 343, 349, 590
Lactate 36
   dehydrogenase 336, 339

Index

Lactulose 468
Lacunar stroke 513
Lassa virus 621
Left atrium 181, 46*f*
Left bundle branch block 100, 129, 236, 237, 240
   aberration 225*f*
Left cardiac sympathetic denervation 257, 260
Left ventricle 51, 83, 129, 133, 143, 240
Left ventricular 25, 30, 44, 46*f*, 48, 87, 100, 110, 181, 187, 217, 236, 250
   assist device 39, 48
   diastolic dysfunction 110*t*
   ejection fraction 24, 30, 43, 82, 83, 85, 100, 101, 103, 133, 179, 187, 199
   end-diastolic pressure 43
   end-systolic diameter 101
   hypertrophy 91
   noncompaction 254*t*
   outflow tract 43, 138
   thrombi, dislodgement of 334
Legionella 432-434
   pneumonia 434
Lethargy 360, 381
Leukemia
   acute myelogenous 382
   chronic 574
Leukotriene
   modifiers 401
   receptor antagonists 401
Levosimendan 40, 71, 72, 121
Levothyroxine, intravenous 561
Lidocaine 266
Lignocaine 277
Linezolid 433
Lipids 370
Lipoprotein, low-density 24
Liver
   cirrhosis 369
   disease 205, 205
      acquired 574
      signs of 462
   function 69
      test 36, 156, 535

Lixivaptan 373
Long QT syndrome 144, 256*t*
   diagnostic score, modified 256*f*
Long-acting beta-agonist 414
   bronchodilator 401
Long-acting muscarinic
   antagonists 401
   agonists 414
Loop diuretics 533
Losartan 92
Low plasma glucose concentration 573
Low-flow nasal cannula 395
Low-molecular weight heparin 312
Lung
   compression, extrinsic 442
   disease 110
   heterogeneous 405
   injury
      acute 424
      ventilator-induced 423, 453
   parenchymal injury 442
   scintigraphy 307
   sliding 61
   ultrasound 60, 119
Lupus
   flare 587
   neonatal 595
Lymphohistiocytosis, hemophagocytic 591
Lymphomatoid granulomatosis 594

M

MACOCHA score 421*t*
Macrobarotraumas 437
Macrophage activation syndrome 591
Macrore-entrant atrial
   arrhythmias 219*t*
   tachycardia 218, 220*fc*, 221, 221*fc*, 222
Magnesium 276
   sulphate 394
Magnetic resonance
   angiography 307
   imaging 58, 102, 135, 195, 516
   venography 516
Major adverse cardiovascular event 24, 26

Index

Malabsorption 383
Malignancies, hematological 621
Malnutrition 383, 579
Marburg virus 621
Mean arterial pressure 41*f*, 598
Mechanical circulatory support 31, 43, 51, 54, 79, 87, 109*t*, 310
Mechanical support device, placement of 288
Mechanical ventilation 33, 78, 308, 383, 394, 398, 416, 424, 436
   initiation of 420*t*
   invasive 389, 420, 413
   noninvasive 413
Meningococcus sepsis 551
Meningoencephalitis 514
Mental status 130
Mepolizumab 402
Meropenem 433
Met acidosis 355
Met alkalosis 355
Meta-analysis global group 104
Metabolic acidosis 353, 356
   signs of 358*t*
   symptoms of 358*t*
Metabolic alkalosis 353, 356, 360*t*
   causes of 361*fc*
   diagnostic clue of 362*fc*
   management of 363*fc*
Metabolism 159
Metallo-beta-lactamase 433
Metastatic calcification 387
Methamphetamine 351
Methimazole 559
Methylprednisolone 394, 403
   intravenous 411
Methylxanthines 394
   intravenous 411
Metolazone 64, 65
Metoprolol 92, 160, 349
   succinate 177
   tartrate 177
Metronidazole 434
Microangiopathy, thrombotic 336, 338, 348
Microvascular resistance index 293
Milrinone 40, 70, 72, 107, 332

Mineralocorticoid
   deficiency 551
   receptor antagonist 24, 67, 90*t*, 104, 114, 115
Minimize expiratory airflow obstruction 440
Mitochondrial permeability transition pore 124
Mitoquinone 124
Mitral regurgitation
   acute 59
   severe 288
Mitral stenosis 42, 59
   moderate 69
   severe 69
Mitral valve 101
   repair, surgical 43
Mometasone 400
Monoarthritis, acute 586
Monomorphic ventricular tachycardia 58
   episode 241*fc*, 248*fc*
Morphine 23, 69
Mortality rate, lower 285
Moxifloxacin 434
Multifocal atrial tachycardia 212, 217*t*
Multiorgan dysfunction 419
Multiple accessory pathways 234*fc*
Multiple intravenous drug infusion facility 33
Multiple myeloma 535
Multivessel coronary artery disease 290
Multivessel disease, management of 44
Murmurs, cardiac 331
Muscle relaxants 422
Myeloma 578
Myocardial contrast echocardiography 293
Myocardial death, risk of 290
Myocardial depression 34
Myocardial infarction 25, 33, 39, 43, 44*fc*, 45*fc*, 162, 187, 280, 290, 337, 374
   acute 32, 34, 38, 48, 278, 359, 573
   transient 5

Myocardial ischemia 79, 113, 438, 443
Myocardial oxygen consumption 118
Myocardial revascularization 6*f*
Myocardial salvage 278
Myocarditis 56, 254*t*
Myoclonus, nature of 131
Myositis, inflammatory 583

N

N-acetylprocainamide 189
Nadolol 177
Narrow QRS tachycardia 212*fc*, 213*f*, 214*fc*
   acute therapy of 215*fc*
Nasogastric tube 561
National Association of EMS Physicians 9, 21
National Early Warning Score 600, 601
National Institute of Health Stroke Score 503
National Institute of Neurological Disorder and Stroke 492
National Institutes of Health Stroke Scale 488
Natriuretic peptide 76, 110, 119
   elevated concentrations of 86*t*
Nausea 84, 338
Nebivolol 92
Necrotizing vasculitis 584
Neoglucogenesis 563
Neoplasms 441
Neoplastic lesions 594
Nephritis, acute interstitial 537
Nervous system 380
Neurologic dysfunction, episode of 490
Neuromuscular blocking agent 460, 632
Neuropeptides 59
Neutropenia 621
Neutrophil gelatin-associated lipocalin 539
New York Heart Association 100, 102, 105-108, 114, 199
   functional class 187

Newcastle protocols 136*t*
Nicardipine 293, 339, 343, 350, 351
Nicorandil 261, 294
Nitric oxide 68
Nitroglycerine 23, 341, 350
Nitroprusside 68, 350, 351
Nonacute respiratory distress syndrome 631
Non-apparent structural heart disease 249*fc*
Noncardiovascular disease 82
Non-catecholamine vasopressor 626
Nondihydropyridine calcium channel blocker 179, 351
Non-infarct artery disease 291
Non-infarct coronary artery lesion, revascularization of 291, 291*fc*
Noninfectious syndrome 604
Non-interventional therapy, acute 492
Noninvasive monitoring 35
Noninvasive positive pressure ventilation 416, 417
   complications of 419
   modes of 416, 418
Noninvasive stress testing 87, 289
Noninvasive ventilation 51, 54, 389, 396, 416, 452, 457, 629
Nonobstructive coronary arteries 25
Nonshockable rhythm 272
Non-ST-elevation myocardial infarction 3, 4, 7, 10, 14, 44
Nonsteroidal anti-inflammatory drugs 154, 377, 338, 462, 537, 583
Non-ST-segment elevation 1*f*, 8, 16, 22
   acute coronary syndrome 2*f*, 7, 10, 14, 18
Nonvariceal upper gastrointestinal bleeding 468, 470*t*
   lesions, Forrest classification of 472*t*
Nonvitamin K antagonists 498
   oral anticoagulant 18, 19*f*, 162, 302, 312, 314
Norepinephrine 40, 71, 107, 277, 319, 624-626, 633

Normothermia 272
N-terminal pro B-type natriuretic
    peptide 85, 110, 123, 309
Nutrition 546, 637

O

Obesity 110, 114
Obliterative bronchiolitis 407
Observatoire Regional Breton sur
    l'Infarctus/du myocarde
    score 31*t*
Obstruction
    large vessel 495
    pulmonary 315
Obstructive coronary artery
    disease 25
Octreotide 467
Omalizumab 402
Omecamtiv mecarbil 121
Opiate 69
    associated emergency 267*fc*
Optic tract 553
Optical coherence tomography 25
Optical medical treatment 80
Organ
    damage, types of 336
    dysfunction, causes of 621
    failure assessment 597
    system involvement 589*t*
Orthodromic atrioventricular
    re-entrant tachycardia 229*f*
Oscillatory ventilation 457
Osmolality, serum 370
Osmotic demyelination 368
Osteoporosis 583
Oxygen
    arterial pressure of 409
    consumption 103, 104, 108
    partial pressure of 598
    saturation 409
    targets 628
    therapy 305, 390, 412
    uptake 103, 104
Oxygenation 274, 310, 429

P

P wave morphology 213*f*
P2Y12 inhibitor, dose of 281
Pacemaker 142
Pain 84, 347, 600
    abdominal 338
    relief, inadequate 440
Panbronchiolitis, diffuse 407
Pancuronium 422
Papillary necrosis 539
Papilledema 342
Paralysis 381
Parameter 309
Pathogenic mutation 261
Pathogens, multidrug-resistant 430
Patient-ventilator dyssynchrony 423
Peak inspiratory pressure 442, 444
Pediatric basic life support 328,
    328*fc*, 329*fc*
Pediatric cardiac
    arrest algorithm 330*fc*
    emergencies 321
Pediatric cardiovascular surgery 321
Pentamidine 375
Penumbra 500
Percutaneous coronary intervention
    6*f*, 7, 9, 14, 16, 18, 18*b*, 21,
    22, 29, 32, 39, 41*f*, 44, 45, 58,
    171*t*, 278, 279, 285, 288, 297,
    302, 351
Percutaneous mechanical support
    devices 46*f*
Pericardial diseases 59
Pericardial tamponade 43
Peripheral capillary oxygen
    saturation 600
Peripheral oxygen saturation 60
Peripheral vascular disease 108
Peripheral vein 381
Periprocedural anticoagulation,
    management of 171*fc*
Permanent junctional reciprocating
    tachycardia 212
Peroxisome proliferator-activated
    receptor gamma
    coactivator 124

P-glycoprotein 189
  substrate 159
Pharmacoinvasive therapy 280
Pharmacology, adjunctive 281
Pharmacotherapy 114, 293
  use of 294*fc*
Phenotypes 457
Phenoxybenzamine 556
Phentolamine 350, 351, 556
Phenylephrine 40, 331
Phenytoin 579
Pheochromocytoma 346*fc*, 347, 555
Phosphodiesterase 40, 68, 71
Phospholamban
    phosphorylation 125
Pigments 537
Piperacillin 432, 433, 616
Pituitary apoplexy 551
Plasma 376
  D-dimer measurement 306
  exchange 589
  neuropeptide 59
  proteins 370
Plasmacytoid cells, prevalence of 594
Plasmapheresis 593
Platelet
  antagonist aspirin 334
  consumption 342
  function testing 296
  glycoprotein 499
  rich thrombi, formation of 342
Pleocytosis 594
Pleural adhesions 61
Pleural effusion 60
  amount of 61
Pneumomediastinum 437
Pneumonia 58, 439, 608
  acute
    cryptogenic organizing 450
    eosinophilic 450
    interstitial 450
  community-acquired 606
  hospital-acquired 435
  nonventilation-associated
      hospital-acquired 434
  risk of 411
  ventilator-associated 429, 430

Pneumothorax 437, 440, 442
  development of 398
Polyangiitis 402, 537
  microscopic 537
Polyarthritis 586
Polycythemia 335
Polyelectrolytes 463
Polymorphic ventricular
    arrhythmia 249*fc*
    tachycardia 260
Polymyxin 433
Positive end-expiratory pressure 420, 423, 424, 457
  adverse effects of 423
  level of 629
Positive pressure ventilation 308, 437
Positron emission tomography 87
Post-cardiac arrest stunning 34
Postresuscitation 271
Postural orthostatic tachycardia
    syndrome 134
Potassium 381, 560, 572
  binders 379*t*
  chloride 560, 572
  iodide, saturated solution of 559
Potential cardiogenic shock care
    pathway 39*t*
Prasugrel 7, 11, 281, 297
Prazosin, oral 556
Prednisolone 394, 403, 579
  oral 411
Prednisone 403
Preeclampsia 336, 343, 344
  severe 343, 344
Pregnancy 203*t*, 234*t*
Premature ventricular complex 239, 250, 251*t*
Pressure
  control 424
    intermittent coronary sinus
        occlusion 295
  support 424
    weaning procedure 458
Primary percutaneous coronary
    intervention 2*f*, 5, 6*f*, 8, 9, 12, 14, 18, 278, 279, 281, 295
  risk stratification of 280

Procainamide 232, 276, 322
Procalcitonin 58, 606-608, 619
Proinflammatory stimuli 606
Propafenone 189, 232
Propranolol times 177
Propylthiouracil 559
Prostaglandin E1 332
Protein 539, 546
    C deficiencies 515
    electrophoresis, serum 535
    kinase A, level of 125
    S deficiencies 515
Prothrombin complex concentrate 168
Proton pump inhibitor 485, 635
Pseudohypoglycemia 574
Pseudohyponatremia 370
Pseudomonas 412
    aeruginosa 432, 609
Pulmonary artery 39, 48, 110, 333
    catheter 34, 36, 43
        use of 445
    diastolic pressure 39
    pressure 122, 123
    pulsatility index 48
    systolic pressure 39, 101
Pulmonary capillary wedge pressure 30, 33, 39, 48, 51, 123
Pulmonary crackles 82
Pulmonary embolism 57, 158, 307, 309, 310, 312, 317*fc*, 319, 636
    acute 38, 50, 304
    high-risk 319*t*
    severity
        classification of 309*t*
        index 309, 310
    thrombolysis trial 315
Pulmonary renal syndrome 592
Pulse
    methylprednisolone 593
    oximetry 35
    rate 309
Pulseless electrical activity 330
Pyelography
    antegrade 539
    retrograde 539
Pyrophosphate 102
Pyruvate kinase 563

Q

QRS complex tachycardia 243*fc*
QT interval prolongation 190
Quick sequential organ failure assessment 597, 600
    score 597*t*

R

Radiography, pulmonary 430
Radionuclide scanning 539
Randomized controlled trial 45, 298*t*
Rapid shallow breathing index 427
Rapid ventricular rate 275
Rash 525
Recanalization therapy, acute 197
Red blood cell 58
    transfusion of 437, 634
Refractory cardiorenal syndrome 532*fc*
Refractory electrolyte abnormalities 546
Regurgitant
    fraction 101
    volume 101
Regurgitation, mitral 42, 101, 101*fc*
Rehabilitation
    cardiac 113
    programs 638
    techniques 503
Renal angiography 539
Renal artery thrombosis 539
Renal biopsy 539
Renal disease 151
    chronic 466
Renal dysfunction 72
Renal excretion 385
Renal failure 359, 381, 579
    acute 370, 385, 520, 523, 623
Renal function 69, 156, 173*t*
    abnormal 154
    impairment of 520
Renal perfusion, adequacy of 524
Renal replacement therapy 51, 80, 532, 541*t*, 546, 603, 619, 623, 636
    indications of 543*t*, 546

medical management of 532*fc*
modalities 540*t*
pathophysiology of 532*fc*
use of 532*fc*
Renal tubular acidosis 382
Renal vein thrombosis 539
Renin-angiotensin system 337, 338, 374, 375, 626
   inhibition 89*t*
Reno-cardiac syndrome
   acute 542
   chronic 542
Reperfusion
   mean 316
   therapy 8*t*
   treatment 315
Respiration
   depth of 328
   volume controlled 423
Respiratory acidosis 354, 356, 413
   acute 355, 356
   chronic 355, 356, 364
   signs of 362*t*
   symptoms of 362*t*
Respiratory alkaloids
   causes of 365*t*
   management of 366*fc*
Respiratory alkalosis
   acute 355, 356
   chronic 355
Respiratory distress, treatment of 417
Respiratory failure 308, 381, 631
   acute 417
   hypoxemic 420, 629
Respiratory rate 35, 309, 409, 420, 423, 444, 468
Respiratory support 305, 412
Respiratory system 442
Respiratory viruses 621
Restrictive transfusion strategy 634
Resuscitation 263, 462, 601
   cardiocerebral 270
   cardiopulmonary 263-265, 320, 327, 328, 330
   goals of 465
Reteplase 20, 316
Retinopathy, hypertensive 342

Retroperitoneal fibrosis 539
Rhabdomyolysis 385, 525
Rheolytic thrombectomy 287
Rheumatoid arthritis 582
Rheumatologic emergency 582, 584
Rheumatological disorders 584
Rhinosinusitis, chronic 402
Rhythm control 180*t*
   strategy 150
Richmond agitation-sedation scale 37
Right atrium 48
Right bundle branch block 129, 236, 237, 240
Right ventricle 51, 129, 310
Right ventricular 43, 44, 48, 100, 103, 309
   cardiomyopathy 131
   dysfunction 83
   failure 39, 313*t*
   outflow tract 240, 250
   pressure overload, assessment of 308*b*
Rituximab 589
Rivaroxaban 170, 173, 302, 313, 498, 509, 589
   safety of 162
Rockall score 471*t*, 473
Rocuronium 422
Rosuvastatin 491
Routine aspiration
   thrombectomy 286

S

Sacubitril 73*t*, 76, 93, 93*t*, 115, 116, 119
Salbutamol 392, 393, 403
   intravenous 395
Salicylate 359
Saphenous vein graft 292
Sarcoidosis 579
   cardiac 255*fc*
Schistocytes 336
Scleroderma renal crisis 590
Sclerosis
   multiple 594
   systemic 583

Sedation 421, 440
   agitation scale 37
Seizures 360, 488, 502, 591
   epileptic 130*t*
   episodes 328
   management 512
   tonic-clonic 338
Selepressin 624, 626
Semaglutide 114
Sensorium 565
Sepsis 597, 606, 607*t*, 608, 608*fc*, 617, 618, 623*t*, 627, 637
   risk of 411
   screening 600*t*
      tools 600*t*
   signs of 604
   survivors of 638
   symptoms of 604
Sequential organ failure assessment 608
   score 598*t*
Serology 535, 585
Serum electrolyte 36
   deficits 562*t*
Severe acute respiratory syndrome coronavirus 2 (SARS-CoV-2) 621
   infection 59
Severe hypertension 342, 351
   management of 346
Shivering ventilator asynchrony 347
Shock 274, 321
   cardiogenic 29, 31-33, 36, 37, 38*t*, 40, 43, 44, 46*f*, 47, 48, 48*fc*, 50, 286, 288
   coordination of 326*t*
   critical cardiogenic 105
   energy 266
   etiology of 38
   index 476*fc*
   normointensive 42
   postcardiotomy 34
   septic 34, 597, 606, 617, 618, 623*t*, 626, 627, 637
Shockable rhythms 324
Short QT syndrome 261, 261*t*

Short-acting bronchodilator reliever medications 403
Simplified pulmonary embolism severity index 309, 310
Simvastatin 491
Sin Nombre virus 621
Single antiplatelet therapy 18, 19*f*
Single-photon emission computed tomography 87, 307
Sinus
   bradycardia 129, 139
   node
      dysfunction 141*fc*, 142*fc*
      recovery time 214
   rhythm 110, 188*t*, 322
      maintenance of 187*fc*
      normal 100
   tachycardia, therapy of 213, 215*fc*
Six-minute walk distance 118
Skin 614
Society for Cardiovascular Angiography and Interventions 9, 21, 31
Sodium 560, 572
   bicarbonate 560
      intravenous 376
   chloride 560, 572
   deficit 371
   glucose cotransporter inhibitor 74, 93, 124
   nitroprusside 293, 339, 341, 556
   polystyrene sulfonate, oral 376
Solid organ transplants 621
Somatostatin 467
Somnolence 338
Sotagliflozin 121
Sotalol 189, 276
Spironolactone 64, 92
Spondyloarthropathy 582
Spontaneous breathing trial, criteria for failure of 428
Spontaneous coronary artery dissection 10, 25
Spot sign 506
Sputum production 405
Stable atrial flutter, acute therapy of 220*fc*

Staphylococcus aureus 432
   methicillin-resistant 432, 606, 608, 609
Statin therapy 514
ST-elevation myocardial infarction 1*f*, 2*f*, 5, 7-9, 13, 18, 21, 24, 44, 246*fc*, 278, 287, 288, 290, 291*fc*, 297
Stenosis 441
   pulmonary 331
Stenotrophomonas 435
   maltophilia 435
Stent thrombosis
   acute 285
   late 285
Steroids 338, 583
   therapy, high-dose 587
Stewart's approach 354
Streptokinase 20, 294, 316
Stress
   bleeding prophylaxis 437
   ulcer prophylaxis 37, 635
Stroke 102, 151, 151*t*, 154, 156, 160*t*, 162, 173, 177*t*, 288, 337, 487
   acute 336, 340
   cardioembolic 157
   hemorrhagic 154, 208, 340
   higher risk of 318
   ischemic 301, 340, 487, 489*t*, 492
   location 500
   mild ischemic 204
   moderate ischemic 204
   prevention 208, 210*fc*, 513
   recognition of 334
   rehabilitation 503
   risk of 153
   seizure 503
   volume 39
Subclinical atrial fibrillation 146, 162
Subendothelium 342
Sudden cardiac
   arrest 242*fc*
   death 133, 239, 247*fc*
      high risk of 139
      prevention 251*t*, 253*t*, 254*t*
Superior vena cava 218, 222

Supraventricular tachycardia 133, 139, 143, 234*t*, 235, 235*t*, 236, 236*t*, 237, 237*t*, 243, 321, 325
   management of 322
   treatment of 323, 323*t*
Surgical aortic valve replacement 43
Surviving sepsis campaign, recommendation of 603, 605, 606, 617, 621, 622, 624, 627-637
Sympathomimetics 338
Synchronized intermittent mandatory ventilation 424
Syncope 127, 129*b*, 130*t*, 131, 134*fc*, 141*fc*, 143*fc*, 144, 328, 488, 524
   causes of 131, 138
   classification of 128*fc*
   reflex 140*fc*
   risk stratification of 132*t*
   treatment of 139
Syndrome of inappropriate antidiuretic hormone 369, 372
Synovial fluid analysis 587
Systemic inflammatory response syndrome 34, 438, 537, 597, 600, 601
Systemic lupus erythematosus 582
Systemic vascular resistance index 33, 40, 43
Systolic pulmonary artery pressure 41*f*

T

Tachyarrhythmia 139
   cardiac 143*fc*
Tachycardia 212, 229*f*, 269*fc*, 331, 408, 468
   complex 237
Tachycardiomyopathy 235*t*, 236
Tachypnea 331, 408, 565
Takotsubo cardiomyopathy cardiac tamponade 38
Tazobactam 432, 433, 616, 617

Temocillin 616
Tenecteplase 20, 294, 316, 494
Tension pneumothorax 267, 442
Terbutaline 403
Terlipressin 467
Tetany 360, 581
Tezepelumab 402
Theophylline 411
Therapeutic drug monitoring 619
Therapeutic subcutaneous enoxaparin 284
Thiazide diuretics 63
Thoracentesis 442
Thrombectomy 286, 287
Thrombocytopenia 313, 343
Thromboembolism 151, 171, 513
   acute venous 314
   apixaban for reduction of 162
   pulmonary 443
Thrombolysis 517
   in myocardial infarction 32
   intravenous 492
   reduced-dose 316
   systemic 315
   trials, meta-analysis of 315
Thrombolytic therapy 315, 493
Thrombophilia, acquired 515
Thrombosis
   catheter-related 284
   pulmonary 268
Thrombotic thrombocytopenic purpura 342, 537
Thrombus aspiration 286, 287, 295
Thyroid
   dysfunction 58
   function test 58, 561
   hormones, rapid replacement of 561
   stimulating hormone 55, 158, 190
   storm 556, 557, 559
      prevention of 560
      treatment of 559t
Thyrotoxic crisis 556
Thyrotoxicosis 558
Thyroxine, oral 561
Ticagrelor 11, 281, 297
   administration of 5

Tidal volume 420, 424
Tilt-table test 136
Tirofiban 12, 294
Tissue
   hypoperfusion 367
   plasminogen activator 294, 496
Tolvaptan 373
Tongue bite 131
Torsades de pointes 189, 190, 232, 276
Torsemide 63
Toxins 268
Tracheal aspirate, culture of 430
Tracheal secretions 429
Tracheostomy 429
   tube 419, 441, 443
Transbronchial biopsy 442
Transcatheter aortic valve replacement 43
Transesophageal echocardiogram 55, 58, 62
Transferrin saturation 85
Transfusion 437
   therapy 467
Transient ischemic attack 102, 127, 151, 171, 195, 490
   management 490
Transjugular intrahepatic portosystemic shunt 468
Transthyretin 102
   amyloid cardiomyopathy 102
   amyloidosis, wild-type 102
Transtubular potassium gradient 377, 382
Triamcinolone 400
Triamterene 64
Tricuspid regurgitation 110, 111
Trimethoprim 375
Troponin 59
Tube migration 439
Tuberculosis 407
Tubular damage 527f
Tubular necrosis, acute 523, 524, 537, 544b
Tumor lysis syndrome 385
Typical atrioventricular nodal re-entrant tachycardia 223f

U

Unconsciousness, duration of 131
Unfractionated heparin 12, 14, 18,
    20, 21, 283, 312, 319, 517,
    594, 636
Unstable atrial fibrillation, acute
    management of 158*fc*
Upper gastrointestinal
    bleeding 467, 485
    endoscopy 468*fc*
    guided management 473*fc*
Urapidil 341, 350
Urea 59, 370
Urinary protein 524*fc*
Urinary tract infections, nosocomial
    616
Urine
    analysis 523*fc*, 524*fc*
    biochemistry 539
    examination 537
    output 35
    sediment 523*fc*, 537
Urokinase 316, 496

V

Vagal maneuvers 322
Vague ill health 522
Valsalva maneuver 134
Valsartan 73*t*, 76, 92, 93, 93*t*, 115, 116,
    119
Valve regurgitation, acute 50
Valvular atrial fibrillation 147
Valvular insufficiency, acute 38
Vancomycin 433
Vascular disease 102, 151
Vascular resistance, pulmonary 40, 43
Vascular smooth muscle 626
Vasculitis 583
    cerebral 594
    systemic
        granulomatous 594
        necrotizing 594
Vasoactive
    agents 624
    drugs 467
    therapy 533

Vasodilators 67, 68*t*
Vasopressin 624-626
    receptor antagonists, use of 372
Vasopressors 40, 70*t*, 72, 107
Vecuronium 422
Vein, pulmonary 195, 213
Venoarterial extracorporeal
    membrane oxygenation 48
Venous thromboembolism 304, 307,
    636
    prophylaxis 511, 635
Venovenous extracorporeal
    membrane oxygenation
    456, 633
Ventilation 274, 632
    complications of 429
    modes of 423
    protective 453, 630
    strategy 425
Ventilator alarm
    interpretation of 444*t*
    sounds 440*fc*
Ventilator bundle 36
Ventilator-associated pneumonia
    429, 430
    empiric treatment of 431*f*
    management of 434
    prevention of 435
Ventricular arrhythmia 244, 251*t*, 257
    management of 246*fc*
    treatment of 253*t*, 254*t*
Ventricular assist device 39
Ventricular drainage, external 509,
    511
Ventricular fibrillation 48, 330
    management of 423
    risk of 324
Ventricular function 38
Ventricular premature complexes 129
Ventricular septal defect 45
Ventricular tachycardia 48, 133, 139,
    143, 189, 236*t*, 237*fc*, 237*t*,
    240, 243, 249*fc*, 250, 250*t*,
    260, 325
    non-sustained 239, 239*fc*
    pulseless 324, 330

Verapamil 178, 217, 232, 293, 322
Vericiguat 92, 94, 121
Vilanterol 401
Viruses 435
Visual acuity 553
Visual analog scale 409
Vitamin
    A intoxication 579
    D 579, 581
        deficiency 579
        intoxication 579
    K antagonist 18, 69, 154, 168, 314
Vomitus, inhalation of 434
von Willebrand factor 342

W

Warfarin 170, 314

Waterhouse-Friderichsen syndrome 551
Weakness 381
Weaning 427, 458
Wegener's granulomatosis 515, 594
Weight loss 113
Whipple's triad 573
Wide complex tachycardia 236t, 237t, 324t
    acute therapy of 238fc
    treatment of 323
Wide QRS tachycardia 221
Wolf-Parkinson-White syndrome 129, 227, 228fc, 235, 322

Z

Zwolle index 280

EU GSPR Authorised Reprsentative
Logos Europe, 9 rue Nicolas Poussin
1700, La Rochelle, France
Phone: +33 (0) 6 67 93 73 78
E-mail: contact@logoseurope.eu

www.ingramcontent.com/pod-product-compliance
Ingram Content Group UK Ltd.
Pitfield, Milton Keynes, MK11 3LW, UK
UKHW021837210426
5322IPUK00021B/340